Evidence-Based
Neurology:
Management of
Neurological Disorders

Second Edition

Evidence-Based Neurology: Management of Neurological Disorders

Second Edition

EDITED BY

Bart M. Demaerschalk, MD, MSc, FRCP(C)

Professor of Neurology
Department of Neurology
Mayo Clinic College of Medicine
Phoenix, AZ
USA

Dean M. Wingerchuk, MD, MSc, FRCP(C)

Professor of Neurology
Department of Neurology
Mayo Clinic College of Medicine
Scottsdale, AZ
USA

WILEY Blackwell

Library of Congress Cataloging-in-Publication Data applied for.

ISBN: 9780470657782

A catalogue record for this book is available from the British Library.

Wiley also publishes its books in a variety of electronic formats. Some content that appears in print may not be available in electronic books.

Cover image: @Svisio/Getty

Set in 9/12pt, MeridienLTStd by SPi Global, Chennai, India

Printed in Singapore by C.O.S. Printers Pte Ltd

1   2015

Contents

Contributors

Amelia K. Adcock, MD
Assistant Professor of Neurology
West Virginia University
Morgantown, West Virginia, USA

Maria I. Aguilar, MD
Associate Professor of Neurology
Cerebrovascular Diseases Center
Mayo Clinic Hospital Phoenix
AZ, USA

Miguel Arango
The University of Western Ontario and
The London Health Sciences Centre
London, Ontario, Canada

Kevin M. Barrett
Department of Neurology
Mayo Clinic
Jacksonville, FL, USA

Jason J.S. Barton, MD, PhD, FRCPC
Professor
Departments of Medicine (Neurology), Ophthalmlogy and
Visual Sciences, Psychology
University of British Columbia
Vancouver, Canada

Andrea J. Boon, MD
Department of Physical Medicine
Mayo Clinic
Rochester, MN, USA

Thomas Brandt, MD, FRCP, FANA
Department of Neurology, German Center for Vertigo and
Balance Disorders and Institute for Clinical Neurosciences
University Hospital Munich
Munich, Germany

Miguel Bussière, MD, PhD, FRCP
Assistant Professor
Neurology and Interventional Neuroradiology, Division of
Neurology
Grey Nuns Hospital
Edmonton, AB, Canada

Richard J. Caselli, MD
Consultant, Professor of Neurology
Department of Neurology, Mayo College of Medicine
Mayo Clinic
Scottsdale, AZ, USA

Nicholas D. Child, MB, ChB
Deep Brain Stimulation Fellow
Department of Neurology
Mayo Clinic College of Medicine
Rochester, MN, USA

Bart M. Demaerschalk, MD, MSc, FRCP(C)
Professor of Neurology
Department of Neurology
Mayo Clinic
Phoenix, AZ, USA

P. James B. Dyck
Department of Neurology
Mayo Clinic
Rochester, MN, USA

William David Freeman, MD
Associate Professor
Departments of Neurology, Neuosurgery, and Critical Care
Mayo Clinic Florida
Jacksonville, FL, USA

Gloria von Geldern
Section of Infections of the Nervous System, NINDS
National Institutes of Health
Bethesda, MD, USA

Brent P. Goodman, MD
Department of Neurology
Mayo Clinic
Scottsdale, AZ, USA

Robin Grant
Consultant Neurologist
Division of Clinical Neurosciences
Western General Hospital
Edinburgh, UK

Gord Gubitz, MD, FRCPC
Division of Neurology, Department of Medicine
Dalhousie University
Halifax, Nova Scotia, Canada

Rashmi B. Halker, MD
Assistant Professors, Department of Neurology
Mayo Clinic
Phoenix, AZ

Michael G. Hart
Neurosurgery Specialty Trainee
Department of neurosurgery
Addenbrooke's Hospital
Cambridge, UK

Nicola M. Kayes
Centre for Person Centred Research, Health and Rehabilitation
Research Institute, School of Clinical Sciences
AUT University
Auckland, New Zealand

Paula Kersten
Centre for Person Centred Research, Health and Rehabilitation
Research Institute, School of Clinical Sciences
AUT University
Auckland, New Zealand

Salah G. Keyrouz, MD
Department of Neurology and Neurological Surgery
Washington University School of Medicine
St. Louis, MO, USA

Bryan T. Klassen, MD
Assistant Professor of Neurology
College of Medicine
Mayo Clinic
Rochester MN, USA

Lawrence Korngut, MD, FRCP
Clinical Assistant Professor (Neurology)
Director, Calgary ALS and Motor Neuron Disease Clinic
Clinical Neurosciences
South Health Campus
Calgary, AB, Canada

Joyce Lee-Iannotti, MD
Vascular Neurology Fellow
Mayo Clinic Arizona
Scottsdale, AZ, USA

E. Anne MacGregor, MD
Centre for Neuroscience & Trauma, BICMS, Barts and
the London School of Medicine and Dentistry
London, UK

Anthony G. Marson
Department of Molecular and Clinical Pharmacology,
Institute of Translational Medicine
University of Liverpool
Liverpool, Merseyside, UK

Kathryn M. McPherson
Centre for Person Centred Research, Health and
Rehabilitation Research Institute, School of
Clinical Sciences
AUT University
Auckland, New Zealand

Avindra Nath
Section of Infections of the Nervous System, NINDS
National Institutes of Health
Bethesda, MD, USA

Cumara B. O'Carroll, MD, MPH
Assistant Professor of Neurology
Department of Neurology,
Mayo Clinic
Phoenix, AZ, USA

Bhavesh M. Patel, MD
Assistant Professor
Department of Critical Care Medicine
Mayo Clinic
Phoenix, AZ, USA

Naresh P. Patel, MD
Associate Professor
Department of Neurological Surgery
Mayo Clinic
Phoenix, AZ, USA

Christopher A. Payne, BS
Trinity College
Dublin, Ireland

Kameshwar Prasad
Department of Neurology
All India Institute of Medical sciences
New Delhi, India

Manya Prasad
Department of Community Medicine
Pandit Bhagwat Dayal Sharma Post Graduate Institute of
Medical Sciences
Rohtak, Haryana, India

Corina Puppo
Emergency Department, Clinics Hospital
University of the Repúblic School of Medicine
Montevideo, Uruguay

Sridharan Ramaratnam
Department of Neurology
SIMS Hospitals
Chennai, Tamil Nadu, India

Bappaditya Ray, MBBS, MD
Department of Neurology
The University of Oklahoma Health Sciences Center
Oklahoma City, OK, USA

Todd J. Schwedt, MD
Associate Professor of Neurology
Mayo Clinic
Phoenix, AZ, USA

Jonathan H. Smith, MD
Assistant Professor of Neurology
University of Kentucky
Lexington, KY, USA

Charlene H. Snyder, DP, NP-BC
Nurse Practitioner, Associate Department of Neurology,
and Assistant Professor of Neurology
Mayo College of Medicine
Mayo Clinic
Scottsdale, AZ, USA

Byron Roderick Spencer
Blue Sky Neurology (Division of Carepoint)
Denver, CO, USA

Michael Strupp, MD, FANA
Department of Neurology
German Center for Vertigo and Balance Disorders and
Institute for Clinical Neurosciences
University Hospital Munich
Munich, Germany

Martin Sutton-Brown, MD, FRCPC
Clinical Assistant Professor
Department of Medicine (Neurology)
University of British Columbia
Vancouver, Canada

Greg Thaera
Mayo Clinic
Scottsdale, AZ, USA

Jennifer A. Tracy
Assistant Professor, Department of Neurology
Mayo Clinic
Rochester, MN, USA

Bert B. Vargas, MD
Assistant Professors, Department of Neurology
Mayo Clinic
Phoenix, AZ

Kenneth A. Vatz
Department of Neurology
Chicago, IL, USA

Joseph L. Verheijde, PhD, MBA, PT
Associate Professor of Biomedical Ethics, College of Medicine
Mayo Clinic
Scottsdale, AZ, USA

Walter Videtta
Intensive Care Unit,
Hospital Posadas,
Buenos Aires, Argentina

Dean M. Wingerchuk, MD, MSc, FRCP(C)
Professor of Neurology
Mayo Clinic
Scottsdale, AZ, USA

Bryan K. Woodruff, MD
Consultant
Assistant Professor of Neurology
Department of Neurology, Mayo College of Medicine
Mayo Clinic
Scottsdale, AZ, USA

PART 1
Evidence-based neurology: introduction

CHAPTER 1

Evidence-based neurology in health education

Lawrence Korngut[1], Miguel Bussière[2], and Bart M. Demaerschalk[3]

[1]*Calgary ALS and Motor Neuron Disease Clinic, Clinical Neurosciences, South Health Campus, Calgary, AB, Canada*
[2]*Neurology and Interventional Neuroradiology, Division of Neurology, Grey Nuns Hospital, Edmonton, AB, Canada*
[3]*Department of Neurology, Mayo Clinic, Phoenix, AZ, USA*

Introduction

Clinical neurology trainees undergo a lengthy and complex process requiring integration of many fundamental skills that coalesce into sound diagnosis and decision making. Beyond the core knowledge of anatomy, physiology, biochemistry, pathology, and the medical sciences, there is an essential requirement for the clinical student, in the arena of evidence-based clinical practice, to acquire skills and expertise in the principles and practice of critical appraisal and to have a working knowledge of the best evidence from the diverse multiple subspecialties that comprise neurology today. Maintaining competence in the current best evidence over a neurologist's career is essential to making accurate diagnoses, providing high-quality neurological care, and selecting appropriate tests and therapies.

Developing the skills necessary for critical appraisal is a difficult process, particularly when competing with the rigorous demands of a residency training program. An evidence-based curriculum in neurology education provides the opportunity for teaching the fundamentals of critical appraisal and engaging in discussion of current clinical questions, hot topics, and continued controversies. Fostering an understanding of what comprises an appropriately comprehensive rigorous literature search, the levels of evidence, the different types of studies, and the methodologies are difficult to consolidate outside of a formalized curriculum or graduate-level training in evidence-based medicine, health research methodology, and clinical epidemiology.

In this chapter, we discuss the development of an evidence-based neurology (EBN) curriculum in health education.

Objectives

Teaching and acquisition of critical appraisal skills is the primary objective of an evidence-based clinical practice curriculum. Fundamental critical appraisal skills include the following: awareness of a clinical knowledge gap, formulation of answerable questions based on clinical uncertainty, performance of a literature search, identification of the highest quality evidence from the search yield, and critical appraisal of the studies to address the original clinical question. Students should become familiar with the different classifications of clinical studies (e.g. prognosis, diagnosis, therapy or harm) and the main methodological and statistical questions that must be addressed in each type of study. The students should also be able to determine whether or not the study findings are worth considering given the methodological quality of the study and its generalizability in reference to the patient population in question.

Students should develop an understanding of both the importance and the limitations of clinical evidence. Emphasis should remain on high-quality patient care and the use of the current best evidence to guide clinical practice within the context of the patient's wishes and the clinician's judgment and reasoning. It must be emphasized that lack of evidence for efficacy does not necessarily mean lack of benefit with treatment, and vice versa for lack of evidence against certain therapies or diagnostic tests.

As a result of the evidence-based medicine, curriculum knowledge about best current evidence practices is accumulated and stored for future use. Owing to the discussion of common clinical scenarios and review of the relevant best evidence, the students develop a working knowledge of the current evidence (Table 1.1).

The following sections describe an example of an EBN curriculum based on two longstanding, mature, and successful programs targeting clinical neurology residents: the EBN curriculum from the Western University (WU) in London, Canada [1–4]; and the Mayo Clinic Evidence-Based Clinical Practice, Research, Informatics, and Training (MERIT)

Evidence-Based Neurology: Management of Neurological Disorders, Second Edition. Edited by Bart M. Demaerschalk and Dean M. Wingerchuk.
© 2015 John Wiley & Sons, Ltd. Published 2015 by John Wiley & Sons, Ltd.

Table 1.1 Objectives of evidence-based neurology curriculum.

1 Students of neurology should develop critical appraisal skills to
  (a) formulate answerable questions based on clinical uncertainty
  (b) perform an appropriate literature search
  (c) identify the best quality evidence from the studies identified
  (d) critically appraise the identified studies to answer the original clinical question
  (e) be familiar with prognostic, diagnostic, and therapeutic clinical studies and the key methodological and statistical questions that should be addressed in each type of study
  (f) determine whether the study findings are valid and useful, considering the methodological quality of the study and the applicability to a particular patient population
2 Students of neurology should develop a working understanding of the importance of high-quality evidence and also realize its limitations
3 Students should accumulate knowledge about best current evidence practices in neurology

Table 1.2 PICO acronym [8].

Patient or population
Intervention, prognostic factor or exposure
Comparison intervention
Outcome to measure or achieve

Curriculum, Mayo Clinic, Phoenix, AZ [5,6]. Another third valuable resource designed to help educators teach students of neurology to understand and use evidence-based medicine is the web-based American Academy of Neurology (AAN) Evidence-Based Medicine Curriculum [7].

Topic selection

Generating the clinical questions
Once annually EBN curriculum facilitators survey all neurology students and faculty members to generate a list of neurological questions for potential review. These clinical questions are then rank ordered by the trainees and facilitators according to multiple factors including clinical importance, relevance, frequency of occurrence, and interest. The most highly ranked questions are reviewed in the upcoming year. The topics are screened to ensure that they are congruent with the educational recommendations of the training program (post-graduate education committee): Royal College of Physicians and Surgeons of Canada Advisory Committee and/or Accreditation Council for Graduate Medical Education – Neurology Residency and American Board of Psychiatry and Neurology [1–6].

Preparing for the tutorial session
Students each select one or two clinical questions per academic year and prepare their critically appraised topic for general discussion with the group. For each clinical topic, a clinical scenario and a focused clinical question are formulated. A focused clinical question should include considerations of the specific patient group, the intervention or exposure, the method of comparison, and the outcome measures. The acronym PICO can serve as a helpful reminder [8] (Table 1.2).

For a given clinical question, the presenting trainee performs a literature search and identifies studies representing the highest level of evidence [9]. Expert librarians and informatics specialists can be called upon to assist in efficient and comprehensive literature searching. Studies are evaluated according to the generally accepted hierarchy of clinical evidence. High-quality meta-analyses, systematic reviews, and randomized clinic trials are preferred over observational studies and case reports. One to four studies are selected for critical appraisal and discussion. A summary of this information is prepared in advance of the discussion in the form of a critically appraised topic (CAT) as described later. One week prior to the session, the presenting trainee circulates copies of the clinical scenario, focusing clinical question, search strategy, and articles for review to the participants. The pre-tutorial process is supervised by one of the facilitators. The faculty often provides instruction and advice on the search strategy and reasons for inclusion or exclusion of studies. Trainees are introduced to different search engines (e.g. PubMed [10], SUMSearch [11], Cochrane Library [12]). Discussions on Medical Subject Headings (MeSH headings), keywords, and their uses are helpful.

Flexibility is available to adjust the clinical topics to suit the needs and training level of the trainees. Semi-annual meetings of the curriculum trainees and facilitators allow for appropriate curriculum content changes and adjustment of group discussion objectives to cover specific epidemiological or biostatistical topics.

Tutorial

Each tutorial session focuses on a trainee presenting one clinical question. The session begins with a 5-min description of the clinical scenario and focused clinical question. This is followed by a 10-min presentation of the background topic including clinical information about the condition, treatment, or diagnostic test. The trainee then presents and discusses the search strategy for 5 min.

The following 45 min is dedicated to critical appraisal of the evidence.

The study type is identified (e.g. prognosis, diagnosis, therapy, or harm), and the appropriate rating scale or worksheet is utilized to assist the presenting trainee and faculty members guide the group through the critical appraisal process. Sample worksheets are available through the Western University Evidence-Based Neurology website [4].

These worksheets were derived from the *Users' Guide to the Medical Literature* [13] and relevant articles contained therein. The rating scales are generally divided into three sections: (1) analysis of the study methodology to determine its validity, (2) assessment of the final results including accuracy and clinical importance, and (3) appraisal of the applicability of these results to the target patient or patient population.

To engage the audience, it is helpful to divide into smaller groups of three or more participants (depending on number of trainees) to each completely assigned portions of a worksheet. For example, for a therapeutic article one group can determine whether the study addressed a focused clinical question, whether treatment allocation was randomized, and whether the randomization list was concealed. A second group could discuss the length of patient follow-up and whether an intention-to-treat analysis was employed. The whole group then discusses the interpretation of results and their applicability to the focus clinical question (5 min). The final conclusions of the group are summarized as "clinical bottom lines" (5 min). The presenting trainee's draft CAT is then reviewed, discussed, and edited. The final CAT reflects the opinion of the entire group.

Post-tutorial

The presenting trainee completes final revisions of the CAT based on the suggestions of the group at the tutorial and submits it for final review to the facilitators. The final CAT is collected and made available for review either in hard copy format, posted to a central repository on the intranet or Internet, or published in peer-reviewed journals.

All trainees are encouraged to utilize their evidence-based skills during their clinical rotations and in teaching sessions. Trainees are encouraged to ask about the evidence underlying their supervising faculty's medical decisions in a collegial manner and to review the literature as appropriate to enhance everyone's knowledge base.

The critically appraised topic (CAT)

The CAT begins with a short summary of the clinical scenario and focused clinical question. The literature search is briefly outlined. The clinical bottom lines are highlighted followed by the most relevant data, typically in table form, and the relevant references. The objective of the CAT is to summarize the tutorial topic and conclusions in a concise manner for future reference. The WU EBN Program maintains an online archive of CATs that assist in clinical decision making and implementation of evidence-based clinical practice [4]. Both the Mayo Clinic MERIT and WU EBN programs have published CATs in peer-reviewed print journals [6,14–26].

Resources

Faculty

Most programs have two full-time neurologists with expertise in evidence-based medicine, clinical epidemiology, and biostatistics who are responsible for coordinating the tutorials and teaching evidence-based care principles and practice. All neurology and neurosurgery faculty are invited to attend tutorials, and special invitations are sometimes extended to other medical and surgical faculty, outside neurology, with particular interest or expertise on the topic of discussion at a given session. Teaching faculty from other departments or other academic institutions are occasionally invited to participate or teach on specific evidence-based medicine topics. Neurosurgery residents attend EBN tutorials when topics relevant to neurosurgical practice are discussed. Neurology residents have graded responsibilities and assume a greater teaching role as they gain experience and skill in EBN. Neurology trainees, residents, and fellows vary in total number from 10 to 14 per year, depending on the institution.

Medical librarians and informatics experts

If available, expert evidence-based medicine librarians and informatics specialists serve as valuable faculty additions and can be called upon to assist in the literature search. They may identify more useful or encompassing search terms, suggest additional specialized databases to search, and help finalize a list of relevant articles.

Time

EBN tutorial sessions range from 60 to 90 min in duration, depending on the program, and are held monthly throughout the typical 4- or 5-year neurology residency training program. Sessions are scheduled into protected educational time for neurology students, thus ensuring mandatory participation. Topics for discussion are generally decided upon early in the academic year, thus allowing ample informal research and preparatory time.

Space

EBN tutorials are generally held in an available university or hospital auditorium. Reference material on evidence-based medicine is made available in the departmental library. Computers, smartphones, and tablets with links to electronic databases are readily available.

Educational resource material

It is helpful to provide an introductory reference book on evidence-based medicine to each new student [27]. Other evidence-based references and educational material can be located in the departmental library. A compilation of all critically appraised topics reviewed is made available in print format (published, peer reviewed, or unpublished) or as a web-based searchable database for intra- or extra-institutional use [4].

Informatics

Students use smartphones, tablets, laptop computers, and digital projection units for presentations and tutorials. With Internet access and links to the commonly used searchable databases of the evidence-based literature, the departmental library based on the real and virtual neurology remains a focal point of the EBN curriculum.

The evidence to support an evidence-based health curriculum

An increasing number of medical residency training programs devote formal educational time to developing evidence-based clinical practice knowledge and skills. One of the core competencies on graduate medical education is *Practice-based learning and improvement*. This requires the clinical student to investigate and evaluate their care of patients, to appraise and assimilate scientific evidence, and to continuously improve patient care based on constant self-evaluation and lifelong learning. Residents/fellows are expected to develop skills and habits to be able to

• Locate, appraise, and assimilate evidence from scientific studies related to their patients' health problems;

• Use information technology to optimize learning.

Other than simply fulfilling a core competency, the question is, "Do these curricula improve knowledge of evidence-based neurology concepts and critical appraisal skills?" "Do they result in a change in clinical practice and patient health outcomes?" Several primarily nonrandomized or quasirandomized studies conducted over the past decade have attempted to address these questions. High-quality evidence is limited as a result of heterogeneity of the teaching method or intervention assessed, small sample sizes, heterogeneity of the outcome instruments or measures, and variability in the duration of the study or timing of the outcome assessment [28–30]. Systematic reviews of the available evidence suggest that post-graduate evidence-based medicine education results in significant improvements in a student's knowledge base but data are lacking, which significantly alter clinical decision making or patient outcomes [28–30].

References

1 Burneo, J.G. & Jenkins, M.E. (2007) Teaching evidence-based clinical practice to neurology and neurosurgery residents. *Clinical Neurology and Neurosurgery*, **109**, 418–421.

2 Burneo, J.G., Jenkins, M.E., Bussière, M. & UWO Evidence-based Neurology Group (2006) Evaluating a formal evidence-based clinical practice curriculum in a neurology residency program. *Journal of the Neurological Sciences*, **250**, 10–19.

3 Demaerschalk, B.M. & Wiebe, S. (2001) *Evidence Based Neurology: an innovative curriculum for post-graduate training in the neurological sciences*. http://www.uwo.ca/cns/ebn (accessed 21 September 2009).

4 *University of Western Ontario's Evidence Based Neurology*. (2001) http://www.uwo.ca/cns/ebn (accessed 21 September 2009).

5 Demaerschalk, B.M. & Wingerchuk, D.M. (2007) The MERITs of evidence-based clinical practice in neurology. *Seminars in Neurology*, **27**(**4**), 303–311.

6 Wingerchuk, D.M. & Demaerschalk, B.M. (2007) The evidence-based neurologist: critically appraised topics. *The Neurologist*, **13**, 1.

7 American Academy of Neurology Evidence Based Medicine Toolkit, http://www.aan.com/education/ebm/ (accessed 21 September 2009).

8 Richardson, W.S., Wilson, M.C., Nishikawa, J. & Hayward, R.S. (1995) The well-built clinical question: a key to evidence-based decisions. *ACP Journal Club*, **123**, A12–A13.

9 University of Oxford Centre for Evidence-Based Medicine. http://www.cebm.net/levels_of_evidence.asp (accessed 23 February 2009)

10 U.S. National Library of Medicine PubMed. http://www.ncbi.nlm.nih.gov/sites/entrez (accessed 23 February 2009)

11 University of Texas Health Science Centre SUMSearch engine. http://sumsearch.uthscsa.edu/ (accessed 23 February 2009).

12 The Cochrane Collaboration. http://www.cochrane.org/index.htm (accessed 23 February, 2009).

13 Guyatt, G.H. & Rennie, D. (2002) *Users' Guides to the Medical Literature. A Manual for Evidence-based Clinical Practice*. AMA Press, Chicago.

14 Zarkou, S., Aguilar, M.I., Patel, N.P., Wellik, K.E., Wingerchuk, D.M. & Demaerschalk, B.M. (2009) The role of corticosteroids in the management of chronic subdural hematomas: a critically appraised topic. *Neurologist*, **15**, 299–302.

15 Wingerchuk, D.M., Spencer, B., Dodick, D.W. & Demaerschalk, B.M. (2007) Migraine with aura is a risk factor for cardiovascular and cerebrovascular disease: a critically appraised topic. *Neurologist*, **13**, 231–233.

16 Demaerschalk, B.M. & Wingerchuk, D.M. (2007) Treatment of vascular dementia and vascular cognitive impairment. *Neurologist*, **13**, 37–41.

17 Hickey, M.G., Demaerschalk, B.M., Caselli, R.J., Parish, J.M. & Wingerchuk, D.M. (2007) "Idiopathic" rapid-eye-movement (REM) sleep behavior disorder is associated with future development of neurodegenerative diseases. *Neurologist*, **13**, 98–101.

18 Halker, R.B., Barrs, D.M., Wellik, K.E., Wingerchuk, D.M. & Demaerschalk, B.M. (2008) Establishing a diagnosis of benign paroxysmal positional vertigo through the dix-hallpike and side-lying maneuvers: a critically appraised topic. *Neurologist*, **14**, 201–214.

19 Hoerth, M.T., Wellik, K.E., Demaerschalk, B.M. *et al.* (2008) Clinical predictors of psychogenic nonepileptic seizures: a critically appraised topic. *Neurologist*, **14**, 266–270.

20 Khoury, J.A., Hoxworth, J.M., Mazlumzadeh, M., Wellik, K.E., Wingerchuk, D.M. & Demaerschalk, B.M. (2008) The clinical utility of high resolution magnetic resonance imaging in

the diagnosis of giant cell arteritis: a critically appraised topic. *Neurologist*, **14**, 330–335.

21 Capampangan, D.J., Wellik, K.E., Aguilar, M.I., Demaerschalk, B.M. & Wingerchuk, D.M. (2008) Does prophylactic postoperative hypervolemic therapy prevent cerebral vasospasm and improve clinical outcome after aneurysmal subarachnoid hemorrhage? *Neurologist*, **14**, 395–398.

22 Almaraz, A.C., Bobrow, B.J., Wingerchuk, D.M., Wellik, K.E. & Demaerschalk, B.M. (2009) Serum neuron specific enolase to predict neurological outcome after cardiopulmonary resuscitation: a critically appraised topic. *Neurologist*, **15**, 44–48.

23 Khoury, J., Wellik, K.E., Demaerschalk, B.M. & Wingerchuk, D.M. (2009) Cerebrospinal fluid angiotensin-converting enzyme for diagnosis of central nervous system sarcoidosis. *Neurologist*, **15**(2), 108–111.

24 Capampangan, D.J., Wellik, K.E., Bobrow, B.J. *et al.* (2009) Telemedicine versus telephone for remote emergency stroke consultations: a critically appraised topic. *Neurologist*, **15**, 163–166.

25 Jenkins, M.E. & Burneo, J.G. (2008) The return of evidence-based neurology to the Journal: It's all about patient care. *The Canadian Journal of Neurological Sciences*, **35**, 273–275.

26 Tartaglia, M.C., Pelz, D.M., Burneo, J.G., Jenkins, M.E. & University of Western Ontario Evidence Based Neurology Group (2009) Cerebral angiography and diagnosis of CNS vasculitis. *The Canadian Journal of Neurological Sciences*, **36**, 93–94.

27 Sackett, D.L., Strauss, S.E. & Richardson, W.S. (2000) *Evidence-based Medicine: How to Practice and Teach EBM*, 2nd edn. Churchill Livingstone, London.

28 Parkes, J., Hyde, C., Deeks, J. & Milne, R. (2001) Teaching critical appraisal skills in health care settings. *Cochrane Database of Systematic Reviews*, (**3**), CD001270 DOI: 10.1002/14651858.CD001270.

29 Coomarasamy, A. & Khan, K.S. (2004) What is the evidence that postgraduate teaching in evidence based medicine changes anything? A systematic review. *BMJ*, **329**, 1–5.

30 Flores-Mateo, G. & Argimon, J.M. (2007) Evidence based practice in postgraduate healthcare education: a systematic review. *BMC Health Services Research*, **7**, 119–127.

2

CHAPTER 2

Evidence-based medicine in health research

Dean M. Wingerchuk

Professor of Neurology, Mayo Clinic, Scottsdale, AZ, USA

Introduction

Evidence-based medical practice combines use of the best available evidence that addresses a particular problem with clinical experience and the patient's values and circumstances [1]. Learning and teaching evidence-based medicine principles have become core components of undergraduate and postgraduate medical curricula, largely with the information "consumer" or "end-user," in mind. That is, evidence-based medicine education largely aims to provide clinicians with fundamental skills that allow critical appraisal of medical literature, interpretation of quantitative evidence, and translation of evidence into practice (see Chapter 1). Clinical investigators provide the data that these practitioners will evaluate and translate to their clinics. Therefore, successful and truly impactful researchers must also possess a thorough understanding of the principles of evidence-based methodology. Such individuals will understand what data the "consumer" will need to change clinical practice with confidence. Possession of poor research design skills leads to undesirable outcomes such as studies with inadequate sample sizes, data marred by biases, and invalid or clinically irrelevant outcome measures. These methodological shortcomings waste both financial and patient resources and have an enormous impact on the effectiveness of global health research [2–6]. The aim of this chapter is to provide an overview of some guiding principles for effective clinical investigators and the implications of evidence-based practice on research publication and subsequent data use.

Using evidence-based principles to develop and answer clinical research questions

In their introductory evidence-based medicine book for clinicians, Straus and colleagues include a chapter entitled "Asking Answerable Clinical Questions" [1]. They suggest that clinicians learn to ask focused questions with four key components (also known as the PICO model): the *patient* (or *problem* or *population*), the *intervention* of interest, *comparison* interventions (if relevant), and the specific *outcome* measure that will be used to interpret the results. This approach provides a template that can be applied to any type of clinical questions, including those that address therapy, diagnosis, prognosis, or causation. The PICO approach has several advantages, a few of which include requiring attention to disease definitions and factors that modify treatment responses or disease course, careful consideration of clinically meaningful outcome measures, and facilitation of literature searches. The goal is to find the best quality evidence that applies to a particular patient and his or her circumstances.

Clinical investigators can also use this schema to guide protocol development. For example, after a thorough, targeted literature search (including systematic reviews published in the *Cochrane Database of Systematic Reviews* and current studies registered at the clinicaltrials.gov website), an investigator may summarize the current status of a therapeutic area and elect to design a new randomized controlled trial to "repurpose" an existing therapy. This approach of combining published literature with registered trials optimizes the chances that the proposed study will address an important knowledge gap and avoid unnecessary duplication. There may be residual uncertainty about the existence of unpublished data. In some instances, this could be mitigated by reviewing conference proceedings for abstracts that report relevant results but have not been followed by a full-text, peer-reviewed publication or by contacting investigators in the field to determine if they know of such studies. The requirement for posting new trials to clinicaltrials.gov promises to gradually reduce this potential bias.

That literature and the PICO framework also guide definition of eligibility criteria, choice of dose and frequency

Evidence-Based Neurology: Management of Neurological Disorders, Second Edition. Edited by Bart M. Demaerschalk and Dean M. Wingerchuk.
© 2015 John Wiley & Sons, Ltd. Published 2015 by John Wiley & Sons, Ltd.

of the study drug, selection of the optimal comparison treatment, and definition of clinically meaningful outcome measures. The details of the protocol are then refined to account for key subgroups, secondary and exploratory outcome measures, and pragmatic considerations necessary for successful trial conduct. This systematic approach provides the greatest likelihood that the study results will contribute meaningfully to clinical practice and guide subsequent research.

Sound research design with the end result in mind

Among the main goals of scientific publication is dissemination of knowledge for use in clinical practice and upon which to build new research. In recent years, many leading academic medical journals have endorsed the use of formal guidelines to ensure transparent research reporting. The most widely known of these is the Consolidated Standards of Reporting Trials (CONSORT) checklist for randomized control trials, which was designed to enable readers to " … understand a trial's design, conduct, analysis and interpretation, and to assess the validity of its results" [7]. Similar requirements have been developed for diagnostic studies (STAR-D) [8] and systematic reviews and meta-analyses (PRISMA) [9]. Although these guidelines have been emphasized for reporting study results, investigators should refer to the pertinent guideline during protocol development to insure that study operations will adequately capture and record the data necessary for future reporting. In other words, the time to be cognizant of the reporting requirements is during protocol development. Some of the key principles of evidence-based research design relevant to therapeutic and diagnostic studies are considered next.

Therapeutic studies

The CONSORT checklist for reporting of therapeutic trials consists of 22 items under several headings: Title and Abstract, Background, Methods, Results, and Discussion [8]. The study author is instructed to include the term "randomized" in the report title if appropriate. The "Methods" section requires reporting of several key elements meant to reassure the consumer that potential sources of bias or threats to validity have been adequately addressed and, importantly, so that a study may be satisfactorily replicated using the reported methods. These key elements include study objectives and hypotheses, how subjects were ascertained (eligibility criteria; setting and location of recruitment), precise details of the study interventions (dose, route of administration, frequency, timing, etc.), clear definitions of primary and secondary outcome measures and any methods to enhance data quality (including training of assessors), and how the study sample size was determined. Details about

subject and investigator blinding are crucial and frequently missing or inadequately described in trial reports [2,3]. These details include randomization method; explicit description of steps taken to conceal treatment allocation; and how blinded status was maintained for subjects, investigators, and other relevant individuals. The consistency of reporting items such as randomization and allocation concealment methods remain mediocre despite use of the CONSORT schema, indicating that peer reviewers and editors have an opportunity for quality improvement.

The "Methods" section of the protocol must contain a description of the statistical analysis plan for the primary and key secondary outcomes. *A priori* definition of secondary or subgroup analyses is also highly desirable. Therefore, consultation with an experienced statistician and, if available, study methodologist is recommended very early in the study design phase.

Planning for eventual study reporting can assist in protocol design because it requires one to consider the sequential operations that govern a subject's progression through the trial process from identification to final evaluation. The CONSORT checklist includes a strong recommendation for use of a flow diagram in the study report. Required variables include the number of participants randomly assigned, receiving intended treatment and completing the protocol, and were included in the primary outcome analysis. The flow diagram allows the reader to easily track those who are lost to follow-up or do not contribute to the outcome analysis, factors that are sometimes not clearly reported.

In addition to completion of the flow diagram, the reporting requirements include recruitment and follow-up dates, baseline demographics and clinical characteristics of study groups, and the number of subjects in each group. It must clear how many subjects contribute to the statistical analyses and whether the analysis was performed by "intention-to-treat" methods; such methods should be specified. The primary and secondary outcomes must be reported with an estimate of the magnitude and precision (e.g. 95% confidence interval) of the effect. Subgroup and adjusted analyses are denoted as pre-planned or exploratory. Adverse event descriptions and rates are required for each intervention group. The CONSORT checklist also includes a section on study interpretation and context, in which investigators should discuss the results and sources of potential bias. Finally, the checklist requires a statement on generalizability (external validity) of the study findings, and that the results be placed in the context of current available evidence, updated from the systematic review conducted before protocol was designed.

Diagnostic studies

The Standards for the Reporting of Diagnostic accuracy studies (STARD) checklist [9] provides for diagnostic studies what CONSORT does for therapeutic trials. It is a guide for investigators reporting results of protocols that evaluate the accuracy of diagnostic tests, ensuring comprehensive description of methods and results. It requires that authors indicate the study population (eligibility criteria and settings for the study), how subjects were recruited (e.g. based on symptoms or results from previous tests), and whether the study was retrospective or prospective. The spectrum of disease included in the study methods consists of rationale for and description of the index diagnostic test (the new test being examined in the study) and the reference ("gold") standard. To insure clarity and potential reproduction of the protocol, investigators should describe the procedures for performing and interpreting each test, including the types of personnel who administer the tests, their training, and cut-off values for the results. Critical issues related to study validity include whether all subjects received both the index test and the reference standard, whether both were evaluated independently and in blinded manner (e.g. if the evaluators of the index and reference tests were blinded to the results of the other). Again, a flow diagram is recommended in the "Results" section to demonstrate the progress of the individuals in the study cohort along different protocol checkpoints and to allow the reader to judge the potential for bias. STARD emphasizes the presentation of results in cross-tabulation form with estimates of diagnostic accuracy (e.g. sensitivity, specificity, likelihood ratios) and with measures of uncertainty (e.g. confidence intervals). As for therapeutic studies, investigators are required to put the results into clinical context.

Resources for clinical investigators

Most medical school curricula and postgraduate training programs now require some formal training in fundamental principles of evidence-based medicine. However, the requirements vary considerably between programs and many clinicians who embark on a clinical research career now elect to pursue certificate or degree programs in clinical epidemiology and methodology in order to establish a methodological foundation for their future research. For those individuals with inadequate time or access to such formal programs, there are numerous resources available to support evidence-based practice and research. A few representative leading resources are described below.

JAMA Evidence (jamaevidence.com)

JAMA evidence a comprehensive reference for investigators and clinicians [10]. Although aimed primarily at the evidence consumer with systematic methods for evidence-based clinical practice (it is divided into sections entitled Assess, Ask, Acquire, Appraise, and Apply), the background knowledge is invaluable for those planning primary research. It also links to the *User's Guide to the Medical Literature*, a leading resource for optimal evaluation and use of the medical literature in clinical practice.

Center for Evidence-Based Medicine (cebm.net)

This program is based at the University of Oxford. In addition to educational resources for evidence-based medicine practitioners and students, it contains an extensive list of online evidence-based medicine resources and links to the contemporary research and publications [11].

EQUATOR Network (equator-network.org)

The enhancing the quality and transparency of health research (EQUATOR) Network is an online resource dedicated to enhancing reporting of research [12]. In addition to the CONSORT and STARD guidelines described earlier, it maintains links to several other reporting guidelines including the following:
• Preferred reporting items for systematic reviews and meta-analyses (PRISMA) for systematic reviews and meta-analyses [9]
• Strengthening the reporting of observational studies in epidemiology (STROBE) Statement for reporting observational studies [13]
• Consolidated criteria for reporting qualitative research (COREQ), a checklist for interviews and focus groups [14]
• SQUIRE, a publication guideline for quality improvement in health care [15]
• Statistical Analyses and Methods in the Published Literature (SAMPLE), which describes basic biomedical statistical reporting [16]
• SPIRIT, which provides checklist guidance on the minimum content that should be included in a clinical trial protocol [17]

The EQUATOR Network website also includes helpful introductory resources for authors and investigators, including planning, conducting, and reporting research.

Summary

A well-equipped clinician uses experience and the best available evidence to make clinical decisions for the welfare of his or her patients. The same skill that makes an evidence-based clinician effective – understanding clinical trial methodology and applied statistics – is germane to every stage of clinical research from asking a relevant research question to designing, executing, and reporting the results of a clinical study. The effective clinical investigator should keep the consumer in mind so that subsequent evaluation of his or her research can achieve the highest possible standards of the evidence appraisal process, and the outcomes stand the greatest chance of resulting in lasting and meaningful impact on healthcare.

References

1 Straus, S.E., Glasziou, P., Richardson, W.S. & Haynes, R.B. (2011) *Evidence-Based Medicine: How to Practice and Teach It*, 4th edn. Churchill Livingstone, Elsevier, pp. 1.

2 Chalmers, I. & Glasziou, P. (2009) Avoidable waste in the production and reporting of research evidence. *Lancet*, **374**, 86–89.

3 McLeod, M.R., Michie, S., Roberts, I. *et al.* (2014) Biomedical research: increasing value, reducing waste. *Lancet*, **383**, 101–104.

4 Ioannidis, J.P.A., Greenland, S., Hlatky, M.A. *et al.* (2014) Increasing value and reducing waste in research design, conduct, and analysis. *Lancet*, **383**, 166–175.

5 Chan, A.-W., Song, F., Vickers, A. *et al.* (2014) Increasing value and reducing waste: addressing inaccessible research. *Lancet*, **383**, 257–266.

6 Glasziou, P., Altman, D.G., Bossuyt, P. *et al.* (2014) Reducing waste from incomplete or unusable reports of biomedical research. *Lancet*, **383**, 267–276.

7 Schulz, K.F., Altman, D.G. & Moher, D. (2010) for the CONSORT Group. CONSORT 2010 Statement: updated guidelines for reporting parallel group randomised trials. *BMJ*, **340**, c332.

8 Bossuyt, P.M., Reitsma, J.B., Bruns, D.E. *et al.* (2003) Toward complete and accurate reporting of studies of diagnostic accuracy: the STARD initiative. *BMJ*, **326**, 41–4.

9 Moher, D., Liberati, A., Tetzlaff, J. & Altman, D.G. (2009) The PRISMA Group. *Preferred Reporting Items for Systematic Reviews and Meta-Analyses: The PRISMA Statement. BMJ*, **339**, b2535.

10 JAMA Evidence. *Available at jamaevidence.com* (accessed 31 March 2014).

11 Centre for Evidence-Based Medicine. *Available at cebm.net* (accessed 31 March 2014).

12 EQUATOR Network. *Available at equator-network.net* (accessed 3 May 2014).

13 von Elm, E., Altman, D.G., Egger, M., Pocock, S.J., Gotzsche, P.C. & Vandenbroucke, J.P. (2007) The Strengthening the Reporting of Observational Studies in Epidemiology (STROBE) Statement: guidelines for reporting observational studies. *Annals of Internal Medicine*, **147**, 573–577.

14 Tong, A., Sainsbury, P. & Craig, J. (2007) Consolidated criteria for reporting qualitative research (COREQ): a 32-item checklist for interviews and focus groups. *International Journal for Quality in Health Care*, **19**, 349–357.

15 Davidoff, F., Batalden, P., Stevens, D., Ogrinc, G. & Mooney, S. (2009) Publication guidelines for quality improvement in health care: evolution of the SQUIRE project. *BMJ*, **338**, a3152.

16 Lang, T.A. & Altman, D.G. (2013) Basic Statistical Reporting for Articles Published in Biomedical Journals: The "Statistical Analyses and Methods in the Published Literature" or The SAMPL Guidelines". In: Smart, P., Maisonneuve, H. & Polderman, A. (eds), *Science Editors' Handbook*. European Association of Science Editors.

17 Chan, A.-W., Tetzlaff, J.M., Altman, D.G. *et al.* (2013) SPIRIT 2013 Statement: Defining standard protocol items for clinical trials. *Annals of Internal Medicine*, **158**, 200–207.

CHAPTER 3
Evidence and ethics

Joseph L. Verheijde

Associate Professor of Biomedical Ethics, College of Medicine, Mayo Clinic, Scottsdale, AZ, USA

Introduction

Ethics and the production and practical use of scientific evidence in the field of neurology intersect minimally at 3 different levels: practical, theoretical, and philosophical. At a practical level, the intersection pertains to selecting the appropriate therapeutic interventions from a variety of available options and conflict resolution regarding the actual or proposed care decisions (clinical ethics), as well as to the establishment of and adherence to ethical guidelines for scientific inquiry involving human subjects (research or investigational ethics). At a theoretical level, they interact with regard to the way evidence is to be applied to the process of medical decision making, and to the formulation of a response to original ethical questions that emanate from the success in medical science and neuroscience in particular of developing new medical and research technologies. These technologies, as we come to realize, profoundly impact how "the good" of medicine, philosophically speaking, is to be appreciated by society. The latter represents the third intersection, which in the ethics literature is now commonly referred to as *neuroethics*. As noted by Farah [1], "[n]ew ethical issues are arising as neuroscience gives us unprecedented ways to understand the human mind and to predict, influence, and even control it." These novel insights into the working of the human mind in many ways raise some fundamental questions such as what behavior should be considered "normal" and to what extent should medicine correct what is believed to be a deviation from the standard of normal? What kind of medicine does society really want? Who decides and by what authority?

In what follows, the origin and features of the biomedical model commonly used in health care, as well as its implications for the ethical conduct of medical research, are discussed. Finally, a brief overview of the new field of neuroethics is presented.

The current ethical framework in health care

Throughout history, the primary intent of physicians has always been to cure disease, minimize suffering, and maximize the well-being of patients. At least since the time of Hippocrates (circa 460 BC– circa 375 BC), normative guidance in clinical practice has been founded on the primacy of the "do-no-harm" principle (primum non nocere); that is, the potential benefits for the patient of any intervention must outweigh its burdens. Although the moral goodness of the physicians' intent in their interactions with patients has been intuitively assumed to be self-evident and clear, the ethical rules that guide medical practice have changed significantly over time. As the medical profession established a stronger organizational structure and a broader academic foundation, subsequently gaining respect and prestige during the 20th century, the notion that "the doctor knows best" became widely accepted in society and thereby provided the appearance of validation of an exclusively paternalistic approach to patient care.

During the later part of the 20th century, the moral nature and tone of medical practice underwent an even more dramatic change from paternalistic to consultative [2], a change that can be exclusively attributed to the introduction of a new model of medical ethics. In the late 1970s, Beauchamp and Childress [3] published what has come to be broadly considered one of the most prominent and important works in contemporary biomedical ethics, *Principles of Biomedical Ethics*. The authors argued that the model based on four principles (i.e. respect for individual autonomy, beneficence, non-maleficence, and justice) would form an appropriate replacement option for the heretofore existing moral theories, and would thus provide a better and more consistent way of dealing with moral problems that arise within medical practice [3]. Some of the main existing normative

Evidence-Based Neurology: Management of Neurological Disorders, Second Edition. Edited by Bart M. Demaerschalk and Dean M. Wingerchuk.
© 2015 John Wiley & Sons, Ltd. Published 2015 by John Wiley & Sons, Ltd.

theories to that date included (1) virtue ethics as proposed by Aristotle [4] and others, that is, a moral theory that focuses on the question of what kind of people we ought to be; (2) deontology (Kant [5]), which requires an action to satisfy the categorical imperative in order for it to be viewed as morally good, acting in such a manner that the reason for the act could/should become a universal law; and (3), consequentialism (Bentham [6] and Mill [7]), which defines the rightness of actions as the one that generates the most intrinsic good for the largest number of people.

In general, a moral theory represents a moral philosophy from which the guiding principles can then be derived. These principles generate rules that are then used to judge the rightness or wrongness of an action [8]. Whether an action can be appreciated as morally correct thus depends to a large degree on which moral theory is being applied. It has been argued that Beauchamp and Childress' *Principles of Biomedical Ethics* was – and still is – superior to traditional normative theories in its ability to deal effectively with biomedical issues because of its universality; it contrasts with moralities that originate from "cultural, religious, and institutional sources, which are not shared universally" [9]. True or not, the "principlist" account of medical ethics has become an influential, if not the dominating, contemporary model in bioethics. Along the way, it has made the notion of respect for autonomy the centerpiece and cornerstone of moral reasoning in medical practice. It has also assisted in constituting the model of "shared decision making," and in cementing the concept of informed consent that now characterizes all interactions between physicians, care providers, and patients.

The term "principlism" was coined by Clouser and Gert in their critique of Beauchamp and Childress' four principle model. Clouser and Gert argued that principlism represents a system of ethics within which "principles seem primarily to name important aspects of morality … [and] are *de facto* the final court of appeal" [8].

Beauchamp and Childress' moral decision-making model originated from a document called the Belmont Report [10], of which Beauchamp was a coauthor. The Belmont Report itself emanated from the American Military Tribunal's criminal proceedings against German physicians and administrators for war crimes and crimes against humanity during the Nuremberg trials that were started in 1946. This report is widely considered to be one of the leading works regarding ethics and healthcare research. Tom Beauchamp, in collaboration with James Childress, inserted the principle of non-maleficence into the three principles that were part of the Belmont Report (autonomy, beneficence, and justice) and transformed this four-principle approach into a comprehensive ethical decision-making model. The principle of respect for autonomy is the first of the four principles the authors described. It encompasses recognizing the patient's right to be self-directing (self-governance).

It correctly presupposes "a capacity for intentional action on the basis of one's own rational deliberations as well as freedom from controlling instances" [11]. In the context of medical practice, the central position must be that patients have the capacity to make decisions about their care. If this capacity is absent, patient autonomy is to be protected by delegating care decisions to a surrogate (i.e. a person preferably designated by the patient to make decisions in circumstances involving severe diminishment or loss of the patient's capacity for informed decision making). The three remaining principles are non-maleficence, beneficence, and justice. To summarize, non-maleficence refers to the physician's obligation not to inflict harm onto the patient. Beneficence in medicine signifies the obligation to act in the best interests of the patient. The fourth principle is justice, which emphasizes the need for all patients to be treated fairly and equitably.

The introduction of principlism in bioethics and medical practice has also resulted in the central positioning of autonomy in healthcare policy making. The Patient Self-Determination Act of 1991 [12] solidified the rights of patients to make autonomous decisions about the medical treatment they prefer, are considered to be entitled to, or want to have withdrawn. The Patient Self-Determination Act was introduced after the 1990 US Supreme Court in Cruzan v. Director, Missouri Dept. of Health ruled in favor of the state to keep Nancy Cruzan on life support (here, medically assisted nutrition and hydration), despite her persistent vegetative state lasting longer than 4 years and her husband's and parents' wishes otherwise [13]. The Court came to this conclusion based on the assessment that an incompetent person's wishes with regard to the withdrawal of life-sustaining treatment be proved by clear and convincing evidence, which the Court found to be unsatisfactory in the Cruzan case.

Respect for patient's rights is not preconditioned either by a physician's agreement with or approval of the patient's decision. However, autonomous decisions made by a patient may also create conflicts with what physicians consider to be their primary duties: to provide care (beneficence), to not inflict harm (non-maleficence), and to contribute toward improving or preserving the fair and equitable distribution of healthcare services (justice).

As a profession, medicine requires its practitioners to have clinical autonomy and independence of judgment [14]. It has been argued that the traditional virtues associated with the role of the physician (compassion in the relief of suffering) can be complementary to principlism. By that view, as Pellegrino [15] has pointed out, virtue ethics becomes an essential element of any moral theory. "How duties, rules, obligations, sentiments, etc., are acted upon, interpreted, given weight, put into priority and with what intention or motives, are all shaped by the character of the moral agent." Or, as Vizcarrondo [16] has argued, principlism by itself "overlooks the moral agent, separates the ethical decisions from the moral sensibilities that shaped them, isolating the decisions from the moral agent" [16].

The centrality and boundaries of autonomy-centered decision making have themselves become contentious medical, moral, and legal issues. Some have argued that taking the older ethic of physician beneficence out of the center of medical ethics and replacing it with patient autonomy has contributed to the prevalence of "certain defensive notions of individualistic rights-based autonomy" at the expense of autonomy understood as part of "a wider morality of relationship and care" [17]. In end-of-life situations, the notion of autonomy has renewed the question of whether the patient's right to self-determination entails the right to die, implicitly challenging the US Supreme Court's 1997 opinion in Washington v. Glucksberg that the right to assisted death is not a fundamental liberty interest protected by the US Constitution [18]. The tremendous advancements in biotechnology have added greater complexity to the moral decision making about whether, and under what specific circumstances (if any), these life-preserving technologies can be discontinued at the patient's request [19–22].

The principle of justice appears problematic for those involved in clinical decision making as well. What is the appropriate concept of justice? Without further explication, Beauchamp and Childress [23] posited that the division of what should be considered obligatory and what is supererogatory is based on a concept of justice that is defined by its realistic possibility. That appears to mean that "the quest for a just society [is placed] within the realm of the supererogatory, and outside of the obligatory" [23]. Such a position would minimize the physician's obligation to contribute to the correction of societal injustices, such as inequality of access to healthcare services, as long as an egalitarian approach to healthcare distribution is not part of the common morality. Nevertheless, others have argued that ensuring equal access to health care should be one of society's moral obligations [24,25].

Beauchamp and Childress' philosophical contributions have also been criticized on theoretical grounds. The notion that the four principles represent a common morality, that is to say, a set of "norms about right and wrong human conduct that are so widely shared that they form a stable (although usually incomplete) social consensus" [26], may lead to the conclusion that their theory is founded on quicksand [27]. Beauchamp and Childress' failure to demonstrate the foundational nature of the four principles has negatively affected their claim to global applicability [28]. Fox and Swacey have rejected the legitimacy of the common morality claim on social scientific grounds. They have pointed toward what they consider to be the most cross-culturally problematic: "the primacy that its paradigm accords to individualism and individual rights" [29]. In addition, the fact that Beauchamp and Childress' framework of bioethics is resolutely secular in nature, constitute an additional source of incompatibility in pluriform societies [29]. Engelhardt has also challenged the central expectation that moral-philosophical reflection can disclose a canonical content-full morality and bioethics because there is "a plurality of moral rationalities among which one cannot through sound rational argument make a principled choice" [30]. As a consequence, secular bioethics "cannot provide uncontroversial, content-full, moral guidance" [30] in resolving issues that arise in medical practice. The plurality of moralities advances "substantively different views as to what is proper in health care and the biomedical sciences" [31]. Or, as Takala [32] has argued, we think that good is good, but "it is what constitutes the good in various circumstances that we cannot agree upon." In "[a] sociological account of the growth of principlism," Evans posited that principlism offers "the lure of calculability and predictability" not offered by more traditional approaches to ethics [33]. He contributes this calculability and predictability to the notion of commensuration, that is, replacing the use of different measurement units for different properties with a single unit that can lead to "discarding information in order to make decisionmaking easier by ignoring aspects of the problem that cannot be translated to the common metric" [33]. Proponents of principlism, on the other hand, have advocated celebrating it as a basis for moral ecumenism and rejecting what they deem to be the mistaken perception that it is an attempt at global moral imperialism [34].

Beauchamp and Childress have made substantial contributions to the field of biomedical ethics, as evidenced by the fact that their model of moral decision making has become firmly integrated into medical practice. In view of the ongoing debate about the concepts, value, and role of principlism, it is no surprise that the jury is still out on the question of whether they were definitively able "to bring some order and coherence to the discussion," something Beauchamp and Childress [3] set out to do in the first edition of their book. Although, as one might expect, the validity of the conceptual foundation of principlism continues to be debated, predominantly among moral philosophers, principlism itself has become deeply integrated into ethical decision making in health care. Considering that the social, political, and economic forces that helped shape a model of moral decision making with autonomy at its center is unlikely to change anytime soon, the dominance of principlism may last far into the foreseeable future. At the same time, as Pellegrino has argued, a new period may have started "in which conceptual conflicts in ethics and the skepticism of moral philosophy challenge the very idea of a universal, normative ethic for medicine" [35].

At least from the perspective of bedside problem resolution, principlism "leaves considerable room for judgment in specific cases" [36]. Within that space, physicians and other healthcare professionals each have an opportunity to exercise their personal responsibility to comply with the core moral value of medicine, beneficence: the act of doing good to another.

The ethical conduct of human subject research

Contemporary medical practice requires physicians to obtain a valid consent for diagnostic testing and subsequent treatment. Such consent is ethically, morally, and legally mandated on the basis of the fiduciary obligations that originate from the physician–patient relationship [2]. In other words, the prerequisite of valid patient consent acknowledges and reinforces the role of respect for the autonomy, dignity, and self-determination of patients seen in a medical practice [37]. Physicians have a moral responsibility to consult with their patients on the best treatment strategy, to provide patients with the information necessary to select a treatment option, to disclose to the best of their knowledge potential risks, and to discuss anticipated benefits, while taking into consideration the patient's preferences and outcome expectations. The amount of information that legally must be disclosed to satisfy the informed consent requirement is frequently based on the so-called prudent patient standard (i.e. all information that a reasonable person would need in order to be able to make a rational, well-informed choice in selecting a particular treatment option must be shared with that patient). In emergency situations, when a delay of treatment while obtaining consent could potentially be harmful to the patient, consent is not required but rather implied.

In general, for an informed consent to be valid, the patient must have the cognitive ability to understand and process the information provided by the physician. But consent must also be given voluntarily, that is, the "patient must not be cognitively impaired by medication, personal emotional stress, or external stress by family members or physicians" [2]. Voluntariness also presumes that patients will not be coerced either directly by threats or indirectly by exaggeration of the risks of not following the physician's preferred treatment plan [37]. Finally, according to the section on the protection of human subjects in the Code of Federal Regulations (CFR) report on public welfare (CFR 46.116(a)), patients can withdraw their consent for treatment at any time, regardless of whether the physician deems their change of heart to be rational or irrational.

Obtaining informed consent is also necessary to comply with the requirements for the ethical conduct of medical research. As Bernat [37] has pointed out, in clinical trials the focus is on producing generalizable knowledge and not necessarily on promoting the welfare of the individual (i.e. the study participant). Therefore, study participants are used as a "means" rather than as an "end." As long as human subjects are deemed essential to the conduct of medical research, the relationship between researcher and study participant must be based on respect, honesty, and trust. National and international ethical research guidelines for informed consent have been developed and continue to be revised. According to Goodman [38], "Valid consent now

enjoys interdisciplinary support, international credibility, and the sort of conceptual traction that gives an idea practical utility in the boardrooms and at the bedside."

The concept of informed consent started to get shape in 1947 with the Nuremberg Code, which, as mentioned earlier, was itself a response to the medical experiments on unwilling humans that were conducted in Europe during the Nazi regime. These experiments were unprecedented in their scope and in the degree of harm to which they subjected human beings. The Nuremberg Code mandated that voluntary and informed consent must be obtained from all human subjects participating in scientific research, that risks must be proportionate to the humanitarian importance of the experiment being studied, and that unnecessary physical and mental suffering and injury must be avoided.

The Nuremberg Code has since become the model for many governmental and professional codes of research conduct. In 1948, the United Nations adopted the Universal Declaration of Human Rights, and in 1953, the first US Federal Policy for Protection of Human Subjects was implemented. This new policy introduced the mechanism of prospective review of proposed research by independent individuals, a model now known as the institutional review board (IRB) system. In 1964, the World Medical Association adopted the Declaration of Helsinki, which has since undergone several revisions, most recently in 2000 [39]. In 1979, the cornerstone document of ethical principles for the protection of research subjects, now known as the Belmont Report [10], was published by the National Commission for the Protection of Human Subjects of Biomedical and Behavioral Research. By this ethics statement, all research involving human subjects must be based on the principles of respect for persons, beneficence (nonmaleficence), and justice.

This requirement points to the investigator's obligation (1) to allow potential study participants to make their own decisions on whether to enroll in the study; and (2) to design study protocols in such a manner that potential benefits are maximized and risks are minimized. In regard to the latter, the notion of clinical equipoise plays an important role. The randomized controlled trial (RCT) is widely considered the "gold standard" for acquiring evidence in medicine and optimizing the soundness of scientific investigations. Like many authors, Sackett et al. [40] based their definition of the RCT on the CFR guidelines, that is, as a clinical study in which "a group of patients is randomized into an experimental group and a control group. These groups are followed up for the variables/outcomes of interest." The belief of investigators that one treatment arm of the study protocol is superior to the other may cause moral conflict. However, as Bernat [37] has pointed out: "Because these clinical judgments may be influenced heavily by nonscientific factors such as last-case bias, physicians should exercise caution about concluding from insufficient evidence which arm may be superior for a given patient." A state of equipoise, as defined by Freedman [41], is a necessary condition for the justification of clinical studies, wherein there can be "an honest, professional disagreement among expert clinicians about the preferred treatment" (i.e. the comparative merits of two or more forms of treatment or condition). Clinical trials can be morally justified only when their scientific rationale "rests in collective equipoise, which means that the medical community as a whole is genuinely uncertain over which treatment is best" [42]. As an RCT is designed to provide an answer to which arm of the protocol is superior, it "should be designed so that at its conclusion, it disturbs the state of clinical equipoise" [37].

The requirement of adequate informed consent also implies that vulnerable populations must be given added protection. The vulnerable category includes, but is not limited to, human fetuses, minors, economically and/or educationally disadvantaged persons, mentally disabled persons, persons with a reduced capacity to make autonomous decisions, and incarcerated prisoners. Added protection includes the requirement that minors can participate in clinical trials only after consent has been obtained from their surrogate decision maker and the minors themselves also assent. The concept of assent refers to what the American Academy of Pediatrics calls "empower[ing] children to the extent of their capacity" [43]. The National Commission for the Protection of Human Subjects of Biomedical and Behavioral Research in its 1977 report indicated that assent should be obtained from children as young as age of 7 years [44]. Surrogate consent is also required for enrollment of patients with cognitive impairment or mental disorders. The American Academy of Neurology and other professional medical organizations have proposed guidelines to limit the use of this vulnerable group to only those research projects that involve no more than minimal risk and from which the subject might benefit directly [45]. The CFR recommendations for the protection of human subjects (45 CFR 46.102(i)) define "minimal risk" as "the probability and magnitude of harm or discomfort anticipated in the research are not greater in and of themselves than those ordinarily encountered in daily life or during the performance of routine physical or psychological examinations or tests" [46].

Added protection further means that all information provided to potential research subjects must be delivered, according to the CFR, in "language understandable to the subject or the representative" (45 CFR 46.116). This might involve translating the information into the subject's native language or adjusting the reading level of consent forms. In specific situations, the need for informed consent might be waived. In clinical settings, this means consent may be waived when the research involves no more than minimal risk, when the waiver or alteration will not adversely affect the right or welfare of the subjects, or when it has been made appropriately clear that the research cannot be carried out practically without the waiver (e.g. research to assess the therapeutic superiority of one drug or intervention over another used in emergency medicine).

The Belmont Report [10] further stipulated that research must be conducted in a just manner, that is, the burdens and benefits of research must be distributed fairly among individuals, groups, and societies. To advance the rights and welfare of human subjects in research, the National Bioethics Advisory Commission was established by presidential order in 1995. In response to public concerns about potential abuses of the privacy of health information, new regulations were enacted in 2003 under the Health Insurance Portability and Accountability Act (HIPAA). The US Department of Health and Human Services later issued the regulations now known as the Privacy Rule (i.e. the Standards for Privacy of Individually Identifiable Health Information), which requires the standard of information disclosure to be the "minimum necessary" [47]. The objective is for covered entities to "make reasonable efforts to limit protected health information (PHI) to the minimum necessary to accomplish the intended purpose of the use, disclosure, or request" (CFR 45.146.502(b)) [47].

Last but not least, the CFR (45 CFR 46.116) defines the IRB and outlines its duties. The role of the IRB is to prospectively review research protocols, to approve or deny the proposed research, and to provide oversight. Most academic medical institutions have their own IRB. Outside of these institutions, so-called independent IRBs have been established. The main function of an IRB is to safeguard the rights and well-being of human subjects involved in the study by ensuring, among other things, that the proposed research activity has been reviewed and approved, that a proper consent process is in place, and that the risks associated with the research protocol have been minimized and are reasonable in relation to the anticipated benefits. IRBs are also required to ensure that the selection of human subjects is equitable, that the privacy of study subjects is protected, and that the confidentiality of data is maintained. The IRB provides continuing oversight by requiring periodic progress reports and pre-approval of any changes to original protocols.

Some categories of human subject research may be exempt from IRB approval as outlined in 45 CFR 46.101(b). However, the IRB, not the investigator, holds the exclusive authority to make such decisions.

The role of empirical evidence in medical practice and ethics

Scientific evidence plays a significant role in at least two different ways: (1) in ensuring that optimal care is provided to the patient, and (2) in enabling clinical decision making through careful ethical analysis whenever there are competing opinions about the most appropriate patient care. Having good scientific evidence not only promotes the practice of good medicine but also assists in the resolution of often difficult moral conflicts.

Since its introduction in 1992 [48], the term "evidence-based medicine" (EBM) has become well established in contemporary medical practice, and it is now an integral part of the standard training of physicians. Before its widespread acceptance, EBM "was a kind of cognitive itch: a troublesome doubt that follows from the realizations that humans are fallible, that scientific knowledge increases and that medical decisions sometimes have very high stakes" [38]. That is not to say that a claim or practice insufficiently supported by evidence is false, but merely that medical professionals may have inadequate grounds to believe it to be true. From this, it can be deduced that physicians have a moral obligation to base the patient care they provide on the best available medical knowledge.

The initial idea of EBM was to exclude or marginalize "the role of implicit or unquantifiable factors such as clinical judgment, experience, qualitative factors, views of patients and the demands of clinical consultation." [49]. However, the definition of EBM evolved over time: "Evidence, whether strong or weak, is never sufficient to make clinical decisions. Individual values and preferences must balance this evidence to achieve optimal shared decision making" [50]. The evolving definition of EBM highlights the idea that its practice should not be hijacked by managers to promote cost-cutting. Some authors have indeed argued that the switch to EBM has involved a takeover of the clinical consultation by administrators [49]. Nevertheless, even in light of the potential misuse of information that originates from EBM, the moral obligation to care for the patient with scientifically validated care ought to be the highest priority and a shared responsibility of both the physician and the healthcare administrator. Equally as important, optimal shared decision making can be accomplished only when the patient's unique values and circumstance are an integral part of the definition of EBM [40,50].

EBM methodologically concerns itself with formulating an answer to the question of whether intervention "X" is safe and effective for condition "Y." In other words, its primary focus is to try to answer epistemological questions. Formulating answers to these questions is a function of research that also extends into the domain of direct patient care. In regard to both the domain of clinical research and the domain of clinical practice, EBM raises ethical issues. The previous section outlined the moral prerequisites to answer clinically relevant epistemological questions. The issue of how to translate research outcomes into the care of individual patients is more complex. How are patient preferences, values, and belief systems to be respected within an evidence-based practice of medicine? What place should the patient's right to make autonomous decisions be awarded in the context of the moral obligation to provide care interventions that are based on the best available evidence? For as Sackett *et al.* [40] stated, even as "population-based 'outcomes research' has repeatedly documented that those patients who do receive evidence-based therapies have better outcomes than those who don't," could patients insist on a therapy less supported by evidence? If providing evidence-based care is expected to reduce the costs of health care, would not providing any other care intervention violate the principle of justice (i.e. fair distribution)? The more fundamental questions then would be how should physicians practice medicine and how would healthcare dollars be best spent [51]. These are normative issues raised within the context of EBM for which answers have yet to be formulated.

Neuroethics

The third intersection between ethics, evidence, and neuroscience pertains to the field of neuroethics. As Farah, who has published extensively on the subject, explained: "New ethical issues are arising as neuroscience gives us unprecedented ways to understand the human mind and to predict, influence, and even control it" [52]. The advancement in functional magnetic resonance imaging (fMRI) technologies introduces new avenues in exploring areas of cognition, emotion, and social processes, making "[a]ny endeavor that depends on being able to understand, assess, predict, control, or improve human behavior … a potential application for neuroscience" [53]. The fMRI identifies and locates certain brain activities by measuring changes in blood flow. This allows scientists to infer which parts of the brain are engaged in cognitive activities or, for that matter, to determine when a person makes different kinds of moral judgments. The greater the knowledge about mental states and human behavior acquired from fMRI, combined with an increased ability to intervene in a person's brain function with the goal of changing these mental states and behaviors, the more complex the ethical, legal, and social challenges will become [53]. Roskies [54] has defined neuroethics, in the words of Al Jonsen, as the "unexplored continent lying between the two populated shores of ethics and of neuroscience." The reason why neuroethics is not just another branch of applied ethics is because in addition to addressing issues such as "the permissibility or advisability of using certain technologies to 'read' minds, enhance capacities, or control behavior …, [it] also questions … what it means to be human, whether we have free will, the nature of knowledge and of self-knowledge" [55].

Farah [53] described the development in brain imaging from its first application for the study of human psychology and the study of cognition to applying these techniques toward the study of human emotions. She concluded that "by demonstrating the existence of physical correlates of our most important human qualities and experiences, neuroimaging has contributed to a fundamental change in how we think of ourselves and our fellow persons" [53]. Much as genetic information reveals a person's physical predispositions, brain imaging results may reveal information about mental and behavioral status without the patient even knowing about it or without the patient ever having acted in accordance with the identified propensities to socially unacceptable behaviors. Although it is unlikely that a single brain region can be identified as the moral center of the brain, there are indications that certain regions in the brain are particularly relevant to moral behavior [56]. In that way, brain imaging may present a potential threat to privacy. Brain imaging, in combination with the increasing options for pharmaceutical interventions, raises questions about conditions under which and to what extent behavior can be modified. In other words, what is the standard of normalcy and who is to decide on it?

Brain imaging technology has also affected the field of ethics itself. It has been shown that changes in the morphological structure of the brain can lead to disruption of a person's moral sensibilities. Damasio [57] described the case of the 19th-century railroad worker Phineas Cage. Cage was working when an accidental explosion occurred that sent a tamping iron rod through his cheek and out of the top of his head. He survived the severe injury to his prefrontal cortex. Although Phineas' cognitive function was unimpaired, he showed significant behavioral changes. Since then, research on the neural foundations to moral reasoning and antisocial behavior has identified regions of the brain that are most commonly activated in moral judgment activities and rule-breaking behaviors. Although Raine and Yang [58] identify "this neurobiological predisposition … [as] likely only one of several biosocial processes involved in the etiology of antisocial behavior, it raises significant moral issues for the legal system and neuroethics," questions arise regarding the notions of "voluntariness" and "responsibility" in human behavior.

The field of neuroethics is fairly new, and research in identifying neural correlates to human behavior is still in the early stages of development. It is reasonable to assume that neuroscientific research will contribute to the better understanding of human behavior, which will have implications for therapeutic medicine, the legal system, and the field of moral philosophy.

To conclude, medicine and ethics have traditionally held a long and close relationship. "To do medicine well, we must start out with the proper ethical norm, what is good for another" [59]. To determine what is good for another, physicians must, among other things, provide care that is supported by the best available evidence. Scientific research is a critical component in obtaining this evidence and increasing our knowledge base. None of this can be accomplished without the strong commitment of all stakeholders in medicine to ethical norms and values.

References

1 Farah, M.J. (2010) Neuroethics: an overview. In: Farah, M.J. (ed), *Neuroethics. An Introduction with Readings*. MIT Press, Cambridge, Massachusetts, pp. 8.

2 Paterick, T.J., Carson, G.V., Allen, M.C. & Paterick, T.E. (2008) Medical informed consent: general considerations for physicians. *Mayo Clinic Proceedings*, **83**(3), 313–319.

3 Beauchamp, T. & Childress, J. (1979) *Principles of Biomedical Ethics*. Oxford University Press, New York.

4 Aristotle (2000). In: Irwin, T. (ed), *Nichomachean Ethics*, 2nd edn. Hackett Publishing Co.

5 Kant, I. (1989) *Foundations of the Metaphysics of Morals*, 2nd Lewis White Beck (translator) edn. Library of Liberal Arts.

6 Bentham, J. (1907) *An Introduction to the Principles of Morals and Legislation*. Clarendon Press, Oxford.

7 Mill, J.S. (2010) *Utilitarianism*. Valde Books.

8 Danner Clouser, K. & Gert, B. (1990) A critique of principlism. *The Journal of Medicine and Philosophy*, **15**, 219–236.

9 Raupich, O. & Vollmann, J. (2011) 30 years principles of biomedical ethics: introduction to a symposium on the 6th edition of Tom L Beauchamp and James F Childress' seminal work. *Journal of Medical Ethics*, **37**, 582–583.

10 Department of Health Education and Welfare (1979) Protection of human subjects; notice of report for public comment. *Federal Register*, **44**(76), 23191–23197.

11 Sjostrand, M., Helgesson, G., Erikson, S. & Juth, N. (2013) Autonomy-based arguments against physician-assisted suicide and euthanasia: a critique. *Medicine, Health Care and Philosophy*, **16**(2), 225–230.

12 Federal Patient Self-Determination Act (1992) Final regulations. *Federal Register*, **57**(45), 8194–8204.

13 US Supreme Court. *Cruzan v. Director MDoH, 497 U.S. 261* (1990) http://supreme.justia.com/us/497/261 and http://www.oyez.org/cases/1980-1989/1989/1989_88_1503 (accessed 16 February 2012).

14 Morreim, E.H. (2002) Professionalism and clinical autonomy in the practice of medicine. *Mount Sinai Journal of Medicine*, **69**(6), 370–377.

15 Pellegrino, E.D. (2002) Professionalism, Profession and the Virtues of the Good Physician. *Mount Sinai Journal of Medicine*, **69**(6), 378–384.

16 Vizcarrondo, F.F. (2012) The return of virtue to ethical medical decision making. *The Linnacre Quarterly*, **79**(1), 73–80.

17 Tauber, A.I. (2003) Sick autonomy. *Perspectives in Biology and Medicine*, **46**(4), 484–495.

18 US Supreme Court. *Washington v. Glucksberg US*. http://supreme.justia.com/us/521/702/ and http://www.oyez.org/cases/1990-1999/1996/1996_96_110 (accessed 16 February 2012).

19 Pellegrino, E.D. (2000) Decisions to withdraw life-sustaining treatment. A moral algorithm. *JAMA*, **283**(8), 1065–1067.

20 Mueller, P.S., Jenkins, S.M., Bramstedt, K.A. & Hayes, D.L. (2008) Deactivating implanted cardiac devices in terminally Ill patients: practices and attitudes. *Pacing and Clinical Electrophysiology*, **31**(5), 560–568.

21 Mueller, P.S., Swetz, K.M. & Freeman, M.R. (2010) Ethical analysis of withdrawing ventricular assist device support. *Mayo Clinic Proceedings*, **85**(9), 791–797.

22 Rady, M.Y. & Verheijde, J.L. (2011) When is deactivating and implanted cardiac device physician-assisted death? Appraisal of

the lethal pathophiology and mode of death. *Journal of Palliative Medicine*, **14**(**10**), 1086–1088.

23 Holm, S. (1995) Not just autonomy - the principles of American biomedical ethics. *Journal of Medical Ethics*, **21**, 332–338.

24 Walzer, M. (1983) *Spheres of Justice: A Defense of Pluralism and Equality*. Basic Books, New York.

25 Verheijde, J.L. (2006) *Managing care: a shared responsibility*. Springer, Dordrecht, The Netherlands.

26 Beauchamp, T. & Childress, J. (2009) *Principles of Biomedical Ethics*, 6th edn. Oxford University Press, New York.

27 Karlsen, J.R. & Solbakk, J.H. (2011) A waste of time: the problem of common morality in Principles of Biomedical Ethics. *Journal of Medical Ethics*, **37**, 588–591.

28 Herissone-Kelly, P. (2011) Determining the common morality's norms in the sixth edition of Principles of Biomedical Ethics. *Journal of Medical Ethics*, **37**, 584–587.

29 Fox, R.C. & Swazey, J.P. (2010) Guest editorial: ignoring the social and cultural context of bioethics is unacceptable. *Cambridge Quarterly of Healthcare Ethics*, **19**(**3**), 278–281.

30 Engelhardt, H.T. Jr., (2011) Confronting moral pluralism in post-traditional Western societies: bioethics critically reassessed. *Journal of Medicine and Philosophy*, **36**, 243–260.

31 Engelhardt, H.T. Jr., (2006) *Global Bioethics: The Collapse of Consensus*. Scrivener Publishing, Salem, MA.

32 Takala, T. (2011) What is wrong with global bioethics? On the limitations of the four principles approach. *Cambridge Quarterly of Healthcare Ethics*, **10**, 72–77.

33 Evans, J.H. (2000) A sociological account of the growth of principlism. *Hastings Center Report*, **30**(**5**), 31–38.

34 Gillon, R. (2003) Ethics needs principles-Four can encompass the rest- and respect for autonomy should be "first among equals". *Journal of Medical Ethics*, **29**, 307–312.

35 Pellegrino, E.D. (1993) The metamorphosis of medical ethics. *JAMA*, **269**(**9**), 1158–1162.

36 Watine, J. (2010) What sort of bioethical values are the evidence-based medicine and the GRADE approaches willing to deal with? *Journal of Medical Ethics*, **37**(**3**), 184–186.

37 Bernat, J.L. (2006) Ethical issues in neurological treatment and clinical trials. In: Noseworthy, J.H. (ed), *Neurological Therapeutics Principles and Practice*, 2nd edn. Vol. **1**. Taylor Fracis, Boca Raton, FL, USA, pp. 73–83.

38 Goodman, K. (2003) *Ethics and Evidence-Based Medicine. Fallibility and Responsibility in Clinical Science*. Cambridge University Press.

39 World Medical Association (2000) World Medical association declaration of Helsinki: ethical principles for medical research involving human subjects. *JAMA*, **284**, 3043–3046.

40 Sackett, D.L., Strauss, S.E., Richardson, W.S., Rosenberg, W. & Haynes, R.B. (2000) *Evidence-Based Medicine. How to Practice and Teach EBM*, 2nd edn. Churchill Livingstone.

41 Freedman, B. (1987) Equipoise and the ethics of clinical research. *NEJM*, **317**(**3**), 141–145.

42 Edwards, S.J.L., Lilford, R.J. & Hewison, J. (1998) The ethics of randomized controlled trials from the perspectives of patients, the public, and healthcare professionals. *BMJ*, **317**, 1209–1212.

43 Committee on Bioethics AAoP (1995) Informed consent, parental permission, and assent in pediatric practice. *Pediatrics*, **95**, 314–317.

44 The National Commission for the Protection of Human Subjects of Biomedical and Behavioral Research. (1977) *Research Involving Children*. http://bioethics.georgetown.edu/pcbe/reports/past_commissions/Research_involving_children.pdf (accessed 20 February 2012).

45 The Ethics and Humanities Subcommittee of the American Academy of Neurology (1998) Ethical issues in neurology: advancing knowledge and protecting human research subjects. *Neurology*, **50**, 592–595.

46 Code of Federal Regulations. *Title 45: Public Welfare, part 46: Protection of Human Subjects. 45 CFR 46.102(i)*.

47 Code of Federal Regulations - *Title 45: Public Welfare 45 CFR 164.502 (b)*.

48 EBM Working Group (1992) Evidence-based medicine. *JAMA*, **268**, 2420–2425.

49 Charlton, B.G. & Miles, A. (1998) The rise and fall of EBM. *QJM*, **91**(**5**), 371–374.

50 Straus, S.E., Haynes, R.B., Glasziou, P., Dickersin, K. & Guyatt, G. (2007) Misunderstandings, misperceptions, and mistakes. *Evidence-Based Medicine*, **12**, 2–3.

51 Sehon, S.R. & Stanley, D.E. (2003) A philosophical analysis of the evidence-based medicine debate. *BMC Health Services Research*, **3**(**14**).

52 Farah, M.J. (2010) *Neuroethics. An Introduction with Readings*. MIT Press, Cambridge, Massachusetts.

53 Farah, M.J. (2012) Neuroethics: the ethical, legal, and societal impact of neuroscience. *Annual Review of Psychology*, **63**, 571–591.

54 Roskies, A. (2002) Neuroethics for the millenium. *Neuron*, **35**(**1**), 21–23.

55 Levy, N. (2011) Neuroethics: a new way of doing ethics. *AJOB Neuroscience*, **2**(**2**), 3–9.

56 Moll, J., de Oliveira-Souza, R. & Eslinger, P. (2003) Morals and the human brain: a working model. *NeuroReport*, **14**(**3**), 299–305.

57 Damasio, A.R. (1994) *Descartes' error: emotion, reason, and the human brain*. G. P. Putnam.

58 Raine, A. & Yang, Y. (2006) Neural foundations to moral reasoning and antisocial behavior. *SCAN*, **1**, 203–213.

59 Dreger, M.D. (2012) Autonomy trumps all. Medicine loses its grounding in science. *Nath Cath Bioethics Q* 2012; **12**(**4**), 653–654.

PART 2

Evidence-based neurology in the hospital

CHAPTER 4
Thunderclap headache

Jonathan H. Smith[1] and Todd J. Schwedt[2]
[1]*Department of Neurology, University of Kentucky, Lexington, KY, USA*
[2]*Department of Neurology, Mayo Clinic, Phoenix, AZ, USA*

Background

In a patient presenting with severe headache, the provider is first tasked with differentiating an idiopathic primary headache from a symptomatic secondary headache [1]. While the majority of patients with severe headache are ultimately determined to have headache attributable to migraine, the failure to recognize a secondary cause for the severe headache can result in significant increases in morbidity and mortality. Among patients presenting with nontraumatic headache, the clinical features of age greater than 50, a sudden onset of headache, and an abnormal neurologic examination are all independently associated with a worrisome underlying cause [2,3]. In fact, without knowledge of any element of the history apart from a sudden, explosive onset of headache, the examiner should already be cognizant to initiate a systematic and careful evaluation.

The term thunderclap headache (TCH) refers to a sudden onset intense and explosive headache, a phenotype well recognized to be associated with multiple dangerous pathologies including aneurysmal subarachnoid hemorrhage (SAH) [4,5]. In a recent analysis of 55 patients presenting to an emergency room or primary care office with chief complaint of headache and then suddenly died, 51% presented with a TCH [6]. While any headache may "appear suddenly" at a nonzero pain intensity on a numerical rating scale (NRS), the headache of TCH invariably reaches a peak intensity (often 10/10) within the time span of 1 min or less [7]. While this definition has not been formally validated, clinical experience of patients imitating the headache onset with a *clap of their hands* suggests that a 1-min time allowance may even be generous [8]. However, in a prospective series of 102 patients, headache peaked within 1–5 min in 19% of patients eventually diagnosed with aneurysmal subarachnoid hemorrhage [9]. Therefore, given the emergent and management-changing implications of this particular component of the history, it is preferable to emphasize sensitivity over specificity at the time of initial assessment.

A diagnostic dilemma may occur if the patient awakens from sleep with a severe headache and thus cannot determine the rate of onset. In this situation, the clinician should err on the side of careful evaluation, especially if there is not a prior history of a recurring primary headache syndrome, and/or the patient is reporting a new type of headache. However, a personal history of migraine and the clinical features of the headache, including response to therapy, do not distinguish among etiologies of TCH [8,10,11]. Finally, it should be noted that recognition of TCH does not depend on the duration of the headache, which can persist for hours to days, depending on the cause.

Case scenario

A 49-year-old musician presents to the emergency room with a chief concern of severe headache that felt like someone had unexpectedly "wacked [me] in the head with a shovel." At the time of evaluation, he was reporting an 8/10 pain intensity on a NRS, whereas it had been 10/10 at the moment of onset, 4 hours earlier. The headache was reported to be holocephalic, pulsating, and worsened by exertion. He was reporting mild nausea, photoallodynia, and associated neck discomfort. Physical examination was revealing for an afebrile patient with a blood pressure of 145/82 and a heart rate of 96. The neurologic examination was normal, and no meningismus was appreciated. A routine noncontrast computed tomography (CT) of the head was normal. On further questioning, he reported a history of occasional "hangover headaches" and migraine headaches during college. He denied current tobacco, alcohol, or illicit substance use. The emergency room physician elected to admit him to the hospital for further evaluation and monitoring.

Framing answerable clinical questions

You are not reassured by his prior history of migraine, and concerned that the current history of TCH suggests a secondary cause not identified by the initial evaluation. In order to best proceed, you frame five basic questions to guide your subsequent diagnostic strategy.

1 In a patient presenting with TCH, what is the likelihood of primary versus secondary TCH? [baseline risk]

2 Among individuals with TCH, what are the most likely causes? [baseline risk]

3 Does the TCH patient with a normal brain CT need to have a lumbar puncture (LP)? [baseline risk]

4 Does the TCH patient with a normal brain CT and normal LP need additional noninvasive diagnostic tests (e.g. CT angiogram (CTA)/MR angiogram (MRA), brain magnetic resonance imaging (MRI))? [baseline risk]

5 Is noninvasive angiography (MRA, CTA) adequate to evaluate the TCH patient with normal CT and LP, or is catheter angiography necessary? [baseline risk]

Critical review of the evidence

Risk of secondary TCH

In a patient presenting with TCH, what is the likelihood of secondary TCH?

All individuals presenting with TCH should be evaluated for secondary etiologies. This is a standard of care [12]. However, the specific risk of secondary TCH and how extensive the evaluation should be is more controversial [13]. The risk of a secondary etiology at the time of initial evaluation has been the topic of several prospective cohort studies, summarized in Table 4.1 [5,8,9,14]. These studies differ in cohort size, referral populations, and diagnostic strategy, which were not always standardized. In these studies, secondary TCH was identified in 27–71.4% of patients, with SAH being most common in all series. Combining the data, secondary TCH was identified in 192/436 (44%) cases. Landtblom *et al.* has estimated the incidence of TCH among individuals >18 years of age to be 43 per 100,000 inhabitants, with 11.3% having SAH [8]. A recent prospective series applied a standardized diagnostic evaluation of CT and LP to 592 patients presenting with acute headache [15]. These authors defined acute headache as reaching a maximal intensity within 1 hour, and allowed inclusion of individuals presenting within 2 weeks of onset. Using this approach, a secondary serious etiology was identified in 69 (11.7%) patients in the cohort.

Among patients presenting for evaluation of TCH, clinical features are not thought to be reliable in distinguishing between primary and secondary forms. This issue has been addressed in several prospective cohort studies [8,9,16]. In the study by Markus, individuals with primary TCH ($n=16$) were ascertained prospectively and compared to a retrospective cohort of individuals with SAH ($n = 37$) [16]. A history of smoking, vomiting at presentation, and elevated blood pressure at presentation were associated with a diagnosis of SAH; however, overlap was seen for all variables. In a larger prospective series ($n=102$), the variables conferring the greatest relative risk for SAH were exertion/Valsalva-like maneuvers at onset (RR 2.3 (95% CI: 1.2–4.6)), and vomiting at onset (RR 1.6 (95% CI: 1.1–2.4)) [9]. Finally, Landtblom *et al.* has compared the clinical features between prospectively identified patients with SAH ($n=23$) and non-SAH TCH ($n=114$) [8]. Nausea, neck stiffness, occipital headache, and impaired consciousness were more likely to occur in the SAH group, but again were not specific for this diagnosis.

Differential diagnosis of TCH

Of those with TCH, what are the most likely causes?

A systematic evaluation of a patient presenting with TCH requires consideration of a broad differential diagnosis, summarized in Table 4.2. In prospective clinical series including all-comers with TCH, the most common diagnoses are presumed primary TCH (62.8%), SAH (16.8–25%), intracerebral hemorrhage (ICH) (6%), cerebral infarction (0.6–3.6%), intracranial infection (i.e. meningoencephalitides) (2.7–2.9%), and cerebral venous sinus thrombosis (CVST) (0.7%) [5,8]. While primary TCH and SAH represent an overwhelming majority of the final diagnoses, this may reflect the diagnostic strategies of the authors, where other etiologies such as the reversible cerebral vasoconstriction syndromes (RCVS), CVST, and cervical artery dissection (CAD) would not have been recognized.

When considering the possible underlying causes for TCH, one should consider the population incidence of each potential etiology along with the likelihood of TCH among individuals with that condition (see Figure 4.1). Certain conditions are both relatively common in the population and likely to present with TCH (i.e. SAH [8,17,18] and ICH [18,19]), whereas others are common, but only uncommonly associated with TCH (i.e. cerebral infarction [18,19]). Likewise, a number of relatively uncommon conditions are known to be associated with TCH in 20% or less of patients (i.e. CVST [20–22], CAD [23,24], and SIH [25]). Therefore, the clinician must assess patient-specific risk factors to determine the pre-test probability of these less common diagnoses.

Among the more common causes of TCH, SAH is the most emergent to recognize [7]. Although clinical outcomes are improving, the overall case fatality rate remains around 50%, with 10% of patients dying prior to presentation, and 25% within 24 hours of onset [26]. The majority of cases are due to rupture of a saccular aneurysm, although other mechanisms are possible (i.e. trauma, vasculitis, coagulopathy). Cigarette smoking, excessive alcohol intake, and hypertension are potentially modifiable risk factors for

Table 4.1 Risk of secondary pathology following evaluation for thunderclap headache

Reference	Study design	Number of patients	Evaluation	Number (%) of patients with secondary TCH	Most common secondary diagnoses (% of total cohort)	Duration of follow-up for patients with presumed primary TCH	Adverse outcomes at last follow-up for patients with presumed primary TCH
Wijdicks et al. [70]	Retrospective study of presumed primary TCH	71	CT and LP. Angiography (n=4)	N.A.	N.A.	Mean 3.3 y, range: 1–7 y (n=71)	SAH (n=0), Recurrent TCH (n=12, 17%)
Harling et al. [14]	Retrospective study of hospitalized TCH	49	CT and LP. Angiography in 8/14 with presumed primary TCH.	35 (71.4%)	1 Subarachnoid hemorrhage (71.4%)	Range: 1.5–2.5 y (n=14)	SAH (n=0)
Markus [16]	Prospective study of presumed primary TCH	16	CT (n=12) and LP (n=16).	N.A.	N.A.	Mean 1.7 y, range: 1.2–2 y (n=16)	SAH (n=0), Recurrent TCH (n=4, 25%)
Linn et al. [5]	Retrospective study of all TCH	148	110 (74%) investigated by CT and LP. Angiogram (n=27)	55 (37% (95% CI 29–45%))	1 Subarachnoid hemorrhage (25%) 2 Intracerebral hemorrhage (6%) 3 Meningoencephalitis (2.7%)	1 y (n=93)	SAH or sudden death (n=0)
Linn et al. [9]	Prospective study of all TCH	102	CT and LP	65 (63.7%)	1 Aneurysmal SAH (41%) 2 Perimesencephalic SAH (23%)	None	N.A.

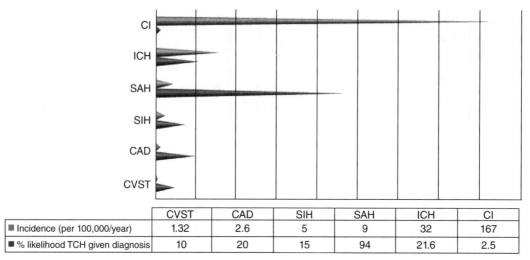

	CVST	CAD	SIH	SAH	ICH	CI
■ Incidence (per 100,000/year)	1.32	2.6	5	9	32	167
■ % likelihood TCH given diagnosis	10	20	15	94	21.6	2.5

Figure 4.1 Likelihood of thunderclap headache (TCH) in selected common and uncommon conditions. Data from epidemiologic studies are of variable quality, but summarized together to demonstrate general principles [17,19,20,23,25]. 95% confidence intervals are not shown. The percent likelihood of TCH given diagnosis refers to best literature estimate [18,22,24,25]. For example, while CI is very common, the likelihood of TCH is low; whereas SAH is much less common, but more likely to present with TCH. CAD cervical artery dissection, CI cerebral infarction, CVST cerebral venous sinus thrombosis, ICH intracerebral hemorrhage, SAH subarachnoid hemorrhage, SIH spontaneous intracranial hypotension.

Table 4.2 Differential diagnosis of thunderclap headache

Initial presentation of TCH	
Vascular	**Non-vascular**
1 Subarachnoid hemorrhage	1 Meningo-encephalitis
2 Cerebral infarction/ intracerebral hemorrhage	2 Spontaneous intracranial hypotension
3 Unruptured intracranial aneurysm ("sentinel headache")	3 Pituitary apoplexy
	4 Colloid cyst
4 Cervical artery dissection	5 Pheochromocytoma
5 Cerebral venous sinus thrombosis	6 Complicated sinusitis
6 Retroclival hematoma	
7 Hypertensive emergency	
8 Reversible cerebral vasoconstriction syndrome (RCVS)	

Primary thunderclap headache (unknown etiology)

Recurrent TCH
1 Subarachnoid hemorrhage
2 Reversible cerebral vasoconstriction syndrome (RCVS)
3 Primary thunderclap headache

SAH [27]. TCH is notoriously reported in the majority of patients with SAH, and may be the isolated manifestation in 1/3 of cases [5]. While the diagnosis of SAH should be pursued in all patients with TCH, exertion prior to onset, loss of consciousness, seizures, vomiting, and meningismus can also be clues to the diagnosis.

Importantly, an estimated 10–43% of patients with aneurysmal SAH will recall a similar sudden onset or other unusual headache in the days to weeks prior to the hemorrhage [28]. These "sentinel headaches" are significantly more likely to occur in patients with aneurysmal SAH compared to patients with nonaneurysmal SAH, cerebral infarction, and ICH [9,18]. The diagnosis of a sentinel headache can only be made retrospectively, and is thought to have the greatest incidence within 24 hours of SAH [7]. The mechanism underlying sentinel headache is presumed to reflect an unstable aneurysm and hemorrhagic leakage too small in volume to be detected by CT and LP evaluation [29]. However, while there is compelling evidence that an unruptured intracranial aneurysm can be associated with TCH, incidental unruptured intracranial aneurysms are also a very common finding, making the relationship difficult to establish [30].

Given that stroke is common, it is not surprising that cerebral infarction and ICH emerge in multiple series as a common cause of secondary TCH [5,8,15]. Overall, headache is common in both ischemic and hemorrhagic strokes, with the exception of most lacunar infarcts [9,31,32]. In a large, prospective study of patients with acute stroke, TCH was reported by 21%, although 60% of the patients could not definitively recall the details of onset [33]. Headache was more likely to be severe, have a thunderclap onset, and precede other neurologic signs in patients with ICH. Headache associated with acute stroke is most likely to be classified as tension type, although this may be confounded by stroke-related nausea and vomiting.

Headache is considered to be a hallmark symptom of meningitis, being present in about 87% of cases of bacterial meningitis [34]. The headache is typically generalized and severe, often associated with photophobia. In patients being evaluated with LP for suspected SAH, approximately 3% will be given an ultimate diagnosis of meningoencephalitis, most often presumed aseptic meningitis [5,8,35]. However, the prospective incidence of TCH among individuals found to have meningoencephalitis is not known.

Among patients investigated with CT and LP for TCH, CVST is only occasionally seen (1 out of 137 cases in one study [8]). The diagnosis is generally considered uncommon, and TCH is present in only 2–10% of patients [20,22]. CVST may present with headache alone in 25% of patients, suggesting that the diagnosis may be overlooked without dedicated investigations [21]. However, unenhanced CT has been reported to have a sensitivity of 73% in the hands of experienced radiologists [36]. In addition, LP may also provide diagnostic clues, including elevation of the opening pressure (present in >80% of patients), cell counts (present in approximately half of patients), and protein (present in about one-third of patients) [22,37,38]. CVST is seen most commonly in women, where pregnancy, puerperium, and oral contraceptives have been identified as risk factors [39].

TCH is present in approximately 20% of patients with CAD [24]. CAD is most often encountered in the setting of other neurologic signs and symptoms, but headache may occur alone in 2–8% of patients [40,41]. The presence of Horner's syndrome on examination is an important clue, being present in 25% of cases. Headache is present in approximately two-thirds of patients with carotid or vertebral artery dissections [42]. Individuals with carotid artery dissection have a slightly greater mean age of 46, are more likely to be men, but less likely to report minor cervical trauma in the month prior to presentation [42]. The diagnosis is important to recognize as the disorder is complicated by stroke in the majority of cases [42].

RCVS are characterized by recurrent TCH, and are associated with diffuse, multifocal narrowing of the cerebral arteries [43]. This disorder is more common in women than in men and has a peak incidence during the 4th to 6th decades of life [23,43]. RCVS often have an identifiable trigger, most commonly pregnancy, or exposure to a vasoactive substance, selective serotonin reuptake inhibitor (SSRI), and cannabis [44]. Although the majority of cases resolve within a several month period, RCVS may be complicated by stroke, seizures, and/or posterior reversible encephalopathy syndrome (PRES). Intracranial vasoconstriction is maximum at an average of 16.3 days after the TCH [45]. The original proposed diagnostic criteria for RCVS stipulated that cerebrospinal fluid (CSF) protein be less than 80 mg/dL and white blood cell count be less than 10/mm^3 [46]. However, recommendations for revised criteria call for CSF protein to be less than 100 mg/dL and a white blood cell count less than 15/mm^3 [47].

Primary TCH is diagnosed when no alternative etiology is identified following a comprehensive evaluation. The International Classification of Headache Disorders (ICHD-3 beta) specifies that the headache must reach maximal intensity within 1 min and persist for at least 5 minutes. The headache may recur within the first week, but should not recur regularly over weeks to months [48]. Given the multitude of potential diagnoses underlying TCH, this diagnosis is understandably controversial in the absence of a systematic evaluation [49]. As will be discussed, the extent of the diagnostic evaluation that is warranted is also a topic of controversy [13].

Lumbar puncture

Does the TCH patient with a normal brain CT need to have a lumbar puncture (LP)?

The current American College of Emergency Physicians (ACEP) guidelines recommend CT, followed by LP if negative as a standard of care in the evaluation of patients with suspected SAH [12]. The sensitivity of CT for the diagnosis SAH depends on the generation of the CT scanner used and the timing of the scan after symptom onset. In an influential 1982 study, a sensitivity of 100% was obtained for the detection of SAH when CT was performed within 24 hours of onset [50]. However, sensitivity declined rapidly to 74% after 3 days and 50% after 1 week [50]. A more recent study using a third-generation CT scanner demonstrated a sensitivity of 100% (95% CI 97–100%) and a specificity of 100% (95% CI 99.9–100%) when patients were scanned within 6 hours [51]. When patients were scanned after 6 hours of onset, the sensitivity dropped considerably to 85.7%, without any change in test specificity [51]. While the results have been criticized on the basis that not all patients with a negative CT underwent LP, similar results have been replicated in a subsequent series [52]. Importantly, all of these studies were performed at high-volume tertiary centers, where the scans were interpreted by an experienced neuroradiologist.

The value of CSF in the detection of xanthochromia also has important time-dependent characteristics. The presence of xanthochromia implies that blood has been present in the CSF for at least 2 hours, and xanthochromia reaches a maximum around 48 hours, persisting for several weeks after a hemorrhage [53]. The sensitivity of CSF analysis is thought to be greatest after 12 hours of onset [53]. Comparing the red blood cell (RBC) count between tubes 1 and 4 is often utilized to differentiate a traumatic (bloody) tap from an SAH. However, even a 25% reduction of RBC count between the first and last tubes does not reliably exclude an aneurysmal SAH [54]. In general, LP confirmation of SAH after a normal or equivocal CT is reported on the order of 2–6% [51,55]. In a retrospective Mayo Clinic study of 152 patients presenting with TCH and a normal head CT, visual identification of xanthochromic CSF was identified in 12% of cases [56]. Subsequent angiography demonstrated a ruptured aneurysm in 72% of these patients [56]. In this study, visual inspection for xanthochromia had a sensitivity of 93% and specificity of 95%. Other authors have demonstrated an improved sensitivity when spectrophotometry is used to identify xanthochromia; however, this comes with a marked reduction in test specificity (as low as 29%) [57]. While most centers do not currently have access to spectrophotometry, some authors have raised concerns that the technique will lead to a rise in unnecessary angiography [57].

Therefore, in the evaluation of TCH, LP is indicated following a negative head CT. While some authors have suggested that LP is not necessary for detection of SAH when a newer generation head CT is performed within 6 hours of onset (and read by an experienced neuroradiologist), one should consider that an LP may still be useful in identifying an alternative cause for the TCH (i.e. meningitis, CVST) [7].

Advanced noninvasive neuroimaging

Does the TCH patient with a normal brain CT and normal LP need additional noninvasive diagnostic tests (e.g. CT angiogram (CTA)/ MR angiogram (MRA), brain magnetic resonance imaging (MRI))?

In deciding whether to pursue advanced diagnostic testing, one is faced with trying to reconcile the supposed benign natural history of CT and LP-negative TCH, with the fairly frequent reporting of a sentinel TCH among individuals with SAH. A meta-analysis of 813 patients all followed for at least 6 months concluded that the risk of SAH in a neurologically intact patient with a negative CT and LP would be less than 0.4% (corresponding to a number needed to the harm of 250 patients) [58]. Not surprisingly, reports have surfaced of unruptured intracranial aneurysms being discovered following negative evaluation of TCH with both CT and LP [4,59]. Raps *et al.* retrospectively studied 111 patients referred with unruptured intracranial aneurysms, of whom 7 had reported a history of TCH [60]. Several of these patients had cranial nerve abnormalities and/or radiographic aneurysmal thrombosis, implicating the unruptured intracranial aneurysms as symptomatic. Perry *et al.* encountered a more common scenario, a 51-year-old woman with a completely normal CT and LP evaluation for TCH, who 1 year later underwent an MRA because of a family history of SAH [15]. She was found to have two small (<7 mm) anterior circulation aneurysms, which were felt to be unruptured, and were repaired by surgical clipping. A similar conundrum of identifying a likely incidental unruptured intracranial aneurysm would be expected in approximately 3% of the general population. While larger aneurysms are both more likely to rupture and/or cause symptoms, the discovery of any aneurysm following a TCH should prompt a careful evaluation [60,61].

A diagnostic approach using a CT and CTA of the head may be considered if an LP cannot be performed or is difficult, as is the case in up to 20% of emergency room patients [62]. CTA has a high sensitivity to detect aneurysms as small as 3 mm, although carries risks of nephrotoxicity, radiation exposure, and the potential for discovery of an incidental aneurysm. There are no comparative studies of CT/LP versus CT/CTA, and it has been estimated that to show equivalence within 0.5%, enrollment of 3,000 patients would be required [63]. In a prospective study of evaluation with CT, CTA, and LP, xanthochromia was identified in only 2/105 patients with a negative CT, both of whom had an aneurysm on CTA [64] Conversely, CTA showed an aneurysm in 3/103 patients who were CT and LP negative for SAH. Using a mathematical probability model, McCormack and Hutson have estimated that CT and CTA approaches would exclude SAH with a greater than 99% posttest probability [63]. Given the relative ease of obtaining a CTA over an LP, the authors suggested that the tests might even be interchangeable. However, it has been pointed out that there may be important unintended consequences of this strategy, including increased identification of incidental aneurysms, missing alternative disorders previously diagnosed by LP, increased CT and contrast-related morbidity, and the observation that "tests beget more tests" (i.e. physicians may be more likely to add-on CTA of the neck) [65].

MRI and MRA are not practically accessible in most emergency room settings, and are relatively time-intensive techniques. The sensitivity of MRI for detecting SAH is greatest when fluid attenuation inversion recovery (FLAIR) and T2 gradient echo or susceptibility-weighted sequences are utilized. In one series including 15 patients scanned after 4 days from onset, the sensitivity of CT, gradient echo, and FLAIR were 75%, 100%, and 89%, respectively [66]. FLAIR was 100% sensitive in another series of 45 patients, irrespective of timing of presentation [67]. MRI also carries the advantage of being able to diagnosis alternative etiologies of TCH, such as SIH, ischemic stroke, pituitary apoplexy, and cerebral edema associated with hypertensive emergency [7]. Similar to CTA, MRA is considered to be highly sensitive in the detection of intracranial aneurysms of 3 mm or larger. In one study evaluating contrast-free 3.0 Tesla MRA and using intra-arterial angiography as a gold standard, a sensitivity of 99.2% (95% CI 98−100%) was reported [68].

In a patient with CT and LP-negative TCH, advanced noninvasive imaging studies have the potential to diagnose alternative causes of TCH. In the diagnosis of RCVS, CTA or MRA may be negative in up to 20% of patients when performed within the first 2 weeks [43]. In these cases, the study should be repeated within 1−2 weeks in search of the characteristic pattern of multifocal, segmental vasoconstriction. Brain MRI in RCVS may demonstrate cortical SAH not visualized on head CT, and/or show findings of PRES.

In the diagnosis of SAH, advanced noninvasive imaging may be especially important in patients with either ultra-early (<2 hours) or late (≥72 hours) presentations, when false-negative results on the LP and CT are more likely, respectively. However, vascular imaging studies are expected to identify an incidental unruptured intracranial aneurysm in approximately 3% of the population.

Invasive angiography

Is noninvasive angiography (magnetic resonance angiography (MRA) and computed tomography angiography (CTA)) adequate to evaluate the TCH patient with normal CT and LP or is catheter angiography necessary?

Intra-arterial digital subtraction angiography is the gold standard test in the diagnosis of intracranial aneurysm. The test is invasive, but may be therapeutic if a ruptured aneurysm amenable to coiling is identified. Similar to noninvasive vascular imaging, angiography may allow for diagnosis of other conditions, such as RCVS and CAD. In a 24-year retrospective analysis of 19,826 consecutive patients undergoing angiography, neurologic complications were seen in 2.63% of cases [69]. SAH as an indication for the test conferred an odds ratio of 2.5 (95% CI: 1.79–3.55) for a neurologic complication, the majority of which were transient in nature. Importantly, the rate of neurologic complications was noted to decline with each 5-year increment of time analyzed. Therefore, while there is a risk for serious morbidity from an angiogram, the rates of neurologic complications are generally low.

In an individual found to have SAH, angiography is indicated, given the potential for intervention on a ruptured aneurysm. However, given the very high sensitivity of noninvasive vascular imaging, catheter angiography cannot be recommended as part of the general evaluation strategy for TCH.

While angiography is also considered the gold standard in the diagnosis of RCVS and CAD, this modality has been largely supplanted given advances in noninvasive imaging modalities. When considering a diagnosis of RCVS or CAD, angiography is generally reserved for suspected, but diagnostically ambiguous cases.

Conclusions

The recognition of TCH should automatically prompt concern for a secondary headache syndrome, with the diagnostic strategy initially directed towards possible SAH. The current guideline recommendations of a brain CT, and then LP, if negative, are supported by the literature. However, in individuals with delayed or atypical presentations and in those with negative CT and LP, brain MRI and noninvasive angiography should be considered.

Future research needs

Common diagnostic tests utilized in the evaluation of TCH have time-dependent characteristics, suggesting that different strategies may be differentially useful at different time points. For example, a strategy of CT/CTA may be most useful for patients with ultra-early (<2 hours from onset), whereas MRI/LP might be better for patients presenting after 72 hours. The prevalent nature of incidental unruptured intracranial aneurysms is an important factor often cited as reason to avoid advanced vascular imaging. Objective biomarkers and risk stratification tools are needed to better assess an unruptured intracranial aneurysm discovered in the evaluation of TCH. Current diagnostic strategies have appropriately focused on excluding SAH; however, have neglected to consider other diagnoses that can cause TCH. Future studies should also specifically assess the risk of CAD, CVST, RCVS and others among patients presenting with TCH, and explore the costs against potential benefits of routinely screening for these conditions. Finally, given that up to 25% of patients with an initial negative evaluation will experience recurrent TCH, a diagnostic strategy needs to be clarified for this subset of patients, who may be more likely to have RCVS, for example.

References

1 De Luca, G.C. & Bartleson, J.D. (2010) When and how to investigate the patient with headache. *Seminars in Neurology*, **30**, 131–144.

2 Locker, T.E., Thompson, C., Rylance, J. & Mason, S.M. (2006) The utility of clinical features in patients presenting with non-traumatic headache: an investigation of adult patients attending an emergency department. *Headache*, **46**, 954–961.

3 Ramirez-Lassepas, M., Espinosa, C.E., Cicero, J.J., Johnston, K.L., Cipolle, R.J. & Barber, D.L. (1997) Predictors of intracranial pathologic findings in patients who seek emergency care because of headache. *Archives of Neurology*, **54**, 1506–1509.

4 Day, J.W. & Raskin, N.H. (1986) Thunderclap headache: symptom of unruptured cerebral aneurysm. *Lancet*, **2**, 1247–1248.

5 Linn, F.H., Wijdicks, E.F., van der Graaf, Y., Weerdesteyn-van Vliet, F.A., Bartelds, A.I. & van Gijn, J. (1994) Prospective study of sentinel headache in aneurysmal subarachnoid haemorrhage. *Lancet*, **344**, 590–593.

6 Lynch, K.M. & Brett, F. (2012) Headaches that kill: a retrospective study of incidence, etiology and clinical features in cases of sudden death. *Cephalalgia*, **32**, 972–978.

7 Schwedt, T.J. (2013) Thunderclap headaches: a focus on etiology and diagnostic evaluation. *Headache*, **53**, 563–569.

8 Landtblom, A.M., Fridriksson, S., Boivie, J., Hillman, J., Johansson, G. & Johansson, I. (2002) Sudden onset headache: a prospective study of features, incidence and causes. *Cephalalgia*, **22**, 354–360.

9 Linn, F.H., Rinkel, G.J., Algra, A. & van Gijn, J. (1998) Headache characteristics in subarachnoid haemorrhage and

benign thunderclap headache. *Journal of Neurology, Neurosurgery and Psychiatry*, **65**, 791–793.

10 Seymour, J.J., Moscati, R.M. & Jehle, D.V. (1995) Response of headaches to nonnarcotic analgesics resulting in missed intracranial hemorrhage. *American Journal of Emergency Medicine*, **13**, 43–45.

11 Pope, J.V. & Edlow, J.A. (2008) Favorable response to analgesics does not predict a benign etiology of headache. *Headache*, **48**, 944–950.

12 Edlow, J.A., Panagos, P.D., Godwin, S.A., Thomas, T.L. & Decker, W.W. (2008) Clinical policy: critical issues in the evaluation and management of adult patients presenting to the emergency department with acute headache. *Annals of Emergency Medicine*, **52**, 407–436.

13 Farzad, A., Radin, B., Oh, J.S. *et al.* (2013) Emergency diagnosis of subarachnoid hemorrhage: an evidence-based debate. *Journal of Emergency Medicine*, **44**, 1045–1053.

14 Harling, D.W., Peatfield, R.C., Van Hille, P.T. & Abbott, R.J. (1989) Thunderclap headache: is it migraine? *Cephalalgia*, **9**, 87–90.

15 Perry, J.J., Spacek, A., Forbes, M. *et al.* (2008) Is the combination of negative computed tomography result and negative lumbar puncture result sufficient to rule out subarachnoid hemorrhage? *Annals of Emergency Medicine*, **51**, 707–713.

16 Markus, H.S. (1991) A prospective follow up of thunderclap headache mimicking subarachnoid haemorrhage. *Journal of Neurology, Neurosurgery and Psychiatry*, **54**, 1117–1118.

17 de Rooij, N.K., Linn, F.H., van der Plas, J.A., Algra, A. & Rinkel, G.J. (2007) Incidence of subarachnoid haemorrhage: a systematic review with emphasis on region, age, gender and time trends. *Journal of Neurology, Neurosurgery and Psychiatry*, **78**, 1365–1372.

18 Gorelick, P.B., Hier, D.B., Caplan, L.R. & Langenberg, P. (1986) Headache in acute cerebrovascular disease. *Neurology*, **36**, 1445–1450.

19 Kleindorfer, D.O., Khoury, J., Moomaw, C.J. *et al.* (2010) Stroke incidence is decreasing in whites but not in blacks: a population-based estimate of temporal trends in stroke incidence from the Greater Cincinnati/Northern Kentucky Stroke Study. *Stroke*, **41**, 1326–1331.

20 Coutinho, J.M., Zuurbier, S.M., Aramideh, M. & Stam, J. (2012) The incidence of cerebral venous thrombosis: a cross-sectional study. *Stroke*, **43**, 3375–3377.

21 Cumurciuc, R., Crassard, I., Sarov, M., Valade, D. & Bousser, M.G. (2005) Headache as the only neurological sign of cerebral venous thrombosis: a series of 17 cases. *Journal of Neurology, Neurosurgery and Psychiatry*, **76**, 1084–1087.

22 de Bruijn, S.F., Stam, J. & Kappelle, L.J. (1996) Thunderclap headache as first symptom of cerebral venous sinus thrombosis. CVST Study Group. *Lancet*, **348**, 1623–1625.

23 Lee, V.H., Brown, R.D. Jr., Mandrekar, J.N. & Mokri, B. (2006) Incidence and outcome of cervical artery dissection: a population-based study. *Neurology*, **67**, 1809–1812.

24 Mitsias, P. & Ramadan, N.M. (1992) Headache in ischemic cerebrovascular disease. Part I: Clinical features. *Cephalalgia*, **12**, 269–274.

25 Schievink, W.I. (2006) Spontaneous spinal cerebrospinal fluid leaks and intracranial hypotension. *JAMA*, **295**, 2286–2296.

26 Broderick, J.P., Brott, T.G., Duldner, J.E., Tomsick, T. & Leach, A. (1994) Initial and recurrent bleeding are the major causes of death following subarachnoid hemorrhage. *Stroke*, **25**, 1342–1347.

27 Feigin, V.L., Rinkel, G.J., Lawes, C.M. *et al.* (2005) Risk factors for subarachnoid hemorrhage: an updated systematic review of epidemiological studies. *Stroke*, **36**, 2773–2780.

28 Polmear, A. (2003) Sentinel headaches in aneurysmal subarachnoid haemorrhage: what is the true incidence? A systematic review. *Cephalalgia*, **23**, 935–941.

29 Ball, M.J. (1975) Pathogenesis of the "sentinel headache" preceding berry aneurysm rupture. *Canadian Medical Association Journal*, **112**, 78–79.

30 Vernooij, M.W., Ikram, M.A., Tanghe, H.L. *et al.* (2007) Incidental findings on brain MRI in the general population. *The New England Journal of Medicine*, **357**, 1821–1828.

31 Arboix, A., Massons, J., Oliveres, M., Arribas, M.P. & Titus, F. (1994) Headache in acute cerebrovascular disease: a prospective clinical study in 240 patients. *Cephalalgia*, **14**, 37–40.

32 Arboix, A., Garcia-Trallero, O., Garcia-Eroles, L., Massons, J., Comes, E. & Targa, C. (2005) Stroke-related headache: a clinical study in lacunar infarction. *Headache*, **45**, 1345–1352.

33 Verdelho, A., Ferro, J.M., Melo, T., Canhao, P. & Falcao, F. (2008) Headache in acute stroke. A prospective study in the first 8 days. *Cephalalgia*, **28**, 346–354.

34 van de Beek, D., de Gans, J., Spanjaard, L., Weisfelt, M., Reitsma, J.B. & Vermeulen, M. (2004) Clinical features and prognostic factors in adults with bacterial meningitis. *The New England Journal of Medicine*, **351**, 1849–1859.

35 Brunell, A., Ridefelt, P. & Zelano, J. (2013) Differential diagnostic yield of lumbar puncture in investigation of suspected subarachnoid haemorrhage: a retrospective study. *Journal of Neurology*, **260(6)**. doi:10.1007/s00415-013-6846-x.

36 Roland, T., Jacobs, J., Rappaport, A., Vanheste, R., Wilms, G. & Demaerel, P. (2010) Unenhanced brain CT is useful to decide on further imaging in suspected venous sinus thrombosis. *Clinical Radiology*, **65**, 34–39.

37 Ferro, J.M., Canhao, P., Stam, J., Bousser, M.G. & Barinagarrementeria, F. (2004) Prognosis of cerebral vein and dural sinus thrombosis: results of the International Study on Cerebral Vein and Dural Sinus Thrombosis (ISCVT). *Stroke*, **35**, 664–670.

38 Saposnik, G., Barinagarrementeria, F., Brown, R.D. Jr. *et al.* (2011) Diagnosis and management of cerebral venous thrombosis: a statement for healthcare professionals from the American Heart Association/American Stroke Association. *Stroke*, **42**, 1158–1192.

39 Coutinho, J.M., Ferro, J.M., Canhao, P. *et al.* (2009) Cerebral venous and sinus thrombosis in women. *Stroke*, **40**, 2356–2361.

40 Silbert, P.L., Mokri, B. & Schievink, W.I. (1995) Headache and neck pain in spontaneous internal carotid and vertebral artery dissections. *Neurology*, **45**, 1517–1522.

41 Arnold, M., Cumurciuc, R., Stapf, C., Favrole, P., Berthet, K. & Bousser, M.G. (2006) Pain as the only symptom of cervical artery

dissection. *Journal of Neurology, Neurosurgery and Psychiatry*, **77**, 1021–1024.

42 Debette, S., Grond-Ginsbach, C., Bodenant, M. *et al.* (2011) Differential features of carotid and vertebral artery dissections: the CADISP study. *Neurology*, **77**, 1174–1181.

43 Yancy, H., Lee-Iannotti, J.K., Schwedt, T.J. & Dodick, D.W. (2013) Reversible cerebral vasoconstriction syndrome. *Headache*, **53**, 570–576.

44 Ducros, A., Boukobza, M., Porcher, R., Sarov, M., Valade, D. & Bousser, M.G. (2007) The clinical and radiological spectrum of reversible cerebral vasoconstriction syndrome. A prospective series of 67 patients. *Brain*, **130**, 3091–3101.

45 Chen, S.P., Fuh, J.L., Wang, S.J. *et al.* (2010) Magnetic resonance angiography in reversible cerebral vasoconstriction syndromes. *Annals of Neurology*, **67**, 648–656.

46 Calabrese, L.H., Dodick, D.W., Schwedt, T.J. & Singhal, A.B. (2007) Narrative review: reversible cerebral vasoconstriction syndromes. *Annals of Internal Medicine*, **146**, 34–44.

47 Ducros, A. (2012) Reversible cerebral vasoconstriction syndrome. *Lancet Neurology*, **11**, 906–917.

48 Headache Classification Committee of the International Headache Society (IHS). *The International Classification of Headache Disorders*, 3rd edition (beta version). *Cephalalgia*. 2013, **33**(**9**), 629–808.

49 Chen, S.P., Fuh, J.L., Lirng, J.F., Chang, F.C. & Wang, S.J. (2006) Recurrent primary thunderclap headache and benign CNS angiopathy: spectra of the same disorder? *Neurology*, **67**, 2164–2169.

50 van Gijn, J. & van Dongen, K.J. (1982) The time course of aneurysmal haemorrhage on computed tomograms. *Neuroradiology*, **23**, 153–156.

51 Perry, J.J., Stiell, I.G., Sivilotti, M.L. *et al.* (2011) Sensitivity of computed tomography performed within six hours of onset of headache for diagnosis of subarachnoid haemorrhage: prospective cohort study. *BMJ*, **343**, d4277.

52 Backes, D., Rinkel, G.J., Kemperman, H., Linn, F.H. & Vergouwen, M.D. (2012) Time-dependent test characteristics of head computed tomography in patients suspected of nontraumatic subarachnoid hemorrhage. *Stroke*, **43**, 2115–2119.

53 Vermeulen, M., Hasan, D., Blijenberg, B.G., Hijdra, A. & van Gijn, J. (1989) Xanthochromia after subarachnoid haemorrhage needs no revisitation. *Journal of Neurology, Neurosurgery and Psychiatry*, **52**, 826–828.

54 Heasley, D.C., Mohamed, M.A. & Yousem, D.M. (2005) Clearing of red blood cells in lumbar puncture does not rule out ruptured aneurysm in patients with suspected subarachnoid hemorrhage but negative head CT findings. *AJNR. American Journal of Neuroradiology*, **26**, 820–824.

55 Gee, C., Dawson, M., Bledsoe, J. *et al.* (2012) Sensitivity of newer-generation computed tomography scanners for subarachnoid hemorrhage: a Bayesian analysis. *Journal of Emergency Medicine*, **43**, 13–18.

56 Dupont, S.A., Wijdicks, E.F., Manno, E.M. & Rabinstein, A.A. (2008) Thunderclap headache and normal computed tomographic results: value of cerebrospinal fluid analysis. *Mayo Clinic Proceedings*, **83**, 1326–1331.

57 Perry, J.J., Sivilotti, M.L., Stiell, I.G. *et al.* (2006) Should spectrophotometry be used to identify xanthochromia in the cerebrospinal fluid of alert patients suspected of having subarachnoid hemorrhage? *Stroke*, **37**, 2467–2472.

58 Savitz, S.I., Levitan, E.B., Wears, R. & Edlow, J.A. (2009) Pooled analysis of patients with thunderclap headache evaluated by CT and LP: is angiography necessary in patients with negative evaluations? *Journal of Neurological Sciences*, **276**, 123–125.

59 Hughes, R.L. (1992) Identification and treatment of cerebral aneurysms after sentinel headache. *Neurology*, **42**, 1118–1119.

60 Raps, E.C., Rogers, J.D., Galetta, S.L. *et al.* (1993) The clinical spectrum of unruptured intracranial aneurysms. *Archives of Neurology*, **50**, 265–268.

61 Wiebers, D.O., Whisnant, J.P., Huston, J. 3rd *et al.* (2003) Unruptured intracranial aneurysms: natural history, clinical outcome, and risks of surgical and endovascular treatment. *Lancet*, **362**, 103–110.

62 Shah, K.H., Richard, K.M., Nicholas, S. & Edlow, J.A. (2003) Incidence of traumatic lumbar puncture. *Academic Emergency Medicine*, **10**, 151–154.

63 McCormack, R.F. & Hutson, A. (2010) Can computed tomography angiography of the brain replace lumbar puncture in the evaluation of acute-onset headache after a negative noncontrast cranial computed tomography scan? *Academic Emergency Medicine*, **17**, 444–451.

64 Carstairs, S.D., Tanen, D.A., Duncan, T.D. *et al.* (2006) Computed tomographic angiography for the evaluation of aneurysmal subarachnoid hemorrhage. *Academic Emergency Medicine*, **13**, 486–492.

65 Edlow, J.A. (2010) What are the unintended consequences of changing the diagnostic paradigm for subarachnoid hemorrhage after brain computed tomography to computed tomographic angiography in place of lumbar puncture? *Academic Emergency Medicine*, **17**, 991–995 discussion 996–997.

66 Mitchell, P., Wilkinson, I.D., Hoggard, N. *et al.* (2001) Detection of subarachnoid haemorrhage with magnetic resonance imaging. *Journal of Neurology, Neurosurgery and Psychiatry*, **70**, 205–211.

67 da Rocha, A.J., da Silva, C.J., Gama, H.P. *et al.* (2006) Comparison of magnetic resonance imaging sequences with computed tomography to detect low-grade subarachnoid hemorrhage: Role of fluid-attenuated inversion recovery sequence. *Journal of Computer Assisted Tomography*, **30**, 295–303.

68 Li, M.H., Li, Y.D., Tan, H.Q. *et al.* (2011) Contrast-free MRA at 3.0 T for the detection of intracranial aneurysms. *Neurology*, **77**, 667–676.

69 Kaufmann, T.J., Huston, J. 3rd, Mandrekar, J.N., Schleck, C.D., Thielen, K.R. & Kallmes, D.F. (2007) Complications of diagnostic cerebral angiography: evaluation of 19,826 consecutive patients. *Radiology*, **243**, 812–819.

70 Wijdicks, E.F., Kerkhoff, H. & van Gijn, J. (1988) Long-term follow-up of 71 patients with thunderclap headache mimicking subarachnoid haemorrhage. *Lancet*, **2**, 68–70.

5

CHAPTER 5

Coma

Bappaditya Ray[1] and Salah G. Keyrouz[2]
[1]*Department of Neurology, The University of Oklahoma Health Sciences Center, Oklahoma City, OK, USA*
[2]*Department of Neurology and Neurological Surgery, Washington University School of Medicine, St. Louis, MO, USA*

Background

The term coma, from Greek, *Kōma*, meaning "deep sleep," describes a pathologic state of unresponsiveness to arousal. An individual's responsiveness depends on the integrity of anatomical, metabolic, and communicative function of ascending reticular activating system (ARAS)-thalamo-cortical pathway in the brain. Disruption in the function of this pathway could result in a comatose state. Conditions causing coma can be varied and are enumerated in Table 5.1. Structural causes include intracranial space-occupying lesions, resulting in brain tissue distortion, shifts, and herniation, whereas metabolic/toxic causes alter the physiology of the ARAS without structural disruptions. In general, the latter results in reversible comatose states, and the former may have permanent sequelae unless reversed in a timely manner.

Traumatic brain injury (TBI), vascular lesions, and hypoxia/anoxia are the three major causes of coma [1]. Of the 1.7 million people who sustain TBI in the United States each year, 275,000 are hospitalized and about 53,000 die [2,3]. Direct and indirect medical costs such as lost productivity from TBI totaled an estimated $76.5 billion in the United States in 2000 [4,5]. Cardiopulmonary arrest (CPA), the most common cause of postanoxic coma, affects 450,000 individuals in the United States every year [6]. Recent data suggest that 300,000 suffer out-of-hospital CPA and 200,000 in-hospital arrests [7,8]. The majority of patients who initially survive a CPA remain comatose for varying lengths of time. The risk-adjusted survival rate to the discharge of in-hospital CPA has improved from 13.7% in 2000 to 22.3% in 2012 [9]. Approximately 40% of the comatose patients progress to a vegetative state (also now known as "unresponsive wakefulness syndrome") [10]. Early identification of patients with a poor prognosis is important in order to reduce uncertainty over goal of care decisions and minimize unnecessary costly and futile care

[1]. Various clinical parameters, neurological examination, biochemical markers, neuroimaging, and electrophysiological studies have been used for the prognostic evaluation of brain function in comatose patients. We address diagnostic, therapeutic, and prognostic issues related to coma by answering the following clinical questions.

Framing clinical questions

How do history, clinical examination, and ancillary tests help in determining the etiology of coma?

How to monitor and treat a comatose patient?

What are the various predictors that help to determine the prognosis of a comatose patient?

How does clinical examination and ancillary tests help in determination of etiology of coma?

When evaluating a comatose patient, both history and neurological examination are of paramount importance. A thorough history can lead to clues to etiological diagnosis. Although often these patients cannot provide a history, every attempt should be made to obtain collateral information from relatives, friends, or emergency medical personnel. Establishing the onset and progression of coma is important. In a previously healthy, young patient, sudden onset of coma may be due to drug poisoning, subarachnoid hemorrhage (SAH), or head trauma [11]. In the elderly, sudden coma is more likely caused by large, critically located cerebrovascular event such as cerebral hemorrhage or infarction. Gradual onset coma with fluctuations in consciousness is the result of metabolic and infective disorders.

Similarly, the neurological examination, which is a vital portion of the initial evaluation, could suggest a structural or a metabolic etiology. In the acute setting, the ability to differentiate between structural and toxic/metabolic causes influence diagnostic and treatment considerations. Assessment of comatose patients requires a working knowledge of examination techniques and clinical anatomic correlation.

Evidence-Based Neurology: Management of Neurological Disorders, Second Edition. Edited by Bart M. Demaerschalk and Dean M. Wingerchuk.
© 2015 John Wiley & Sons, Ltd. Published 2015 by John Wiley & Sons, Ltd.

Table 5.1 Common etiologies of coma

Structural lesions
  Vascular
    Anoxic/hypoxic-ischemic encephalopathy
    Bilateral thalamic infarction
    Large stroke with edema
    Basilar artery territory infarction
    Cerebellar infarction with edema
    Intracerebral hemorrhage with mass effect
    Pontine hemorrhage
  Traumatic
    Diffuse axonal injury
    Penetrating head trauma
    Multiple contusions
    Extra-axial hematoma (e.g. subdural, epidural) with mass effect
  Demyelinating disorders
    Adult demyelinating encephalopathy
    Central pontine myelinolysis
  Neoplastic
    Lymphoma
    Brain tumor/metastasis with edema

Metabolic or infectious
  Substrate deficiency
    Hypoxia
    Hypoglycemia
    Hyponatremia
    Hypocalcemia
    Hypotension/hypertensive encephalopathy
    Cofactor deficiency: thiamine, niacin, pyridoxine
  Disorder in homeostasis
    Organ dysfunction – hepatic, uremic, hypercapnic
      encephalopathy
    Endocrine dysfunction – diabetic ketoacidosis, nonketotic
      hyperglycemic coma, hyperthyroid, myxedema coma,
      Addisonian crisis
    Serotonin syndrome, neuroleptic malignant syndrome
  Exogenous poisons
    Drug overdose with barbiturates, benzodiazepines, alcohol,
      opioids, sedative/hypnotics, pyschotropics
  Infectious – e.g. encephalitis
Pyschiatric disorders – e.g. catatonia

General physical exam

The physical examination of a comatose patient should include vital signs and a general medical exam. Fever noted on vital signs may indicate infectious etiology while hypothermia may be suggestive of myxedema coma. An emaciated individual with icteric sclera and altered consciousness may suggest hepatic encephalopathy. The triad of bradycardia, hypertension, and irregular respirations known as the Cushing reflex may be an indication of elevated intracranial pressure (ICP). Evidence of incontinence can be associated with seizure, whereas presence of vomitus may indicate elevated ICP. As trauma is one of the leading causes of coma, a patient should be examined for signs of head trauma, such as postauricular ecchymosis, hemotympanum, or periorbital hematomas indicating a basilar skull fracture. Neck stiffness on exam is indicative of meningeal irritation that may be due to infection, carcinomatous meningitis, inflammatory, or chemical (i.e. subarachnoid hemorrhage) process. A fundoscopic exam can reveal subhyaloid hemorrhages noticed in SAH, papilledema indicative of elevated ICP, or embolic material suggestive of carotid disease and stroke.

Neurologic exam

The commonly used scales to assess disorders of consciousness in acute care setting, Glasgow Coma Score (GCS) and full outline of unresponsiveness (FOUR) score scales use facets of the neurologic examination to rate the severity of alteration of consciousness, but both are incomplete for localization purposes.

Mental status: Before evaluating mental status, one should be certain that the patient has been off narcotic/sedative and paralytic medications for a reasonable time period to allow recovery from central nervous system depression and regain the ability to move. Level of consciousness can be assessed in a comatose patient by first observing for spontaneous eye opening followed by an attempt to elicit a response to loud voice and external stimulation. Care should be taken to assess for a locked-in state by asking a patient to blink or look up before administering painful stimuli. Clear withdrawal or localization indicates more preserved function than reflexive responses such as posturing or triple flexion, or no response to a painful stimulus.

Cranial nerves: The cranial nerve examination in a comatose patient usually begins with an assessment of eye movements, first observing for any spontaneous movements. While roving eye movements are seen in varied etiology, they usually disappear in severe brainstem injury. Ocular bobbing is seen in pontine lesions, whereas reverse bobbing (or ocular dipping) is seen in acute thalamic or midbrain pathology. Rhythmic eye movements may be a subtle presentation of seizures. Next, one should note whether the eyes are deviated to one side, and whether they are conjugate or disconjugate. Stroke or dysfunction of the frontal eye-field area will cause deviation of the eyes to the ipsilateral side, whereas seizure affecting similar area or thalamic dysfunction would cause contralateral conjugate eye deviation. Internuclear pathways of the brain stem can be evaluated with the oculocephalic maneuver in patients who do not have cervical spine injury. Otherwise, or in patients in whom the oculocephalic maneuver produces unclear results, the vestibulo-ocular reflex should be tested. Vertical eye movements (especially in patients suspected of locked-in syndrome) should also be tested with the oculocephalic maneuver by moving the head vertically or with cold calorics by irrigating both ears simultaneously; this normally produces tonic downward deviation of the eyes. Pupils should be examined for size and reaction to light. Anisocoria is a difference in pupil size of >1 mm. Compression of cranial nerve III (CN III), such as in transtentorial herniation, may lead to a unilateral dilated pupil with loss of the pupillary light reflex. Bilateral fixed mid-position pupils localize lesions to midbrain while bilateral pin-point reactive pupils indicate pontine lesion or narcotic overdose. The corneal reflex tests the integrity of CN V and VII, and is performed by touching a cotton swab to the cornea. Tracheal suctioning assesses the cough reflex, whereas stimulation of the posterior pharynx assesses the gag reflex, both of which test the integrity of CN IX and X.

Motor exam: In the comatose patient, the motor exam overlaps significantly with the mental status exam. It should be observed for symmetric and rhythmic spontaneous or involuntary movements, whether purposeful, myoclonic, or tonic–clonic in nature. Classically, flexor (decorticate) posture is most commonly associated with the damage to the thalamus or the upper midbrain above the level of the red nucleus, and extensor (decerebrate) posture is associated with severe damage to the midbrain or upper pons. Severe metabolic disorders as well as bilateral deep hemispheric lesions can also result in extensor posturing. In clinical practice, extensor posturing is regarded as a manifestation of a catastrophic injury.

Respirations: Cheyne–Stokes respirations (alternating progressive hyperpnea and apnea) are seen with the bilateral cerebral dysfunction, increased ICP and metabolic disturbances. Central neurogenic hyperventilation (rapid, deep breathing) results from damage to the midbrain tegmentum. Ataxic breathing is irregular, uneven breaths in no identifiable pattern, and can be due to lesions in the reticular formation of the dorsomedial medulla. Kussmaul breathing is deep regular inspirations accompanying metabolic acidosis.

Ancillary testing

All comatose patients should have basic laboratory studies including complete blood count, serum electrolytes, urine analysis, urine drug screening, liver function, arterial blood gas, and serum lactate. These test results, along with history and physical exam, are often adequate to identify the etiology of a coma and initiate therapy. Almost every comatose patient, especially those with focal neurologic findings, should also undergo an urgent noncontrast computed tomography (CT) brain scan to assess for, or exclude structural lesions (e.g. intracranial bleeding). A lumbar puncture (LP) should be performed in patients where there is a suspicion of meningitis or SAH despite an unremarkable CT scan. Evidence of intracranial compartmental pressure differences that could potentially lead to brain herniation is a contraindication for proceeding with an LP. An electroencephalogram (EEG) is critical for any patient who presents with seizure activity, even after cessation to rule

out nonconvulsive seizures. Magnetic resonance imaging (MRI) can be useful in identifying strokes, especially in the posterior fossa, and characterizing mass lesions. MRA, CTA, or cerebral angiography can be used to identify the source of an aneurysmal SAH or diagnose basilar artery thrombosis.

How to monitor and treat a comatose patient?

Bedside clinical examination remains a fundamental monitoring tool in any acutely neurologically injured patients, especially those comatose. Advances in technology, however, have brought many technological monitoring tools to the clinical arena. Tools that have scientific evidence-based support are listed in Table 5.2. In coma of acute onset, the aim of management is to prevent or limit secondary brain injury since the etiology of primary brain injury is rarely reversible (except in cases of acute subdural or epidural hematoma, superficial intracerebral hemorrhage, etc.). Hence, in order to prevent such damage, the purpose of invasive and noninvasive neuromonitoring techniques is to detect potential scarcity in substrate delivery, prevent substrate–demand mismatch and direct therapies to prevent such scarcities and mismatches.

Monitoring of a comatose patient

Intracranial pressure (ICP) monitoring

ICP monitoring is mostly utilized in patients with TBI. It is commonly performed by placing devices in the cranium, such as a ventriculostomy catheter or an intraparenchymal fiberoptic monitor. The main reasons for ICP monitoring in patients with TBI are to provide early warning of the development of an intracranial hemorrhage requiring intervention, and to offer guidance for the targeted use of medication or other measures to lower increased ICP (in order to maintain a goal cerebral perfusion pressure, CPP). Acceptance of ICP monitoring has increased since the publication of the Brain Trauma Foundation (BTF) recommendations for ICP monitoring in comatose patients [12]. The primary aim of monitoring ICP is to prevent secondary brain injury from cerebral ischemia. The first evidence that maintaining CPP above a predetermined target (>70 mm Hg) is beneficial came from a single centered nonrandomized study [13]. Though increasing CPP may increase oxygen delivery to the brain, it also leads to loss of vascular autoregulation in the injured brain. Hence, increasing CPP can lead to passive increases in blood vessel diameter, increasing cerebral blood volume and consequently ICP. Increased hydrostatic pressure across the cerebral capillary bed can also lead to vasogenic edema, which again increases ICP. An alternative approach, one dubbed the Lund protocol, has been suggested; it aims to minimize the CPP target to a level (>50 mm Hg) that avoids frank ischemia but does not lead to further cerebral insults [14]. Despite reports of lower

Table 5.2 Commonly used tools for neurologic monitoring

	Type	Monitors	Parameters	Advantages	Drawbacks
ICP	Global	Intracranial pressure	ICP < 20 mm Hg	Commonly used; easy to interpret; both diagnostic and therapeutic especially with EVD	Invasive; Infection risk
$PbtO_2$	Regional	Partial pressure of oxygen in tissue	Goal: $PbtO_2$ > 15–20 mmHg	Easy to insert, may help to ascertain correct CPP	Poor data if tissue hematoma, air bubble or placed in infarcted tissue
$SjvO_2$	Global	Saturation of venous blood returning from brain	Goal: 50–80%	Can help identify episodes of ischemia	Frequent recalibration; requires trained nursing staff; risk of thrombosis
Microdialysis	Regional	Biochemical composition of extracellular fluid in brain	Glucose, lactate, pyruvate, glutamate	Information about metabolic state of brain tissue	Costly; labor intensive; not validated
EEG	Global and regional	Electrophysiologic activity and abnormal patterns	Disease related	Noninvasive; can provide continuous data	Difficult in agitated patients; trained technicians required to perform; artefacts in ICU environment

EEG, electroencephalography; EVD, external ventricular drain; ICP, intracranial pressure; $PbtO_2$, partial brain tissue oxygenation; $SjvO_2$, jugular venous oxygen saturation.

mortality at centers in which ICP monitoring is widely used [15,16], there was no class I evidence supporting routine use of ICP monitoring in TBI. This is likely because monitoring alone, without accepted effective therapies implemented in response to the results of such monitoring, is unlikely to impact outcome. Moreover, increased CPP and hence increased blood flow may facilitate increased substrate delivery; however, this does not guarantee substrate utilization by the injured brain.

The outcome benefit of ICP/CPP-based TBI management has not been convincingly proven. Clinical studies done in 1970s and 1980s showed lower mortality in patients undergoing ICP monitoring [17–20]. In a paper reviewing clinical trials published after 1970, mortality rate was approximately 12% ($P < 0.001$) lower among patients in the intense ICP treatment group [16]. However, similar benefit could not be replicated in other studies; to the contrary, it leads to patients in the ICP monitoring group spending more days on mechanical ventilation, without a favorable impact on outcome or mortality rates [21]. A recent multicenter study from Latin America compared ICP-directed versus imaging/clinical directed care in 324 patients with severe TBI showed no statistical difference in morbidity and mortality [22]. The lack of a consistent benefit of ICP monitoring suggests that refractory elevation of ICP may be a mere marker of severity of brain injury. A recent Cochrane database review could not identify appropriate studies to assess the role of ICP monitoring on mortality or severe disability following TBI [23].

The role of ICP monitoring in nontraumatic brain injury, such as status epilepticus, intracerebral hemorrhage, cerebral infarction, fulminant hepatic failure, Reye's syndrome, diffuse cerebritis, and metabolic encephalopathies, is even less clear than that in TBI. Decisions to monitor ICP in such patients should be made on a case-by-case basis, depending on the clinical scenario and while weighing the advantages and disadvantages of the invasive procedure.

Jugular bulb oximetry ($SjvO_2$)

Cannulation of the internal jugular vein allows measurement of $SjvO_2$, a global cerebral marker for balance between cerebral oxygen delivery and utilization. The normal range for $SjvO_2$ is 60–75%, and desaturation to less than 50% is regarded as indicative of cerebral ischemia. $SjvO_2$ also decreases when there is disproportionately high metabolism compared to cerebral blood flow (CBF) (e.g. seizure or hyperthermia). Elevated $SjvO_2$ > 80% is seen when oxygen demand decreases secondary to mitochondrial dysfunction or cell death (e.g. brain death), or there is luxury perfusion/cerebral hyperemia [24].

In TBI, $SjvO_2$ monitoring provides an early indication of ischemia resulting from either intracranial or systemic causes [25]. Small series have shown that $SjvO_2$ monitoring may improve outcome after TBI [26,27]. $SjvO_2 \leq 50\%$ reflects cerebral ischemia and should be avoided. Immediate correction is important since hypoxic/ischemic $SjvO_2$ values are associated with metabolic derangements reflected by increased lactate and glutamate levels [28] as well as increased mortality and morbidity [29]. Level III evidence of BTF guidelines advocates maintenance of a $SjvO_2 > 50\%$. But positron emission tomography (PET) and microdialysis studies questioned the sensitivity of $SjvO_2$, showing that

$SjvO_2$ does not decrease by <50% until 13% of the brain becomes ischemic [30]. It should also be noted that $SjvO_2$ is a global measure and has a poor correlation with regional tissue oxygenation in the areas of focal pathology.

Brain tissue oxygen tension ($PbtO_2$) monitoring

$PbtO_2$ monitoring provides a measure of focal cerebral oxygenation. The principle of $PbtO_2$ monitoring has been reviewed recently [31]. A significant relationship between $PbtO_2$ and the product of CBF and cerebral arteriovenous oxygen tension difference exists [32]. This indicates a strong association between $PbtO_2$ and diffusion of dissolved plasma oxygen across the blood–brain barrier. $PbtO_2$ value in patients with normal ICP and CPP is 25–30 mm Hg, and the critical threshold for ischemic damage is around 10–15 mm Hg. Hypoxia at a threshold of 10 mm Hg is associated with increased extracellular glutamate if not corrected within 30 min [33,34]. Such ischemic episodes were associated with neuropsychological deficits in survivors [35].

$PbtO_2$ was also monitored in clinical studies involving patients receiving osmotic therapy, decompressive craniectomy, those developing vasospasm, and to study the effect of spontaneous hyperventilation in TBI [36–39]. Although low $PbtO_2$ was associated with poor outcome, it is unclear whether interventions aimed at altering $PbtO_2$ can have a positive impact on overall outcome. Single-centered studies have compared $PbtO_2$-based therapy with ICP/CPP-based therapy in patients with TBI [38,40,41]. In one case, mortality in patients with similar ICP and CPP levels was higher in the conventional ICP/CPP management group as compared to the $PbtO_2$ group (44% vs. 25%. $P<0.05$) [38]. Overall, 40% of patients receiving ICP/CPP-guided management and 64.3% of those receiving $PbtO_2$-guided management had a favorable short-term outcome ($P=0.01$). In a study of 139 patients treated using a $PbtO_2$-guided protocol, elevated ICP and persistently low $PbtO_2$ at 2 hours were associated with higher odds of death [odds ratio (OR) 14.3]. Patients with favorable outcomes had significantly higher mean daily $PbtO_2$ and CPP values compared to nonsurvivors [40,42]. To the contrary, in their study, Adamides et al. showed that although $PbtO_2$-guided therapy was associated with a decreased duration of episodes of cerebral hypoxia, there was no significant improvement in outcome [43]. In a larger study of 629 patients with severe TBI, $PbtO_2$ monitoring did not reduce mortality; the procedure was associated with poorer neurological outcome and increased hospital resource utilization [44]. An ongoing phase 2 clinical trial (BOOST-2) comparing $PbtO_2$ and ICP/CPP-based therapies for TBI could quell the dilemma generated by the conflicting results of prior studies [45].

Microdialysis

Cerebral microdialysis allows continuous monitoring of changes in brain tissue chemistry. The benefit of this monitoring technique is based on the underlying principle that biochemical changes occur before low CPP is detected [46]. However, it should also be noted that due to dialysis duration (~60 minutes), metabolic changes reflect derangements that have already occurred. Hence, it is recommended that all monitoring parameters such as ICP, CPP, $SjvO_2$, and $PbtO_2$ are taken into consideration when initiating corrective treatment. The substances that can be analyzed from the dialysate are glucose, lactate, pyruvate, glutamate, aspartate, gamma amino butyric acid, and glycerol [42]. Lactate and the lactate/pyruvate index (LPI) are markers commonly used to detect brain tissue hypoxia. Elevated extracellular glutamate reflects excessive neuronal excitation or indicates neuronal damage with release of intracellular glutamate store. Decreased glucose levels may be due to increased cellular uptake and metabolism and/or insufficient supply due to hypoglycemia, impaired perfusion, or insufficient expression of glucose transporter. In TBI, cerebral microdialysis has been used to guide CPP targets [33]. Derangement of metabolism during periods of intracranial hypertension has been associated with a reduction in brain glucose and elevation of the LPI. A recent study showed that low glucose and elevated LPI is a significant independent predictor of mortality [47]. Metabolic changes observed by microdialysis may even be used as an early warning system to unmask pathological alterations that precede increased ICP by 12 hours [34,46]. Moreover, energy metabolism may be impaired in severe TBI even in the presence of adequate cerebral oxygen transport. In a recent article, microdialysis identified new biomarkers of cellular injury (proteomic analysis revealing peptides of cytoarchitectural, blood breakdown, and mitochondrial proteins) in TBI [48]. Intracranial monitoring after CPA undergoing therapeutic hypothermia (TH) is usually not a standard practice but has been investigated in small case series [49]. The patients showed early peak in LPI and glutamate concentration with near normalization of LPI by the end of monitoring period, and transient increase occurred during the rewarming phase. All of them had good clinical outcome with recovery of consciousness. Despite the enthusiasm that it generated, microdialysis is not widely available or used. Some experts believe that the local chemistry is weakly correlated to ICP and CPP. Furthermore, there remains a lack of definitive evidence linking the use of microdialysis and improved outcome [50].

Electroencephalography (EEG)

EEG offers a continuous, real time, noninvasive measure of the brain function. Continuous EEG (cEEG) has been used in different settings in the intensive care unit for early detection of cerebral ischemia secondary to decreased CBF or decreased energy utilization, and nonconvulsive status epilepticus. Indications of cEEG are listed in Table 5.3, and its utility has been recently reviewed [51].

Table 5.3 Indications for continuous electroencephalogram (cEEG) monitoring

---

1 Detection of nonconvulsive seizures and characterization of spells in patients with altered mental status with:

   A history of epilepsy

   Fluctuating level of consciousness

   Acute brain injury

   Recent convulsive status epilepticus

   Stereotyped activity such as paroxysmal movements, nystagmus, twitching, jerking, hippus, autonomic variability

2 Monitoring of ongoing therapy

   Induced coma for elevated intracranial pressure or refractory status epilepticus

   Assessing level of sedation

3 Ischemia detection

   Vasospasm in subarachnoid hemorrhage

   Cerebral ischemia in other patients at high risk for stroke

4 Prognosis

   Following cardiac arrest

   Following acute brain injury

Source: Adapted from Friedman [51].

This monitoring technique is being promoted as a mean for continuous real-time monitoring of the brain at the bedside to improve neurological outcome through early detection and appropriate intervention for "at risk" brain.

With increased frequency of cEEG being adopted in clinical practice in the neurocritical care unit, nonconvulsive seizures (NCSz) and nonconvulsive status epilepticus (NCSE) are increasingly recognized, with 8–48% of comatose patients reported to have NCSz, depending on case series [52–55]. Incidence of NCSz in these studies may be spuriously high because of selection bias; therefore, the occurrence of NCSz is thought to be lower in a general comatose population. In a prospective study, where patients were monitored with cEEG for 24 hours after termination of convulsive SE, 48% and 14% had NCSz and NCSE, respectively [55]. Patients with NCSE after convulsive SE had more than a twofold greater mortality compared with patients whose seizures ended with convulsive activity [55,56]. In a retrospective series of 570 patients who underwent cEEG for mental status change or suspicion of seizures, 19% had seizures, with 101 patients having NCSz [52]. Three to 19% of patients with intracerebral hemorrhage (ICH) experience in-hospital convulsive seizures [57–60]. Conversely, two recent studies using cEEG found 18–21% of patients with ICH had NCSz [57,61]. Similarly, although the rate of acute clinical seizures after ischemic stroke ranges between 2% and 9% in population and hospital-based studies [58,60,62], using cEEG the Columbia series reported 11% of 56 patients with ischemic stroke had seizures [52].

The incidence of seizures during the first week after TBI has decreased to <1% [63] from 4 to 14% [64–66] since the routine use of prophylactic antiepileptic agents during the first week following trauma. Two recent studies using cEEG in TBI report the incidence of seizures of any kind (NCSz or NCSE) to be around 18–22% [52,67]. Similarly, the incidence of seizures after cardiac arrest is reported to be as high as 35% [68–70]. In a case series of comatose patients diagnosed with NCSE, 42% had hypoxic/anoxic injury [54]. Twenty percent of patients with hypoxic-ischemic injury monitored in the Columbia series had seizures, mostly NCSz [52]. With more frequent use of TH for neuroprotection after cardiac arrest, the role of cEEG is becoming more important because most patients are sedated and paralyzed for maintenance of hypothermia. Therefore, more overt and subtle electrographic seizures in this group of comatose patients will likely be detected. In patients with toxic-metabolic encephalopathy monitored with cEEG, the incidence of NCSz has been reported to be 21% [52]. In medical intensive care unit population without known brain injury who underwent cEEG, 11–22% of patients had periodic epileptiform discharges or electrographic seizures mostly associated with sepsis, metabolic disturbances, or respiratory failure significantly contributing to such findings [71,72].

The current literature supports a role of cEEG in diagnosing and monitoring comatose patients. The unresolved questions are when and for how long to monitor. Pandian *et al.* found that routine EEGs (30 minutes) detected seizures in 11% of patients, whereas subsequent cEEG did so in 28% [53]. In 110 critically ill patients with seizures detected by cEEG, Claassen *et al.* found that half of patients had their first seizure within the first hour of monitoring [52]. Although 95% of noncomatose patients had their first seizure within 24 hours, only 80% of those who were comatose had a seizure by this time. Extending the monitoring to 48 hours, 98% of noncomatose and 87% of comatose patients had their first seizure. Hence, some advocate monitoring for 24 hours to exclude NCSz in noncomatose, while longer periods may be necessary for comatose patients. But there is still debate among clinicians and electroencephalographers regarding the implications of detection of electrographic seizures, and some authorities consider such discharges as mere bystander of severely injured brain. Whether aggressively treating such electrographic seizures would confer better clinical outcome is unknown.

Management

Osmotic therapy

The use of osmotic agents is commonplace in coma-inducing conditions that result in brain tissue shifts, cerebral edema and herniation, and elevated ICP. Both mannitol and hypertonic saline solutions are available and used in emergency department and intensive care units. Mannitol is a metabolically inert hexose that is infused intravenously and excreted unchanged by kidneys. It produces an osmotic diuresis that helps decrease intracranial content volume [73,74], thus lowering intracranial pressure [75]. Other potential mechanism of action includes improving microvascular flow via its effect on hematocrit and viscosity. Almost immediately following infusion, mannitol is effective in reducing ICP [76–78]. Hypertonic saline solutions vary in their concentrations of sodium chloride. The most commonly used solutions have 3%, 7.5%, or 23.4% sodium chloride. They are too infused intravenously and act by inducing a water shift down an osmotic gradient resulting in reduction of ICP. The osmotic diuretic effect of mannitol could result in hypotension, an adverse effect not encountered when using hypertonic saline.

There is evidence for using either one of these agents to reduce ICP in a myriad of conditions such as subarachnoid and intracerebral hemorrhage, cerebral infarction, mass lesion, trauma, and fulminant liver failure [36,75,79–82]; however, evidence for an effect on outcome is lacking. Trials to study such effect would be difficult to conduct, given that not intervening in the face of malignant elevation of ICP or clinical evidence of cerebral herniation is hardly an option. Despite the lack of adequate class I studies, mannitol is regarded as the gold standard therapy for reducing elevated ICP [83]. However, more recent retrospective studies and large case series are suggesting that hypertonic saline solutions might be as or more effective in reducing ICP with less adverse events than typically seen with mannitol such as hypotension, electrolytes imbalance, renal failure, and rebound elevation in ICP; the latter being linked to idiogenic osmole production in the brain [82,84].

Hypothermia
Cardiopulmonary arrest
TH was proven beneficial in comatose patients following successful resuscitation from ventricular fibrillation cardiopulmonary arrest. Two randomized controlled studies are worth mentioning. The study by Bernard *et al.* randomized 77 patients (43 to TH and 34 to normothermia), with TH initiated in the prehospital setting. Temperature was maintained at 33°C for 12 hours. Good outcome measured at hospital discharge with the Cerebral Performance Category (CPC) scale was significantly more likely in patients treated with TH (49% vs. 26%; $P = 0.046$) [85]. Subsequently, the Hypothermia After Cardiac Arrest (HACA) study randomized 273 patients (136 to TH and 137 to normothermia) [86]. Temperature was maintained at 33°C for 24 h in the TH group. This study had long-term follow-up, with CPC scores reported at 6 months. Good outcomes were seen in 55% of hypothermia-treated patients compared to 39% of the normothermia controls ($P = 0.009$ for favorable neurological outcome). Current recommendations by the American Heart Association (AHA) and International Liaison Committee on Resuscitation (ILCOR) suggest treating unconscious patients with spontaneous circulation after out-of-hospital

CPA due to VF/VT with moderate hypothermia (32–34°C) for 12–24 h. It is unclear whether TH is beneficial for CPA caused by other rhythms or in-hospital arrests, though recent retrospective case series show benefits in other rhythms and etiologies too [87,88]. Both the 2002 trials have been criticized for their methodology and improper treatment of control population (e.g. not treating fever that is known to worsen neurological outcome). A recent multicenter randomized controlled trial was completed [89]. A total of 939 patients were randomized to receive targeted temperature of 33°C or 36°C for 36 hours with gradual rewarming starting at 28 hours; temperature was not allowed to reach > 37.5°C up to 72 hours. At the 180-day follow-up, 54% of patients in the 33°C group had died or had a poor neurologic outcome according to the CPC, as compared with 52% of patients in the 36°C group (risk ratio, 1.02; 95% CI, 0.88–1.16; $P = 0.78$). The study has led to questioning of the exact role that TH has in cardiac arrest.

Traumatic brain injury
Although animal studies demonstrated beneficial effect of induced moderate hypothermia following TBI, the evidence supporting its routine use in humans with severe TBI remain controversial. Numerous clinical studies have been completed since 1990 [90–95], and three meta-analyses have been published on the efficacy of moderate hypothermia (32–34°C) for TBI [96–98]. The largest study conducted in the United States included 392 patients with GCS of 3–8, randomized to hypothermia or normothermia within 8 hours of injury [99]. Hypothermia was maintained for 48 hours after which patients were actively rewarmed. A poor outcome (GOS of 1–3) was seen in 57% of patients in both groups; mortality was also equal (28% in hypothermic group vs. 26% in controls, $P = 0.79$). In a single center study by Zhi *et al.*, 396 patients with TBI were randomized to hypothermia or normothermia within 24 hours of trauma [100]. In this study, patients were kept hypothermic until ICP had remained normal for 24 h. Mortality was 36.4% in the normothermic patients compared to 25.7% in the hypothermic group ($P < 0.05$). Little information, however, was provided regarding randomization, blinding, and medical management.

In an effort to integrate the results of many published studies into a single assessment, three meta-analyses have been carried out and published. Published studies varied considerably in method of blinding, randomization, and management of ICP as well as the care of control subjects. The Cochrane Review included 10 trials with 771 patients and did not find evidence of benefit with respect to death or severe disability. Hypothermia seemed to be associated with an increased risk for pneumonia [96]. Similarly, another meta-analysis that included three trials with a total of 748 patients failed to find evidence of benefit in favor of hypothermia [98]. A larger number of studies were included in the third meta-analysis with 12 trials and 1069 patients [97]. It concluded that hypothermia following TBI was associated with a reduction in death (relative risk [RR] of 0.81 (95% confidence interval [CI] 0.69–0.96) as well as improved neurologic outcome (RR was 0.78 for Glasgow Outcome Scale [GOS] 1–3 [95% CI 0.63–0.98]). Subgroup analysis also suggested that cooling for a longer period of time (>48 hours) had an even greater beneficial effect. These conflicting results have led to TH being relegated to a secondary order in the management of patients with TBI. TH is used in settings of refractory elevation of ICP when other therapies fail.

Pharmacologic agents in coma

Corticosteroids were used after TBI since it was thought that the anti-inflammatory effect of steroids would lead to improved clinical outcome. A multicenter randomized trial (MRC CRASH) was aborted after enrollment of ~10,000 patients due to increased morbidity and mortality in the intervention arm [101]. In that cohort, 3944 patients had severe TBI (i.e. GCS 3–8). Mortality was 39.8% in the steroid, as compared to 34.8% in the placebo group ($P < 0.05$). Another putative agent promoted to improve neurological outcome after TBI is progesterone. Cochrane database analyzing the effect of progesterone administration acutely after TBI concluded that there is evidence from three small randomized trials indicating potential benefit on morbidity [102]. A planned phase III clinical trial is aimed at uncovering a similar potential benefit [103].

What are the various predictors that help in determination of prognosis of a comatose patient?

Functional outcome and prognosis of a comatose patient depend on the etiology of the insult, the early identification of the cause, and how soon a structural or functional derangement is reversed. Bedside clinical examination provides information regarding initial and long-term prognoses. As a part of the clinical examination, the GCS has high inter-rater predictability. It was first developed in 1974 for use in patients with acute TBI. Since then it has been used in various clinical settings not only to initially assess a comatose patient but also to reliably communicate among healthcare providers about the degree and progression of coma.

Clinical examination and scales

Comatose TBI patients

Families of patients with TBI are usually dissatisfied because they rarely receive accurate prognostic information [104–106]. Subjective prognostic estimates based on the clinician's personal experience are far from accurate [107–109]. BTF reviewed studies on closed head injury and identified older age, lower GCS at presentation, large

unreactive pupils, and hypotension as clinical predictors of poor functional outcome. Similarly, more recent studies showed that older age and low GCS scores are associated with poor outcome [110–112]. In addition, severe disability was unlikely whether length of coma <2 weeks or posttraumatic amnesia less than 2 months. Conversely, good recovery was unlikely if coma lasted longer than 4 weeks or posttraumatic amnesia more than 3 months.

Among the clinical scales for predicting recovery from coma, the FOUR scale was recently validated against GCS and found to be even superior to it [113]. The FOUR score is a clinical grading scale designed for use by medical professionals in the assessment of patients with impaired level of consciousness. It is a 17-point scale; scores range from 0 to 16, with lower numbers suggesting a poor level of consciousness. The FOUR score assesses four domains of neurological function: eye responses, motor responses, brainstem reflexes, and breathing pattern. Sadaka et al. prospectively collected data on 51 patients, 15 had poor functional outcome [113]. For every 1-point increase in the total FOUR score, the odds of in-hospital mortality were reduced by an estimated 36%. The odds of a poor functional outcome were reduced by 29% when defined as a modified Rankin scale (mRS) of 3–6, and 33% when defined as a GOS of 1–3.

Comatose postcardiac arrest patients

Certain variables, such as age, duration of arrest and of coma, have been investigated as predictors of functional outcome in postcardiac arrest. Studies showed a significant difference in survival between patients under 60 and those over the age of 80 [114]; in addition, younger patients were twice more likely to survive at 30 and 180 days [115]. However, another prospective study of 255 in-hospital CPA demonstrated that age was not an independent predictor of survival [116]. Similarly, in another prospective study of 774 patients, old age did not nullify good neurologic outcome after cardiac arrest [117].

The duration of cardiac arrest correlates with the extent of brain damage [117,118]. As many as 80% of patients are comatose after CPA. Of those patients destined to awaken, over 90% will do so within the first 72 hours [119]. Thereafter, the probability of awakening decreases significantly to the extent that recovery after 3 months of unresponsiveness becomes unlikely [120]. Survival rates of 48% and 2% correlate with periods of arrest of less than and longer than 10 min, respectively [114,119]. The pupillary light reaction, corneal response, and motor responses have been analyzed for prediction of outcome following CPA. The *American Academy of Neurology* published guidelines on this topic are widely used by clinicians seeking guidance when prognosticating in this patient population [121]. An absent pupillary or corneal reflex reaction to light after 72 hours portends practically no chance for awakening

(100% specificity) [122,123]. Absence of motor responses to noxious stimuli after 3 days of coma correlates, similarly, with a poor outcome with a specificity of 100% [124]. Moreover, in the Brain Resuscitation Clinical Trials I, lack of motor responses after 72 hours was the only independent predictor of poor outcome [125]. In two prospective studies, absence of the corneal reflex at 72 hours was associated with strongly predicted poor outcome [126,127].

With the worldwide acceptance of TH after CPA, the guidelines that help predict neurological outcome have been questioned and were recently reviewed [128]. The effects of sedatives and paralytics used during TH are prolonged because of decreased metabolism, affecting clinical examination even after rewarming. In a prospective study of 111 patients who underwent TH, among the 45 survivors, 25 had good outcomes (CPC = 1–2, with two participants lost to follow-up) [129]. Two patients with absent pupillary, oculocephalic, or corneal reflexes 36–72 hours postarrest achieved good outcomes, and 11 patients with poor motor responses survived, four with good outcomes. In another study of 72 patients, the presence of a good motor response in 44 patients within 24 hours of discontinuation of sedation predicted good outcome with 100% specificity [130]. A meta-analysis of 1,153 TH-treated patients from 10 studies found that a motor response of 1–2 on the GCS had a high false-positive ratio for predicting poor outcome compared with bilaterally absent corneal or pupillary responses [131]. Hence, traditional clinical outcome predictors can no longer be reliably used at standard time points [128]. In a cohort of 200 CPA patients (TH-treated = 32, non-TH-treated = 168), absent pupillary and corneal reflexes on days 3 and 7 postarrest were 100% specific for predicting poor outcome; however, of 74 patients with poor motor responses on day 3 (three of whom underwent TH), 8.1% achieved good outcomes [132]. To summarize, absence of corneal and pupillary reflexes at least 72 hours post-rewarming seem to be highly reliable indicator of poor outcome. Motor responses were inconsistent and less reliable [128].

Neuroimaging

Neuroimaging following acute brain injury is a valuable resource used to determine prognosis and counsel family members regarding long-term functional outcome of a comatose patient. An ideal neuroimaging examination for a comatose patient should assess all structures involved in arousal and awareness functions. MRI of the brain is usually the imaging modality that is most commonly used. When performed in the acute phase (first 24 hours), it can provide information about reversible lesions such as edema but can miss secondary insults. An examination performed late after the injury (e.g. more than 3 weeks) may only detect sequelae such as nonspecific global atrophy, and will have less impact on medical management or prognosis.

An early subacute examination (first 2 weeks) would be best to evaluate brain damage critical for therapeutic and prognostic decisions (i.e. to determine outcome, cognitive, and behavioral deficits) [133].

Traumatic brain injury
Conventional MRI
In patients with TBI, the total number of lesions detected by FLAIR and T2*-gradient echo are inversely correlated with GOS scores [134,135]. Studies on traumatic coma patients with conventional MRI showed that lesions of the pons, midbrain, and basal ganglia, especially when bilateral, are predictive of poor outcome [136–141]. Nevertheless, these studies fail to explain why some patients in minimal conscious state, unresponsive wakefulness syndrome, or with long-term marked cognitive impairments have no or minimal lesions on conventional MRI examination. Hence, lack of specificity and insufficient sensitivity of conventional MR sequences in predicting outcome after coma is of concern as it fails to reveal lesions like ischemic axonal injuries. Thus, morphological MRI alone cannot be considered as a reliable tool to assess consciousness disorders severity or to predict their evolution [133].

Advanced imaging modalities
Diffusion tensor imaging (DTI) is based on the principle of restriction of water movement by barriers to diffusion in the brain depending on tissue organization. The diffusion of water protons is higher along fiber tracts in the white matter. Therefore, DTI can track fibers and compute the fractional anisotropy. In TBI, a significant negative correlation has been shown between fractional anisotropy in the splenium of the corpus callosum and the internal capsule and GCS scores at discharge [139]. In an imaging study performed on 43 TBI patients during the subacute phase (24±11 days) predicted nonrecovery after 1 year with up to 86% sensitivity and 97% specificity when taking into account both DTI and magnetic resonance spectroscopy (MRS) values [142]. Nonrecovery of traumatic patients was also shown to correlate with decreased fractional anisotropy in cerebral peduncles, posterior limb of the internal capsule, posterior corpus callosum, and inferior longitudinal fasciculus [143]. These results suggest that DTI could be used as a surrogate biomarker for poor functional outcome in patients with TBI and disordered consciousness.

Proton MRS is an imaging method that provides useful metabolic information on brain damage that is not evident on other morphologic imaging. The exploration of disorders of consciousness is performed at intermediate or long echo time (135–288 ms), and the metabolites analyzed are choline (for membrane synthesis and catabolism); creatine (Cr), a marker for aerobic metabolism; N-acetylaspartate (NAA), a marker for neuronal density and viability that is produced in the mitochondria, and lactate, which is a marker for anaerobic metabolism. In a case–control study, comparing 10 TBI patients with 10 healthy controls, lower NAA/Cr ratio correlated with poor GOS [144]. In yet another study, NAA levels were decreased and correlated with the initial GCS and outcome at 3 months [145]. Several other studies showed a significant correlation between NAA/Cr ratio and outcome of TBI patients in gray and white matter of occipito-parietal [146,147], and frontal lobes [148], splenium of corpus callosum [149], and thalamic brain regions [150]. NAA/Cr ratio seems to be more reliable than NAA/Cho for predicting outcome in patients with TBI [151]. The NAA decreases within a few minutes after TBI and reaches its minimum within 48 hours. Its level remains stable within the first month after the injury, supporting the usefulness of MRS assessments during the second or third week after injury [152,153].

Functional magnetic resonance imaging (fMRI) is capable of measuring brain activity, at rest, during passive stimulation and in response to commands [154,155]. Most of the studies using fMRI are performed in patients with chronic disorders of consciousness because of the practical difficulty in obtaining meaningful results during the acute stage of TBI. Some of these difficulties are related to intracranial hypertension, agitation and motor restlessness, use of sedatives, and hemodynamic instability. There are three broad categories of fMRI imaging sequences that can be used for prognostication purposes – task-based fMRI, resting-state fMRI, and arterial spin labeling MRI. Interested readers are referred to a recent review for details regarding its applicability [155]. Most feasible in the acute–subacute stage after TBI is the resting state fMRI that is based on the principle of spontaneous fluctuations in brain activity being temporally correlated in functionally related brain regions at rest. Of these, the most recognized and studied is the concept of "default mode network" (DMN) of brain function, proposed by Raichle et al. to describe a number of brain regions encompassing the precuneus, posterior parietal lobe, and medial prefrontal cortex that are more active at rest than when we are involved in attention-demanding cognitive tasks [156]. Using resting-state fMRI, strong association was reported for quantitative preservation of posterior cingulate cortex/precuneus network and recovery of consciousness [157]. Hence, this technique tests the functional integrity of major brain structures and could be useful to distinguish unconscious–vegetative from conscious–minimally conscious patients. However, future large multicenter standardized studies are needed to give a full characterization of DMN connectivity in vegetative state and minimal conscious state patients and its potential use in outcome prediction [133].

Anoxic-ischemic brain injury
Conventional imaging modalities
Computed tomography (CT) performed immediately after CPA is usually normal; however, by day 3 it might show brain swelling and reversal of the gray/white matter density

in patients with a poor outcome [158]. Two small studies showed that gray matter/white matter (GM/WM) ratio using Hounsfield units (HU) at the basal ganglia level of <1.18 within 48 hours of arrest [158], or <1.22 within 24 hours of ROSC [159], was 100% specific for predicting poor outcome. In a larger cohort of 240 patients (70% underwent TH), an average GM/WM ratio of <1.2 predicted death with a sensitivity of 36% (95% CI 29–45%) and specificity of 98% (95% CI 91–100%) [160]. In a retrospective cohort of 98 patients who underwent TH, CT performed within 7 days of CPA (median 5 hours; interquartile range 2–24 hours) was analyzed for GM/WM ratio (at basal ganglia and cortical levels). A value of <1.16 predicted poor outcome with 38% sensitivity and 100% specificity [161].

MRI brain is also routinely used to determine prognosis after CPA; however, there is limited data available on its reliability. Moreover, the frequent use of TH after CPA has led to altered temporal evolution of MRI characteristics [128]. Four case series used MRI at variable time points after cardiac arrest; two of them showed that widespread abnormal findings on diffusion-weighted imaging (DWI) and fluid-attenuated inversion recovery (FLAIR) correlated with a poor outcome [162,163]. Preliminary studies using quantitative MRI showed that none of the patients with >10% of brain tissue with an apparent diffusion coefficient (ADC) value $<650 \times 10^{-6}$–700×10^{-6} mm^2/s regained consciousness [164,165]. These studies of whole-brain quantitative DWI analyses suggested that the ideal time window for prognostication appears to be between 49 and 108 hours after the arrest, when the ADC reductions are most apparent. Conversely, patients who regain consciousness exhibit increased diffusion involving the temporal and occipital lobes, corona radiata, and hippocampus; in addition, qualitative changes in the deep gray nuclei alone are common in these patients. In a prospective cohort of 20 patients undergoing TH who remained in coma 72 hours after reaching normothermia, patients who died tended to exhibit larger numbers of lesions on DWI, particularly in the parietal region and thalamus [166]. In another MRI study that was performed on a comatose patient after CPA showed progressive DWI changes in different areas of the brain with highly energy-dependent areas (e.g. cortical areas) affected early compared to later involvement of the white matter regions [167]. Patients imaged in the first 1–2 days postarrest often showed DWI changes confined to the cerebellum and basal ganglia, which subsequently moved to the cortex around days 3–5, and then affected the subcortical white matter on days 6–12. It is also reported that patients with pronounced hippocampal abnormalities on DWI – the so-called bright hippocampus sign – invariably had poor outcomes [168].

Advanced imaging modalities
MRS (e.g. for pH and NAA) has been reported to correlate with a poor outcome in comatose patients after CPA [165].

In a recent review of 15 positron emission tomography and fMRI studies involving 48 published cases, where findings were categorized as "absent cortical activation," "typical activation" (involving low-level primary sensory cortices), and "atypical activation" (corresponding to higher-level associative cortices), atypical patterns of activity predicted recovery from the vegetative state with 93% specificity and 69% sensitivity [169]. In a study using somatosensory evoked potential (SSEP) and blood-oxygen-level-dependent (BOLD) contrast fMRI, patients with good outcome were noted to have better BOLD signal in the primary somatosensory cortex contralateral to the stimulated hand, when compared with patients with an unfavorable outcome and without SSEP responses [170]. Similar to TBI, functional alteration in brain connectivity is also reported using resting-state fMRI study in patients with anoxic brain injury that showed multiple disconnections in primary areas and in high-order associative areas [171]. Such studies using fMRI may have potential to predict functional outcome in this population of patients, but their validity in larger cohorts is awaited.

Electrophysiology

EEG

EEG monitoring can provide information about brain activity after anoxic injury from CPA that can help clinicians to prognosticate, though the AAN practice parameters caution that despite the correlation between electrographic seizures or burst-suppression patterns and poor outcome, the prognostic accuracy remain insufficient [121]. Prolonged monitoring can provide information on EEG reactivity, sleep architecture, and epileptiform discharges, all of which could help with prognostication [172]. In the pre-TH era, burst-suppression patterns after hypoxic-ischemic injury have been associated with lack of neurologic recovery [173]. Invariant EEG patterns that are not modulated by stimulation, such as alpha coma, are associated with an 88% likelihood of persistent vegetative state or death after anoxia [174]. However, this and other patterns, such as theta and alpha-theta coma, may be transient; up to 20% of patients with such patterns who subsequently developed EEG reactivity recovered consciousness in one series [173]. In the TH era, in a retrospective case series of six patients with status epilepticus, one returned to baseline functioning, three remained moderately impaired and, one dependent, and one died due to pneumonia [175]. In a prospective series, 79 patients diagnosed with status myoclonus, 9 (12%) had good functional outcome [176]. In addition, quantitative EEG tools, such as amplitude-integrated EEG, can also be used to predict outcome after CPA, mostly by identifying burst suppression patterns [177]. Burst-suppression pattern, alpha coma, clinical seizures with noncontinuous background were all associated with poor neurological outcome, whereas all patients with initially continuous EEG pattern regained consciousness [177]. In yet another prospective

cohort of 56 patients treated with TH who were monitored with cEEG during the first 5 days after admission, 43% of patients with good outcome showed continuous, diffuse, slow EEG rhythms, compared to none in the poor outcome group [178]. Perhaps the most promising EEG feature for prediction of clinical outcome is the presence or absence of reactivity of background to external stimuli [128].

EEG has also provided useful prognostic information in other clinical settings. After convulsive status epilepticus, normalization of the EEG background was associated with good clinical outcome, whereas patterns such as burst suppression and continued electrographic seizures portended mortality rates of more than 50% [179]; most of the survivors with these patterns remained debilitated. Similarly, periodic discharges also increased the risk of poor outcome. In a study of 116 patients with poor grade SAH, absence of sleep architectures and presence of periodic lateralized epileptiform discharges (PLEDs) were independent risk factors for poor outcome [180]. All patients with absent EEG reactivity, generalized periodic epileptiform discharges, bilaterally independent PLEDs, or NCSE had poor outcomes. In patients with TBI, the absence of normal sleep architecture is also a predictor of poor outcome [181].

Evoked potentials

SSEPs are noninvasive, reproducible, and simple to perform and interpret, and are less susceptible to electrical interference. Most importantly, they are less affected by metabolic disturbances or medications. The N20 component is the evoked potential waveform best studied as a prognostic indicator. The primary cortical SSEP component following median nerve stimulation, N20, is recorded as a near-field potential over the parietal area contralateral to the stimulated median nerve. While a thalamic or subcortical origin for N20 has been suggested, most authors believe that N20 predominantly reflects activity of neurons in the hand area of the primary somatosensory cortex. In the pre-TH era, absence of N20, after stimulation of the median nerve, has been shown to be a reliable predictor of poor outcome in comatose patients after CPA [127,172,182]. A systematic review of 18 studies analyzing the predictive ability of SSEPs in 1136 adult comatose patients following cardiac arrest found that all 336 patients with bilaterally absent cortical N20 peaks did not awaken [183]. Two other clinical trials also showed that absence of cortical SSEP peaks was associated with poor prognosis, with a specificity of 100% [184,185]. Presence of cortical N20 responses, however, does not necessarily predict awakening from coma [184,186]. In a cohort of 185 patients treated with TH, 36 patients showed bilaterally absent N20 responses at 72 hours (i.e. 48 hours after rewarming was started). Of these 36 patients only one had good functional outcome [187]. In another multicenter prospective cohort of 391 patients, SSEP performed during TH and 48 hours after rewarming showed false-positive rate (FPR) of 3% (95% CI 1–7%) during TH and 0% (95% CI

0–18%) after normothermia was achieved [188]. Another potential of SSEP, long-latency N70 peaks have also been studied in a case series of 66 patients. N70 latency was less than 118 milliseconds in all patients who had a good recovery and was absent or greater than 118 milliseconds in patients with a poor outcome [189].

Endogenous evoked potential (e.g. P300) in comatose patients was also effective in predicting awakening in small patient series, but its absence does not necessarily predict a good prognosis [190,191]. Since the P300 is thought to be associated with attention or expectancy and is dependent on the level of vigilance, it is preferable to record mismatch negativity (MMN), which does not require awareness [1]. The presence of MMN in a comatose patient is highly predictive of evolution toward awakening [192,193]. In summary, absent exogenous EPs are established prognosticators of poor outcome, whereas the presence of endogenous components, notably the MMN and P300, appears to predict a favorable outcome [1,194].

Biomarkers

Several serum biomarkers have been evaluated for their prognostic value after CPA, neuron-specific enolase (NSE) has the most robust data especially in the era preceding TH [127]. NSE, used as a marker for neuronal injury, is found in neurons, and elevated levels are detected in the blood or cerebrospinal fluid [195]. In the PROPAC study, in which investigators were blinded to all blood tests, all 138 patients with NSE values >33 µg/l at any time had poor outcomes [127]. The AAN Practice Parameters published in 2006 recommended an NSE level >33 µg/l as a reliable predictor of poor outcome when measured on days 1–3 [121]. Hypothermia attenuates NSE levels, potentially leading to misinterpretation of results when measurements are taken at standard time points in TH-treated patients [128]. Both maximum levels of NSE and changes in levels over time have been investigated for correlation with outcome in TH-treated patients [128]. NSE levels that decline temporally seem to correlate with good outcome [196], whereas progressive increase in levels seems to predict poor outcome [197,198]. In a prospective observational cohort of 123 TH-treated patients, NSE level measured 72 hours after arrest needed to surpass 78.9 µg/l to have 100% specificity for predicting poor outcome [199]. In another cohort, 4 out of 42 patients regained consciousness and achieved a good outcome despite NSE levels >33 µg/l [200]. In yet another prospective cohort of more than 300 patients, NSE level of >33 µg/l had FPR of 10% (95% CI 6–16%) at admission, 9% (95% CI 5–14%) at 36 hours and 7% (95% CI 4–12%) at 48 hours [188]. Hence, NSE level cannot be recommended as an independent marker for poor prognosis after CPA treated with TH, and should be combined with other predictors to increase its reliability (see later). S100B was not regarded as an accurate predictor of outcome in the pre-TH era but recent reports on its predictive value after TH is promising. In a prospective cohort of 37 patient who underwent TH, S100B levels at the time of admission were significantly lower in those eventually achieving good outcome at 14 days [201]. In another multicenter, prospective observational study from Japan, S100B performed better than NSE for prediction of poor outcome, with 100% specificity when levels were >1.41 ng/ml on admission, >0.21 ng/ml at 6 hours, and >0.05 ng/ml at 24 hours [153].

Combining various parameters to predict outcome

Several studies have looked at combining the values of the above tests to increase the reliability of outcome predictions [202,203]. In one study, clinical examination correctly predicted outcome in 58%, SSEPs in 59%, EEG in 41%, while combining the three increased the rate of correct predictions to 82% [202]. A single center study on 134 patients undergoing TH that combined clinical examination, EEG reactivity and NSE yielded the best predictive performance (receiving operator characteristic areas: 0.89 for mortality and 0.88 for poor outcome), with 100% positive predictive value [204].

Conclusion

Coma is not a disease, but a symptomatic presentation of many diseases. The pathophysiology of coma lies in dysfunction of the ARAS and/or its connections, and the clinical examination is aimed at identifying the insult and its location. Neuromonitoring techniques are being refined, with an ultimate goal of identifying "at risk" brain in a timely manner, so appropriate therapy can be instituted. Eventually, all of this should improve our means to predict outcome, specifically recovery.

References

1 Stanziano, M., Foglia, C., Soddu, A., Gargano, F. & Papa, M. (2011) Post-anoxic vegetative state: imaging and prognostic perspectives. *Functional Neurology*, **26**(1), 45–50.

2 Faul, M.D., Xu, L., Wald, M.M. & Coronado, V.G. (2010) *Traumatic Brain Injury in the United States: Emergency Department Visits, Hospitalizations and Deaths.* Centers for Disease Control and Prevention, National Center for Injury Prevention and Control, Atlanta, GA.

3 Coronado, V.G., Xu, L., Basavaraju, S.V. *et al.* (2011) Surveillance for traumatic brain injury-related deaths–United States, 1997-2007. *MMWR Surveillance Summaries*, **60**(5), 1–32.

4 Finkelstein, E., Corso, P., Miller, T. & Associates (2006) *Incidence and economic burden of injuries in the United States, 2000.* Oxford University Press, New York.

5 Corso, P.S., Mercy, J.A., Simon, T.R., Finkelstein, E.A. & Miller, T.R. (2007) Medical costs and productivity losses due to interpersonal and self-directed violence in the United States. *American Journal of Preventive Medicine*, **32**(**6**), 474–482.

6 Callans, D.J. (2004) Out-of-hospital cardiac arrest–the solution is shocking. *The New England Journal of Medicine*, **351**(**7**), 632–634.

7 McNally, B., Robb, R., Mehta, M. *et al.* (2011) Out-of-hospital cardiac arrest surveillance—Cardiac Arrest Registry to Enhance Survival (CARES), United States, October 1, 2005–December 31, 2010. *MMWR Surveillance Summaries*, **60**(**8**), 1–19.

8 Merchant, R.M., Yang, L., Becker, L.B. *et al.* (2011) Incidence of treated cardiac arrest in hospitalized patients in the United States. *Critical Care Medicine*, **39**(**11**), 2401–2406.

9 Girotra, S., Nallamothu, B.K., Spertus, J.A., Li, Y., Krumholz, H.M. & Chan, P.S. (2012) Trends in survival after in-hospital cardiac arrest. *The New England Journal of Medicine*, **367**(**20**), 1912–1920.

10 Madl, C. & Holzer, M. (2004) Brain function after resuscitation from cardiac arrest. *Current Opinion in Critical Care*, **10**(**3**), 213–217.

11 Posner, J.B., Saper, C.B., Schiff, N.D. & Plum, F. (2007) *Plum and Posner's - Diagnosis of Stupor and Coma*, 4th edn. Oxford University Press, Oxford, UK.

12 Brain Trauma, F., American Association of Neurological S & Congress of Neurological S (2007) Guidelines for the Management of Severe Traumatic Brain Injury. *Journal of Neurotrauma*, **24**(**Suppl. I**), S1–S106.

13 Rosner, M.J., Rosner, S.D. & Johnson, A.H. (1995) Cerebral perfusion pressure: management protocol and clinical results. *Journal of Neurosurgery*, **83**(**6**), 949–962.

14 Eker, C., Asgeirsson, B., Grande, P.O., Schalen, W. & Nordstrom, C.H. (1998) Improved outcome after severe head injury with a new therapy based on principles for brain volume regulation and preserved microcirculation. *Critical Care Medicine*, **26**(**11**), 1881–1886.

15 Patel, H.C., Bouamra, O., Woodford, M., King, A.T., Yates, D.W. & Lecky, F.E. (2005) Trends in head injury outcome from 1989 to 2003 and the effect of neurosurgical care: an observational study. *Lancet*, **366**(**9496**), 1538–1544.

16 Stein, S.C., Georgoff, P., Meghan, S., Mirza, K.L. & El Falaky, O.M. (2010) Relationship of aggressive monitoring and treatment to improved outcomes in severe traumatic brain injury. *Journal of Neurosurgery*, **112**(**5**), 1105–1112.

17 Saul, T.G. & Ducker, T.B. (1982) Effect of intracranial pressure monitoring and aggressive treatment on mortality in severe head injury. *Journal of Neurosurgery*, **56**(**4**), 498–503.

18 Marshall, L.F., Smith, R.W. & Shapiro, H.M. (1979) The outcome with aggressive treatment in severe head injuries. Part I: the significance of intracranial pressure monitoring. *Journal of neurosurgery*, **50**(**1**), 20–25.

19 Becker, D.P., Miller, J.D., Ward, J.D., Greenberg, R.P., Young, H.F. & Sakalas, R. (1977) The outcome from severe head injury with early diagnosis and intensive management. *Journal of Neurosurgery*, **47**(**4**), 491–502.

20 Jennett, B., Teasdale, G., Galbraith, S. *et al.* (1977) Severe head injuries in three countries. *Journal of Neurology, Neurosurgery and Psychiatry*, **40**(**3**), 291–298.

21 Cremer, O.L., Moons, K.G., Bouman, E.A., Kruijswijk, J.E., de Smet, A.M. & Kalkman, C.J. (2001) Long-term propofol infusion and cardiac failure in adult head-injured patients. *Lancet*, **357**(**9250**), 117–118.

22 Chesnut, R.M., Temkin, N., Carney, N. *et al.* (2012) A trial of intracranial-pressure monitoring in traumatic brain injury. *The New England Journal of Medicine*, **367**(**26**), 2471–2481.

23 Forsyth, R.J., Wolny, S. & Rodrigues, B. (2010) Routine intracranial pressure monitoring in acute coma. *The Cochrane Database of Systematic Reviews*, **2**, CD002043.

24 Stover, J.F. (2011) Actual evidence for neuromonitoring-guided intensive care following severe traumatic brain injury. *Swiss Medical Weekly*, **141**, w13245.

25 Murr, R. & Schurer, L. (1995) Correlation of jugular venous oxygen saturation to spontaneous fluctuations of cerebral perfusion pressure in patients with severe head injury. *Neurological Research*, **17**(**5**), 329–333.

26 Chieregato, A., Marchi, M., Zoppellari, R. *et al.* (2002) Detection of early ischemia in severe head injury by means of arteriovenous lactate differences and jugular bulb oxygen saturation. Relationship with CPP, severity indexes and outcome. Preliminary analysis. *Acta Neurochirurgica Supplement*, **81**, 289–293.

27 Macmillan, C.S., Andrews, P.J. & Easton, V.J. (2001) Increased jugular bulb saturation is associated with poor outcome in traumatic brain injury. *Journal of Neurology, Neurosurgery and Psychiatry*, **70**(**1**), 101–104.

28 Chan, M.T., Ng, S.C., Lam, J.M., Poon, W.S. & Gin, T. (2005) Re-defining the ischemic threshold for jugular venous oxygen saturation–a microdialysis study in patients with severe head injury. *Acta Neurochirurgica. Supplement*, **95**, 63–66.

29 Gopinath, S.P., Robertson, C.S., Contant, C.F. *et al.* (1994) Jugular venous desaturation and outcome after head injury. *Journal of Neurology, Neurosurgery and Psychiatry*, **57**(**6**), 717–723.

30 Gupta, A.K., Hutchinson, P.J., Al-Rawi, P. *et al.* (1999) Measuring brain tissue oxygenation compared with jugular venous oxygen saturation for monitoring cerebral oxygenation after traumatic brain injury. *Anesthesia and Analgesia*, **88**(**3**), 549–553.

31 Maloney-Wilensky, E. & Le Roux, P. (2010) The physiology behind direct brain oxygen monitors and practical aspects of their use. *Child's Nervous System : ChNS : Official Journal of the International Society for Pediatric Neurosurgery*, **26**(**4**), 419–430.

32 Rosenthal, G., Hemphill, J.C. 3rd,, Sorani, M. *et al.* (2008) Brain tissue oxygen tension is more indicative of oxygen diffusion than oxygen delivery and metabolism in patients with traumatic brain injury. *Critical Care Medicine*, **36**(**6**), 1917–1924.

33 Sarrafzadeh, A.S., Sakowitz, O.W., Callsen, T.A., Lanksch, W.R. & Unterberg, A.W. (2002) Detection of secondary insults by brain tissue pO2 and bedside microdialysis in severe head injury. *Acta Neurochirurgica. Supplement*, **81**, 319–321.

34 Meixensberger, J., Kunze, E., Barcsay, E., Vaeth, A. & Roosen, K. (2001) Clinical cerebral microdialysis: brain metabolism and

brain tissue oxygenation after acute brain injury. *Neurological Research*, **23**(8), 801–806.

35 Meixensberger, J., Renner, C., Simanowski, R., Schmidtke, A., Dings, J. & Roosen, K. (2004) Influence of cerebral oxygenation following severe head injury on neuropsychological testing. *Neurological Research*, **26**(4), 414–417.

36 Oddo, M., Levine, J.M., Frangos, S. *et al.* (2009) Effect of mannitol and hypertonic saline on cerebral oxygenation in patients with severe traumatic brain injury and refractory intracranial hypertension. *Journal of Neurology, Neurosurgery and Psychiatry*, **80**(8), 916–920.

37 Shahlaie, K., Boggan, J.E., Latchaw, R.E., Ji, C. & Muizelaar, J.P. (2009) Posttraumatic vasospasm detected by continuous brain tissue oxygen monitoring: treatment with intraarterial verapamil and balloon angioplasty. *Neurocritical Care*, **10**(1), 61–69.

38 Stiefel, M.F., Heuer, G.G., Smith, M.J. *et al.* (2004) Cerebral oxygenation following decompressive hemicraniectomy for the treatment of refractory intracranial hypertension. *Journal of Neurosurgery*, **101**(2), 241–247.

39 Weiner, G.M., Lacey, M.R., Mackenzie, L. *et al.* (2010) Decompressive craniectomy for elevated intracranial pressure and its effect on the cumulative ischemic burden and therapeutic intensity levels after severe traumatic brain injury. *Neurosurgery*, **66**(6), 1111–1118 discussion 1118-1119.

40 Narotam, P.K., Morrison, J.F. & Nathoo, N. (2009) Brain tissue oxygen monitoring in traumatic brain injury and major trauma: outcome analysis of a brain tissue oxygen-directed therapy. *Journal of Neurosurgery*, **111**(4), 672–682.

41 Spiotta, A.M., Stiefel, M.F., Gracias, V.H. *et al.* (2010) Brain tissue oxygen-directed management and outcome in patients with severe traumatic brain injury. *Journal of Neurosurgery*, **113**(3), 571–580.

42 Rao, G.S. & Durga, P. (2011) Changing trends in monitoring brain ischemia: from intracranial pressure to cerebral oximetry. *Current Opinion in Anaesthesiology*, **24**(5), 487–494.

43 Adamides, A.A., Cooper, D.J., Rosenfeldt, F.L. *et al.* (2009) Focal cerebral oxygenation and neurological outcome with or without brain tissue oxygen-guided therapy in patients with traumatic brain injury. *Acta Neurochirurgica (Wien)*, **151**(11), 1399–1409.

44 Martini, R.P., Deem, S., Yanez, N.D. *et al.* (2009) Management guided by brain tissue oxygen monitoring and outcome following severe traumatic brain injury. *Journal of Neurosurgery*, **111**(4), 644–649.

45 *Brain Tissue Oxygen Monitoring in Traumatic Brain Injury (TBI) (BOOST 2)* http://clinicaltrials.gov/ct2/show/NCT00974259.

46 Belli, A., Sen, J., Petzold, A., Russo, S., Kitchen, N. & Smith, M. (2008) Metabolic failure precedes intracranial pressure rises in traumatic brain injury: a microdialysis study. *Acta Neurochirurgica (Wien)*, **150**(5), 461–469 discussion 470.

47 Timofeev, I., Carpenter, K.L., Nortje, J. *et al.* (2011) Cerebral extracellular chemistry and outcome following traumatic brain injury: a microdialysis study of 223 patients. *Brain*, **134**(Pt 2), 484–494.

48 Lakshmanan, R., Loo, J.A., Drake, T. *et al.* (2010) Metabolic crisis after traumatic brain injury is associated with a novel microdialysis proteome. *Neurocritical Care*, **12**(3), 324–336.

49 Nordmark, J., Rubertsson, S., Mortberg, E., Nilsson, P. & Enblad, P. (2009) Intracerebral monitoring in comatose patients treated with hypothermia after a cardiac arrest. *Acta Anaesthesiologica Scandinavica*, **53**(3), 289–298.

50 Nelson, D.W., Thornquist, B., MacCallum, R.M. *et al.* (2011) Analyses of cerebral microdialysis in patients with traumatic brain injury: relations to intracranial pressure, cerebral perfusion pressure and catheter placement. *BMC Medicine*, **9**, 21.

51 Friedman, D., Claassen, J. & Hirsch, L.J. (2009) Continuous electroencephalogram monitoring in the intensive care unit. *Anesthesia and Analgesia*, **109**(2), 506–523.

52 Claassen, J., Mayer, S.A., Kowalski, R.G., Emerson, R.G. & Hirsch, L.J. (2004) Detection of electrographic seizures with continuous EEG monitoring in critically ill patients. *Neurology*, **62**(10), 1743–1748.

53 Pandian, J.D., Cascino, G.D., So, E.L., Manno, E. & Fulgham, J.R. (2004) Digital video-electroencephalographic monitoring in the neurological-neurosurgical intensive care unit: clinical features and outcome. *Archives of Neurology*, **61**(7), 1090–1094.

54 Towne, A.R., Waterhouse, E.J., Boggs, J.G. *et al.* (2000) Prevalence of nonconvulsive status epilepticus in comatose patients. *Neurology*, **54**(2), 340–345.

55 DeLorenzo, R.J., Waterhouse, E.J., Towne, A.R. *et al.* (1998) Persistent nonconvulsive status epilepticus after the control of convulsive status epilepticus. *Epilepsia*, **39**(8), 833–840.

56 Treiman, D.M., Meyers, P.D., Walton, N.Y. *et al.* (1998) A comparison of four treatments for generalized convulsive status epilepticus. Veterans Affairs Status Epilepticus Cooperative Study Group. *The New England Journal of Medicine*, **339**(12), 792–798.

57 Claassen, J., Jette, N., Chum, F. *et al.* (2007) Electrographic seizures and periodic discharges after intracerebral hemorrhage. *Neurology*, **69**(13), 1356–1365.

58 Bladin, C.F., Alexandrov, A.V., Bellavance, A. *et al.* (2000) Seizures after stroke: a prospective multicenter study. *Archives of Neurology*, **57**(11), 1617–1622.

59 Faught, E., Peters, D., Bartolucci, A., Moore, L. & Miller, P.C. (1989) Seizures after primary intracerebral hemorrhage. *Neurology*, **39**(8), 1089–1093.

60 Szaflarski, J.P., Rackley, A.Y., Kleindorfer, D.O. *et al.* (2008) Incidence of seizures in the acute phase of stroke: a population-based study. *Epilepsia*, **49**(6), 974–981.

61 Vespa, P.M., O'Phelan, K., Shah, M. *et al.* (2003) Acute seizures after intracerebral hemorrhage: a factor in progressive midline shift and outcome. *Neurology*, **60**(9), 1441–1446.

62 Camilo, O. & Goldstein, L.B. (2004) Seizures and epilepsy after ischemic stroke. *Stroke; A Journal of Cerebral Circulation*, **35**(7), 1769–1775.

63 Temkin, N.R., Anderson, G.D., Winn, H.R. *et al.* (2007) Magnesium sulfate for neuroprotection after traumatic brain injury: a randomised controlled trial. *Lancet Neurology*, **6**(1), 29–38.

64 Annegers, J.F., Grabow, J.D., Groover, R.V., Laws, E.R. Jr., Elveback, L.R. & Kurland, L.T. (1980) Seizures after head trauma: a population study. *Neurology*, **30**(7 Pt 1), 683–689.

65 Lee, S.T., Lui, T.N., Wong, C.W., Yeh, Y.S. & Tzaan, W.C. (1995) Early seizures after moderate closed head injury. *Acta Neurochirurgica (Wien)*, **137**(3-4), 151–154.

66 Temkin, N.R., Dikmen, S.S., Wilensky, A.J., Keihm, J., Chabal, S. & Winn, H.R. (1990) A randomized, double-blind study of phenytoin for the prevention of post-traumatic seizures. *The New England Journal of Medicine*, **323**(8), 497–502.

67 Vespa, P. (2005) Continuous EEG monitoring for the detection of seizures in traumatic brain injury, infarction, and intracerebral hemorrhage: "to detect and protect". *Journal of Clinical Neurophysiology*, **22**(2), 99–106.

68 Wijdicks, E.F., Wiesner, R.H. & Krom, R.A. (1995) Neurotoxicity in liver transplant recipients with cyclosporine immunosuppression. *Neurology*, **45**(11), 1962–1964.

69 Krumholz, A., Stern, B.J. & Weiss, H.D. (1988) Outcome from coma after cardiopulmonary resuscitation: relation to seizures and myoclonus. *Neurology*, **38**(3), 401–405.

70 Wright, W.L. & Geocadin, R.G. (2006) Postresuscitative intensive care: neuroprotective strategies after cardiac arrest. *Seminars in Neurology*, **26**(4), 396–402.

71 Oddo, M., Carrera, E., Claassen, J., Mayer, S.A. & Hirsch, L.J. (2009) Continuous electroencephalography in the medical intensive care unit. *Critical Care Medicine*, **37**(6), 2051–2056.

72 Kamel, H., Betjemann, J.P., Navi, B.B. *et al.* (2013) Diagnostic yield of electroencephalography in the medical and surgical intensive care unit. *Neurocritical Care*, **19**(3), 336–341.

73 Cascino, T., Baglivo, J., Conti, J., Szewczykowski, J., Posner, J.B. & Rottenberg, D.A. (1983) Quantitative CT assessment of furosemide- and mannitol-induced changes in brain water content. *Neurology*, **33**(7), 898–903.

74 Bell, B.A., Smith, M.A., Kean, D.M. *et al.* (1987) Brain water measured by magnetic resonance imaging. Correlation with direct estimation and changes after mannitol and dexamethasone. *Lancet*, **1**(8524), 66–69.

75 Wise, B.L. & Chater, N. (1962) The value of hypertonic mannitol solution in decreasing brain mass and lowering cerebro-spinal-fluid pressure. *Journal of Neurosurgery*, **19**, 1038–1043.

76 Marshall, L.F., SMith, R.W., Rauscher, L.A. & Shapiro, H.M. (1978) Mannitol dose requirements in brain-injured patients. *Journal of Neurosurgery*, **48**(2), 169–172.

77 Sorani, M.D. & Manley, G.T. (2008) Dose-response relationship of mannitol and intracranial pressure: a metaanalysis. *Journal of Neurosurgery*, **108**(1), 80–87.

78 James, H.E., Langfitt, T.W., Kumar, V.S. & Ghostine, S.Y. (1977) Treatment of intracranial hypertension. Analysis of 105 consecutive, continuous recordings of intracranial pressure. *Acta Neurochirurgica (Wien)*, **36**(3-4), 189–200.

79 Bereczki, D., Liu, M., Prado, G.F. & Fekete, I. (2000) Cochrane report: A systematic review of mannitol therapy for acute ischemic stroke and cerebral parenchymal hemorrhage. *Stroke; A Journal of Cerebral Circulation*, **31**(11), 2719–2722.

80 Schwarz, S., Georgiadis, D., Aschoff, A. & Schwab, S. (2002) Effects of hypertonic (10%) saline in patients with raised intracranial pressure after stroke. *Stroke; A Journal of Cerebral Circulation*, **33**(1), 136–140.

81 Bentsen, G., Breivik, H., Lundar, T. & Stubhaug, A. (2006) Hypertonic saline (7.2%) in 6% hydroxyethyl starch reduces intracranial pressure and improves hemodynamics in a placebo-controlled study involving stable patients with subarachnoid hemorrhage. *Critical Care Medicine*, **34**(12), 2912–2917.

82 Vialet, R., Albanese, J., Thomachot, L. *et al.* (2003) Isovolume hypertonic solutes (sodium chloride or mannitol) in the treatment of refractory posttraumatic intracranial hypertension: 2 mL/kg 7.5% saline is more effective than 2 mL/kg 20% mannitol. *Critical Care Medicine*, **31**(6), 1683–1687.

83 Wakai, A., Roberts, I.G. & Schierhout, G. Mannitol for acute traumatic brain injury. *Cochrane Database of Systematic Reviews*, 2007;1: CD001049. doi:10.1002/14651858.CD001049.pub4.

84 Freshman, S.P., Battistella, F.D., Matteucci, M. & Wisner, D.H. (1993) Hypertonic saline (7.5%) versus mannitol: a comparison for treatment of acute head injuries. *Journal of Trauma*, **35**(3), 344–348.

85 Bernard, S.A., Gray, T.W., Buist, M.D. *et al.* (2002) Treatment of comatose survivors of out-of-hospital cardiac arrest with induced hypothermia. *The New England Journal of Medicine*, **346**(8), 557–563.

86 2002) Mild therapeutic hypothermia to improve the neurologic outcome after cardiac arrest. *The New England Journal of Medicine*, **346**(8), 549–556.

87 Dumas, F. & Rea, T.D. (2012) Long-term prognosis following resuscitation from out-of-hospital cardiac arrest: role of aetiology and presenting arrest rhythm. *Resuscitation*, **83**(8), 1001–1005.

88 Mehta, C. & Brady, W. (2012) Pulseless electrical activity in cardiac arrest: electrocardiographic presentations and management considerations based on the electrocardiogram. *American Journal of Emergency Medicine*, **30**(1), 236–239.

89 Nielsen, N., Wetterslev, J., Cronberg, T. *et al.* (2013) Targeted temperature management at 33 degrees C versus 36 degrees C after cardiac arrest. *The New England Journal of Medicine*, **369**(23), 2197–2206.

90 Clifton, G.L., Allen, S., Barrodale, P. *et al.* (1993) A phase II study of moderate hypothermia in severe brain injury. *Journal of Neurotrauma*, **10**(3), 263–271 discussion 273.

91 Aibiki, M., Maekawa, S. & Yokono, S. (2000) Moderate hypothermia improves imbalances of thromboxane A2 and prostaglandin I2 production after traumatic brain injury in humans. *Critical Care Medicine*, **28**(12), 3902–3906.

92 Jiang, J., Yu, M. & Zhu, C. (2000) Effect of long-term mild hypothermia therapy in patients with severe traumatic brain injury: 1-year follow-up review of 87 cases. *Journal of Neurosurgery*, **93**(4), 546–549.

93 Jiang, J.Y., Xu, W., Li, W.P. *et al.* (2006) Effect of long-term mild hypothermia or short-term mild hypothermia on outcome of

patients with severe traumatic brain injury. *Journal of Cerebral Blood Flow and Metabolism*, **26**(**6**), 771–776.

94 Shiozaki, T., Hayakata, T., Taneda, M. *et al.* (2001) A multicenter prospective randomized controlled trial of the efficacy of mild hypothermia for severely head injured patients with low intracranial pressure. Mild Hypothermia Study Group in Japan. *Journal of Neurosurgery*, **94**(**1**), 50–54.

95 Polderman, K.H., Tjong Tjin Joe, R., Peerdeman, S.M., Vandertop, W.P. & Girbes, A.R. (2002) Effects of therapeutic hypothermia on intracranial pressure and outcome in patients with severe head injury. *Intensive Care Medicine*, **28**(**11**), 1563–1573.

96 Gadkary, C.A., Alderson, P. & Signorini, D.F. Therapeutic hypothermia for head injury. *The Cochrane Database of Systematic Reviews*, 2002;**1**: CD001048. doi:10.1002/14651858.CD001048

97 McIntyre, L.A., Fergusson, D.A., Hebert, P.C., Moher, D. & Hutchison, J.S. (2003) Prolonged therapeutic hypothermia after traumatic brain injury in adults: a systematic review. *JAMA*, **289**(**22**), 2992–2999.

98 Henderson, W.R., Dhingra, V.K., Chittock, D.R., Fenwick, J.C. & Ronco, J.J. (2003) Hypothermia in the management of traumatic brain injury. A systematic review and meta-analysis. *Intensive Care Medicine*, **29**(**10**), 1637–1644.

99 Clifton, G.L., Miller, E.R., Choi, S.C. *et al.* (2001) Lack of effect of induction of hypothermia after acute brain injury. *The New England Journal of Medicine*, **344**(**8**), 556–563.

100 Zhi, D., Zhang, S. & Lin, X. (2003) Study on therapeutic mechanism and clinical effect of mild hypothermia in patients with severe head injury. *Surgical Neurology*, **59**(**5**), 381–385.

101 Roberts, I., Yates, D., Sandercock, P. *et al.* (2004) Effect of intravenous corticosteroids on death within 14 days in 10008 adults with clinically significant head injury (MRC CRASH trial): randomised placebo-controlled trial. *Lancet*, **364**(**9442**), 1321–1328.

102 Ma, J., Huang, S., Qin, S. & You, C. (2012) Progesterone for acute traumatic brain injury. *The Cochrane database of systematic reviews*, **10**, CD008409.

103 *Progesterone for the Treatment of Traumatic Brain Injury (ProTECT III)* https://clinicaltrials.gov/ct2/show/NCT00822900?term=ProTECT+III&rank=1.

104 1999) Consensus conference. Rehabilitation of persons with traumatic brain injury. NIH Consensus Development Panel on Rehabilitation of Persons With Traumatic Brain Injury. *JAMA*, **282**(**10**), 974–983.

105 Holland, D. & Shigaki, C.L. (1998) Educating families and caretakers of traumatically brain injured patients in the new health care environment: a three phase model and bibliography. *Brain Injury*, **12**(**12**), 993–1009.

106 Junque, C., Bruna, O. & Mataro, M. (1997) Information needs of the traumatic brain injury patient's family members regarding the consequences of the injury and associated perception of physical, cognitive, emotional and quality of life changes. *Brain Injury*, **11**(**4**), 251–258.

107 Perkins, H.S., Jonsen, A.R. & Epstein, W.V. (1986) Providers as predictors: using outcome predictions in intensive care. *Critical Care Medicine*, **14**(**2**), 105–110.

108 Poses, R.M., Bekes, C., Copare, F.J. & Scott, W.E. (1989) The answer to "What are my chances, doctor?" depends on whom is asked: prognostic disagreement and inaccuracy for critically ill patients. *Critical Care Medicine*, **17**(**8**), 827–833.

109 Chang, R.W., Lee, B., Jacobs, S. & Lee, B. (1989) Accuracy of decisions to withdraw therapy in critically ill patients: clinical judgment versus a computer model. *Critical Care Medicine*, **17**(**11**), 1091–1097.

110 Kothari, S. (2007) Prognosis after severe TBI: a practical, evidence-based approach. In: Zesler, N., Katz, D. & Zafonte, R. (eds), Brain Injury Medicine: Principles and Practice. Demos Medical Publishing, New York, pp. 169–199.

111 Kothari, S. (2011) Practical guidelines for prognostication after traumatic brain injury. In: Zollman, F.S. (ed), Manual of Traumatic Brain Injury Management. Demos Medical Publishing, New York, pp. 271–276.

112 Walker, W.C., Ketchum, J.M., Marwitz, J.H. *et al.* (2010) A multicentre study on the clinical utility of post-traumatic amnesia duration in predicting global outcome after moderate-severe traumatic brain injury. *Journal of Neurology, Neurosurgery and Psychiatry*, **81**(**1**), 87–89.

113 Sadaka, F., Patel, D. & Lakshmanan, R. (2012) The FOUR score predicts outcome in patients after traumatic brain injury. *Neurocritical Care*, **16**(**1**), 95–101.

114 Schultz, S.C., Cullinane, D.C., Pasquale, M.D., Magnant, C. & Evans, S.R. (1996) Predicting in-hospital mortality during cardiopulmonary resuscitation. *Resuscitation*, **33**(**1**), 13–17.

115 Roest, A., van Bets, B., Jorens, P.G., Baar, I., Weyler, J. & Mercelis, R. (2009) The prognostic value of the EEG in postanoxic coma. *Neurocritical Care*, **10**(**3**), 318–325.

116 Berger, R. & Kelley, M. (1994) Survival after in-hospital cardiopulmonary arrest of noncritically ill patients. A prospective study. *Chest*, **106**(**3**), 872–879.

117 Rogove, H.J., Safar, P., Sutton-Tyrrell, K. & Abramson, N.S. (1995) Old age does not negate good cerebral outcome after cardiopulmonary resuscitation: analyses from the brain resuscitation clinical trials. The Brain Resuscitation Clinical Trial I and II Study Groups. *Critical Care Medicine*, **23**(**1**), 18–25.

118 Grubb, N.R. (2001) Managing out-of-hospital cardiac arrest survivors: 1. Neurological perspective. *Heart*, **85**(**1**), 6–8.

119 Saklayen, M., Liss, H. & Markert, R. (1995) In-hospital cardiopulmonary resuscitation. Survival in 1 hospital and literature review. *Medicine (Baltimore)*, **74**(**4**), 163–175.

120 1994) Medical aspects of the persistent vegetative state (1). The Multi-Society Task Force on PVS. *The New England Journal of Medicine*, **330**(**21**), 1499–1508.

121 Wijdicks, E.F., Hijdra, A., Young, G.B., Bassetti, C.L. & Wiebe, S. (2006) Practice parameter: prediction of outcome in comatose survivors after cardiopulmonary resuscitation (an evidence-based review): report of the Quality Standards Subcommittee of the American Academy of Neurology. *Neurology*, **67**(**2**), 203–210.

122 Jorgensen, E.O. & Holm, S. (1999) Prediction of neurological outcome after cardiopulmonary resuscitation. *Resuscitation*, **41**(**2**), 145–152.

123 Zandbergen, E.G., de Haan, R.J., Stoutenbeek, C.P., Koelman, J.H. & Hijdra, A. (1998) Systematic review of early prediction of poor outcome in anoxic-ischaemic coma. *Lancet*, **352**(**9143**), 1808–1812.

124 Codazzi, D., Pifferi, S., Savioli, M. & Langer, M. (1997) Neurologic prognosis after cardiocirculatory arrest outside the hospital. *Minerva Anestesiologica*, **63**(**11**), 353–364.

125 Edgren, E., Hedstrand, U., Kelsey, S., Sutton-Tyrrell, K. & Safar, P. (1994) Assessment of neurological prognosis in comatose survivors of cardiac arrest. BRCT I Study Group. *Lancet*, **343**(**8905**), 1055–1059.

126 Berek, K., Lechleitner, P., Luef, G. *et al.* (1995) Early determination of neurological outcome after prehospital cardiopulmonary resuscitation. *Stroke; A Journal of Cerebral Circulation*, **26**(**4**), 543–549.

127 Zandbergen, E.G., Hijdra, A., Koelman, J.H. *et al.* (2006) Prediction of poor outcome within the first 3 days of postanoxic coma. *Neurology*, **66**(**1**), 62–68.

128 Greer, D.M., Rosenthal, E.S. & Wu, O. (2014) Neuroprognostication of hypoxic-ischaemic coma in the therapeutic hypothermia era. *Nature reviews Neurology*, **10**(**4**), 190–203. doi:10.1038/nrneurol.2014.36.

129 Rossetti, A.O., Oddo, M., Logroscino, G. & Kaplan, P.W. (2010) Prognostication after cardiac arrest and hypothermia: a prospective study. *Annals of Neurology*, **67**(**3**), 301–307.

130 Schefold, J.C., Storm, C., Kruger, A., Ploner, C.J. & Hasper, D. (2009) The Glasgow Coma Score is a predictor of good outcome in cardiac arrest patients treated with therapeutic hypothermia. *Resuscitation*, **80**(**6**), 658–661.

131 Kamps, M.J., Horn, J., Oddo, M. *et al.* (2013) Prognostication of neurologic outcome in cardiac arrest patients after mild therapeutic hypothermia: a meta-analysis of the current literature. *Intensive Care Medicine*, **39**(**10**), 1671–1682.

132 Greer, D.M., Yang, J., Scripko, P.D. *et al.* (2013) Clinical examination for prognostication in comatose cardiac arrest patients. *Resuscitation*, **84**(**11**), 1546–1551.

133 Tshibanda, L., Vanhaudenhuyse, A., Boly, M. *et al.* (2010) Neuroimaging after coma. *Neuroradiology*, **52**(**1**), 15–24.

134 Yanagawa, Y., Tsushima, Y., Tokumaru, A. *et al.* (2000) A quantitative analysis of head injury using T2*-weighted gradient-echo imaging. *Journal of Trauma*, **49**(**2**), 272–277.

135 Carpentier, A., Galanaud, D., Puybasset, L. *et al.* (2006) Early morphologic and spectroscopic magnetic resonance in severe traumatic brain injuries can detect "invisible brain stem damage" and predict "vegetative states". *Journal of Neurotrauma*, **23**(**5**), 674–685.

136 Hoelper, B.M., Soldner, F., Chone, L. & Wallenfang, T. (2000) Effect of intracerebral lesions detected in early MRI on outcome after acute brain injury. *Acta Neurochirurgica. Supplement*, **76**, 265–267.

137 Paterakis, K., Karantanas, A.H., Komnos, A. & Volikas, Z. (2000) Outcome of patients with diffuse axonal injury: the significance and prognostic value of MRI in the acute phase. *Journal of Trauma*, **49**(**6**), 1071–1075.

138 Karantanas, A. & Paterakis, K. (2000) Magnetic resonance imaging and brainstem injury. *Journal of Neurosurgery*, **92**(**5**), 896–897.

139 Schaefer, P.W., Huisman, T.A., Sorensen, A.G., Gonzalez, R.G. & Schwamm, L.H. (2004) Diffusion-weighted MR imaging in closed head injury: high correlation with initial glasgow coma scale score and score on modified Rankin scale at discharge. *Radiology*, **233**(**1**), 58–66.

140 Galanaud, D., Naccache, L. & Puybasset, L. (2007) Exploring impaired consciousness: the MRI approach. *Current Opinion in Neurology*, **20**(**6**), 627–631.

141 Weiss, N., Galanaud, D., Carpentier, A. *et al.* (2008) A combined clinical and MRI approach for outcome assessment of traumatic head injured comatose patients. *Journal of Neurology*, **255**(**2**), 217–223.

142 Tollard, E., Galanaud, D., Perlbarg, V. *et al.* (2009) Experience of diffusion tensor imaging and 1H spectroscopy for outcome prediction in severe traumatic brain injury: Preliminary results. *Critical Care Medicine*, **37**(**4**), 1448–1455.

143 Perlbarg, V., Puybasset, L., Tollard, E., Lehericy, S., Benali, H. & Galanaud, D. (2009) Relation between brain lesion location and clinical outcome in patients with severe traumatic brain injury: a diffusion tensor imaging study using voxel-based approaches. *Human Brain Mapping*, **30**(**12**), 3924–3933.

144 Choe, B.Y., Suh, T.S., Choi, K.H., Shinn, K.S., Park, C.K. & Kang, J.K. (1995) Neuronal dysfunction in patients with closed head injury evaluated by in vivo 1H magnetic resonance spectroscopy. *Investigative Radiology*, **30**(**8**), 502–506.

145 Marino, S., Zei, E., Battaglini, M. *et al.* (2007) Acute metabolic brain changes following traumatic brain injury and their relevance to clinical severity and outcome. *Journal of Neurology, Neurosurgery and Psychiatry*, **78**(**5**), 501–507.

146 Ross, B.D., Ernst, T., Kreis, R. *et al.* (1998) 1H MRS in acute traumatic brain injury. *Journal of Magnetic Resonance Imaging: JMRI*, **8**(**4**), 829–840.

147 Friedman, S.D., Brooks, W.M., Jung, R.E. *et al.* (1999) Quantitative proton MRS predicts outcome after traumatic brain injury. *Neurology*, **52**(**7**), 1384–1391.

148 Garnett, M.R., Blamire, A.M., Corkill, R.G., Cadoux-Hudson, T.A., Rajagopalan, B. & Styles, P. (2000) Early proton magnetic resonance spectroscopy in normal-appearing brain correlates with outcome in patients following traumatic brain injury. *Brain*, **123**(**Pt 10**), 2046–2054.

149 Sinson, G., Bagley, L.J., Cecil, K.M. *et al.* (2001) Magnetization transfer imaging and proton MR spectroscopy in the evaluation of axonal injury: correlation with clinical outcome after traumatic brain injury. *AJNR. American Journal of Neuroradiology*, **22**(**1**), 143–151.

150 Uzan, M., Albayram, S., Dashti, S.G., Aydin, S., Hanci, M. & Kuday, C. (2003) Thalamic proton magnetic resonance spectroscopy in vegetative state induced by traumatic brain injury. *Journal of Neurology, Neurosurgery and Psychiatry*, **74**(**1**), 33–38.

151 Cecil, K.M., Lenkinski, R.E., Meaney, D.F., McIntosh, T.K. & Smith, D.H. (1998) High-field proton magnetic resonance

spectroscopy of a swine model for axonal injury. *Journal of Neurochemistry*, **70**(**5**), 2038–2044.

152 Holshouser, B.A., Tong, K.A., Ashwal, S. *et al.* (2006) Prospective longitudinal proton magnetic resonance spectroscopic imaging in adult traumatic brain injury. *Journal of Magnetic Resonance Imaging : JMRI*, **24**(**1**), 33–40.

153 Signoretti, S., Marmarou, A., Fatouros, P. *et al.* (2002) Application of chemical shift imaging for measurement of NAA in head injured patients. *Acta Neurochirurgica. Supplement*, **81**, 373–375.

154 Giacino, J.T., Hirsch, J., Schiff, N. & Laureys, S. (2006) Functional neuroimaging applications for assessment and rehabilitation planning in patients with disorders of consciousness. *Archives of Physical Medicine and Rehabilitation*, **87**(**12 Suppl 2**), S67–76.

155 Edlow, B.L., Giacino, J.T. & Wu, O. (2013) Functional MRI and outcome in traumatic coma. *Current Neurology and Neuroscience Reports*, **13**(**9**), 375.

156 Raichle, M.E., MacLeod, A.M., Snyder, A.Z., Powers, W.J., Gusnard, D.A. & Shulman, G.L. (2001) A default mode of brain function. *Proceedings of the National Academy of Sciences of the United States of America*, **98**(**2**), 676–682.

157 Vanhaudenhuyse, A., Noirhomme, Q., Tshibanda, L.J. *et al.* (2010) Default network connectivity reflects the level of consciousness in non-communicative brain-damaged patients. *Brain*, **133**(**Pt 1**), 161–171.

158 Torbey, M.T., Selim, M., Knorr, J., Bigelow, C. & Recht, L. (2000) Quantitative analysis of the loss of distinction between gray and white matter in comatose patients after cardiac arrest. *Stroke; A Journal of Cerebral Circulation*, **31**(**9**), 2163–2167.

159 Choi, S.P., Park, H.K., Park, K.N. *et al.* (2008) The density ratio of grey to white matter on computed tomography as an early predictor of vegetative state or death after cardiac arrest. *Emergency Medicine Journal : EMJ*, **25**(**10**), 666–669.

160 Metter, R.B., Rittenberger, J.C., Guyette, F.X. & Callaway, C.W. (2011) Association between a quantitative CT scan measure of brain edema and outcome after cardiac arrest. *Resuscitation*, **82**(**9**), 1180–1185.

161 Scheel, M., Storm, C., Gentsch, A. *et al.* (2013) The prognostic value of gray-white-matter ratio in cardiac arrest patients treated with hypothermia. *Scandinavian Journal of Trauma, Resuscitation and Emergency Medicine*, **21**(**1**), 23.

162 Arbelaez, A., Castillo, M. & Mukherji, S.K. (1999) Diffusion-weighted MR imaging of global cerebral anoxia. *AJNR. American Journal of Neuroradiology*, **20**(**6**), 999–1007.

163 Wijdicks, E.F., Campeau, N.G. & Miller, G.M. (2001) MR imaging in comatose survivors of cardiac resuscitation. *AJNR. American Journal of Neuroradiology*, **22**(**8**), 1561–1565.

164 Wijman, C.A., Mlynash, M., Caulfield, A.F. *et al.* (2009) Prognostic value of brain diffusion-weighted imaging after cardiac arrest. *Annals of Neurology*, **65**(**4**), 394–402.

165 Wu, O., Sorensen, A.G., Benner, T., Singhal, A.B., Furie, K.L. & Greer, D.M. (2009) Comatose patients with cardiac arrest: predicting clinical outcome with diffusion-weighted MR imaging. *Radiology*, **252**(**1**), 173–181.

166 Jarnum, H., Knutsson, L., Rundgren, M. *et al.* (2009) Diffusion and perfusion MRI of the brain in comatose patients treated with mild hypothermia after cardiac arrest: a prospective observational study. *Resuscitation*, **80**(**4**), 425–430.

167 Greer, D., Scripko, P., Bartscher, J. *et al.* (2011) Serial MRI changes in comatose cardiac arrest patients. *Neurocritical Care*, **14**(**1**), 61–67.

168 Greer, D.M., Scripko, P.D., Wu, O. *et al.* (2013) Hippocampal magnetic resonance imaging abnormalities in cardiac arrest are associated with poor outcome. *Journal of Stroke and Cerebrovascular Diseases : The Official Journal of National Stroke Association*, **22**(**7**), 899–905.

169 Di, H., Boly, M., Weng, X., Ledoux, D. & Laureys, S. (2008) Neuroimaging activation studies in the vegetative state: predictors of recovery? *Clinical Medicine (London, England)*, **8**(**5**), 502–507.

170 Gofton, T.E., Chouinard, P.A., Young, G.B. *et al.* (2009) Functional MRI study of the primary somatosensory cortex in comatose survivors of cardiac arrest. *Experimental Neurology*, **217**(**2**), 320–327.

171 Achard, S., Kremer, S., Schenck, M. *et al.* (2011) Global Functional Disconnections in Post-anoxic Coma Patient. *The Neuroradiology Journal*, **24**(**2**), 311–315.

172 Koenig, M.A., Kaplan, P.W. & Thakor, N.V. (2006) Clinical neurophysiologic monitoring and brain injury from cardiac arrest. *Neurologic Clinics*, **24**(**1**), 89–106.

173 Young, G.B., Blume, W.T., Campbell, V.M. *et al.* (1994) Alpha, theta and alpha-theta coma: a clinical outcome study utilizing serial recordings. *Electroencephalography and Clinical Neurophysiology*, **91**(**2**), 93–99.

174 Kaplan, P.W., Genoud, D., Ho, T.W. & Jallon, P. (1999) Etiology, neurologic correlations, and prognosis in alpha coma. *Clinical Neurophysiology : Official Journal of the International Federation of Clinical Neurophysiology*, **110**(**2**), 205–213.

175 Rossetti, A.O., Oddo, M., Liaudet, L. & Kaplan, P.W. (2009) Predictors of awakening from postanoxic status epilepticus after therapeutic hypothermia. *Neurology*, **72**(**8**), 744–749.

176 Bouwes, A., van Poppelen, D., Koelman, J.H. *et al.* (2012) Acute posthypoxic myoclonus after cardiopulmonary resuscitation. *BMC Neurology*, **12**, 63.

177 Rundgren, M., Rosen, I. & Friberg, H. (2006) Amplitude-integrated EEG (aEEG) predicts outcome after cardiac arrest and induced hypothermia. *Intensive Care Medicine*, **32**(**6**), 836–842.

178 Cloostermans, M.C., van Meulen, F.B., Eertman, C.J., Hom, H.W. & van Putten, M.J. (2012) Continuous electroencephalography monitoring for early prediction of neurological outcome in postanoxic patients after cardiac arrest: a prospective cohort study. *Critical Care Medicine*, **40**(**10**), 2867–2875.

179 Jaitly, R., Sgro, J.A., Towne, A.R., Ko, D. & DeLorenzo, R.J. (1997) Prognostic value of EEG monitoring after status epilepticus: a prospective adult study. *Journal of Clinical Neurophysiology*, **14**(**4**), 326–334.

180 Claassen, J., Hirsch, L.J., Frontera, J.A. *et al.* (2006) Prognostic significance of continuous EEG monitoring in patients with

poor-grade subarachnoid hemorrhage. *Neurocritical Care*, **4**(**2**), 103–112.

181 Bergamasco, B., Bergamini, L., Doriguzzi, T. & Fabiani, D. (1968) EEG sleep patterns as a prognostic criterion in post-traumatic coma. *Electroencephalography and Clinical Neurophysiology*, **24**(**4**), 374–377.

182 Zandbergen, E.G., de Haan, R.J., Koelman, J.H. & Hijdra, A. (2000) Prediction of poor outcome in anoxic-ischemic coma. *Journal of Clinical Neurophysiology*, **17**(**5**), 498–501.

183 Robinson, L.R., Micklesen, P.J., Tirschwell, D.L. & Lew, H.L. (2003) Predictive value of somatosensory evoked potentials for awakening from coma. *Critical Care Medicine*, **31**(**3**), 960–967.

184 Logi, F., Fischer, C., Murri, L. & Mauguiere, F. (2003) The prognostic value of evoked responses from primary somatosensory and auditory cortex in comatose patients. *Clinical Neurophysiology : Official Journal of the International Federation of Clinical Neurophysiology*, **114**(**9**), 1615–1627.

185 Zingler, V.C., Krumm, B., Bertsch, T., Fassbender, K. & Pohlmann-Eden, B. (2003) Early prediction of neurological outcome after cardiopulmonary resuscitation: a multimodal approach combining neurobiochemical and electrophysiological investigations may provide high prognostic certainty in patients after cardiac arrest. *European Neurology*, **49**(**2**), 79–84.

186 Rothstein, T.L. (2009) The utility of median somatosensory evoked potentials in anoxic-ischemic coma. *Reviews in the Neurosciences*, **20**(**3-4**), 221–233.

187 Leithner, C., Ploner, C.J., Hasper, D. & Storm, C. (2010) Does hypothermia influence the predictive value of bilateral absent N20 after cardiac arrest? *Neurology*, **74**(**12**), 965–969.

188 Bouwes, A., Binnekade, J.M., Kuiper, M.A. *et al.* (2012) Prognosis of coma after therapeutic hypothermia: a prospective cohort study. *Annals of Neurology*, **71**(**2**), 206–212.

189 Madl, C., Kramer, L., Domanovits, H. *et al.* (2000) Improved outcome prediction in unconscious cardiac arrest survivors with sensory evoked potentials compared with clinical assessment. *Critical Care Medicine*, **28**(**3**), 721–726.

190 Yingling, C.D., Hosobuchi, Y. & Harrington, M. (1990) P300 as a predictor of recovery from coma. *Lancet*, **336**(**8719**), 873.

191 De Giorgio, C.M., Rabinowicz, A.L. & Gott, P.S. (1993) Predictive value of P300 event-related potentials compared with EEG and somatosensory evoked potentials in non-traumatic coma. *Acta Neurologica Scandinavica*, **87**(**5**), 423–427.

192 Fischer, C., Luaute, J., Adeleine, P. & Morlet, D. (2004) Predictive value of sensory and cognitive evoked potentials for awakening from coma. *Neurology*, **63**(**4**), 669–673.

193 Fischer, C., Luaute, J., Nemoz, C., Morlet, D., Kirkorian, G. & Mauguiere, F. (2006) Improved prediction of awakening or nonawakening from severe anoxic coma using tree-based classification analysis. *Critical Care Medicine*, **34**(**5**), 1520–1524.

194 Daltrozzo, J., Wioland, N., Mutschler, V. & Kotchoubey, B. (2007) Predicting coma and other low responsive patients outcome using event-related brain potentials: a meta-analysis. *Clinical Neurophysiology : Official Journal of the International Federation of Clinical Neurophysiology*, **118**(**3**), 606–614.

195 Schmechel, D., Marangos, P.J., Zis, A.P., Brightman, M. & Goodwin, F.K. (1978) Brain endolases as specific markers of neuronal and glial cells. *Science*, **199**(**4326**), 313–315.

196 Tiainen, M., Roine, R.O., Pettila, V. & Takkunen, O. (2003) Serum neuron-specific enolase and S-100B protein in cardiac arrest patients treated with hypothermia. *Stroke; A Journal of Cerebral Circulation*, **34**(**12**), 2881–2886.

197 Oksanen, T., Tiainen, M., Skrifvars, M.B. *et al.* (2009) Predictive power of serum NSE and OHCA score regarding 6-month neurologic outcome after out-of-hospital ventricular fibrillation and therapeutic hypothermia. *Resuscitation*, **80**(**2**), 165–170.

198 Rundgren, M., Karlsson, T., Nielsen, N., Cronberg, T., Johnsson, P. & Friberg, H. (2009) Neuron specific enolase and S-100B as predictors of outcome after cardiac arrest and induced hypothermia. *Resuscitation*, **80**(**7**), 784–789.

199 Steffen, I.G., Hasper, D., Ploner, C.J. *et al.* (2010) Mild therapeutic hypothermia alters neuron specific enolase as an outcome predictor after resuscitation: 97 prospective hypothermia patients compared to 133 historical non-hypothermia patients. *Critical Care*, **14**(**2**), R69.

200 Samaniego, E.A., Mlynash, M., Caulfield, A.F., Eyngorn, I. & Wijman, C.A. (2011) Sedation confounds outcome prediction in cardiac arrest survivors treated with hypothermia. *Neurocritical Care*, **15**(**1**), 113–119.

201 Derwall, M., Stoppe, C., Brucken, D., Rossaint, R. & Fries, M. (2009) Changes in S-100 protein serum levels in survivors of out-of-hospital cardiac arrest treated with mild therapeutic hypothermia: a prospective, observational study. *Critical Care*, **13**(**2**), R58.

202 Bassetti, C., Bomio, F., Mathis, J. & Hess, C.W. (1996) Early prognosis in coma after cardiac arrest: a prospective clinical, electrophysiological, and biochemical study of 60 patients. *Journal of Neurology, Neurosurgery and Psychiatry*, **61**(**6**), 610–615.

203 Sherman, A.L., Tirschwell, D.L., Micklesen, P.J., Longstreth, W.T. Jr. & Robinson, L.R. (2000) Somatosensory potentials, CSF creatine kinase BB activity, and awakening after cardiac arrest. *Neurology*, **54**(**4**), 889–894.

204 Oddo, M. & Rossetti, A.O. (2014) Early multimodal outcome prediction after cardiac arrest in patients treated with hypothermia. *Critical Care Medicine*, **42**(**6**), 1340–1347. doi:10.1097/CCM.0000000000000211

CHAPTER 6

Acute ischemic stroke and transient ischemic attack

Maria I. Aguilar

Department of Neurology, Cerebrovascular Diseases Center, Mayo Clinic Hospital, Phoenix, AZ, USA

Background

Stroke refers to the clinical syndrome of sudden onset of focal or global disturbance of central nervous system function, with no apparent cause other than a vascular cause [1]. Ischemic stroke is responsible for about 80% of all strokes, intracerebral hemorrhage (ICH) for 15%, and subarachnoid hemorrhage (SAH) for 5%. A transient ischemic attack (or TIA) has the same symptom complex as a stroke, but with a resolution of these symptoms within 24 hours [2]. Most TIAs though resolve within 1 hour. It is increasingly understood that TIAs and minor strokes represent a continuum of disease; some now suggest that the time-based definition of TIA yield to a tissue-based definition, as approximately one-third of people with clinically diagnosed TIAs will actually have structural changes visible on neuroimaging, such as diffusion-weighted MRI scanning (DWI) [3,4].

Mechanism and pathophysiology

Strokes and TIAs occur when the blood supply to the brain is disrupted, usually for one of the following reasons:
• Large vessel disease because of the occlusion of the lumen of an artery by a blood clot that develops as a local thrombus, often in relation to atherosclerotic plaque rupture and endothelial injury, with the activation of the local coagulation cascade.
• Distal occlusion of the lumen of an artery by a blood clot that has embolized from the heart (atrial fibrillation), aortic arch, or arterial system.
• Narrowing of smaller arteries due to arteriosclerosis (small vessel cerebrovascular disease).
• Local or embolic blood clots related to hypercoagulable states (hereditary or secondary to systemic disease or malignancy).

• Occlusion of the arterial lumen following the dissection of the arterial wall.
• Rupture of a blood vessel wall (artery or vein), leading to hemorrhage.
• Hypotension secondary to cardiac arrest or decreased circulating blood volume.

During stroke or TIA, normal cellular function is lost in the affected area of the brain, leading to the presenting symptoms. If normal blood flow is not restored promptly, an infarct core of dead cells will form; these cells do not recover. In many cases, there is also an area of tissue around the infarct core (the ischemic penumbra), which is tissue at risk, metabolically threatened, but still viable [5]. If blood flow is restored quickly, this penumbral tissue may be salvageable, resulting in a better clinical.

Epidemiology

Each year, about 15 million people worldwide suffer a stroke; of these, 5 million die and 5 million are left permanently disabled. In developed countries, stroke is a leading cause of death and dementia, and is the primary cause of adult disability [6]. In general, stroke is a disease of the elderly, and so these trends will increase over the next several decades as the result of an aging population combined with the disturbing persistence of many well-understood "modifiable" risk factors, including hypertension, dyslipidemia, smoking, diabetes, obesity, sleep-related breathing disorders, physical inactivity, excessive alcohol intake, and diets high in saturated fats and low in fruits and vegetables.

Clinical scenario

A 67-year-old woman is brought to the local emergency room by ambulance. Her family informs that exactly 1 hour

---

Evidence-Based Neurology: Management of Neurological Disorders, Second Edition. Edited by Bart M. Demaerschalk and Dean M. Wingerchuk.
© 2015 John Wiley & Sons, Ltd. Published 2015 by John Wiley & Sons, Ltd.

and 15 minutes ago, she experienced, suddenly, complete paralysis of her left arm and leg, with an associated facial droop, while having her evening meal. There was no associated loss of consciousness, and the patient is not aware that anything in particular is the matter, apart from a slight headache. Her physical examination confirms a dense left-sided hemiparesis, with associated neglect phenomena, including a left visual field cut. She has hypertension, dyslipidemia, and smokes one package of cigarettes per day. She is not taking aspirin or any antithrombotic agents; her only medication is a diuretic. An emergency computed tomography [7] head scan does not demonstrate any obvious abnormality. An electrocardiograph (ECG) shows her to be in atrial fibrillation.

Framing clinical questions and general approach to searching evidence

In general, four goals for the management of the patient with acute stroke can be defined: (1) minimize brain damage and restore perfusion, (2) restore functional independence, (3) prevent complications, and (4) reduce the risk of stroke recurrence.

This chapter will address the following main clinical questions:

1 Among patients with hyperacute ischemic stroke, how do intravenous (IV) thrombolysis, intra-arterial (IA) thrombolysis, and mechanical clot retrieval within the first few hours affect the probability of long-term outcomes such as death or dependency and of short-term adverse events such as death and symptomatic intracranial hemorrhage (ICH)?

2 Among patients with acute ischemic stroke, how does the pharmacological treatment, the management of complications, and the organization of care affect the probability of long-term outcomes, such as death or dependence, and of short-term adverse events?

3 Among patients with acute ischemic stroke with brain edema, what treatment options affect the probability of long-term outcomes, such as death or dependence, and of short-term adverse events?

4 Among patients with acute hemorrhagic stroke, are there surgical treatments or drug therapies that influence the probability of long-term outcomes, such as death or dependence, and of short-term adverse events?

5 What can be done to prevent further strokes in stroke survivors?

The search strategy conducted to provide the best available evidence to answer these questions included a review of the Cochrane Library (using standard search terms) for completed systematic reviews and randomized controlled trials, as well as a search of the Internet Stroke Center's Stroke Trials Directory (http://www.strokecenter.org/trials/) for completed clinical trials not yet included in relevant systematic reviews, as well as ongoing clinical trials.

Critical review of the evidence
Thrombolysis and clot retrieval
Among patients with hyperacute ischemic stroke, how do IV thrombolysis, IA thrombolysis, and mechanical clot retrieval within the first few hours affect the probability of long-term outcomes such as death or dependency and of short-term adverse events such as death and symptomatic ICH?

IV thrombolysis
A Cochrane Systematic Review has demonstrated that thrombolytic therapy with recombinant tissue plasminogen activator (rt-PA) administered IV within 3 hours of stroke onset for highly selected patients who meet strict eligibility criteria has been shown to save lives and reduce disability despite an early risk of intracerebral hemorrhage [8]. The systematic review included 26 randomized controlled trials with 7152 patients. The trials tested urokinase, streptokinase, recombinant tissue plasminogen activator, recombinant pro-urokinase, or desmoteplase. Four trials used intra-arterial administration; the rest used the intravenous route. Most data come from trials that started treatment up to 6 hours after stroke; three trials started treatment up to 9 hours and one small trial up to 24 hours after stroke. About 55% of the data (patients and trials) come from trials testing intravenous tissue plasminogen activator. Very few of the patients (0.5%) were aged over 80 years. Overall, thrombolytic therapy, administered up to 6 hours after ischemic stroke, significantly reduced the proportion of patients who were dead or dependent (modified Rankin 3–6) at the end of follow-up at 3–6 months (odds ratio (OR) 0.81, 95% confidence interval (CI) 0.73–0.90). This was in spite of a significant increase in the following: the odds of death within the first 10 days (OR 1.81, 95% CI 1.46–2.24) and the main cause of which was fatal ICH (OR 4.34, 95% CI 3.14–5.99). Symptomatic ICH was increased following thrombolysis (OR 3.49, 95% CI 2.81–4.33). Thrombolytic therapy also increased the odds of death at the end of follow-up at 3–6 months (OR 1.33, 95% CI 1.15–1.53). For patients treated within 3 hours of stroke, thrombolytic therapy appeared more effective in reducing death or dependency (OR 0.71, 95% CI 0.52–0.96), with no statistically significant adverse effect on death (OR 1.13, 95% CI 0.86–1.48). There was heterogeneity between the trials that could have been due to many trial features including the following: thrombolytic drug used, variation in the use of aspirin and heparin, severity of the stroke (both between trials and between treatment groups within trials), and time to treatment. It was the opinion of the authors of the systematic review that the data are strong and justify the use of thrombolytic therapy with IV recombinant tissue plasminogen activator in selected patients. A subsequent individual patient data meta-analysis suggested that the time window for IV rt-PA may extend beyond 3 hours [9].

In 2008, the NEJM published the results of the European Cooperative Acute Stroke Study III [10], which evaluated the efficacy and safety of administering intravenous rt-PA to acute ischemic stroke patients 3–4.5 hours after the onset of stroke symptoms. The study assessed outcomes 90 days after the stroke occurred and reported a modest, statistically significant increased likelihood of having normal or near normal recovery in favor of rt-PA treatment compared to placebo. The symptomatic ICH rate was similar to that observed in prior trials, although the definition used by the ECASS III investigators (which more closely examined whether the ICH was the likely cause of the deterioration) yielded a rate of 2.4%. Mortality at 90 days was similar between treatment and placebo groups in ECASS III (7.7% and 8.4%, respectively), and was lower than the older tPA stroke trials in which mortality was around 20% in treatment and placebo groups.

In early 2009, the AHA/ASA guidelines for the administration of rt-PA following acute stroke were revised to expand the window of treatment from 3 to 4.5 hours to provide more patients with an opportunity to receive benefit from this effective therapy [11]. Eligibility criteria for treatment in the 3–4.5 hours after acute stroke are similar to those for treatment at earlier time periods, with any one of the following additional exclusion criteria:

- Patients older than 80 years
- All patients taking oral anticoagulants are excluded regardless of the international normalized ratio [12]
- Patients with baseline NIHSS score > 25
- Patients with a history of stroke and diabetes

IA thrombolysis

One systematic review was identified [13], including 10 trials involving 1641 patients. Only one trial ($n = 35$) compared IV plus IA rt-PA versus IA rt-PA alone, unfortunately the data were inconclusive. The practice is presently of limited clinical application, except in highly specialized centers where research continues. Results of the endovascular therapy after intravenous t-PA versus t-PA alone for Stroke Trial (IMS-3) [14] were presented at the International Stroke Conference in February 2013 and subsequently published on the NEJM in March 2013, showing similar safety outcomes and no significant difference in functional independence with endovascular therapy after intravenous rt-PA, as compared with intravenous t-PA alone among 434 patients in the endovascular group and 222 in the intravenous group. Similar results were reproduced in a smaller study (362 patients) conducted in Italy [15]. Imaging selection (penumbral pattern) failed to identify patients that would benefit from endovascular therapy [16].

Mechanical clot retrieval

Mechanical embolectomy has also been studied in the acute stroke population, but no systematic review or randomized controlled trials have been published.

There are currently four devices available: the MERCI retrieval system, the PENUMBRA system, and most recently the SOLITAIRE Flow Restoration Device and the TREVO Retriever. The last two are retrievable stents [17].

The Mechanical Embolus Removal in Cerebral Ischemia trial [18], a phase II non-randomized study, involved 141 patients treated within 8 hours of symptom onset with MERCI retriever device; patients were not eligible for rt-PA. The primary outcomes were recanalization and safety. In the study, recanalization of treatable vessels with the study device was achieved in 48% ($p = 0.0001$) patients treated. Investigators used adjuvant therapy in 51 instances after deployment of the device. Clinically significant procedural complications occurred in 10 of 141 (7%) patients; symptomatic ICH was observed in 11 of 141 (7.8%) patients. Three percent of the devices used during the trial fractured, possibly causing the death of two patients. The MERCI retriever device gained FDA approval in 2005 based on the above trial [18].

In March 2012, the FDA approved the SOLITAIRE device, based on the results of the industry-sponsored noninferiority SWIFT trial (http://clinicaltrials.gov/ct2/show/NCT01054560. Accessed January 3, 2012), which compared SOLITAIRE nondetachable microcatheter-based stent-like device ($n = 58$) versus MERCI retriever device ($n = 55$). SOLITAIRE was superior to MERCI in terms of successful recanalization (68.5% vs. 30.2%, $p < 0.001$), good neurologic outcome at 90 days (58.2% vs. 33.3%, $p = 0.017$), mortality at 90 days (17.2% vs. 38.2%, $p = 0.020$), and intracerebral hemorrhage rates (1.7% vs. 10.9%, $p < 0.0001$ for noninferiority). This trial was stopped early because of robust interim results (http://www.medscape.com/viewarticle/758087).

The 2013 American Heart Association (AHA) Guidelines recommend the use of stent retrievers (SOLITAIRE and TREVO) over the coil retrievers as MERCI [17], with the caveat that their ability to improve patient outcomes has not yet been established.

Organization of care

Among patients with acute ischemic stroke, how does the organization of care affect the probability of long-term outcomes such as death or dependence and of short-term adverse events?

Reliable evidence from systematic reviews of randomized trials strongly supports a policy of caring for *all* patients with acute stroke on a geographically defined stroke unit with a coordinated multidisciplinary team [19]. Organized stroke unit care is provided by multidisciplinary teams that either manage stroke patients in a dedicated ward (stroke ward), with a mobile team (stroke team), or within a generic disability service (a mixed rehabilitation ward). Twenty-three trials were included in the systematic review. Compared with alternative services, stroke unit care showed reductions in the odds of death recorded at final (median

1 year) follow-up (OR 0.86, 95% CI 0.71–0.94, $p = 0.005$), the odds of death or institutionalized care (0.80, 0.71–0.90, $p = 0.0002$), and death or dependency (0.78, 0.68–0.89, $p = 0.0003$). Subgroup analyses indicated that the observed benefits remained when the analysis was restricted to truly randomized trials with blinded outcome assessment. Outcomes were independent of patient age, sex, and stroke severity but appeared to be better in stroke units based in a discrete ward. There was no indication that organized stroke unit care resulted in increased hospital stay. The authors concluded that patients who receive organized inpatient care in a stroke unit are more likely to be alive, independent, and living at home 1 year after the stroke. The benefits were most apparent in units based in a discrete ward. No systematic increase was observed in the length of inpatient stay.

Treatment of acute ischemic stroke

Among patients with acute ischemic stroke, how does the pharma-cological treatment affect the probability of long-term outcomes such as death or dependence and of short-term adverse events?

Antiplatelet agents (predominantly aspirin)

The use of antiplatelet agents in the acute stroke period has been evaluated in one Cochrane Systematic Review [20]. Twelve involving 43,041 patients were included. Two trials testing aspirin 160–300 mg once daily started within 48 hours of onset contributed 94% of the data. The maximum follow-up was 6 months. With treatment, there was a significant decrease in death or dependency at the end of follow-up (OR 0.95, 95% CI 0.91–0.99). In absolute terms, 13 more patients were alive and independent at the end of follow-up for every 1000 patients treated (NNT 79). Further-more, treatment increased the odds of making a complete recovery from the stroke (OR 1.06, 95% CI 1.01–1.11). In absolute terms, 10 more patients made a complete recovery for every 1000 patients treated. Antiplatelet therapy was associated with a small but definite excess of 2 symptomatic ICH for every 1000 patients treated, but this was more than offset by a reduction of 7 recurrent ischemic strokes and about 1 pulmonary embolus for every 1000 patients treated. The authors concluded that antiplatelet therapy with aspirin 160–300 mg daily, given orally (or per rectum in patients who cannot swallow), and started within 48 hours of onset of presumed ischemic stroke reduces the risk of early recurrent ischemic stroke without a major risk of early hemorrhagic complications and improves long-term out-come. Further information regarding the appropriate dose of aspirin has been provided by a non-Cochrane meta-analysis, which had suggested that a policy of administering aspirin (75–150 mg/day) within the first few days after stroke will reduce the RR of stroke (and other adverse vascular events) by about 20% [21].

Anticoagulants

The use of anticoagulants in acute stroke has been evaluated in one Cochrane Systematic Review [22]. Twenty-two trials involving 23,547 patients were included in the review. The quality of the trials varied considerably. The anticoagulants tested were standard unfractionated heparin (UFH), low molecular-weight heparins, heparinoids, oral anticoagu-lants, and thrombin inhibitors. Based on nine trials (22,570 patients), there was no evidence that anticoagulant therapy reduced the odds of death from all causes (OR 1.05, 95% CI 0.98–1.12) at the end of follow-up. Similarly, based on six trials (21,966 patients), there was no evidence that anticoagulants reduced the odds of being dead or dependent at the end of follow-up (OR 0.99, 95% CI 0.93–1.04). Although anticoagulant therapy was associated with about 9 fewer recurrent ischemic strokes per 1000 patients treated (OR 0.76, 95% CI 0.65–0.88), it was also associated with a similar sized 9 per 1000 increase in symptomatic ICH (OR 2.52, 95% CI 1.92–3.30). Similarly, anticoagulants avoided about 4 pulmonary emboli per 1000 (OR 0.60, 95% CI 0.44–0.81), but this benefit was offset by an extra 9 major extracranial hemorrhages per 1000 (OR 2.99, 95% CI 2.24–3.99).

Sensitivity analyses did not identify a particular type of anticoagulant regimen or patient characteristic associated with net benefit, including those with cardioembolic stroke, "stroke in progression," vertebrobasilar territory stroke, or following thrombolysis for acute ischemic stroke to prevent rethrombosis of the treated cerebral artery. The authors concluded that immediate anticoagulant therapy in patients with acute ischemic stroke is not associated with net short- or long-term benefit. The data from this review do not support the routine use of any type of anticoagulant in acute ischemic stroke. It was also suggested that people treated with anticoagulants had less chance of developing deep vein thrombosis (DVT) and pulmonary embolism (PE) following their stroke, but these sorts of blood clots are not very common, and may be prevented in other ways.

HMG CoA reductase inhibitors (statins)

The role that statins might play within the first hours of acute stroke was addressed to some degree by the pilot trial Fast Assessment of Stroke and Transient ischemic attack to prevent Early Recurrences [23], a multicenter, randomized, double-blind, controlled trial involving 392 patients over the age of 40 with reported or ongoing symptoms lasting at least 5 minutes and having included either weakness and/or language disturbance at time of TIA/minor stroke, randomized to clopidogrel (300 mg loading dose then 75 mg daily; 198 patients) or placebo (194 patients), and simvastatin (40 mg daily; 199 patients) or placebo (193 patients). The primary outcomes were stroke at 90 days and stroke severity. The trial was stopped early due to a failure to recruit patients at the prespecified minimum enrollment rate because of increased use of statins. Fourteen (7.1%) patients on clopidogrel had a stroke within 90 days compared with 21 (10.8%) patients on placebo (RR 0.7 [95% CI 0.3–1.2]; absolute risk reduction −3.8% [95% CI −9.4 to 1.9]; $p = 0.19$). Twenty-one (10.6%) patients on simvastatin had a stroke within 90 days compared with 14 (7.3%) patients on placebo (RR 1.3 [0.7–2.4]; absolute risk increase 3.3% [−2.3–8.9]; $p = 0.25$). The interaction between clopidogrel and simvastatin was not significant ($p = 0.64$). Two patients on clopidogrel had intracranial hemorrhage compared with none on placebo (absolute risk increase 1.0% [−0.4–2.4]; $p = 0.5$). There was no difference between groups for the simvastatin safety outcomes. The authors concluded that immediately after TIA or minor stroke, patients are at high risk of stroke, which might be reduced by using clopidogrel in addition to aspirin. The hemorrhagic risks of the combination of aspirin and clopidogrel do not seem to offset this potential benefit. We were unable to provide evidence of the benefit of simvastatin in this setting.

One systematic review was identified [24], including 8 trials and 625 patients. There were insufficient published data from the eight studies for all planned primary and secondary outcomes; only one study was judged as "low risk" of bias. Statin treatment did not reduce all-cause mortality (OR 1.51, 95% CI 0.60–3.81). No cases of rhabdomyolysis occurred in 274 patients enrolled in three studies. The authors concluded insufficient data were available from randomized trials to establish whether statins are safe and effective in cases of acute ischemic stroke and transient ischemic attack.

Neuroprotective agents
A number of different agents acting at various points in the ischemic cascade to potentially protect vulnerable neurons or salvage the ischemic penumbra have been developed. Cochrane Systematic Reviews have evaluated excitatory amino acid antagonists [25], gangliosides [26], calcium channel antagonists [27], lubeluzole [28], methylxanthine derivatives [29], and tirilazad [30]. Unfortunately, none of these agents has been proven to be effective in the treatment of acute ischemic stroke, and some of them may actually cause harm. A number of clinical trials involving agents with different suspected neuroprotective mechanisms are ongoing (http://www.strokecenter.org/trials/). Most recently, cerebrolysin showed a favorable outcome trend in severely affected patient with acute ischemic stroke when compared to placebo [31].

Cooling
Hyperthermia has been associated with poor outcome after stroke. One Cochrane Systematic Review has evaluated the role of cooling in patients with acute stroke [32]. The objective of the systematic review was to assess the effects of cooling when applied to patients with acute ischemic stroke or primary intracerebral hemorrhage (PICH). Five pharmacological temperature reduction trials and three physical cooling trials were included, involving a total of 423 patients. Neither intervention had a statistically significant effect in reducing the risk of death or dependency. Both interventions were associated with a nonsignificant increase in the occurrence of infections. The authors concluded there is currently no evidence from randomized trials to support the routine use of physical or pharmacological strategies to reduce temperature in patients with acute stroke, and large randomized clinical trials are needed to study the effect of such strategies.

The Nordic Cooling Stroke Study (NOCSS), a multicenter randomized controlled trial with an anticipated recruitment of 1000 patients (current study size 44 participants), is presently evaluating the safety and possible neuroprotective efficacy of induced mild hypothermia in non-anesthetized patients who present within 6 hours of a moderate-to-severe acute hemispheric stroke (http://www.strokeconference.org/sc_includes/pdfs/CTP8.pdf).

Management of complications
Among patients with acute ischemic stroke, how does the management of complications affect the probability of long-term outcomes such as death or dependence, and of short-term adverse events?

People with acute stroke are at higher risk of complications, such as deep venous thrombosis, PE, infection, pneumonia, and skin breakdown. In general, all of these are preventable with excellent nursing care. In addition, there is at least some evidence supporting the maintenance adequate oxygenation, treating fevers with antipyretics, and maintaining a normal blood glucose level [7].

Prevention of deep venous thrombosis
One area that has been studied in more detail is involving the prevention of deep venous thrombosis and PE. One Cochrane Review evaluated the effectiveness and safety of physical methods of preventing the onset of DVT and fatal or nonfatal PE in patients with recent stroke [33]. Symptomatic DVT and resulting PE are uncommon but important complications of stroke. There is good evidence that anticoagulants can reduce the risk of DVT and PE after stroke, but this benefit is offset by a small but definite risk of serious hemorrhages. Physical methods to prevent DVT and PE (such as compression stockings applied to the legs) are not associated with any bleeding risk and are effective in some categories of medical and surgical patients. Two trials (2615 patients) evaluated graduated compression stockings (GCS), and two trials (177 patients) evaluated intermittent pneumatic compression (IPC) applied to the legs. Overall, physical methods were not associated with a

significant reduction in DVTs during the treatment period (odds ratio (OR) 0.85, 95% confidence interval (CI) 0.70 to 1.04) or deaths (OR 1.12, 95% CI 0.87–1.45). Use of GCS was not associated with any significant reduction in risk of DVT (OR 0.88, 95% CI 0.72–1.08) or death (OR 1.13, 95% CI 0.87–1.47) at the end of follow-up. IPC was associated with a nonsignificant trend toward a lower risk of DVTs (OR 0.45, 95% CI 0.19–1.10) with no evidence of an effect on deaths (OR 1.04, 95% CI 0.37–2.89). The authors concluded that there was insufficient evidence from randomized trials to support the routine use of physical methods for preventing DVT in acute stroke. Clots in legs or TEDS after stroke (CLOTS) [34], was a two-part, multicenter, randomized, partially blinded, controlled trial of 3114 immobile patients hospitalized with acute stroke between January 2002 and May 2009. A total of 1552 patients received thigh-length stockings and 1562 patients received below-knee stockings to wear while they were in the hospital. The primary outcome (DVT detected on either Doppler ultrasound or venography) occurred in 98 patients (6.3%) who received thigh-length and 138 (8.8%) who received below-knee stockings, an absolute difference of 2.5 percentage points (95% CI, 0.7–4.4 percentage points; $P = 0.008$), an odds reduction of 31% (CI, 9% to 47%). Seventy-five percent of patients in both groups wore the stockings for 30 days or until they were discharged, died, or regained their mobility. Skin breaks occurred in 61 patients who received thigh-length (3.9%) and 45 (2.9%) who received below-knee stockings. Blinding was incomplete, two scans were not obtained for all enrolled patients, and the trial was stopped before target accrual was reached. In conclusion, proximal DVT occurs more often in patients with stroke who wear below-knee stockings than in those who wear thigh-length stockings.

The PREVAIL study [35] (efficacy and safety of enoxaparin vs. unfractionated heparin for the prevention of venous thromboembolism after acute ischaemic stroke) compared, open-label, enoxaparin 40 mg subcutaneously once per day to UFH 5000 U subcutaneously every 12 hours. Primary end points included symptomatic and asymptomatic DVT, symptomatic or fatal pulmonary embolism, symptomatic intracranial hemorrhage (sICH), major extracranial hemorrhage, and all-cause mortality. Enoxaparin was associated with a significant relative risk reduction in VTE events compared with unfractionated heparin of 43%, representing approximately 8 fewer events per 100 patients treated (number needed to treat for benefit: 13). Those with more severe strokes, defined in the trial as NIHSS score ≥14, were twice as likely to have VTE but were also at higher risk of bleeding complications, and the absolute risk among less severe strokes (NIHSS < 14) in the enoxaparin group remained high at 8.3%.

There was no difference in the rate of sICH (1% in each group), but the rate of major extracranial bleeding was higher with enoxaparin (7 [1%] vs. 0, $p = 0.015$).

One Cochrane review [36] compared the effects of low-molecular-weight heparins (LMWH) with those of UFH in acute ischemic stroke. Nine trials involving 3137 people were included. Four trials compared a heparinoid (danaparoid), four trials compared LMWH (enoxaparin or certoparin), and one trial compared an unspecified low-molecular-weight heparin with standard UFH. Allocation to LMWH or heparinoid was associated with a significant reduction in the odds of deep vein thrombosis compared with standard UFH (odds ratio (OR) 0.55, 95% confidence interval (CI) 0.44–0.70). However, the number of more major events (pulmonary embolism, death, intracranial or extracranial hemorrhage) was too small to provide a reliable estimate of the benefits and risks of LMWH or heparinoids compared with UFH for these, arguably more important, outcomes. Insufficient information was available to assess effects on recurrent stroke or functional outcome. In conclusion, treatment with an LMWH or heparinoid after acute ischemic stroke appears to decrease the occurrence of deep vein thrombosis compared with standard UFH, but there are too few data to provide reliable information on their effects on other important outcomes, including death and intracranial hemorrhage.

Blood pressure

Acute blood pressure (BP) alteration has been evaluated in one Cochrane Systematic Review [37], which sought to assess the effect of lowering or elevating BP in people with acute stroke, and the effect of different vasoactive drugs on BP in acute stroke. Data were obtained for 12 trials (1153 patients; 603 assigned to active therapy and 550 to placebo/control). Calcium channel blockers (CCBs), clonidine, glyceryl tinitrate (GTN), thiazide diuretic, and mixed antihypertensive therapy were tested. One trial tested phenylephrine. At 24 hours after randomization, ACEIs reduced systolic blood pressure (SBP, mean difference, MD −6 mmHg, 95% confidence interval, CI −22 to 10) and diastolic blood pressure (DBP, MD −5 mmHg, 95% CI −18 to 7), ARA-reduced SBP (MD −3, 95% CI −7 to 2) and DBP (MD −3, 95% CI −6 to 0.4), iv CCBs reduced SBP (MD −32 mmHg, 95% CI −65 to 1) and DBP (MD −13 mmHg, 95% CI −31 to 6), oral CCBs reduced SBP (MD −13 mmHg, 95% , CI −43 to 17) and DBP (MD −6 mmHg, 95% CI −14 to 2), GTN reduced SBP (MD −10 mmHg, 95% CI −18 to 3) and DBP (MD −1 mmHg, 95% CI −5 to 3) while phenylephrine, nonsignificantly increased SBP (MD 21 mmHg, 95% CI −13 to 55) and DBP (MD 1 mmHg, 95% CI −15 to 16). Functional outcome and death were not altered by any of the drugs. The authors concluded that there is insufficient evidence to evaluate the effect of altering blood pressure on outcome during the acute phase of stroke. In patients with acute stroke, CCBs, ACEI, ARA and GTN each lower blood pressure while phenylephrine probably increases blood pressure.

The Continue or Stop post-Stroke Antihypertensives Collaborative Study (COSSACS [38], a multicenter, prospective, randomized, open, blinded-endpoint trial, included patients older than 18 years who were taking antihypertensive drugs, enrolled within 48 hours of stroke, and the last dose of antihypertensive drug. Patients were assigned (1:1) to either continue or stop pre-existing antihypertensive drugs for 2 weeks. The primary endpoint was death or dependency at 2 weeks. Seven hundred and sixty-three patients were assigned to continue ($n=379$) or stop ($n=384$) pre-existing antihypertensive drugs. Seventy-two of 379 patients in the continue group and 82 of 384 patients in the stop group reached the primary endpoint (relative risk 0.86, 95% CI 0.65–1.14; $p=0.3$). The difference in systolic blood pressure at 2 weeks between the continue group and the stop group was 13 mm Hg (95% CI 10–17), and the difference in diastolic blood pressure was 8 mm Hg (6–10; difference between groups $p<0.0001$). No substantial differences were observed between groups in rates of serious adverse events, 6-month mortality, or major cardiovascular events. The study was terminated early and as consequence probably underpowered.

The Controlling Hypertension and Hypotension Immediately Post-Stroke Trial [39] (CHHIPPS) randomized 179 hypertensive (SBP >160 mmHg) patients to receive oral labetalol, lisinopril, or placebo if they were nondysphagic, or intravenous labetalol, sublingual lisinopril, or placebo if they had dysphagia, within 36 hours of symptom onset. Target SBP (145–155 mmHg) or a reduction in SBP of 15 mmHg was compared with SBP at randomization. Mean age was 74 [SD 11] years; SBP 181 [SD 16] mmHg; diastolic blood pressure [DBP] 95 [SD 13] mm Hg; median National Institutes of Health Stroke Scale [NIHSS] score 9 [IQR 5–16] points. Subjects were randomly assigned to receive labetolol ($n=58$), lisinopril ($n=58$), or placebo ($n=63$). The primary outcome – death or dependency at 2 weeks – occurred in 61% ($n=69$) of the active and 59% ($n=35$) of the placebo group (relative risk [RR] 1·03, 95% CI 0·80–1·33; $p=0.82$). There was no evidence of early neurological deterioration with active treatment (RR 1.22, 0.33–4.54; $p=0.76$) despite the significantly greater fall in SBP within the first 24 hours in this group compared with placebo (21 [17–25] mm Hg vs. 11 [5–17] mm Hg; $p=0.004$). No increase in serious adverse events was reported with active treatment (RR 0.91, 0.69–1.12; $p=0.50$) but 3-month mortality was halved (9.7% vs. 20.3%, hazard ratio [HR] 0.40, 95% CI 0.2–1.0; $p=0.05$). The authors concluded that labetalol and lisinopril are effective antihypertensive drugs in acute stroke that do not increase serious adverse events. Early lowering of blood pressure with lisinopril and labetalol after acute stroke seems to be a promising approach to reduce mortality and potential disability. However, in view of the small sample size, care must be taken when these results are interpreted.

Blood glucose control

Hyperglycemia is associated with poor outcome after stroke, suggesting that may be beneficial. One Cochrane Systematic Review [40] proposed to determine whether maintaining serum glucose within a specific normal range (4–7.5 mmol/L) in the first 24 hours of acute ischemic stroke influenced outcome. Seven trials involving 1296 participants (639 participants in the intervention group and 657 in the control group) were included. There was no difference between treatment and control groups in the outcome of death or disability and dependence (OR 1.00, 95% CI 0.78–1.28) or final neurological deficit (SMD – 0.12, 95% CI – 0.23 to 0.00). The rate of symptomatic hypoglycemia was higher in the intervention group (OR 25.9, 95% CI 9.2–72.7). In the subgroup analyses of diabetes mellitus [41] versus non-DM, there was no difference for the outcomes of death and dependency or neurological deficit. The authors concluded the administration of intravenous insulin with the objective of maintaining serum glucose within a specific range in the first hours of acute ischemic stroke does not provide benefit in terms of functional outcome, death, or improvement in final neurological deficit and significantly increased the number of hypoglycemic episodes.

The Stroke Hyperglycemia Insulin Network Effort Trial (SHINE) will open enrollment soon: multicenter, randomized, controlled clinical trial of 1400 patients. The hypotheses are that treatment of hyperglycemic acute ischemic stroke patients with targeted glucose concentration (80–130 mg/dL) will be safe and result in improved 3-month outcome after stroke. More information can be found at http://clinicaltrials.gov/ct2/show/study/NCT01369069? show_locs=Y#locn.

Brain edema

Among patients with acute ischemic stroke and significant brain edema, what treatment options affect the probability of long-term outcomes such as death or dependence and of short-term adverse events?

Several treatment strategies have been identified that attempt to deal specifically with brain edema in the early stages of ischemic stroke, but support for their routine use has not been confirmed by the evidence.

Mannitol

One Cochrane Systematic Review evaluated the use of mannitol in acute ischemic stroke [42]. It has been theorized that since mannitol is an osmotic agent and a free radical scavenger, it might decrease edema and tissue damage in stroke. Three trials involving 226 patients were included. Although no statistically significant differences were found between the mannitol-treated and control groups, the confidence intervals for the treatment effect estimates were wide and included both clinically significant benefits and clinically significant harms as possibilities. The authors concluded that there is currently not enough evidence to decide whether the routine use of mannitol in acute stroke would result in any beneficial or harmful effect.

Glycerol

One Cochrane Systematic Review evaluated the role of IV glycerol treatment in acute stroke [43]. A 10% solution of glycerol is a hyperosmolar agent that is thought to reduce brain edema. The review sought to determine whether IV glycerol treatment in acute stroke, either ischemic or hemorrhagic, influences death rates and functional outcome in the short or long term, and whether the treatment is safe. Eleven completed, randomized trials comparing IV glycerol and control were considered. Analysis of death during the scheduled treatment period for acute ischemic and/or hemorrhagic stroke was possible in 10 trials where 482 glycerol-treated patients were compared with 463 control patients. Glycerol was associated with a nonsignificant reduction in the odds of death within the scheduled treatment period (OR 0.78, 95% CI 0.58–1.06). Among patients with definite or probable ischemic stroke, glycerol was associated with a significant reduction in the odds of death during the scheduled treatment period (OR 0.65, 95% CI 0.44–0.97). However, at the end of the scheduled follow-up period, there was no significant difference in the odds of death (OR 0.98, 95% CI 0.73–1.31). Functional outcome was reported in only two studies, but there were nonsignificantly more patients who had a good outcome at the end of scheduled follow-up (OR 0.73, 95% CI 0.37–1.42). Hemolysis seems to be the only relevant adverse effect of glycerol treatment. The authors concluded that there was the suggestion of a favorable effect of glycerol treatment on short-term survival in patients with probable or definite ischemic stroke, but the CIs were wide and the magnitude of the treatment effect may be only minimal. The lack of evidence of benefit in long-term survival does not support the routine or selective use of glycerol treatment in patients with acute stroke.

Corticosteroids

Corticosteroids have been used to reduce brain swelling to help limit damage and speed recovery. Although studies of their use in acute stroke have been disappointing, many physicians continue to treat stroke with corticosteroids. One Cochrane Systematic Review [44] included eight trials involving 466 people. No difference was shown in the odds of death within 1 year (OR 0.87, 95% CI 0.57–1.34). Treatment did not appear to improve functional outcome in survivors. Seven trials reported neurological impairment, but pooling the data was impossible because no common scale or time interval was used. The results were inconsistent between individual trials. The only adverse effects reported were small numbers of gastrointestinal bleeds, infections, and deterioration of hyperglycemia across both groups. There is not enough evidence to evaluate corticosteroid treatment for people with acute presumed ischemic stroke.

Craniectomy

The high mortality that follows large cerebral infarctions is in part due to brain edema, with mass effect leading to herniation. Craniectomy is sometimes performed on patients with massive infarcts whose level of consciousness is declining in an attempt to improve survival and hopefully longer term outcome. One Cochrane Systematic Review [45] evaluated the role of decompressive surgery with medical therapy alone on the outcomes death and "death or dependency" in patients with an acute ischemic stroke complicated by clinical and radiologically confirmed cerebral edema. Over 9000 citations were retrieved and inspected for relevance in this systematic review. No randomized controlled trials were identified to include in a meta-analysis. Five observational studies reporting comparative data were found along with a number of small series and single case reports. The authors concluded that there was no evidence from randomized controlled trials to support the use of decompressive surgery for the treatment of cerebral edema in acute ischemic stroke.

More recently, randomized controlled trials (RCTs), decompressive craniectomy in malignant middle cerebral artery infarction [46] (DECIMAL), and decompressive surgery for the treatment of malignant infarction of the middle cerebral artery [47] (DESTINY) suggest that decompression within 36 hours of stroke onset reduces case fatality compared to best medical treatment. Hofmeijer and colleagues conducted the HAMLET [48] trial, a multicenter, open, randomized controlled trial and an updated meta-analysis that suggests that surgical decompression reduces case fatality and poor outcome when performed within 48 hours of stroke onset.

Surgical decompression within 4 days of stroke onset did not reduce poor outcome (ARR 0%, 95% CI − 21 to 21), although it did reduce case fatality (ARR 38%, 95% CI 15–60). The group updated the existing pooled analysis [49], and in this paper they present an updated meta-analysis including data from HAMLET [48], DECIMAL [46], and DESTINY [47] for patients who had surgical intervention within 48 hours. The earlier pooled analysis included 93 patients (23 patients from the then-ongoing HAMLET trial) and showed positive effects on both mortality and functional outcome when decompressive craniectomy was performed within 48 hours of stroke onset. The updated meta-analysis ($n = 109$, 39 from HAMLET) demonstrated similar results, with a substantial reduction in risk of poor outcome and case fatality in the patients who underwent surgical decompression within 48 hours of stroke onset. The ARR for poor outcome (mRS > 4) is 42% (23–56 95% CI), with a number needed to treat (NNT) of 2 (4 to 2 95% CI). The ARR for case fatality is 50% (32–64 95% CI) with an NNT of 2 (3 to 2 95% CI). Apart from the above risk reduction in case fatalities, the other secondary outcome measures were essentially not significant. However, this data was skewed because of the large difference in fatalities between the two groups. In addition, two patients in the surgical decompression arm had such severe aphasia that their quality of life or mood could not be evaluated. Subgroup analyses were performed according to age, presence of aphasia, and time between stroke and randomization, which did not demonstrate any significant differences. Thus, the authors concluded that surgical decompression performed within 48 hours of stroke onset reduced the risk of poor outcome as defined by the mRS and case fatality. When including all HAMLET subjects (not limited to randomization within 48 hours) there is a nonsignificant trend toward benefit in all three trials with an ARR of 13% (95% CI − 2 to 28) for the combined outcome of death and severe disability [50].

Transient ischemic attack

Transient ischemic attack [51] is a sudden, focal neurological deficit that lasts less than 24 hours, resolves completely, is presumed to be of vascular origin, and is confined to an area of the brain or eye perfused by a specific artery [52]. However, it is known that most TIAs usually last less than 60 minutes, most resolving within 30 minutes. The vascular neurology community has then proposed new criteria, where by definition the clinical symptoms would be transient (without a specific time frame defined), and most importantly there would be no evidence of infarction. By using "tissue" rather than "time," this revised definition recognized TIA as a pathophysiological entity. The AHA endorsed revised definition is as follows: "Transient ischemic attack [51]: a transient episode of neurological dysfunction caused by focal brain, spinal cord, or retinal ischemia, without acute infarction" [41]. The "old" definition included a time frame of 24 hours, although it is known that most TIAs usually last less than 60 minutes, most resolving within 30 minutes [53–55].

TIAs are caused by different clinical situations, that is, ipsilateral carotid artery stenosis, cardiac embolism, intracranial atherosclerosis, small vessel cerebrovascular disease, among others. The causes of TIA are identical to those of stroke, so secondary prevention strategies are similar for both entities.

Epidemiology

The estimated annual incidence of TIA in the United States is 200,000–500,000. Many episodes never come to medical attention and the above is probably an underestimate. It is presumed that about 5 million Americans have been given the diagnosis of TIA [41,52–56].

Diagnosis

The 2006 guidelines make strong emphasis on prompt evaluation, within 24–48 hours [57]. The diagnostic evaluation is divided into four groups: general evaluation, brain imaging, carotid imaging, and cardiac evaluation.

Evaluation

General evaluation should include electrocardiogram (EKG), full blood count, serum electrolytes and creatinine, fasting blood sugar, and lipids.

Although the diagnosis of TIA is clinical, brain imaging may reveal infarcts or other pathologies that can mimic TIA. Computed tomography [7] or magnetic resonance imaging (MRI) of the head should be included in the initial diagnostic evaluation. Conventional angiography (CA) of the cerebral vessels remains the gold standard diagnostic modality to assess the presence and to quantify the location and degree of carotid stenosis. CA is invasive, expensive, and not free of risk (contrast exposure, risk of arterial vasospasm, plaque embolization). Doppler ultrasonography (DUS) is a useful screening tool that provides accurate information [58]. It is noninvasive and inexpensive when compared to other imaging modalities such as magnetic resonance angiography (MRA) or computed tomographic angiography (CTA). MRA has better discriminatory power than DUS recognizing 70–99% stenosis and its sensitivity and specificity is comparable to CA [59,60]. CTA has high sensitivity and high negative predictive value for carotid disease [61]; however, it is unable to reliably distinguish between moderate (50–69%) and severe (70–99%) stenosis [62], and tends to underestimate clinically relevant grades of stenosis [63]. The 2006 guidelines [57] recommend DUS for screening, MRA or CTA, if DUS does not yield reliable results or endarterectomy is seriously considered. CA is recommended for cases where DUS and MRA/CTA yield discordant results.

The most recent AHA 2009 guidelines [41] emphasize again the importance of prompt evaluation (as soon as possible after an event) and recommend the following imaging studies (class I recommendations):

1 Neuroimaging within 24 hours of symptom onset, MRI with DWI preferred. CT is an alternative (Level of Evidence B).

2 Routine noninvasive imaging of cervicocephalic vessels (Level A).

3 Noninvasive testing of the intracranial vasculature, when knowledge of intracranial steno-occlusive disease will alter management (Level A).

If a cardioembolic mechanism is suspected, transthoracic echocardiography (TTE) is indicated. Transesophageal echocardiography (TEE) is recommended for patients younger than 45 years, when brain, carotid, and general evaluation provide no clue to the cause of TIA.

The need for admission to the hospital is a topic of great debate, especially in this era of financial grief.

Clinical case example

A 54-year-old woman present to the emergency department after a 15-minute episode of numbness involving the left side of her face and her left arm. She has no vascular risk factors and is currently on no prescription medications. On clinical examination her blood pressure (BP) is elevated (150/95) and her neurological examination reveals no focal abnormalities.

Framing clinical questions and general approach to searching evidence

1 Should this woman be admitted to the hospital for observation, management, and further evaluation?
2 What is this woman's risk of suffering a stroke in the near future?

The search strategy conducted to provide the best available evidence to answer these questions included a review of the Cochrane Library (using standard search terms) for completed systematic reviews and randomized controlled trials, as well as a search of the Internet Stroke Center's Stroke Trials Directory (http://www.strokecenter.org/trials/) for completed clinical trials not yet included in relevant systematic reviews as well as ongoing clinical trials.

No randomized-controlled trials were identified. When deciding if a patient who has just suffered a TIA needs to be institutionalized for work up and management, the first step is to determine the patient's risk of stroke. From Johnston's cohort study [64], it is well known that TIAs carry short-term risk of stroke and other adverse events. A significant proportion of strokes (~50%) preceded by a TIA take place in the first 48 hours after the TIA. Multiple prediction models have been proposed to help clinicians risk-stratify these patients, and the unified ABCD^2 score [65] has been shown to be the most predictive of short-term recurrence [64–66]. This score takes into account the patient's age, BP during evaluation, clinical features (motor deficit and speech, carry higher risk, respectively, than sensory symptoms), and history of diabetes (Table 6.1).

Based on the ABCD^2 score, the risk of stroke or an adverse event in the subsequent 90 days can be estimated (Table 6.2).

Back to the clinical case, this woman's ABCD^2 score is 2 due to symptom duration 10–59 minutes and elevated BP. She then belongs in the low-risk group, and she probably does not require inpatient evaluation. She should expeditiously though undergo general evaluation, brain and carotid imaging and cardiac evaluation. The higher the score on the ABCD^2 risk stratification model, the higher the risk of an adverse event. Also the higher the score, the higher the likelihood that the episode was indeed a TIA [67].

Table 6.1 ABCD^2 risk stratification score

	Score	Feature
Age	1	≥60
BP	1	SBP >140 or DBP >90
Clinical features	2	Unilateral weakness
	1	Speech impairment
Duration	2	>60 minutes
	1	10–59 minutes
	0	<10 minutes
DM	1	

Source: Rothwell et al. [65]. Reproduced by permission of Elsevier.

Table 6.2 Risk of stroke after TIA based on ABCD^2 score

ABCD^2 score	2-day risk (%)	7-day risk (%)	90-day risk (%)
0–3 (low risk)	1.0	1.2	3.1
4–5 (moderate risk)	4.2	5.9	9.8
6–7 (high risk)	8.1	11.7	17.8

Source: Rothwell et al. [65]. Reproduced by permission of Elsevier.

The AHA guidelines [41] consider hospitalization reasonable for TIA victims who present within 72 hours of the event and meet any of the following criteria (class II recommendations):

1 ABCD^2 score of ≥ 3 (Level of Evidence C).
2 ABCD^2 score 0–2, and uncertainty that diagnostic workup can be completed within 48 hours in the out-patient setting (Level C).
3 ABCD^2 score 0–2, and other evidence indicating that the event was caused by focal ischemia (Level C).

Treatment

Treatment after a TIA is directed toward stroke and cardiovascular disease prevention. The specific treatment depends on the etiology, but overall every effort should be made to modify the individual's vascular risk factors (i.e. HTN, DM, dyslipidemia, atrial fibrillation, smoking cessation)

Noncardioembolic TIA

Daily long-term antiplatelet therapy should be prescribed immediately [57]. The 2006 guidelines recommend aspirin-plus extended-release dypiridamole as the firstline agent. The evidence to support this comes mainly for the ESPIRIT trial [68]. Clopidogrel is indicated when aspirin alone or in combination with dypiridamole is not tolerated. The recent PRoFESS trial though [69], published two years after the guidelines, has shown that clopidogrel is somewhat better than previous evidence suggests, and probably aspirin-plus extended-release dypiridamole is somewhat worse than previous evidence suggests [70].

Cardioembolic TIA

For patient with paroxysmal or sustained atrial fibrillation (valvular or nonvalvular) who have had a cardioembolic TIA long-term anticoagulation with warfarin is indicated to a goal INR of 2.5 (2.0–3.0). Regarding future risk of stroke, not every patient who has AF must be anticoagulated. The risk of stroke should be addressed and balanced against the benefit and the risk inherent to long-term anticoagulation. Risk stratification schemes are available when addressing the use of anticoagulation versus antiplatelet therapy in this patient population [57,71].

In 2000, Pearce and colleagues [72] compared three-stroke risk stratification schemes (AFI, ACCPC, SPAF) in nonvalvular atrial fibrillation. The CHADS^2 score was then implemented [73]. The acronym stands for

- C = congestive heart failure (1 point)
- H = hypertension (1 point)
- A = age older than 75 (1 point)
- D = DM (1 point)
- S^2 = history of stroke or transient ischemic attack [51] (2 points).

The estimated annual risk of stroke based on the CHADS^2 score varies from 1.9% to 18.2% as more risk factors are added.

Clinical case example

While undergoing evaluation at the emergency department, the above-mentioned 54-year-old woman goes into atrial fibrillation and has a second TIA, this time with left-sided hemiparesis and dysarthria. Symptoms resolved within 10 minutes.

Her ABCD^2 score is now a 5, 2 points added for unilateral weakness and 1 for speech impairment. She is now in the "moderate risk" group, and the decision is made to admit her to the hospital. CT of the brain is unremarkable, CTA shows no significant stenosis at either carotid bifurcation or intracranial vasculature. TTE shows normal ejection fraction and severe left atrial enlargement. AF is documented on EKG.

Should she be treated with intravenous (IV) heparin while warfarin therapy is initiated and her INR becomes therapeutic?

Ovid MEDLINE database was searched from 1996 to February week 1 2012, no randomized trials addressed our clinical question. One randomized single-blinded trial addressed the use of a heparin bolus versus no bolus [74] and found no difference in outcome. In the absence of evidence, information is extrapolated from trials regarding the use of IV heparin after a cardioembolic stroke (not TIA). A meta-analysis of seven trials involving almost 5000 patients [75] showed that early anticoagulation in this clinical scenario is associated with a nonsignificant reduction in recurrence of ischemic stroke, no substantial reduction in death and disability and an increased risk of intracranial bleeding. We then recommend against the use of IV heparin after cardioembolic stroke or TIA as either acute therapy or as bridging therapy to long-term anticoagulation.

In summary TIA is a neurological emergency, and as such mandates prompt evaluation with the goal to identify the etiologic cause of the event and implement early therapy to prevent TIA recurrence, stroke, cardiovascular events, and death.

References

1 Warlow, C.P., Dennis, M.S. & van Gijn, J. (2001) *What caused this transient or persisting ischaemic event?* Blackwell Science.

2 Special Report from the National Institute of Neurological Disorders and Stroke (1990) Classification of cerebrovascular diseases III. *Stroke*, **21**(4), 637–676.

3 Albers, G.W., Caplan, L.R., Easton, J.D. *et al.* (2002) Transient ischemic attack—proposal for a new definition. *New England Journal of Medicine*, **347**(21), 1713–1716.

4 Warach, S. & Kidwell, C.S. (2004) The redefinition of TIA. *Neurology*, **62**(3), 359–360.

5 1990) Pathophysiology of brain ischemia as it relates to the therapy of acute ischemic stroke. *Clinical Neuropharmacology* Review, **13**(**Suppl 3**), S1–S8.

6 World Health Organization. *The Atlas of Heart Disease and Stroke [database on the Internet].* http://www.who.int/cardiovascular_diseases/resources/atlas/en/, [cited 04/16/2012].

7 Langhorne, P. & Pollock, A. (2002) Collaboration iCwTSUT. What are the components of effective stroke unit care? *Age and Ageing*, **31**(5), 365–371.

8 Wardlaw, J.M., Murray, V., Berge, E. & del Zoppo, G.J. (2009) Thrombolysis for acute ischaemic stroke. *Cochrane Database of Systematic Reviews*,(**4**). doi:10.1002/14651858

9 2004) Association of outcome with early stroke treatment: pooled analysis of ATLANTIS, ECASS, and NINDS rt-PA stroke trials. *The Lancet*, **363**(**9411**), 768–774.

10 Hacke, W., Kaste, M., Bluhmki, E. *et al.* (2008) Thrombolysis with alteplase 3 to 4.5 hours after acute ischemic stroke. *New England Journal of Medicine*, **359**(13), 1317–1329.

11 del Zoppo, G.J., Saver, J.L., Jauch, E.C. & Adams, H.P. (2009) Council obotAHAS. Expansion of the time window for treatment of acute ischemic stroke with intravenous tissue plasminogen activator. *Stroke*, **40**(8), 2945–2948.

12 Ezekowitz, M.D., Bridgers, S.L., James, K.E. *et al.* (1992) Warfarin in the prevention of stroke associated with nonrheumatic atrial fibrillation. Veterans Affairs Stroke Prevention in Nonrheumatic Atrial Fibrillation Investigators. [see comment] [erratum appears in N Engl J Med 1993 Jan 14;328(2):148]. *New England Journal of Medicine*, **327**(20), 1406–1412.

13 2000) Thrombolysis (different doses, routes of administration and agents) for acute ischaemic stroke. *Cochrane Database of Systematic Reviews*,(**2**), CD000514.

14 Broderick, J.P., Palesch, Y.Y., Demchuk, A.M. *et al.* (2013) Endovascular therapy after intravenous t-PA versus t-PA alone for stroke. *The New England Journal of Medicine* Research Support, N.I.H., Extramural Research Support, Non-U.S. Gov't, **368**(10), 893–903.

15 Ciccone, A., Valvassori, L., Nichelatti, M. *et al.* (2013) Endovascular treatment for acute ischemic stroke. *The New England Journal of Medicine* Research Support, Non-U.S. Gov't, **368**(10), 904–913.

16 Kidwell, C.S., Jahan, R., Gornbein, J. *et al.* (2013) A trial of imaging selection and endovascular treatment for ischemic stroke. *The New England Journal of Medicine* Research Support, N.I.H., Extramural 17Research Support, Non-U.S. Gov't, **368**(10), 914–923.

17 Jauch, E.C., Saver, J.L., Adams, H.P. Jr. *et al.* (2013) Guidelines for the early management of patients with acute ischemic stroke: a guideline for healthcare professionals from the american heart

association/american stroke association. *Stroke; A Journal of Cerebral Circulation*, **44**(**3**), 870–947.

18 Smith, W.S., Sung, G., Starkman, S. *et al.* (2005) Safety and efficacy of mechanical embolectomy in acute ischemic stroke. *Stroke*, **36**(**7**), 1432–1438.

19 Collaboration SUT (2007) Organised inpatient (stroke unit) care for stroke. *Cochrane Database of Systematic Reviews*,(**4**).

20 Sandercock, P., Counsell, C., Gubitz, G. & Tseng, M. (2008) Antiplatelet therapy for acute ischaemic stroke. *Cochrane Database of Systematic Reviews*,(**3**).

21 2002) Collaborative meta-analysis of randomised trials of antiplatelet therapy for prevention of death, myocardial infarction, and stroke in high risk patients. *BMJ*, **324**(**7329**), 71–86.

22 Sandercock, P., Counsell, C. & Kamal, A. (2008) Anticoagulants for acute ischaemic stroke. *Cochrane Database of Systematic Reviews*,(**4**).

23 Kennedy, J., Hill, M.D., Ryckborst, K.J., Eliasziw, M., Demchuk, A.M. & Buchan, A.M. (2007) Fast assessment of stroke and transient ischaemic attack to prevent early recurrence (FASTER): a randomised controlled pilot trial. *The Lancet Neurology*, **6**(**11**), 961–969.

24 Squizzato, A., Romualdi, E., Dentali, F. & Ageno, W. (2012) Statins for acute ischemic stroke. *Stroke*, **43**(**2**), e18–e19.

25 Muir, K. & Lees, K. (2003) Excitatory amino acid antagonists for acute stroke. *Cochrane Database of Systematic Reviews*,(**3**).

26 Candelise, L. & Ciccone, A. (2002) Gangliosides for Acute Ischemic Stroke. *Stroke*, **33**(**9**), 2336.

27 2000) Calcium antagonists for acute ischemic stroke. *Cochrane Database of Systematic Reviews* Review,(**2**), CD001928.

28 2002) Lubeluzole for acute ischaemic stroke. *Cochrane Database of Systematic Reviews*,(**1**), CD001924.

29 2004) Pentoxifylline, propentofylline and pentifylline for acute ischaemic stroke. *Cochrane Database of Systematic Reviews*,(**3**), CD000162.

30 Tirilazad International Steering Committee (2000) Tirilazad mesylate in acute ischemic stroke: a systematic review. *Stroke*[Comparative Study Meta-Analysis Research Support, Non-U.S. Gov't], **31**(**9**), 2257–2265.

31 Heiss, W.-D., Brainin, M., Bornstein, N.M., Tuomilehto, J. & Hong, Z. (2012) Cerebrolysin in patients with acute ischemic stroke in Asia. *Stroke*, **43**(**3**), 630–636.

32 2009) Cooling therapy for acute stroke. *Cochrane Database of Systematic Reviews*[Meta-Analysis Review], **1**(**1**), CD001247.

33 2010) Physical methods for preventing deep vein thrombosis in stroke. *Cochrane Database of Systematic Reviews*[Meta-Analysis Review], **4**(**8**), CD001922.

34 Collaboration TCT (2010) Thigh-length versus below-knee stockings for deep venous thrombosis prophylaxis after stroke. *Annals of Internal Medicine*, E-280.

35 Sherman DG, Albers GW, Bladin C, Fieschi C, Gabbai AA, Kase CS, et al. The efficacy and safety of enoxaparin versus unfractionated heparin for the prevention of venous thromboembolism after acute ischaemic stroke (PREVAIL Study): an open-label randomised comparison. *The Lancet*. 2007 **369**(**9570**):1347–1355.

36 2008) Low-molecular-weight heparins or heparinoids versus standard unfractionated heparin for acute ischaemic stroke. *Cochrane Database of Systematic Reviews*[Review], **16**(**3**), CD000119.

37 2008) Interventions for deliberately altering blood pressure in acute stroke. *Cochrane Database of Systematic Reviews* Meta-Analysis Review, **8**(**4**), CD000039.

38 Robinson, T.G., Potter, J.F., Ford, G.A. *et al.* (2010) Effects of antihypertensive treatment after acute stroke in the Continue Or Stop post-Stroke Antihypertensives Collaborative Study (COSSACS): a prospective, randomised, open, blinded-endpoint trial. *The Lancet Neurology*, **9**(**8**), 767–775.

39 2009) Controlling hypertension and hypotension immediately post-stroke (CHHIPS): a randomised, placebo-controlled, double-blind pilot trial. *Lancet Neurology* Randomized Controlled Trial Research Support, Non-U.S. Gov't, **8**(**1**), 48–56 Epub 2008 Dec 4.

40 Bellolio, M., Gilmore, R. & Stead, L. (2011) Insulin for glycaemic control in acute ischaemic stroke. *Cochrane Database of Systematic Reviews*,(**9**).

41 Easton, J.D., Saver, J.L., Albers, G.W. *et al.* (2009) Definition and evaluation of transient ischemic attack: a scientific statement for healthcare professionals from the American Heart Association/American Stroke Association Stroke Council; Council on Cardiovascular Surgery and Anesthesia; Council on Cardiovascular Radiology and Intervention; Council on Cardiovascular Nursing; and the Interdisciplinary Council on Peripheral Vascular Disease: The American Academy of Neurology affirms the value of this statement as an educational tool for neurologists. *Stroke*, **40**(**6**), 2276–2293.

42 Bereczki, D., Liu, M., Fernandes do Prado, G. & Fekete, I. (2007) Mannitol for acute stroke. *Cochrane Database of Systematic Reviews*,(**3**).

43 Righetti, E., Celani, M.G., Cantisani, T.A., Sterzi, R., Boysen, G. & Ricci, S. (2005) Glycerol for acute stroke. *Stroke*, **36**(**1**), 171–172.

44 Sandercock, P. & Soane, T. (2011) Corticosteroids for acute ischaemic stroke. *Cochrane Database of Systematic Reviews*,(**9**).

45 Morley, N.C.D., Berge, E., Cruz-Flores, S. & Whittle, I.R. (2003) Surgical decompression for cerebral edema in acute ischemic stroke. *Stroke*, **34**(**5**), 1337.

46 Vahedi, K., Vicaut, E., Mateo, J. *et al.* (2007) Sequential-design, multicenter, randomized, controlled trial of early decompressive craniectomy in malignant middle cerebral artery infarction (DECIMAL Trial). *Stroke*, **38**(**9**), 2506–2517.

47 Juttler, E., Schwab, S., Schmiedek, P. *et al.* (2007) Decompressive Surgery for the Treatment of Malignant Infarction of the Middle Cerebral Artery (DESTINY): a randomized, controlled trial. *Stroke*, **38**(**9**), 2518–2525.

48 Hofmeijer, J., Kappelle, L.J., Algra, A. *et al.* (2009) Surgical decompression for space-occupying cerebral infarction (the Hemicraniectomy After Middle Cerebral Artery infarction with Life-threatening Edema Trial [HAMLET]): a multicentre, open, randomised trial. *Lancet Neurology*, **8**(**4**), 326–333.

49 Vahedi, K., Hofmeijer, J., Juettler, E. *et al.* (2007) Early decompressive surgery in malignant infarction of the middle cerebral artery: a pooled analysis of three randomised controlled trials. *Lancet Neurology*, **6**(3), 215–222.

50 2009) Reassessment of the HAMLET study. *Lancet Neurology* Comment Letter, **8**(7), 602–623 author reply 3–4.

51 Diener, H.C., Bogousslavsky, J., Brass, L.M. *et al.* (2004) Aspirin and clopidogrel compared with clopidogrel alone after recent ischaemic stroke or transient ischaemic attack in high-risk patients (MATCH): randomised, double-blind, placebo-controlled trial.[see comment]. *Lancet*, **364**(9431), 331–337.

52 Johnston, S.C. (2002) Clinical practice. Transient ischemic attack. *The New England Journal of Medicine*, **347**(21), 1687–1692.

53 Levy, D.E. (1988) How transient are transient ischemic attacks? *Neurology*, **38**(5), 674–677.

54 Pessin, M.S., Duncan, G.W., Mohr, J.P. & Poskanzer, D.C. (1977) Clinical and angiographic features of carotid transient ischemic attacks. *New England Journal of Medicine*, **296**(7), 358–62.

55 Weisberg, L.A. (1991) Clinical characteristics of transient ischemic attacks in black patients. *Neurology*, **41**(9), 1410–4.

56 Bots, M.L., van der Wilk, E.C., Koudstaal, P.J., Hofman, A. & Grobbee, D.E. (1997) Transient neurological attacks in the general population : prevalence, risk factors, and clinical relevance. *Stroke*, **28**(4), 768–773.

57 Johnston, S.C., Nguyen-Huynh, M.N., Schwarz, M.E. *et al.* (2006) National Stroke Association guidelines for the management of transient ischemic attacks.[see comment]. *Annals of Neurology*, **60**(3), 301–313.

58 Fürst, G., Saleh, A., Wenserski, F. *et al.* (1999) Reliability and validity of noninvasive imaging of internal carotid artery pseudo-occlusion. *Stroke*, **30**(7), 1444–1449.

59 Nederkoorn, P.J., van der Graaf, Y. & Hunink, M.G.M. (2003) Duplex ultrasound and magnetic resonance angiography compared with digital subtraction angiography in carotid artery stenosis. *Stroke*, **34**(5), 1324–1331.

60 Forsting, M. & Wanke, I. (2003) Editorial Comment—Funeral for a Friend. *Stroke*, **34**(5), 1331–1332.

61 Josephson, S.A., Bryant, S.O., Mak, H.K., Johnston, S.C., Dillon, W.P. & Smith, W.S. (2004) Evaluation of carotid stenosis using CT angiography in the initial evaluation of stroke and TIA. *Neurology*, **63**(3), 457–460.

62 Anderson, G.B., Ashforth, R., Steinke, D.E., Ferdinandy, R. & Findlay, J.M. (2000) CT angiography for the detection and characterization of carotid artery bifurcation disease. *Stroke*, **31**(9), 2168–2174.

63 Silvennoinen, H.M., Ikonen, S., Soinne, L., Railo, M. & Valanne, L. (2007) CT angiographic analysis of carotid artery stenosis: comparison of manual assessment, semiautomatic vessel analysis, and digital subtraction angiography. *American Journal of Neuroradiology*, **28**(1), 97–103.

64 Johnston, S.C., Gress, D.R., Browner, W.S. & Sidney, S. (2000) Short-term prognosis after emergency department diagnosis of TIA. *JAMA*, **284**(22), 2901–2906.

65 Rothwell, P.M., Giles, M.F., Flossmann, E. *et al.* (2005) A simple score (ABCD) to identify individuals at high early risk of stroke after transient ischaemic attack. *Lancet*, **366**(9479), 29–36.

66 Johnston, S.C., Rothwell, P.M., Nguyen-Huynh, M.N. *et al.* (2007) Validation and refinement of scores to predict very early stroke risk after transient ischaemic attack. [see comment]. *Lancet*, **369**(9558), 283–292.

67 Josephson, S.A., Sidney, S., Pham, T.N., Bernstein, A.L. & Johnston, S.C. (2008) Higher ABCD2 score predicts patients most likely to have true transient ischemic attack. *Stroke*, **39**(11), 3096–3098.

68 2006) Aspirin plus dipyridamole versus aspirin alone after cerebral ischaemia of arterial origin (ESPRIT): randomised controlled trial. *The Lancet*, **367**(9523), 1665–1673.

69 Sacco, R.L., Diener, H.C., Yusuf, S. *et al.* (2008) Aspirin and extended-release dipyridamole versus clopidogrel for recurrent stroke.[see comment]. *New England Journal of Medicine*, **359**(12), 1238–51.

70 Kent, D.M. & Thaler, D.E. (2008) Stroke prevention--insights from incoherence.[comment]. *New England Journal of Medicine*, **359**(12), 1287–1289.

71 Sacco, R.L., Adams, R., Albers, G. *et al.* (2006) Guidelines for prevention of stroke in patients with ischemic stroke or transient ischemic attack: a statement for healthcare professionals from the American Heart Association/American Stroke Association Council on Stroke: co-sponsored by the Council on Cardiovascular Radiology and Intervention: the American Academy of Neurology affirms the value of this guideline. [see comment]. *Stroke*, **37**(2), 577–617.

72 Pearce, L.A., Hart, R.G. & Halperin, J.L. (2000) Assessment of three schemes for stratifying stroke risk in patients with non-valvular atrial fibrillation. *American Journal of Medicine*, **109**(1), 45–51.

73 Gage, B.F., Waterman, A.D., Shannon, W., Boechler, M., Rich, M.W. & Radford, M.J. (2001) Validation of clinical classification schemes for predicting stroke: results from the National Registry of Atrial Fibrillation. *JAMA*, **285**(22), 2864–2870.

74 Toth, C. (2003) The use of a bolus of intravenous heparin while initiating heparin therapy in anticoagulation following transient ischemic attack or stroke does not lead to increased morbidity or mortality. *Blood Coagulation & Fibrinolysis*, **14**(5), 463–468.

75 Paciaroni, M., Agnelli, G., Micheli, S. & Caso, V. (2007) Efficacy and safety of anticoagulant treatment in acute cardioembolic stroke. *Stroke*, **38**(2), 423–430.

CHAPTER 7
Spinal cord compression

Naresh P. Patel[1], Christopher A. Payne[2], and Bhavesh M. Patel[3]

[1] *Department of Neurological Surgery, Mayo Clinic, Phoenix, AZ, USA*
[2] *Trinity College, Dublin, Ireland*
[3] *Department of Critical Care Medicine, Mayo Clinic, Phoenix, AZ, USA*

Introduction

The spine functions to carry loads and to allow a wide range of motion while protecting the spinal cord. Compression of the spinal cord may occur when the spine is compromised by tumor, infection, degenerative disease, or trauma. Spinal cord compression is often a medical emergency, which may result in devastating outcomes such as permanent disability and even death, highlighting the need for immediate appropriate medical and/or surgical management [1,2].

In developed countries, traumatic spinal cord injury (TSCI) occurs predominantly in males aged 18–32 years with a second peak occurring among males and females aged over 65 years. Global incidence is estimated to be approximately 23 cases per million per year with a higher incidence in the United States of 38 cases per million per year. In the United States, 47% of these injuries occur due to motor vehicle accidents, 22% result from falls, 16% are associated with violence and self-harm, and 10% with sport and recreation. Low falls make up a large proportion of the TSCI occurring in the population aged over 65 years, and it is thought this will increase as the population ages [3]. The reporting of nontraumatic spinal cord injury (NTSCI) is not as well documented, and high-quality incidence reports of NTSCI are not as readily available. It can be noted however that developed countries tend to have predominantly NTSCI associated with tumors and degenerative disease, whereas developing countries report higher incidence associated with infection. The overall incidence of NTSCI is also expected to increase as the population ages [4,5].

Spinal cord compression due to tumor – metastatic spinal cord compression

The spine is the most common bony site of metastatic tumor spread. The most common primary tumor types are the prostate, breast, and lung with metastasis most commonly occurring in the thoracic spine [6–8]. Metastatic spinal cord compression (MSCC) occurs in 10–20% of all patients with cancer. It is expected that the incidence of MSCC will increase as cancer care improves and patients live longer with their disease. Metastasis to the spine often presents with severe pain and, if left untreated, may progress to paralysis and sensory loss. Magnetic resonance imaging (MRI) remains the imaging of choice for diagnosing MSCC. Radiographic confirmation of this disease process should prompt neurosurgical consultation within 24 hours [6].

Clinical questions: management of acute metastatic spinal cord compression

1 *For adults with acute MSCC, does surgical management improve clinical outcomes?*

Surgery with or without radiotherapy (RT) should be considered first as this is associated with the highest rates of neurological preservation, restoration of ambulation, and pain control. It is of particular benefit in patients with a good overall prognosis and a single area of spinal cord compression. The goal of surgery in cases of MSCC is to decompress the cord by removing tumor and to stabilize the spine [6–8]. A randomized trial by Patchel *et al.* in 2005 comparing surgery in combination with RT to radiotherapy alone demonstrated that 84% of patients undergoing surgery were able to ambulate after treatment, compared with 57% in the radiotherapy alone group (OR 6.2; 95% CI 2.0–19.8, $p = 0.001$) [9]. A systematic review and analysis of the literature by Kim *et al.* in 2012 further supported the benefit of surgery showing that of nonambulatory patients receiving surgery, 64% were able to regain the ability to ambulate compared to only 29% of patients receiving RT alone ($p < 0.001$). Of note, though the survival among these patients was strongly influenced by tumor type, ambulatory

Evidence-Based Neurology: Management of Neurological Disorders, Second Edition. Edited by Bart M. Demaerschalk and Dean M. Wingerchuk.
© 2015 John Wiley & Sons, Ltd. Published 2015 by John Wiley & Sons, Ltd.

patients regardless of tumor type had a five- to six-fold greater median survival than those who were unable to ambulate, supporting the importance of ambulation as a valuable prognostic indicator. Pain relief was also significantly higher among patients receiving surgery at 88% compared with 74% in patients treated with RT alone ($p < 0.001$) [7]. Prophylactic decompression may also be considered in patients without neurological signs but who are likely to progress toward spinal cord compression.

2 *For adults with acute MSCC, does the use of high-dose corticosteroids improve clinical outcomes?*

A Cochrane review identified three trials examining the role of corticosteroids in the management of MSCC and noted that high-dose corticosteroids were likely *not of benefit* to these patients (Overall ambulation RR 0.91; CI 0.68–1.23). Among the relevant trials reviewed in this Cochrane report, high doses of corticosteroids were instead associated with an increase in adverse effects such as adverse drug reactions and death because of infection, and such events were noted in 17% of patients receiving high-dose steroids compared with 0% in those patients on moderate- or low-dose corticosteroids (RR 0.12; 95% CI 0.02–0.97) [10]. Steroids not given in high doses are, however, recommended for patients with confirmed or suspected MSCC with neurological deficits as well as those with no neurological deficit but undergoing six or more fractions of RT [6,8]. Appropriate dosing for adult patients with symptomatic MSCC included dexamethasone 10 mg intravenous bolus followed by 16 mg/day in divided doses [6].

3 *For adults with acute MSCC, does radiotherapy improve clinical outcomes?*

Radiotherapy alone is indicated in patients who are unfit to undergo surgery, those who have an expected survival of less than 3 months, patients with radiosensitive tumors, those with neurological deficit for longer than 24–48 hours, or patients with multilevel disease[8]. The Cochrane Review identified one randomized multicenter trial by Maranzano et al. in 2005 comparing radiotherapy of 30 Gy in eight fractions with 16 Gy in two fractions and reported no difference in outcome between the two treatment regimens [10,11]. Regardless of whether surgery or RT is performed, appropriate follow-up is recommended to monitor for local recurrence.

4 *For adults with acute MSCC, does radiosurgery improve clinical outcomes?*

Stereotactic radiosurgery (SRS) has the ability to deliver radiation to a more focused area and potentially limit the total dose of radiation the spinal cord is exposed to. This form of treatment may have a role in the large number of patients who present with MSCC and disease at multiple spinal levels or who are inoperable at presentation [12]. A pilot study using SRS for the treatment of patients with confirmed metastasis to the spine with epidural compression demonstrated a significant increase in thecal sac patency after radiosurgery with mean patency at 55% before SRS compared with 76% after radiosurgery ($p < 0.001$). Additionally, an improvement in neurological function was noted in 81% of these patients [13]. Although radiation-induced myelopathy is of concern when delivering high doses of radiation in close proximity to the spinal cord and the tolerance of the spinal cord to a single dose of radiation has not been adequately defined, only rare reports of radiation-induced myelopathy exist in the literature [14–16]. At this time, we do not know whether radiosurgery provides a benefit over conventional RT. The Radiation Therapy Oncology Group is currently conducting a randomized controlled trial comparing SRS to RT for cord compression. In most radiation oncology centers, SRS is limited in the acute setting of MSCC due to the extended time required for planning and execution of SRS [6,8].

Spinal cord compression due to infection – spondylodiscitis

Most cases of infection of the spine arise from the disk space and adjacent vertebra. Spondylitis, discitis, osteomyelitis, and epidural abscess represent a spectrum of the same disease process and can be referred to collectively as spondylodiscitis. Spondylodiscitis may occur by hematogenous spread or from contiguous spread of infection from adjacent tissue. Spondylodiscitis represents a rare infection, affecting between 4 and 10 persons per million per year with a higher incidence reported in the elderly and in males [17–19]. Spinal infection should be suspected in any febrile patient presenting with new onset localized pain along the vertebral column. White blood cell count, erythrocyte sedimentation rate (ESR), and C-reactive protein (CRP) are useful initial tests for baseline levels and for monitoring response to treatment while blood cultures or biopsy can be used to determine microbiological etiology. Diagnosis is best achieved with contrast-enhanced spinal MRI [19–21]. Risk factors for spondylodiscitis include diabetes mellitus, immunosuppression, alcoholism, or long-term steroid use. Further risk factors include rheumatoid arthritis, polytrauma, malignant tumor, and any procedure or surgery involving the spine. A 7-year prospective study of patients with spondylodiscitis demonstrated two poor prognostic factors: the presence of neurological symptoms (relative risk (RR) 2.87; 95% confidence interval (CI) 1.02–8.07) and prolonged duration of symptoms (>60 days) before diagnosis (RR 2.65; 95% CI 0.92–7.59). This study also reported that the most commonly isolated microorganism was *Staphylococcus aureus* and that more than half of all cases of spondylodiscitis were hospital-acquired [17]. Although the lumbar spine is the most frequently affected, spondylodiscitis involving the thoracic spine is most likely to lead to neurological symptoms. Spinal cord compression in spondylodiscitis may occur by direct compression of the spinal cord either with infective material (e.g. phlegmon or abscess) or with dorsal displacement of bone fragments or disk into the canal as the integrity of the spine is compromised by infection [18]. Of epidural abscesses, a 10-year review of patients at a single center demonstrated neurological compromise more frequently in patients who had a dorsally located spinal epidural abscess compared to a ventrally located abscess. Paraplegia or quadriplegia was reported in 30.6% of dorsal epidural abscesses in comparison to only 7.3% with ventral epidural abscesses ($p = 0.003$). It has been suggested that this may be due to dorsal epidural abscesses presenting later [22].

Clinical questions: management of spinal cord compression due to infection

1 *For adults with spinal cord compression due to infection, what is the role of surgical management?*

Any infective process leading to symptomatic spinal cord compression carries the same need for emergent treatment as other forms of acute spinal cord compression. These cases should be treated ideally within the first 24 hours to avoid permanent neurological disability [18,19]. Currently, surgical decompression, which is most often achieved by laminectomy, hemilaminectomy, or interlaminar fenestration, remains the standard of care for these patients [19]. Further stabilization by instrumentation of the spine is performed as needed and may be done immediately, if instability is considered a factor in neurological compromise, or in a delayed manner to avoid the risk of hardware infection [18–20,23,24]. Surgery is also indicated in any scenario where spinal cord compression is imminent. Such scenarios include cases of infection leading to unstable pathological fractures [18]. Patients experiencing complete paresis for longer than 72 hours are unlikely to obtain an improvement in neurological function after surgery [19]. Surgery may be needed in any case of spondylodiscitis, regardless of the duration of symptoms, when the infective process is not controlled with adequate antibiotic treatment [18,20,23,24].

2 *For adults with spinal cord compression due to infection, what minimally invasive procedures exist for management?*

For small abscesses without significant bony destruction, less invasive techniques have been advocated. These include computed tomography (CT) guided percutaneous abscess drainage and percutaneous endoscopic debridement [20]. A number of case reports as well as a retrospective analysis by Siddiq *et al.* reported successful control of spondylodiscitis with percutaneous needle drainage of abscesses [25–28]. Percutaneous endoscopic debridement may also provide an effective means of management with Yang *et al.*, reporting an 87% success rate after the treatment of 15 patients with infectious spondylitis [29]. A retrospective analysis of 52 patients with spondylitis reported that percutaneous endoscopic discectomy and drainage was significantly more effective than CT-guided biopsy in not only diagnosing spondylodiscitis (90% vs. 47%, $p = 0.002$) but also controlling infection (75% vs. 44%, $p = 0.027$) [30]. In all cases, intravenous antibiotic therapy targeted to the infectious organism is paramount.

3 *For adults with spinal cord compression due to infection, what is the role of corticosteroids in management?*

At this time, there is no conclusive evidence as to whether steroids should be utilized in the management of cases of SD. However, level III evidence from a retrospective review of 35 cases of spinal epidural abscess demonstrated that steroids were associated with poor outcome with only 4 of 13 patients receiving treatment with steroids recovering completely compared with 15 of the 22 patients not receiving steroids ($p < 0.05$) [31]. This is likely due to the suppressive effect steroids have on the immune response, wound healing, and bone fusion [23].

Spinal cord compression due to degenerative disease – cervical and thoracic spondylotic myelopathy

The most serious complication of degenerative disease of the spine is spinal cord compression with resultant neurological deficit (spondylotic myelopathy). Spondylotic myelopathy occurs primarily in the cervical spine, as opposed to the thoracic spine, due to its greater range of motion. It is the most common cause of myelopathy in adults [32–35]. Cervical spondylosis is commonly seen with increasing age, but not all patients with cervical spondylosis present with symptoms. Approximately 10–15% of patients with spinal spondylosis present with symptoms of root or cord compression [36]. The exact prevalence and incidence of cervical spondylotic myelopathy (CSM) or thoracic spondylotic myelopathy (TSM) is not known [35,37]. Estimates place the prevalence of presentations of CSM requiring surgical intervention to at least 1.6 per 100,000 of the population [37]. Various developmental factors such as a person's spinal canal size as well as other developmental and genetic factors may predispose patients with cervical or thoracic degenerative disease to progress to CSM or TSM [33,38]. Patients with CSM or TSM may present with gait disturbance, sensory loss, and weakness in the upper and/or lower extremities and bowel or bladder symptoms. On examination, loss of coordination of the upper and/or lower extremities, hyperreflexia, clonus, Hoffman sign, and Babinski sign may be present [34]. MRI remains the most useful imaging modality in patients with CSM and TSM with electromyography, and nerve conduction studies used as adjuncts to rule out other possible diagnoses [34,39]. Harrop *et al.* demonstrated a significant correlation between myelopathy and radiographic evidence of cord compression ($p < 0.0001$) as well as T2 hyperintense signal within the cord ($p < 0.0001$) [40]. A blinded prospective, observational study by Arvin *et al.* reported features on MR spinal cord imaging, which could predict poorer preoperative neurological baseline as well as poorer postoperative response to surgery. These included the presence of low T1 signal, focal increased T2 signal, and segmentation of T2 signal changes within the spinal cord [41].

Clinical questions: management of spinal cord compression due to degenerative disease

1 *For adults with spinal cord compression due to degenerative disease, what are the preferred means of management?*

A Cochrane Review in 2010 identified a need for large-scale randomized control trials to examine the role of surgery compared with conservative management in patients with CSM. This study concluded that the available evidence comparing conservative with surgical treatment could not reliably allow a definitive conclusion be made regarding a preferred means of treatment [36]. The decision to manage patients with CSM or TSM conservatively or more aggressively with surgery should be made on a case-by-case basis with careful consideration of the clinical and radiographic presentation [39].

2 *For adults with spinal cord compression due to degenerative disease, what is the role of conservative management?*

Conservative management involves neck stabilization and protection of the spinal cord from further injury as well as symptom control. Neck stabilization may be achieved with the use of a cervical collar. Patients should also be counseled regarding the avoidance of activities that may promote further neurological compromise during this time of increased spinal cord vulnerability. Isolated upper and lower extremity strengthening exercises may be used to improve function while gait training may be utilized to improve balance and avoid falls. Pain control may be achieved with analgesics, muscle relaxants, or with neuromodulating medications such as gabapentin and pregabalin [34,39]. A prospective cohort study following 60 patients with *mild* CSM demonstrated that conservative treatment was adequate to avoid clinical progression of the disease in 70% of patients at 147 months of follow-up. This study also noted, however, that among patients with clinically mild presentations, certain radiographic features such as an "angular-edged deformity" may predispose to progression of CSM and may indicate a need for more aggressive management with surgery [42]. Patients managed conservatively should be followed up every 6–12 months or in the event of any progression of symptoms [39].

3 *For adults with spinal cord compression due to degenerative disease, what is the role of surgery in management?*

CSM may be addressed by a number of surgical treatment options. There is ongoing debate as to the ideal surgical approach. The goal of surgical treatments is to decompress the cervical spinal cord, prevent further spinal cord damage, stabilize the bony spine, and improve symptoms and quality of life. Cheung *et al.* prospectively followed 55 consecutive patients with CSM managed surgically and reported neurological improvement of patients up to 6 months postoperatively with 71% of patients experiencing neurological improvement after surgery [43]. Furlan *et al.* conducted a similar prospective study following 81 consecutive patients managed surgically for CSM and showed that a significant improvement from baseline was noted at 6 months ($p < 0.01$) but further noted that older patients ($p < 0.002$) and those with a higher number of comorbidities ($p < 0.01$) were significantly less likely to show functional improvement. This study reported no significant advantage regarding anterior versus posterior surgical approach in terms of functional outcome [44]. A prospective study by Karpova *et al.* demonstrated better recovery in younger patients ($p = 0.005$) [45]. A large prospective study examining 302 patients surgically treated for CSM reported a perioperative complication rate of 15.6% and noted higher complications associated with older age ($p = 0.006$) and operative time ($p = 0.009$). This study concluded, however, that the vast majority of the complications reported were treatable and had no long-term impact on patient outcome [46]. Currently, there exists considerable equipoise in the medical literature regarding appropriate timing of surgery for CSM and TSM [35,44,45,47,48]. For example, Karpova *et al.* reported no significant difference in postoperative outcome when comparing duration of symptoms of less than or equal to 12 months compared with treatment after 12 months [45]. Aizawa *et al.* however reported a significant difference in recovery rate between patients treated at less than or equal to 6 months compared with the treatment of patients who had symptoms for 6 months to 1 year ($p < 0.05$) [35]. Unfortunately these studies compared different time periods in which treatment was initiated and such discrepancies may explain variations in outcome within the literature. At this time, the ideal time window within which surgical treatment should take place is not known.

Spinal cord compression due to trauma – traumatic spinal cord injury

The guidelines for the management of acute cervical spine and spinal cord injuries published in 2013 in Neurosurgery represent the most up-to-date evidence-based guideline for the management of these conditions and are the primary source of the recommendations for this section [49]. This section will discuss the management of patients with TSCI *after* arrival at an acute care facility. A meaningful clinical assessment of patients with spinal cord injury both in the acute setting and long term should include assessment with both a neurological scale and a functional outcome scale. Level II evidence supports that the most consistent, reliable, and valid scoring system for the neurological assessment of patients with TSCI remains the American Spinal Injury Association (ASIA) Standards [50]. Level I medical evidence demonstrates that with regard to the assessment of functional outcome, the Spinal Cord Independence Measure III (SCIM III) is the tool with greatest validity, reliability and sensitivity [50]. Level I evidence recommends radiographic imaging with high-quality CT for patients with potential head trauma who are awake and symptomatic as well as for those with altered mental status. If this is not available, assessment with three-view cervical spine radiography (anteroposterior, lateral, and odontoid views) should be performed [51].

Clinical questions: management of spinal cord compression due to traumatic injury

1 *For adults with spinal cord injury due to trauma, what is the role of methylprednisolone and GM-1 ganglioside in the management of these patients?*

Multiple medical publications have reported adverse effects with high-dose steroid administration such as increased risk of infections, hyperglycemia, GI hemorrhage, and even death due to respiratory failure [52]. Although there exists level III evidence reporting some neuroprotective effect of methylprednisolone in patients with TSCI, this is not supported by any level I or level II medical evidence [52]. Level I evidence against the use of methylprednisolone in TSCI included a randomized control trial by Pointillart *et al.*, which demonstrated no difference in neurological outcome between patients receiving methylprednisolone and those receiving no steroid treatment after spinal cord injury [53]. Furthermore, a randomized trial by Matsumoto *et al.* demonstrated a significantly higher complication rate after high-dose methylprednisolone therapy compared with no steroid treatment after cervical spinal cord injury [54]. GM-1 ganglioside is a pharmacological agent thought to have anti-excitotoxic activity and was proposed as a potential agent that could benefit patients with TSCI. Because of a lack of medical evidence to support this treatment, it is not recommended for use in the management of TSCI [52].

2 *For adults with spinal cord injury due to trauma, what is the role of surgical management of these patients?*

The goal of treatment for subaxial spine fractures and dislocations is to adequately decompress the spinal cord and restore stability of the spine thus preventing further injury. This allows safe mobilization and rehabilitation to begin. Current guidelines report that surgical treatment appears to achieve these goals at a faster rate and with greater reliability than nonsurgical treatments such as traction and use of orthoses [55]. Both anterior and posterior surgical approaches are appropriate to address cord compression and instability [55].

3 *For patients with spinal cord injury without radiographic abnormality (SCIWORA), how should management be carried out?*

SCIWORA most commonly occurs in the pediatric population. This is described in patients who demonstrate signs or symptoms, either transient or persistent, of TSCI but show no radiographic evidence of spine abnormality despite adequate CT or three-view cervical spine radiography. Such patients should undergo MRI evaluation and assessment of spinal stability with flexion-extension radiographs. Management involves external immobilization of the injured spinal segment for up to 12 weeks. Patients and families should be counseled regarding the avoidance of activities, which may lead to further spinal cord compromise [56].

4 *For adults with spinal cord injury due to trauma, what other considerations in patient management should be taken?*

Spinal cord injury is frequently associated with respiratory, ventilatory, and cardiovascular dysfunction. The current guidelines have identified a number of studies, which report that management in a monitored setting leads to lower rates of morbidity and mortality [57]. Monitored management of these patients should be carried out in the intensive care unit (ICU) where issues such as hypotension or respiratory insufficiency may be detected and managed early [57]. Venous thromboembolism (VTE) is also a significant complication in patients with TSCI. Restricted mobilization associated with management, as well as the inability to ambulate after spinal cord injury, contributes to this complication. It is recommended that patients with TSCI undergo early VTE prophylaxis with low-molecular-weight heparin, pneumatic compression, or other forms of effective VTE prophylaxis utilized by the care facility [58].

Summary

Spinal cord compression may result from a number of pathological processes. Tumor, infection, trauma, and degenerative disease may all lead to direct spinal cord damage and/or secondary bony instability with resultant spinal cord injury. The guiding principle for treatment is decompression of the spinal cord with appropriate stabilization before irreversible neurological damage occurs. Modalities for treatment include surgery, radiation, minimally invasive percutaneous procedures, and pharmacological therapy. The goal is to avoid the severe morbidity and mortality associated with injury to the spinal cord. The time period within which a compressed spinal cord must be decompressed depends on the etiology of the compression. Symptomatic spinal cord compression due to tumor and infection should prompt urgent neurosurgical consultation. In these cases, implementation of treatment should be sought ideally within 24 hours of presentation. Similarly, spinal cord compression due to acute trauma should be addressed as soon as possible. Chronic cord compression due to degenerative disease, on the other hand, does not appear to require immediate aggressive management with treatment usually initiated based on progression of symptoms.

References

1 Stokes, O.M. & Arnold, F.J.L. (2012) Spinal emergencies. *Surgery (Oxford)*, **30**(**3**), 122–128.

2 Harktopp, H., Bronnum-Hansen, H., Seidenschnur, A.-M. & Biering-Sorensen, F. (1997) Survival and cause of death after traumatic spinal cord injury A long-term epidemiological survey from Denmark. *Spinal Cord.*, **35**, 76–85.

3 Lee, B.B., Cripps, R.A., Fitzharris, M. & Wing, P.C. (2014) The global map for traumatic spinal cord injury epidemiology: update 2011, global incidence rate. *Spinal Cord*, **52**(**2**), 110–116.

4 New, P.W., Cripps, R.A. & Bonne, L.B. (2014) Global maps of non-traumatic spinal cord injury epidemiology: towards a living data repository. *Spinal Cord*, **52**(**2**), 97–109.

5 New, P.W. & Marshall, R. (2014) International Spinal Cord Injury Data Sets for non-traumatic spinal cord injury. *Spinal Cord*, **52**(**2**), 123–132.

6 Loblaw, D.A., Mitera, G., Ford, M. & Laperriere, N.J. (2012) A 2011 updated systematic review and clinical practice guideline for the management of malignant extradural spinal cord compression. *International Journal of Radiation Oncology, Biology, Physics*, **84**(**2**), 312–317.

7 Kim, J.M., Losina, E., Bono, C.M. *et al.* (2012) Clinical outcome of metastatic spinal cord compression treated with surgical excision ± radiation versus radiation therapy alone. *Spine*, **37**(**1**), 78–84.

8 Bhatt, A.D., Schuler, J.C., Boakye, M. & Woo, S.Y. (2013) Current and emerging concepts in non-invasive and minimally invasive management of spine metastasis. *Cancer Treatment Reviews*, **39**(**2**), 142–152.

9 Patchell, R.A., Tibbs, P.A., Regine, W.F. *et al.* (2005) Direct decompressive surgical resection in the treatment of spinal cord compression caused by metastatic cancer: a randomised trial. *The Lancet*, **366**(**9486**), 643–648.

10 George R, Jeba J, Ramkuma G, Chacko A, Leng M, Tharyan P. Interventions for the treatment of metastatic extradural spinal cord compression in adults. *Cochrane Database of Systematic Reviews.* 2008;**4**: CD006716. doi: 10.1002/14651858. CD006716.pub2.

11 Maranzano, E., Bellavita, R., Rossi, R. *et al.* (2005) Short-course versus split-course radiotherapy in metastatic spinal cord compression: results of a phase III, randomized, multicenter trial. *Journal of Clinical Oncology*, **23**(**15**), 3358–3365.

12 Regine, W.F., Ryu, S. & Chang, E.L. (2011) Spine radiosurgery for spinal cord compression: the radiation oncologist's perspective. *Journal of Radiosurgery and SBRT.*, **1**, 55–61.

13 Ryu, S., Rock, J., Jain, R. *et al.* (2010) Radiosurgical decompression of metastatic epidural compression. *Cancer*, **116**(**9**), 2250–2257.

14 Bilsky, M.H., Angelov, L., Rock, J. *et al.* (2011) Spinal radiosurgery: a neurosurgical perspective. *Journal of Radiosurgery and SBRT.*, **1**, 47–54.

15 Gibbs, I.C., Patil, C., Gerszten, P.C., Adler, J.R.J. & Burton, S.A. (2009) Delayed radiation-induced myelopathy after spinal radiosurgery. *Neurosurgery*, **64**(**2**), A67–A72. doi:10.1227/ 01.NEU.0000341628.98141.B6

16 Ryu, S., Jin, J.-Y., Jin, R. *et al.* (2007) Partial volume tolerance of the spinal cord and complications of single-dose radiosurgery. *Cancer*, **109**(**3**), 628–636.

17 D'Agostino, C., Scorzolini, L., Massetti, A.P. *et al.* (2010) A seven-year prospective study on spondylodiscitis: epidemiological and microbiological features. *Infection*, **38**(**2**), 102–107.

18 Di Martino, A., Papapietro, N., Lanotte, A., Russo, F., Vadalà, G. & Denaro, V. (2012) Spondylodiscitis: standards of current treatment. *Current Medical Research and Opinion*, **28**(**5**), 689–699.

19 Sendi, P., Bregenzer, T. & Zimmerli, W. (2007) Spinal epidural abscess in clinical practice. *Qjm*, **101**(**1**), 1–12.

20 Guerado, E. & Cerván, A.M. (2012) Surgical treatment of spondylodiscitis. *An update. International Orthopaedics*, **36**(**2**), 413–420.

21 Reihsaus, E., Waldbaur, H. & Seeling, W. (2000) Spinal epidural abscess: a meta-analysis of 915 patients. *Neurosurg Rev*, **23**(**4**), 175–204.

22 Karikari, I.O., Powers, C.J., Reynolds, R.M., Mehta, A.I. & Isaacs, R.E. (2009) Management of a spontaneous spinal epidural abscess. *Neurosurgery*, **65**(**5**), 919–924.

23 Pradilla, G., Ardila, G., Hsu, W. & Rigamonti, D. (2009) Epidural abscesses of the CNS. *Lancet Neurology*, **8**, 292–300.

24 Pola E, Logroscino CA, Gentiempo M, Colangelo D, Mazzotta V, Di Meco E, et al. (2012) Medical and surgical treatment of pyogenic spondylodiscitis. *Eur Rev Med Pharmacol Sci.***16** Suppl **2**: 35–49.

25 Cwikiel, W. (1991) Percutaneous drainage of abscess in psoas compartment and epidural space. *Acta Radiologica*, **32**(**2**), 159–161.

26 Lyu, R.-K., Chen, C.-J., Tang, L.-M. & Chen, S.-T. (2002) Spinal epidural abscess successfully treated with percutaneous, computed tomography-guided, needle aspiration and parenteral antibiotic therapy: case report and review of the literature. *Neurosurgery*, **51**(**2**), 509–512.

27 Tabo, E., Ohkuma, Y., Kimura, S., Nagaro, T. & Aral, T. (1994) Successful percutaneous drainage of epidural abscess with epidural needle and catheter. *Anesthesiology*, **80**(**6**), 1393–1395.

28 Siddiq, F., Chowfin, A., Tight, R., Sahmoun, A.E. & Smego, R.A. Jr., (2004) Medical vs surgical management of spinal epidural abscess. *Archives of Internal Medicine*, **164**(**22**), 2409–2412.

29 Yang, S.-C., Fu, T.-S., Chen, L.-H., Niu, C.-C., Lai, P.-L. & Chen, W.-J. (2007) Percutaneous endoscopic discectomy and drainage for infectious spondylitis. *International Orthopaedics*, **31**(**3**), 367–373.

30 Yang, S.-C., Fu, T.-S., Chen, L.-H., Chen, W.-J. & Tu, Y.-K. (2008) Identifying pathogens of spondylodiscitis: percutaneous endoscopy or CT-guided biopsy. *Clin Orthop Relat Res*, **466**(**12**), 3086–3092.

31 Danner, R. & Hartman, B. (1987) Update of spipinal epidural abscess: 35 cases and review of the literature. *Review of infectious diseases*, **9**(**2**), 265–274.

32 Sanghvi, A., Chhabra, H., Mascarenhas, A., Mittal, V. & Sangondimath, G. (2011) Thoracic myelopathy due to ossification of ligamentum flavum: a retrospective analysis of predictors of surgical outcome and factors affecting preoperative neurological status. *European Spine Journal*, **20**(**2**), 205–215.

33 Fehlings, M. & Skaf, G. (1998) A review of the pathophysiology of cervical spondylotic myelopathy with insights for potential novel mechanisms drawn from traumatic spinal cord injury. *Spine*, **23**, 2730–2737.

34 Tracy, J.A. & Bartleson, J.D. (2010) Cervical spondylotic myelopathy. *The Neurologist*, **16**(**3**), 176–187.

35 Aizawa, T., Sato, T., Sasaki, H. *et al.* (2007) Results of surgical treatment for thoracic myelopathy: minimum 2-year follow-up study in 132 patients. *Journal of Neurosurgery: Spine*, **7**(**1**), 13–20.

36 Ioannis N, Ioannis FP, Peter SAG, Patrick SF. Surgery for cervical radiculopathy or myelopathy. *Cochrane Database of Systematic Reviews*. 2010;**1**: CD001466. doi: 10.1002/14651858. CD001466.pub3.

37 Boogaarts, H.D. (2013) *Bartels RHMA*. Prevalence of cervical spondylotic myelopathy, European Spine Journal.

38 Patel, A.A., Spiker, W.R., Daubs, M., Brodke, D.S. & Cannon-Albright, L.A. (2012) Evidence of an inherited predisposition for cervical spondylotic myelopathy. *Spine*, **37**(**1**), 26–29.

39 Toledano, M. & Bartleson, J.D. (2013) Cervical spondylotic myelopathy. *Neurologic Clinics*, **31**(**1**), 287–305.

40 Harrop, J.S., Naroji, S., Maltenfort, M. *et al.* (2010) Cervical myelopathy: a clinical and radiographic evaluation and correlation to cervical spondylotic myelopathy. *Spine*, **35**(**6**), 620–624. doi:10.1097/BRS.0b013e3181b723af

41 Arvin, B., Kalsi-Ryan, S., Mercier, D., Furlan, J.C., Massicotte, E.M. & Fehlings, M.G. (2013) Preoperative magnetic resonance imaging is associated with baseline neurological status and can predict postoperative recovery in patients with cervical spondylotic myelopathy. *Spine*, **38**(**14**), 1170–1176.

42 Sumi, M., Miyamoto, H., Suzuki, T., Kaneyama, S., Kanatani, T. & Uno, K. (2012) Prospective cohort study of mild cervical spondylotic myelopathy without surgical treatment. *Journal of Neurosurgery: Spine*, **16**(**1**), 8–14.

43 Cheung, W.Y., Arvinte, D., Wong, Y.W., Luk, K.D.K. & Cheung, K.M.C. (2008) Neurological recovery after surgical decompression in patients with cervical spondylotic myelopathy - a prospective study. *International Orthopaedics*, **32**(**2**), 273–278.

44 Furlan, J.C., Kalsi-Ryan, S., Kailaya-Vasan, A., Massicotte, E.M. & Fehlings, M.G. (2011) Functional and clinical outcomes following surgical treatment in patients with cervical spondylotic myelopathy: a prospective study of 81 cases. *Journal of Neurosurgery: Spine*, **14**(**3**), 348–355.

45 Karpova, A., Arun, R., Davis, A.M. *et al.* (2013) Predictors of surgical outcome in cervical spondylotic myelopathy. *Spine*, **38**(**5**), 392–400.

46 Fehlings, M.G., Smith, J.S., Kopjar, B. *et al.* (2012) Perioperative and delayed complications associated with the surgical treatment of cervical spondylotic myelopathy based on 302 patients from the AOSpine North America Cervical Spondylotic Myelopathy Study. *Journal of Neurosurgery: Spine*, **16**(**5**), 425–432.

47 Saunders, R.L., Bernini, P.M., Shirrefks, T.G. & Reeves, A.G. (1991) Central corpectomy for cervical spondylotic myelopathy: a consecutive series with long-term follow-up evaluation. *Journal of Neurosurgery*, **74**(**2**), 163–170.

48 Ebersold, M.J., Pare, M.C. & Quast, L.M. (1995) Surgical treatment for cervical spondylitic myelopathy. *Journal of Neurosurgery*, **82**(**5**), 745–751.

49 Hadley, M.N. & Walters, B.C. (2013) Introduction to the guidelines for the management of acute cervical spine and spinal cord injuries. *Neurosurgery*, **72**, 5–16 0.1227/NEU. 0b013e3182773549.

50 Hadley, M.N., Walters, B.C., Aarabi, B. *et al.* (2013) Clinical assessment following acute cervical spinal cord injury. *Neurosurgery*, **72**, 40–53.

51 Ryken, T.C., Hadley, M.N., Walters, B.C. *et al.* (2013) Radiographic assessment. *Neurosurgery*, **72**, 54–72.

52 Hurlbert, R.J., Hadley, M.N., Walters, B.C. *et al.* (2013) Pharmacological therapy for acute spinal cord injury. *Neurosurgery*, **72**, 93–105.

53 Pointillart, V., Petitjean, M.E., Wiart, L. *et al.* (2000) Pharmacological therapy of spinal cord injury during the acute phase. *Spinal Cord*, **38**(**2**), 71–76.

54 Matsumoto, T., Tamaki, T., Kawakami, M., Yoshida, M., Ando, M. & Yamada, H. (2001) Early complications of high-dose methylprednisolone sodium succinate treatment in the follow-up of acute cervical spinal cord injury. *Spine*, **26**(**4**), 426–430.

55 Gelb, D.E., Aarabi, B., Dhall, S.S. *et al.* (2013) Treatment of subaxial cervical spinal injuries. *Neurosurgery*, **72**, 187–194.

56 Rozzelle, C.J., Aarabi, B., Dhall, S.S. *et al.* (2013) Spinal cord injury without radiographic abnormality (SCIWORA). *Neurosurgery*, **72**, 227–233.

57 Ryken, T.C., Hurlbert, R.J., Hadley, M.N. *et al.* (2013) The acute cardiopulmonary management of patients with cervical spinal cord injuries. *Neurosurgery*, **72**, 84–92.

58 Dhall, S.S., Hadley, M.N., Aarabi, B. *et al.* (2013) Deep venous thrombosis and thromboembolism in patients with cervical spinal cord injuries. *Neurosurgery*, **72**, 244–254.

CHAPTER 8
Delirium

William D. Freeman

Departments of Neurology, Neuosurgery, and Critical Care, Mayo Clinic Florida, Jacksonville, FL 32224, USA

Introduction

Delirium is an extremely common problem, especially in hospitalized settings [1]. From the 2002 National Hospital Discharge survey, 13 million hospitalized patients aged 65 and older, delirium occurred in up to half of patients [2]. Delirium is also associated with a 10–26% rate of in-hospital mortality [3] when delirium is the admitting diagnosis. When delirium occurs during hospitalization, the mortality is higher at 22–76% [4] and continues after hospital discharge. The increased mortality occurs regardless of adjustment for severity of illness, age, and pre-existing history of dementia [1]. Patients with delirium have a longer length of stay, increased hospitalization costs, and complications [4].

Delirium is also known as an acute confusional state and is not a disease per se, but a syndrome with multiple causes. Delirium results in a similar constellation of symptoms and must be distinguished from other phenotypic mimics such as dementia with memory impairment and psychosis, psychiatric disease such as bipolar disease [5]. Delirium may occur from an underlying medical disorder, infection, medication effect, postoperative state, or develop during the intensive care unit (ICU) stay due to critical illness and the sedative effects on brain physiology [1].

The diagnosis of delirium is fundamental to recognition and earlier treatment. The main diagnostic criteria for delirium as described in the Diagnostic and Statistical Manual of Mental disorders version 5 (DSM-V) can be summarized as follows:
- Disturbed awareness and reduced levels of concentration
- Disorientation and lapses of cognitive ability.
- Rapidly developing disturbance that fluctuates in severity.
- Empirical evidence supports a medical condition as cause of disturbance.

Other nonkey diagnostic indicators include disrupted sleep cycle, psychomotor perceptual or emotional disturbance, delusions, labile affect, dysarthria, and abnormal EEG output [5,6]. Delirium can also be classified into different clinical subtypes based on whether or not the patient has "hyperactive" or "hypoactive" symptoms [7]. In this study of 325 elderly patients using a structured instrument, they found about 15% of delirium patients were "hyperactive type" (15%), 19% were hypoactive, 52% were of a "mixed type" (52%), and 14% fell into no category (14%). This underscores the clinical variation in presentation and fluctuating course of delirium. Obtaining a thorough history is essential from the patient, caregiver, the patient's medical record or other healthcare providers to proper diagnosis. Patients with dementia typically have a chronic progressive history of memory or cognitive impairment. Most patients with dementia are docile unless they have an agitated progressive dementia such as frontotemporal dementia or a superimposed agitated delirium or psychosis. Delirium may even complicate hospitalization after stroke [8] and carries similar increased mortality and longer hospitalization similar to other literature. After the history is collected, a physical examination is typically performed with cognitive evaluation including orientation and basic neurological examination. Tremulousness, myoclonus, and even asterixis (bilateral) are often seen in acute delirium. Laboratory tests may be performed such as thyroid, renal, or hepatic function if there are historical or examination findings to suggest organic impairment. Drug screening of the urine or blood can be performed in those suspected of a toxic ingestion or drug overdose. Sometimes, drug or alcohol withdrawal (delirium tremens) is suggested by the history. If the patient is febrile or there is suspicion of infection, often urine analysis or culture, chest radiograph for pneumonia or blood cultures are performed if the patient has elevated serum white blood cell count. Serum glucose can be assessed readily and can exclude hypoglycemia or hyperglycemia as the cause of delirium especially in diabetics. In patients with an abnormal neurological examination or lateralizing weakness, neglect, or aphasia, neuroimaging such as a CT without contrast of the brain or MRI may be indicated. Electroencepahlogram (EEG) is usually nonspecific and

Evidence-Based Neurology: Management of Neurological Disorders, Second Edition. Edited by Bart M. Demaerschalk and Dean M. Wingerchuk.
© 2015 John Wiley & Sons, Ltd. Published 2015 by John Wiley & Sons, Ltd.

shows slowing and diminished cerebral activity or triphasic waves, especially with liver disease. Pulse oximetry (SpO2) may disclose hypoxia in some patients in which case may be the cause of delirium from an underlying pulmonary cause such as pneumonia. Lumbar puncture may be indicated if there is concern about CNS infection as the cause of delirium, such as meningitis.

Methodology

We performed PubMed database literature searches using the search terms, "delirium," with limits set for controlled clinical trials, clinical guidelines, systematic reviews, and meta-analyses specific to this topic. The GRADE system was performed [9] ranking the quality of the level of evidence with the following definitions: *high*, further research is very unlikely to change the confidence in the estimate of effect; *moderate*, further research is likely to impact the confidence in the estimate of effect and may change the estimate of effect; *low*, further research is very likely to have important changes on the confidence and estimate of effect; and *very low*, any estimate of effect is uncertain.

Recommendations were defined by the GRADE system using a weighted and operationally defined system, where *net benefit* is defined as when the intervention clearly does more good than harm; *trade-offs* defined when there are important considerations that must be taken into account between benefits and harms; *uncertain trade-offs* defined when it is unclear whether the intervention does more good than harm; and *no net benefit* defined when the intervention does not result in more good than harm.

Clinical questions and evidence

Clinical question (#1): What is the best approach to diagnose delirium?

Delirium is a clinical diagnosis. Therefore, the "gold standard" diagnosis reported in the literature is by clinical criteria and by a delirium expert [10]. However, there is a limited availability of such experts outside of research trials. In the absence of such a clinical expert, there is considerable and growing amounts of literature investigating the use of nonexpert screening tests to diagnose delirium compared to expert diagnosis that are effective. The Confusion Assessment Method (CAM) is an effective screening tool to help diagnose delirium [11]. For ICU patients, a recent meta-analysis by Neto *et al.* of 1,523 participants and five screening tools was reviewed [10]. The authors found the pooled sensitivities and specificities of Confusion Assessment Method for the Intensive Care Unit (CAM-ICU) tool for detection of delirium in critically ill patients in these studies to be 75.5% and 95.8%, respectively. Another method called the Intensive Care Delirium Screening Checklist had a sensitivity of 80.1% and specificity of 74.6%, respectively.

The reviewers pointed out that all measures had some heterogeneity of measurement, and all but one of these studies was performed in a research setting, with the one nonresearch study detecting only half of delirium cases.

(a) *GRADE level of evidence*: The quality of the evidence is *high* for expert clinical diagnosis of delirium, and the CAM has fairly high specificity for diagnosis of delirium in the research setting.

(b) *GRADE level of recommendation*: Further research is needed to validate the CAM method of delirium diagnosis in the clinical setting use outside of clinical trials for delirium diagnosis. There are *uncertain trade offs* that should be considered such as the benefits and costs of delirium screening and interventions, and pharmacological therapies such as antipsychotics that have side-effects. Future studies should measure the impact of delirium screening and intervention on patient outcomes.

Clinical question (#2): Once delirium is diagnosed, what is the best pharmacologic intervention?

Several consensus papers, systematic reviews, and guidelines suggest that once delirium is diagnosed that no single intervention, pharmacologic, and nonpharmacologic be implemented, but rather a multipronged approach should be utilized [1,12–15]. Of the pharmacologic interventions studied to reduce delirium severity, low-dose haloperidol (<3.0 mg per 24 hours) was compared to atypical antipsychotics olanzapine and risperdal and showed no difference in reduction in delirium severity [12]. Higher dose haloperidol >4.5 mg per 24 hours was associated with a higher association of extrapyramidal side-effects such as parkinsonism than atypical agents. Low-dose haloperidol is however effective when compared to placebo decreasing the degree and duration of postoperative delirium. The risks of haloperidol and other antipsychotic agents should be mentioned and include ECG effects such as potential QTc prolongation, extrapyramidal side-effects such as parkinsonism, and tardive dyskinesia. Additional caution should be applied in patients with pre-existing Parkinson's disease or parkinsonism since these patients are known to be especially sensitive. Benzodiazepines are not recommended for delirium unless it is associated with alcohol withdrawal [13]. Cholinergic agents such as donepezil and rivastigamine were ineffective in reducing severity of delirium [16,17].

(a) *GRADE level of evidence*: The quality of the evidence is *moderate* that low-dose haloperidal, and risperdal or olanzapine lessen the severity and shorten duration of delirium. In addition, there is a *moderate* amount of evidence by guidelines that suggest a multipronged approach to delirium patients should be employed beyond just pharmacologic therapy and includes frequent nursing assessments, and supportive care interventions.

(b) *GRADE level of recommendation*: There are *trade offs* to be considered in treating delirium patients pharmacologically, as well as overall cost and outcome benefits that need to be defined based on clinical outcomes of such interventions such as overall mortality. There is a moderate amount of evidence that benzodiazepines are not recommended for delirium unless it is associated with alcohol withdrawal. Additionally, cholinergic agents such as donepezil and rivastigamine are not effective in treating delirium in most patients. There is insufficient evidence to know whether or not removal of these agents in patients with Alzheimer's dementia taking them is harmful or not. Individual clinical judgment should prevail and be tailored to such patients.

Clinical question (#3): What are other evidence-based interventions are recommended in treating delirium?

Beyond pharmacological interventions, what other interventions can be used to treat delirium patients? Several systematic reviews and guidelines suggest a multi-interventional approach to delirium that combines screening for the disorder, as well as multiple interventions used to treat it are suggested [1,14,15]. For example, the NICE (National Institute for Health and Clinical Excellence) guidelines suggest a list of interventions to lessen delirium [14] and optimize patient outcomes (Table 8.1). For patients with delirium in the intensive care unit, adaptation of the CAM (ICU) screening assessment has been proposed, as well as daily sedation cessation in those it is safe to perform [18–20]. Additional strategies for ICU patients based on systematic reviews include early mobilization and minimizing sleep deprivation [21,22]. Additionally, one randomized trial demonstrated that simple earplugs in ICU patients reduced delirium by minimizing the effects of noise especially when used within the first 48 hours [23] (Hazard Ratio of 0.47 (95% confidence interval (CI) 0.27–0.82).

(a) *GRADE level of evidence*: The quality of the evidence is *moderate* for nonpharmacologic multiple interventions on delirium. Further research is likely to impact the confidence and estimate of effect.

(b) *GRADE level of recommendation*: There are *trade offs* to consider for multiple nonpharmacologic and protocolized interventions such as the costs and overall benefits of developing a hospitalized team that can screen for delirium and provide the multidisciplinary interventions proposed.

Clinical question (#4): How does delirium affect outcome?

A systematic review by Zhang [24] demonstrated that in 14 studies involving 5891 patients, delirious patients had higher mortality rate than nondelirious patients (OR: 3.22; 95% CI: 2.30–4.52), higher rate of complications (OR: 6.5; 95% CI: 2.7–15.6), and longer length of stay. Similar findings are reported in the systematic review by Khan *et al.* [1]. Unfortunately, we could not find a study in which an intervention was studied in a randomized controlled manner on delirium patients in terms on eventual patient outcomes.

Table 8.1 2010 National Institute for Health and Clinical Excellence (NICE). Recommendations for prevention of delirium in at-risk adults

1 Delirium patients should be cared for by a team of healthcare professionals who are familiar with delirium and persons at risk.

2 Screen within 24 hours of hospitalization patients at risk for delirium, and if detected provide a patient-specific, multipronged interventions for delirium.

3 Delirium patients should be care for by a multidisciplinary team trained and competent in delirium prevention and intervention.

4 Provide cognitive reorientation strategies by providing appropriate lighting, a clearly visible and easy to read clock, calendar and signage, talking with the patient to reorient them to the date, location, and recent events that can be facilitated by regular visits from family and friends.

5 Ensure adequate hydration and nutrition, and avoiding constipation, and possibly offering intravenous (or even subcutaneous) fluids keeping in mind comorbidities of heart failure or chronic kidney disease.

6 Optimize homeostasis such as preventing hypoxia, providing supplemental oxygen saturation if needed.

7 Prevent and treat infection, avoid unnecessary urinary catheterization, and implement infection-control procedures such as hand hygiene of medical personnel, sterile access of central venous catheters, and decontamination procedures for patient bodily fluids or feces.

8 Promote mobilization consulting physical therapists or equivalent to walk patients after surgery (providing walking aids if needed and fall precautions) or during hospitalization.

9 Monitor and treat pain as needed.

10 Identify and optimize communication. Identify communication impediments such as hearing or learning impairments by providing hearing aids or speaking clearly and slowly with unsophisticated terminology. Identify language impairments or differences and if needed obtain a translator. For patients with a tracheostomy consider a communication board for them to write or communicate their needs.

11 Review medications for appropriateness because some medications are known to worsen delirium and reduce polypharmacy.

12 Screen for other sensory impairments such as hearing deficits from ear wax, lack of hearing aids, vision impairment due to lack of corrective lenses by providing them.

13 Promote normal day and night light and sleep patterns. Minimize nursing checks, vital sign, laboratory draws, and other medical procedures during sleeping hours if possible. Minimize noise during the night.

Source: Modified from O'Mahony 2011 [14].

(a) *GRADE level of evidence*: The quality of the evidence is *high* that delirium increases mortality, prolongs hospital and ICU length of stay, as well as hospitalized complications.

(b) *GRADE level of recommendation*: There are *uncertain trade-offs* based on the risks of the interventions proposed due to the lack of randomized or comparative outcomes trials. Expert guidelines and systematic reviews suggest, however, a multidisciplinary screening and interventional response to delirium to optimize patient outcomes. Future prospective trials evaluating these methods against nonprotocolized interventions are need to measure difference in outcomes.

Summary

Delirium is a common syndrome caused by various medical conditions that requires prompt recognition. Delirium is associated with increased mortality, hospital length of stay, and complications. Expert guidelines and systematic reviews suggest that a multidisciplinary team of nurses and medical professionals should screen for this delirium, and when diagnosed it should be treated with a multi-interventional approach (both supportive and possibly pharmacologic). Future research is needed to validate the sensitivity of the delirium screening tools such as the CAM method against expert clinician diagnosis outside of research trials. Further research is needed on specified antidelirium interventions on patient outcomes such as mortality.

Acknowledgments/Disclosures

The author reports no conflict of interest or funding for this manuscript.

References

1 Khan, B.A., Zawahirii, M., Campbell, N.L., Fox, G.C. *et al.* (2012) Delirium in hospitalized patients: implications of current evidence on clinical practice and future avenues for research—a systematic evidence review. *Journal of Hospital Medicine*, **7**, 580–589.

2 DeFrances, C.J. & Hall, M.J. (2004) 2002 National Hospital Discharge Survey. *Advance Data*, **342**, 1–29.

3 McCusker, J., Cole, M., Abrahamowicz, M., Primeau, F. & Belzile, E. (2002) Delirium predicts 12-month mortality. *Archives of Internal Medicine*, **162**(**4**), 457–463.

4 Marcantonio, E.R., Kiely, D.K., Simon, S.E. *et al.* (2005) Outcomes of older people admitted to postacute facilities with delirium. *Journal of American Geriatrics Society*, **53**(**6**), 963–969.

5 Blazer, D.G. & van Nieuwenhuizen, A.O. (2012) Evidence for the diagnostic criteria of delirium: an update. *Current Opinion in Psychiatry*, **25**(**3**), 239–243 doi: 10.1097/YCO.0b013e3283523ce8.

6 American Psychiatric Association (APA). (2010) *Diagnostic and Statistical Manual of mental disorders, version 5 (DSM-V)*. www.dsm5 .org. Document link at http://www.dsm5.org/Proposed%20

Revision%20Attachments/APA%20Neurocognitive%20 Disorders%20Proposal%20for%20DSM-5.pdf.

7 Liptzin, B. & Levkoff, S.E. (1992) An empirical study of delirium subtypes. *The British Journal of Psychiatry*, **161**, 843–845.

8 Shi, Q., Presutti, R., Selchen, D. & Saposnik, G. (2012) Delirium in acute stroke: a systematic review and meta-analysis. *Stroke*, **43**(**3**), 645–649 doi: 10.1161/STROKEAHA.111.643726. Epub 2012 Jan 19.

9 Atkins, D., Best, D., Briss, P.A., Eccles, M. *et al.* (2004) Grading quality of evidence and strength of recommendations. *BMJ*, **328**(**7454**), 1490.

10 Neto, A.S., Nassar, A.P. Jr., Cardoso, S.O. *et al.* (2012 Jun) Delirium screening in critically ill patients: a systematic review and meta-analysis. *Critical Care Medicine*, **40**(**6**), 1946–1951 doi: 10.1097/CCM.0b013e31824e16c9.

11 Inouye, S.K., Van Dyck, C.H., Alessi, C.A., Balkin, S., Siegal, A.P. & Horwitz, R.I. (1990) Clarifying delirium: the confusion assessment method. A new method for detection of delirium. *Annals of Internal Medicine*, **113**(**12**), 941–948.

12 Lonergan, E., Britton, A.M., Luxenberg, J. & Wyller, T. (2007) Antipsychotics for delirium. *Cochrane Database of Systematic Reviews*, **2**, CD005594.

13 Mayo-Smith, M.F. (1997) Pharmacological management of alcohol withdrawal. A meta-analysis and evidence-based practice guideline. American Society of Addiction Medicine Working Group on Pharmacological Management of Alcohol Withdrawal. *JAMA*, **278**(**2**), 144–151.

14 O'Mahony, R., Murthy, L., Akunne, A., Young, J. & Guideline Development Group (2011) Synopsis of the National Institute for Health and Clinical Excellence guideline for prevention of delirium. *Annals of Internal Medicine*, **154**(**11**), 746–51 doi: 10.1059/0003-4819-154-11-201106070-00006.

15 Inouye, S.K., Bogardus, S.T., Charpentier, P.A. *et al.* (1999) A multicomponent intervention to prevent delirium in hospitalized older patients. *The New England Journal of Medicine*, **340**(**9**), 669–676.

16 Overshott, R., Karim, S. & Burns, A. (2008) Cholinesterase inhibitors for delirium. *Cochrane Database of Systematic Reviews*, CD005317.

17 van Eijk, M.M., Roes, K.C., Honing, M.L., Kuiper, M.A., Karakus, A. & van der Jagt, M. (2010) Effect of rivastigamine as an adjunct to usual care with haloperidol on duration of delirium and mortality in critically ill patients: a multicentre, double-blind, placebo-controlled randomised trial. *Lancet*, **376**(**9755**), 1829–1837. doi:10.1016/S0140-6736(10)61855-7.

18 Ely, E.W., n, S.K. & Bernard, G.R. (2001) Delirium in mechanically ventilated patients: validity and reliability of the confusion assessment method for the intensive care unit (CAM-ICU). *JAMA*, **286**(**21**), 2703–2710.

19 Kress, J.P., Pohlman, A.S., O'Connor, M.F. & Hall, J.B. (2000) Daily interruption of sedative infusions in critically ill patients undergoing mechanical ventilation. *The New England Journal of Medicine*, **342**, 1471–1477.

20 Jacobi, J., Fraser, G.L., Coursin, D.B., Riker, R.R. Task Force of the American College of Critical Care Medicine (ACCM) of the

Society of Critical Care Medicine (SCCM), American Society of Health-System Pharmacists (ASHP), American College of Chest Physicians *et al.* (2002) Clinical practice guidelines for the sustained use of sedatives and analgesics in the critically ill adult. *Critical Care Medicine*, **30**, 119–141.

21 Kamdar, B.B., Needham, D.M. & Collop, N.A. (2012) Sleep deprivation in critical illness: its role in physical and psychological recovery. *Journal of Intensive Care Medicine*, **27**(**2**), 97–111.

22 Truong, A.D., Fan, E., Brower, R.G. & Needham, D.M. (2009) Bench-to-bedside review: mobilizing patients in the intensive care unit–from pathophysiology to clinical trials. *Critical Care*, **13**(**4**), 216. doi:10.1186/cc7885.

23 Van Rompaey, B., Elseviers, M.M., Van Drom, W., Fromont, V. & Jorens, P.G. (2012) The effect of earplugs during the night on the onset of delirium and sleep perception: a randomized controlled trial in intensive care patients. *Critical Care*, **16**(**3**), R73. doi:10.1186/cc11330.

24 Zhang, Z., Pan, L. & Ni, H. (2013) Impact of delirium on clinical outcome in critically ill patients: a meta-analysis. *Gen Hosp Psychiatry*, **35**(**2**), 105–111. doi:10.1016/j.genhosppsych.2012.11.003.

CHAPTER 9

Status epilepticus

Kameshwar Prasad[1], Manya Prasad[2], Sridharan Ramaratnam[3], and Anthony G. Marson[4]

[1]*Department of Neurology, All India Institute of Medical Sciences, New Delhi, India*

[2]*Department of Community Medicine, Pandit Bhagwat Dayal Sharma Post Graduate Institute of Medical Sciences, Rohtak, Haryana, India*

[3]*Department of Neurology, SIMS Hospitals, Chennai, Tamil Nadu, India*

[4]*Department of Molecular and Clinical Pharmacology, Institute of Translational Medicine, University of Liverpool, Liverpool, Merseyside, UK*

Background

Status epilepticus is defined as a condition in which either there is more than 30 minutes of continuous seizure activity or two or more sequential seizures without recovery of full consciousness between the seizures. Status epilepticus is a medical emergency. It is associated with an overall mortality of 8% in children and 30% in adults [1]. An additional 5–10% of people experiencing this condition have permanent sequelae, such as a permanent vegetative state or cognitive difficulties. Approximately 12–30% of adults with a new diagnosis of epilepsy are present in status epilepticus [2]. Some authors, depending on the duration of seizure activity, stipulate three stages of the condition: early, established and refractory. Early status epilepticus consists of the first 30 minutes of the epileptic state during which physiological mechanisms compensate for the greatly enhanced metabolic activity.

Established status epilepticus is defined as the stage beyond 30 minutes, where the status continues despite early stage treatment. It is during this phase that physiological compensation mechanisms begin to fail. If seizures continue for 60–90 minutes after the initiation of therapy, the stage of refractory status is said to have been reached. Status epilepticus may be convulsive or non-convulsive. Although convulsive status epilepticus is associated with a higher mortality and morbidity than non-convulsive status epilepticus, both require prompt and effective treatment. However, the most effective treatment regimen is not clear from the literature. Different experts give different recommendations regarding the best treatment regimen for status epilepticus [1–3], and the evidence base of many of these recommendations is often unclear. We conducted a systematic review of all the randomised controlled trials that we could identify to summarise the existing evidence, to delineate the reasons for disagreements and to highlight areas requiring further research.

Framing clinical questions and search for evidence

Clinically relevant questions in status epilepticus may include the following:

- Patient population: patients with early, established or refractory status epilepticus.
  - *Early* status epilepticus consists of the first 30 minutes of the epileptic state during which physiological mechanisms compensate for the greatly enhanced metabolic activity.
  - *Established* status epilepticus is defined as the stage beyond 30 minutes, where the status continues despite early stage treatment. It is during this phase that physiological compensation mechanisms begin to fail.
  - *Refractory* – if seizures continue for 60–90 minutes after the initiation of therapy, the stage of *refractory* status is said to have been reached.
- Interventions: all injectable anti-convulsants given intramuscular or intravenously, or in children, administered rectally or intranasally.
- Outcomes:
  - Outcomes in early or established status epilepticus:
    1 Death.
    2 Continuation of status epilepticus requiring use of a different drug or general anaesthesia for control.
    3 Long-term disabling sequelae, defined as persistent neurological deficits severe enough to require

dependence on some other person for activities of daily living (walking, toileting, bathing, dressing and eating) at 6 months after randomisation.

4 Need for ventilatory support.

5 Incomplete recovery before discharge, defined as inability to attain pre-status epilepticus state at the time of discharge. This outcome was included because most people attain their pre-status epilepticus state before discharge and are not followed up subsequently. People who do not recover need to be followed up in order to judge recovery or persistent deficit.

○ Outcomes in refractory status epilepticus:

1 Death.

2 Long-term sequelae defined as dependence for activities of daily living (walking, toileting, bathing, dressing and eating) assessed at 6 months or beyond, but if studies reported only 1 or 3 months after onset, this was treated as long-term outcome.

We searched the following databases:

1 Cochrane Epilepsy Group Specialized Register (December 2009);

2 Cochrane Central Database of Controlled Trials (CENTRAL) (The Cochrane Library Issue 4, 2009) using the strategy outlined in Appendix 1;

3 MEDLINE (1950 to December week 4, 2009) using the strategy outlined in Appendix 2.

In addition, we searched EMBASE (1966–January 2003) for the original version of this review.

Critical review of the evidence for each question

What is the pre-hospital treatment for status epilepticus? Is intramuscular midazolam non-inferior or superior to intravenous lorazepam?

There was a single RCT [4] with 893 participants. The study reported statistically significant difference favouring midazolam for cessation of seizures (329/448 vs. 282/445; RR 1.16 (1.06–1.27), for requirement for ICU admission (128/448 vs. 161/445 participants; RR 0.79, 95% CI 0.65–0.96) and for requirement for hospitalisation (258/448 vs. 292/445 participants; RR 0.88, 95% CI 0.79–0.97). There was no statistically significant difference between the two groups for following outcomes; endotracheal intubation (63/448 vs. 64/445 participants; RR 0.98, 95% CI 0.71–1.35); recurrence of seizures (51/448 vs. 47/445 participants; RR 1.08, 95% CI 0.74–1.57); adverse effects (16/448 vs. 18/445 participants; RR 0.88, 95% CI 0.46–1.71): for ICU stay (mean difference 1.60, CI −0.23 to 3.43, p =0.09); and length of hospital stay (mean difference 1.20, CI −0.24 to 2.64, p = 0.10).

In patients with early or established status epilepticus, what are the effects of treatment with lorazepam versus placebo?

We found one systematic review [5].

There was one RCT [6] with 137 participants. Compared to placebo, lorazepam had a statistically significant lower risk of non-cessation of seizures (27/66 vs. 56/71 participants; RR 0.52, 95% CI 0.38–0.71) and of continuation of status epilepticus requiring a different drug or general anaesthesia (27/66 vs. 56/71 participants; RR 0.52, 95% CI 0.38–0.71). There was a statistically non-significant but strong trend favouring lorazepam for the following outcomes: death (5/66 vs. 11/71 participants; RR 0.49, 95% CI 0.18–1.33); requirement for ventilatory support (7/66 vs. 16/71 participants; RR 0.47, 95% CI 0.21–1.07) and adverse effects (7/66 vs. 16/71 participants; RR 0.47, 95% CI 0.21–1.07).

There was a statistically non-significant trend favouring lorazepam for reducing requirement for ventilatory support (12/130 v 17/134 participants; RR 0.73; 95% CI 0.36–1.49) and adverse effects (7/130 vs. 11/134 participants; risk difference −0.03, 95% CI −0.10 to 0.03).

In patients with early or established status epilepticus, is lorazepam more effective or safer than diazepam?

We found two systematic reviews [5,7].

The first systematic review [7] included four trials involving 383 participants. It included only one quasi-randomised trial comparing IV lorazepam with IV diazepam. It revealed that IV lorazepam is as effective as IV diazepam in the treatment of acute tonic-clonic convulsions, 19/27 (70%) versus 22/34 (65%), RR 1.09 (95% CI 0.77–1.54), has fewer adverse events and rectal lorazepam may be more effective than rectal diazepam, 6/6 versus 6/19 (31%), RR 3.17 (95% CI 1.63–6.14).

In the second systematic review [5], there were three RCTs with 289 participants [6,8,9]. The outcome of death was available in two studies (203 participants). There was no statistically significant difference in deaths between the two groups (5/103 vs. 3/100 participants; risk difference 0.02; 95% CI −0.04 to 0.08). Compared to diazepam, lorazepam had statistically significant lower risk of non-cessation of seizures (32/130 vs. 51/134 participants; RR 0.64, 95% CI 0.45–0.90) and of continuation of status epilepticus requiring a different drug or general anaesthesia (32/130 participants vs. 52/134; RR 0.63, 95% CI 0.45–0.88).

In patients with early or established status epilepticus, is lorazepam IV more effective or safer than diazepam plus phenytoin IV?

We found one systematic review [5].

There were two RCTs [10,11] with 370 participants. The outcome of non-cessation of seizures and adverse effects were available in both the studies. There was a statistically non-significant trend favouring lorazepam for both non-cessation of seizures (34/185 vs. 42/185 participants; risk difference −0.04; CI −0.35 to 0.26) and adverse effects (46/187 vs. 53/183 participants; RR 0.85,

95% CI 0.63–1.15). The outcome of death and requirement of ventilatory support were available in one study. There was no statistically significant difference in outcome of death (0/88 vs. 0/90 participants and requirement of ventilatory support (0/88 vs. 0/90).

In patients with early or established status epilepticus, is lorazepam IV more effective or safer than phenobarbitone IV?

We found one systematic review [5].

A single RCT [11] with 188 participants showed no statistically significant difference in the risk of non-cessation of seizures (34/97 vs. 38/91 participants; RR 0.84, 95% CI 0.58–1.21) or adverse effects (42/97 vs. 46/91 participants; RR 0.86, 95% CI 0.63–1.16) between the two drugs.

In patients with early or established status epilepticus, is lorazepam IV more effective or safer than phenytoin IV?

We found one systematic review [5].

There was only one RCT [11] with 198 participants. Risk of non-cessation of seizures was less with lorazepam compared to phenytoin (34/97 vs. 57/101, RR 0.62, 95% CI 0.45–0.86). There was no statistically significant difference between the two groups regarding adverse effects (42/97 vs. 44/101, RR 0.99, 95% CI 0.72–1.37).

In patients with early or established status epilepticus, is lorazepam more effective or safer than levetiracetam?

We found no systematic reviews. We found one randomised controlled trial [12].

In the RCT [12], results are based on 79 patients. Both levetiracetam (LEV) and lorazepam (LOR) were equally effective. In the first instance, the SE was controlled by LEV in 76.3% (29/38) and by LOR in 75.6% (31/41) of patients. In those resistant to the above regimen, LEV controlled SE in 70.0% (7/10) and LOR in 88.9% (8/9) patients. The 24-hour freedom from seizure was also comparable by LEV in 79.3% (23/29) and LOR in 67.7% (21/31). LOR was associated with significantly higher need of artificial ventilation and insignificantly higher frequency of hypotension. For the treatment of SE, LEV is an alternative to LOR and may be preferred in patients with respiratory compromise and hypotension.

In patients with early or established status epilepticus, is lorazepam intranasal more effective or safer than paraldehyde I/M?

We found two systematic reviews [7] and [5]. One includes studies on children [7], and second includes studies on adults [5].

The first systematic review [7] included four trials involving 383 participants were included. There is moderate evidence that intranasal lorazepam is more effective than intramuscular paraldehyde for acute tonic-clonic convulsions and patients treated with intranasal lorazepam are significantly

less likely to require further anti convulsants to control continuing seizures, 8/80 (10%) versus 21/80 (26%), RR 0.58 (95% CI 0.42–0.79).

In the second systematic review [5], there was a single RCT [13] with 160 participants. There was no statistically significant difference between two groups for cessation of seizures (60/80 vs. 49/80 participants; RR 1.15, 95% CI 0.59–2.27). There was no statistically significant difference between two groups for deaths (15/80 vs. 13/80 participants; RR 1.15, 95% CI 0.59–2.27).

In patients with early or established status epilepticus, is midazolam IV more effective or safer than lorazepam IV?

We found one systematic review [5].

There was a single small RCT [14] with 27 participants. This study reported a statistically non-significant trend favouring midazolam regarding the following outcomes: non-cessation of seizures (1/15 vs. 4/12 participants; RR 0.2, 95% CI 0.03–1.56); requirement for ventilatory support (1/15 vs. 2/12 participants; RR 0.40, 95% CI 0.04–3.90) and adverse effects (1/15 vs. 2/12 participants; RR 0.40, 95% CI 0.04–3.90); and continuation of status epilepticus requiring a different drug or general anaesthesia (1/15 vs. 4/12 participants; RR 0.2, 95% CI 0.03–1.56).

In patients with early or established status epilepticus, is midazolam IV more effective or safer than diazepam IV?

We found one systematic review [5].

There was a single RCT [15] with 40 participants. There was no statistically significant difference between the two groups regarding the following outcomes: non-cessation of seizures (3/21 vs. 2/19 participants; RR 1.36, 95% CI 0.25–7.27); requirement for ventilatory support (11/21 vs. 9/19 participants; RR 1.11, 95% CI 0.59–2.07); and adverse effects (8/21 vs. 9/19 participants; RR 0.80, 95% CI 0.39–1.66). There was a statistically non-significant trend favouring diazepam for the outcome of death (8/21 vs. 2/19 participants; RR 3.62, 95% CI 0.87–14.97).

In patients with early or established status epilepticus, is midazolam IM more effective or safer than diazepam IV?

We found one systematic review [5].

A small single RCT [16] of 24 participants showed no statistically significant difference between the two groups for the following outcomes: non-cessation of seizures (1/13 vs. 1/11 participants; RR 0.85, 95% CI 0.06–12.01); requirement for ventilatory support (1/13 vs. 1/11 participants; RR 0.85, 95% CI 0.06–12.01); adverse effects (1/13 vs. 1/11 participants; RR 0.85, 95% CI 0.06–12.01); and continuation of status epilepticus requiring a different drug or general anaesthesia (1/13 vs. 1/11 participants; RR 0.85, 95% CI 0.06–12.01).

In patients with early or established status epilepticus is intranasal midazolam more effective or safer than diazepam IV?

We found one systematic review [7].

In the systematic review, four trials involving 383 participants were included. Intranasal midazolam is as effective as intravenous diazepam in the treatment of prolonged febrile convulsions, 23/26 (88%) versus 24/26 (92%), RR 0.96 (95% CI 0.8–1.14).

In patients with early or established status epilepticus, what are the effects of treatment with diazepam IV versus placebo IV?

We found one systematic review [5].

One hundred and thirty-nine participants in a single study [6] were analysed. Most of the outcomes significantly favoured diazepam: non-cessation of seizures (39/68 vs. 56/71 participants; RR 0.73, 95% CI 0.57–0.92); death (3/68 vs. 11/71 participants; RR 0.28, 95% CI 0.08–0.98); requirement for ventilatory support (6/68 vs. 16/71 participants; RR 0.39, 95% CI 0.16–0.94); and continuation of status requiring a different drug or general anaesthesia (39/68 vs. 56/71 participants; RR 0.73, 95% CI 0.57–0.92). There was a non-significant trend favouring diazepam for adverse effects (7/68 vs. 16/71 participants; RR 0.46, 95% CI 0.20–1.04).

In patients with early or established status epilepticus, what are the effects of treatment with rectal diazepam gel versus placebo gel?

We found one systematic review [5].

There were two RCTs [17,18] with a total of 165 participants. The risk of non-cessation of seizures was significantly less with diazepam gel compared to placebo gel (24/77 vs. 63/88 participants; RR 0.43, 95% CI 0.30–0.62). For adverse effects there was a strong but statistically non-significant trend towards the placebo gel (29/77 vs. 22/88 participants; RR 1.50, 95% RR 0.94–2.37).

In patients with early or established status epilepticus, is diazepam plus phenytoin IV more effective or safer than phenobarbitone IV?

We found one systematic review [5].

There were two RCTs [19,11] with a total of 222 participants. For the outcomes of death and requirement for ventilatory support, data were available in only one study (36 participants). There was no statistically significant difference between the two groups for the following outcomes: requirement for ventilatory support (6/18 vs. 6/18 participants; RR 1.00, 95% CI 0.40–2.52); adverse effects (57/113 vs. 55/109 participants, RR 1.00, 95% CI 0.77–1.30); and death (0/18 vs. 0/18 participants; risk difference 0.00, 95% CI −0.10 to 0.10). For non-cessation of seizures, the test for heterogeneity was significant and the type of status epilepticus studied was different, hence the two studies were analysed separately for this outcome. There was a weak statistically non-significant trend favouring phenobarbitone in one of the studies [19] (8/18 vs. 2/18 participants; RR

4.00, 95% CI 0.98–16.30). In the other larger study [11], there was no statistically significant difference between the two groups for non-cessation of seizures (42/95 vs. 38/91 participants; RR 1.06, 95% CI 0.76–1.47).

In patients with early or established status epilepticus, is diazepam plus phenytoin more effective or safer than phenytoin IV?

We found one systematic review [5].

There was a single RCT [11] with 196 participants. The study reported a statistically non-significant trend favouring diazepam plus phenytoin for non-cessation of seizures (42/95 vs. 57/101 participants; RR 0.78, 95% CI 0.59–1.04). There was no statistically significant difference between the two groups for adverse effects (48/95 vs. 44/101 participants, RR 1.16, 95% CI 0.86–1.56).

In patients with established status epilepticus, what is the safety and efficacy of pentobarbital versus midazolam versus propofol?

We found one systematic review [20].

The systematic review found that compared to midazolam or propofol, pentobarbital treatment was associated with a lower frequency of short-term treatment failure (8 vs. 23%; $p < 0.01$), breakthrough seizures (12 vs. 42%; $p < 0.001$), changes to a different cIV-AED (3 vs. 21%; $p < 0.001$) and a higher frequency of hypotension (systolic blood pressure <100 mm Hg; 77 vs. 34%; $p < 0.001$). Compared with seizure suppression ($n = 59$), titration of treatment to EEG background suppression ($n = 87$) was associated with a lower frequency of breakthrough seizures (4 vs. 53%; $p < 0.001$) and a higher frequency of hypotension (76 vs. 29%; $p < 0.001$).

In patients with early or established status epilepticus, is phenobarbitone IV more effective or safer than phenytoin IV?

We found one systematic review [5].

There was a single RCT [11] with 186 participants. There was a statistically non-significant trend favouring phenobarbitone for non-cessation of seizures (38/91 vs. 51/95 participants; RR 0.78, 95% CI 0.57–1.06). There was no statistically significant difference between the two groups for adverse effects (46/91 vs. 44/95 participants; RR 1.09, 95% CI 0.81–1.47).

In patients with early or established status epilepticus, is valproate more effective or safer than phenytoin?

We found two systematic reviews [21,22].
We found one randomised controlled trial [23].
The first systematic review [21] found that compared with diazepam, sodium valproate had a statistically significant lower risk of time interval for control of refractory status epilepticus (RSE) after having drugs; however, there was

no statistically significant difference in SE controlled within 30 minutes between the two groups. There was no statistically significant difference in cessation from status between intravenous sodium valproate and levetiracetam. Intravenous sodium valproate was as effective as intravenous phenytoin for SE controlled and risk of seizure continuation.

The second systematic review [22] found in a single RCT that compared with PHT, VPA had statistically lower risk of adverse effects (RR 0.31, 95% CI 0.12–0.85), with no differences in GCSE cessation after drug administration (RR 1.31, 95% CI 0.93–1.84) and in seizure freedom at 24 hours (RR 0.96, 95% CI 0.88–1.06). This review suggests that IV VPA has a better tolerability than PHT in treatment of GCSE, without any statistically significant differences in terms of efficacy. More rigorous RCTs of VPA versus an appropriate comparator, in a well-defined population with a systematic definition of SE, are however required to conclude about efficacy and tolerability of VPA in clinical practice.

In the RCT [24] found that valproate IV was successful in 88% and phenytoin IV in 84% ($p > 0.05$) of patients of SE with a significantly better response in patients of SE <2 hours ($p < 0.05$). The total number of adverse events did not differ significantly between the two groups ($p > 0.05$). There were no differences among the treatments with respect to recurrence after 12-hours study period or the outcome at 7 days.

In patients with early or established status epilepticus, is valproate IV more effective or safer than phenytoin IV or diazepam IV infusion or levetiracetam?

We found four systematic reviews [25,21,22,5].

The first systematic review [25] included only six RCTs, which were already included in earlier systematic reviews [5,21,22].

The second systematic review [21] found that compared with diazepam, sodium valproate had a statistically significant lower risk of time interval for control of RSE after having drugs; however, there was no statistically significant difference in SE controlled within 30 minutes between the two groups. There was no statistically significant difference in cessation of status between intravenous sodium valproate and levetiracetam. Intravenous sodium valproate was as effective as intravenous phenytoin for control of SE and risk of seizure continuation.

The third systematic review [22] found that compared with PHT, VPA had statistically lower risk of adverse effects (RR 0.31, 95% CI 0.12–0.85), with no differences in GCSE cessation after drug administration (RR 1.31, 95% CI 0.93–1.84) and in seizure freedom at 24 hours (RR 0.96, 95% CI 0.88–1.06). This review suggests that IV VPA has a better tolerability than PHT in treatment of GCSE, without any statistically significant differences in terms of efficacy. More rigorous RCTs of VPA versus an appropriate comparator, in a well-defined population with a systematic

definition of SE, are however required to conclude about efficacy and tolerability of VPA in clinical practice.

The fourth systematic review [5] included a single RCT [24] with 66 participants comparing intravenous valproate with diazepam infusion. There was a no statistically significant difference between two groups for effective control of seizures (15/30 vs. 20/36 participants; RR 0.90, 95% CI 0.57–1.43).

In patients with established status epilepticus, is propofol IV more effective or safer than barbiturates I/V?

We found one systematic review [5].

There was a single RCT [26] with 23 participants comapring propofol with barbiturates. There was no statistically significant difference between the two groups in any of the following outcomes: RSE controlled with first course of drug (6/14 vs. 2/9 participants; RR 1.93, 95% CI 0.49–7.54); RSE treated subsequently (4/8 vs. 5/7 participants; RR 0.7, 95% CI 0.3–1.62); thrombotic/embolic complication (0/14 vs. 0/9 participants); mortality (6/14 vs. 3/9 participants; RR 1.29, 95% CI 0.43–3.88); functional outcome at three weeks (5/14 vs. 3/9 participants; RR 1.07, 95% CI 0.34–3.42); infection requiring antibiotics (7/14 vs. 6/9 participants; RR 0.75, 95% CI 0.37–1.51).

Summary

Status epilepticus is a life-threatening emergency. Aim of treatment is to achieve cessation of seizures as early as possible without serious adverse effects. Buccal midazolam, rectal diazepam and intramuscular midazolam are effective in controlling seizures and may be used out-of-hospital. In early or established status, intravenous lorazepam is more effective and safer than intravenous diazepam in cessation of seizures, but for maintaining seizure-free status, intravenous phenytoin, phenobarbitone, valproate or levetiracetam are effective and safe. More randomised controlled comparative trials are needed to study drugs for the established and refractory stages of status epilepticus.

Acknowledgements

We thank All India Institute of Medical Sciences, New Delhi, India, and the editorial board of the Cochrane Epilepsy Review Group, Liverpool, UK, for all the support extended to us in completing this chapter.

References

1 Treatment of convulsive status epilepticus. (1993) Recommendations of the Epilepsy Foundation of America's Working Group on Status Epilepticus. *JAMA, the Journal of the American Medical Association,* **270**(**7**), 854–859.

2 Lowenstein, D.H. & Alldredge, B.K. (1998) Status epilepticus. *The New England Journal of Medicine,* **338**(**14**), 970–976.

3 Prasad, K. (1995) Management of convulsive status epilepticus. In: Chaubey, P.C. (ed), Current Practice in Emergency Care. Saurabh Publishers, New Delhi, pp. 170–173.

4 Silbergleit, R., Durkalski, V., Lowenstein, D. et al. (2012 Feb 16) Intramuscular versus intravenous therapy for prehospital status epilepticus. *The New England Journal of Medicine*, **366(7)**, 591–600.

5 Prasad, K., Al-Roomi, K., Krishnan, P.R. & Sequeira, R. (2005) Anticonvulsant therapy for status epilepticus. *Cochrane Database of Systematic Reviews*, **(4)**, CD003723.

6 Alldredge, B.K., Gelb, A.M., Isaacs, S.M. et al. (2001) A comparison of lorazepam, diazepam, and placebo for the treatment of out-of-hospital status epilepticus. *The New England Journal of Medicine*, **345(9)**, 631–637.

7 Appleton, R., Macleod, S. & Martland, T. (2008) Drug management for acute tonic-clonic convulsions including convulsive status epilepticus in children. *Cochrane Database of Systematic Reviews*, **(3)**, CD001905.

8 Appleton, R., Sweeney, A., Choonara, I., Robson, J. & Molyneux, E. (1995) Lorazepam versus diazepam in the acute treatment of epileptic seizures and status epilepticus. *Developmental Medicine and Child Neurology*, **37(8)**, 682–688.

9 Leppik, I.E., Derivan, A.T., Homan, R.W., Walker, J., Ramsay, R.E. & Patrick, B. (1983) Double-blind study of lorazepam and diazepam in status epilepticus. *JAMA, the Journal of the American Medical Association*, **249(11)**, 1452–1454.

10 Sreenath, T.G., Gupta, P., Sharma, K.K. & Krishnamurthy, S. (2010) Lorazepam versus diazepam-phenytoin combination in the treatment of convulsive status epilepticus in children: a randomized controlled trial. *European Journal of Paediatric Neurology*, **14(2)**, 162–168.

11 Treiman, D.M., Meyers, P.D., Walton, N.Y. et al. (1998) A comparison of four treatments for generalized convulsive status epilepticus. Veterans Affairs Status Epilepticus Cooperative Study Group. *The New England Journal of Medicine*, **339(12)**, 792–798.

12 Misra, U.K., Kalita, J. & Maurya, P.K. (2012) Levetiracetam versus lorazepam in status epilepticus: a randomized, open labeled pilot study. *Journal of Neurology*, **259(4)**, 645–648.

13 Ahmad, S., Ellis, J.C., Kamwendo, H. & Molyneux, E. (2006) Efficacy and safety of intranasal lorazepam versus intramuscular paraldehyde for protracted convulsions in children: an open randomised trial. *Lancet*, **367(9522)**, 1591–1597.

14 McCormick, E.M., Lieh-lai, M., Knazik, S. & Negro, M. (1999) A prospective comparison of midazolam and lorazepam in the initial treatment of status epilepticus in the pediatric patient. *Epilepsia*, **40(7)**, 160.

15 Singhi, S., Murthy, A., Singhi, P. & Jayashree, M. (2002) Continuous midazolam versus diazepam infusion for refractory convulsive status epilepticus. *Journal of Child Neurology*, **17(2)**, 106–10.

16 Chamberlain, J.M., Altieri, M.A., Futterman, C., Young, G.M., Ochsenschlager, D.W. & Waisman, Y. (1997) A prospective, randomized study comparing intramuscular midazolam with intravenous diazepam for the treatment of seizures in children. *Pediatric Emergency Care*, **13(2)**, 92–94.

17 Cereghino, J.J., Cloyd, J.C., Kuzniecky, R.I. & North American Diastat Study Group (2002) Rectal diazepam gel for treatment of acute repetitive seizures in adults. *Archives of Neurology*, **59(12)**, 1915–1920.

18 Pellock, J.M. (1998) Treatment of seizures and epilepsy in children and adolescents. *Neurology*, **51(5 Suppl 4)**, S8–S14.

19 Shaner, D.M., McCurdy, S.A., Herring, M.O. & Gabor, A.J. (1988) Treatment of status epilepticus: a prospective comparison of diazepam and phenytoin versus phenobarbital and optional phenytoin. *Neurology*, **38(2)**, 202–207.

20 Claassen, J., Hirsch, L.J., Emerson, R.G. & Mayer, S.A. (2002) Treatment of refractory status epilepticus with pentobarbital, propofol, or midazolam: a systematic review. *Epilepsia*, **43(2)**, 146–153.

21 Liu, X., Wu, Y., Chen, Z., Ma, M. & Su, L. (2012) A systematic review of randomized controlled trials on the therapeutic effect of intravenous sodium valproate in status epilepticus. *International Journal of Neuroscience*, **122(6)**, 277–283.

22 Brigo, F., Storti, M., Del Felice, A., Fiaschi, A. & Bongiovanni, L.G. (2012) IV Valproate in generalized convulsive status epilepticus: a systematic review. *Official Journal of the European Paediatric Neurology Society*, **19(9)**, 1180–1191.

23 Agarwal, P., Kumar, N., Chandra, R., Gupta, G., Antony, A.R. & Garg, A. (2007) Randomized study of intravenous valproate and phenytoin in status epilepticus. *Seizure*, **16(6)**, 527–532.

24 Rossetti, A.O. & Lowenstein, D.H. (2011) Management of refractory status epilepticus in adults: still more questions than answers. *Lancet Neurology*, **10(10)**, 922–930.

25 Trinka, E., Höfler, J., Zerbs, A. & Brigo, F. (2014) Efficacy and safety of intravenous valproate for status epilepticus: a systematic review. *CNS Drugs*, **28(7)**, 623–639.

26 Chen, W.B., Gao, R., Su, Y.Y. et al. (2011) Valproate versus diazepam for generalized convulsive status epilepticus: a pilot study. *European Journal of Neurology*, **18(12)**, 1391–1396.

10 CHAPTER 10
Raised intracranial pressure

William David Freeman

Departments of Neurology and Critical Care, Mayo Clinic Florida, Jacksonville, FL 32224, USA

Introduction

Normal intracranial pressure (ICP) is typically greater than 0 mmHg but less than 15 mmHg. Raised ICP also known as intracranial hypertension is defined as an ICP, which is sustained higher than 20 mmHg. ICP must be measured through an invasively placed brain catheter. The two most common types of ICP monitoring probes are either an intraventricular catheter (IVC), which can drain cerebrospinal fluid (CSF) and detects ICP, or a parenchymal ICP probe. IVC have the ability to drain CSF and thus can be diagnostic and therapeutic in conditions in which there is hydrocephalus or build up of CSF. Table 10.1 lists the main pathophysiologic categories of raised intracranial pressure.

Regardless of the underlying cause, elevations in ICP reduce cerebral perfusion pressure (CPP) because the equation for CPP = MAP−ICP, where mean arterial pressure (MAP). If ICP equals MAP (e.g. if ICP = MAP), then CPP = 0. If CPP = 0 for more than a few minutes, intracranial circulation arrest occurs, which causes global brain ischemia from lack of cerebral blood flow (CBF). If this is not immediately corrected, this leads to global brain ischemia, edema, and subsequent brain death. The clinical manifestations of elevated intracranial pressure depend on the acuity of the disease. For example, if ICP is chronic, mild, and progressive, then headache, nausea, and papilledema can occur. In contrast, when an abrupt ICP crisis occurs (i.e. >60 mmHg), a patient may present comatose or in stupor due to reduced CPP and CBF.

Other causes of raised ICP include massive ischemic stroke with secondary cytotoxic brain edema (most commonly from middle cerebral artery occlusion) or carotid occlusion, or intracranial bleeding (intraparenchymal and/or intraventricular). Secondary brain injury can occur when elevations in ICP lead to drops in CPP, causing more cerebral ischemia and edema. This can lead to more elevations in ICP and drops in CPP, causing a vicious cycle –and if unchecked – leading to possible brain death. For example, in severe TBI with global brain edema or large middle cerebral artery (MCA) infarction, progressive brain edema can lead to uncontrolled ICP, very low CPP, cerebral herniation, and brain death. Management of ICP is, therefore, aimed at alleviating ICP but also optimizing CPP by raising MAP as well. This chapter reviews the evidence-based treatments for raised intracranial pressure. Table 10.2 provides an overview of the methods discussed as well as major risks of therapy.

Methodology

We performed PubMed and Cochrane database literature searches using the search terms, "intracranial pressure," with limits set for randomized controlled trials, clinical guidelines, systematic reviews, controlled clinical trials, and meta-analyses specific to this topic. We also reviewed any review articles on the subject. The GRADE system was utilized to rank the level of evidence [10], which uses the following definitions in grading the quality of the evidence: *high*, further research is very unlikely to change the confidence in the estimate of effect; *moderate*, further research is likely to impact the confidence in the estimate of effect and may change the estimate of effect; *low*, further research is very likely to have important changes on the confidence and estimate of effect; *very low*, any estimate of effect is uncertain. Recommendations are weighted and operationally defined by the GRADE system, where the *net benefit* is defined as when the intervention clearly does more good than harm; *trade-offs* defined as when important considerations must be taken into account between benefits and harms; *uncertain trade-offs* defined as when it is unclear whether the intervention does more good than harm; and *no net benefit* defined when the intervention does not result in more good than harm.

Evidence-Based Neurology: Management of Neurological Disorders, Second Edition. Edited by Bart M. Demaerschalk and Dean M. Wingerchuk.
© 2015 John Wiley & Sons, Ltd. Published 2015 by John Wiley & Sons, Ltd.

Table 10.1 Major pathophysiologic categories of raised intracranial pressure (ICP)

Stroke
- Intracranial hemorrhage (ICH) with or without intraventricular hemorrhage (IVH),
- Supratentorial large ischemic infarct (malignant middle cerebral artery (MCA) or internal carotid artery (ICA) infarction)
- Subarachnoid hemorrhage (SAH) with hydrocephalus and/or IVH
- Posterior fossa infarction or ICH 3 cm or greater

Mass lesion
- Brain tumor – astrocytoma (infratentorial/supratentorial, e.g. glioblastoma multiforme), glioma, meningioma, oligodendroglioma, metastatic brain tumor (e.g., small cell carcinoma or adenocarcinoma, renal cell carcinoma, melanoma)
- Abscess – bacterial (endocarditis, staphylococcus, or gram negative), fungal (e.g., most common in immunocompromised patients (HIV/AIDS, transplant recipients)

Hydrocephalus
- Communicating – microscopic obstruction of the arachnoid granulations that filter CSF exiting the subarachnoid space and drain into the cerebral venous sinuses and into the jugular vein. For example, SAH, meningitis, and other processes that cause build up of debris that clog the arachnoid granulations.
- Non-communicating (obstructive) – blockage of one of the ventricular CSF pathways (lateral ventricles → foramen of Monro → 3rd ventricle → cerebral aqueduct → 4th ventricle → foramen of Magendie (medial) and Luschka (lateral)

Brain edema
- Cytotoxic – traumatic brain injury (TBI) with diffuse axonal injury (DAI), hypoxic-ischemic brain injury (HIBI) with global cerebral edema (GCE, subarachnoid hemorrhage (SAH) with GCE, acute liver failure (ALF) with global brain edema
- Vasogenic – brain tumor

Venous obstruction
- Sagittal sinus thrombosis (SST) or cortical vein thrombosis (CVT) leading to venous hypertension, build up of hydrostatic CSF pressure within the ventricle or region of brain with venous obstruction

Idiopathic
- Pseudotumor cerebri

Table 10.2 Overview of methods to control ICP

Treatment	Side effects
Mannitol 20%	Dehydration, hypernatremia, hyperosmolar state, osmotic diuresis, electrolyte and volume depletion, and hypotension. Caution in renal failure and congestive heart failure
Hypertonic saline (HTS)	Hypernatremia, hyperosmolar state, volume and sodium overload (anasarca) with repeated use, central pontine myelinolysis (rare), red blood cell lysis
Sedation and analgesia	Depressed neurologic examination
Neuromuscular blockade	Respiratory arrest, need for mechanical ventilation, neuromuscular weakness, CNS toxicity at high doses, loss of neurological exam (except pupils)
Barbiturates	Cardiac depressant, hemodynamic instability, immune depression, prolonged barbiturate cognitive depression with high-dose, long-duration use
Hypothermia	Bradycardia and QT prolongation proportionate to in-depth of hypothermia, immune suppression, glucose elevation because of increased insulin requirements in hypothermia, which are reversed when rewarmed. Shiver
Craniectomy	Surgical bleeding, infection

Clinical question (#1): What is the best initial medical therapy in reducing intracranial pressure?

One of the most widely available agents for raised ICP is mannitol, an osmotic diuretic. Mannitol has demonstrated efficacy in three randomized controlled trials in reducing ICP compared to pentobarbital (RR for death = 0.85; 95% CI 0.52–1.38), mannitol compared to hypertonic saline (RR for death = 1.25; 95% CI 0.47–3.33), and mannitol compared to conservative therapy (RR for death = 0.83; 95% CI 0.47–1.46) [1]. These data suggest that mannitol when used for treatment of raised ICP may reduce mortality when compared to pentobarbital and conservative therapy, but mannitol's effect may be inferior to hypertonic saline effect on mortality. One prospective study in humans demonstrated that 20% mannitol against equimolar osmotic methods of 30% urea and 10% glycerol worked similar to reducing ICP [2]. Barbiturates are reported effective in reducing ICP in TBI patients in guidelines, but the benefits must be weighed against cardiac depressant effects, reduced systemic vascular resistance, added cerebral dysautoregulatory effects, and possibly negative immune system effects [3]. Modest hyperventilation ($PaCO_2$ ~30–35) is effective in reducing ICP but should only be used as an early, transient intervention until another method of ICP control is obtained. Prolonged hyperventilation and aggressive hyperventilation ($PaCO_2$ ~25 or less) is harmful on patient outcomes [4]. Sedation and neuromuscular blockade are reported to control ICP in refractory or severe ICP cases, but there is no outcome data [5].

More recently hypertonic saline (HTS) has been studied of varying concentrations including 3%, 7.5%, or 23.4% in reducing ICP. It should be noted that 20% mannitol can be given through a peripheral IV, whereas hypertonic saline (>3%) is typically administered through a central venous catheter (CVC) or line [5,6]. The risks of CVC placement must be weighed against the benefits of such catheter placement and in emergent situations, the risks of the delay in ICP treatment of ICP considered until such a line is placed. In a prospective randomized study of 20 TBI patients, 20% mannitol (1160 mOsm/kg/H(2)O) was compared against 7.5% hypertonic saline ((2400 mOsm/kg/H(2)O) using an infusion based on 2 ml/kg body weight for ICP elevations. The data showed that both agents reduced ICP, but HTS was more effective by virtue of less subsequent ICP elevations over several days compared to mannitol [7], as well as less "treatment failure" in reducing ICP with repeated use of HTS compared to mannitol. A criticism of the study is lack of equimolar comparison of the two agents and relative small sample size. However, subsequent meta-analyses of eight prospective randomized trials comparing mannitol and HTS demonstrate that both agents reduce ICP, but that HTS (7.5% boluses or 23.4% boluses) may work longer than mannitol and have less treatment failure [8–10]. There are a number of physiological factors, however, that need to be considered in choosing a hyperosmotic agent, such as serum sodium, intravascular volume status (since mannitol is an osmotic diuretic and can induce diuresis), systemic hemodynamics, and mannitol's effect on improved blood rheology. HTS however has a reflection coefficient of 1.0, which is better than mannitol being 0.9, meaning there is less theoretical risk of extravasation of mannitol across the blood brain barrier and exacerbating brain edema. However, this is a theoretical risk that is poorly substantiated in clinical trials.

Indomethacin is another medical therapy reported for ICP reduction. A randomized, placebo-controlled study investigated 30 patients with supratentorial mass lesions who underwent craniotomy and received either indomethacin (IV bolus of 0.2 mg/kg followed by an infusion of 0.2 mg/kg/h) or placebo. The study showed that indomethacin did not reduce ICP but did significantly decrease cerebral blood flow velocity compared to placebo [11]. This drug however in a separate prospective, controlled study by Puppo et al. in 16 severe TBI patients showed the drug did reduce ICP, providing conflicting data [12]. Indomethacin also carries risks especially with repeated use of gastrointestinal (GI) mucosal injury, GI bleeding, and renal failure.

(a) *GRADE level of evidence*: There is a *moderate* level of evidence that the interventions of mannitol and hypertonic saline reduce raised ICP as compared to other medical therapies or when compared to conservative therapy. There are limitations in the evidence of mannitol compared to other equivalent medical therapies other than the therapies listed earlier, requiring further comparative randomized controlled trials. Furthermore, there are limited data about equimolar mannitol compared to HTS in terms of eventual clinical outcomes. Other therapies reported to reduce ICP include barbiturates, glycerol, urea, and possibly indomethacin.

(b) *GRADE recommendations*: Both mannitol and HTS have *trade-offs* in terms of benefits in reducing ICP weighed against risks. Both mannitol and HTS when used in equimolar doses appear equally effective in reducing ICP. Mannitol remains a widely available and efficacious agent for emergent ICP crises and can be given via a peripheral IV line. This treatment should be weighed against subsequent diuretic effects, electrolyte depletion if repeated therapy is needed since significant hemodynamic intravascular volume depletion can occur after therapy. These side effects can be offset by physiological saline and electrolyte replacement. Mannitol should be used with caution and potentially avoided in patients with severe congestive heart failure and renal failure. In patients who have a central venous catheter or central line, HTS boluses (7.5%, 23.4%) or a 3% HTS infusion appear at least equally effective in reducing ICP compared to mannitol and may provide more prolonged benefit. Future prospective randomized trials of larger sample size in comparison with equimolar concentrations of mannitol and HTS and with similar study methodology comparing clinical outcomes in a homogeneous patient population are needed. Barbiturates are effective in reducing ICP, but the risks of prolonged sedation, need for mechanical ventilation, immune and cardiac depression weighed against the benefits.

Clinical question (#2): What is the role for corticosteroids in elevated ICP?

Corticosteroids have been studied in acute cerebral infarction, and acute intracerebral hemorrhage in two controlled studies. Both studies were negative in terms of any statistical significance in terms of outcome or change in cerebral spinal fluid pressure [13,14]. Corticosteroids were also studied in TBI and found to be ineffective and are no longer recommended in national guidelines [15,16]. Corticosteroids are effective in reducing vasogenic brain edema with brain tumors, however [17].

(a) *GRADE level of evidence*: There is a *moderate* level of evidence that the intervention of corticosteroids is ineffective in controlling ICP in TBI, cerebral edema from acute cerebral hemorrhage, and acute cerebral infarction. Corticosteroids are temporarily effective in vasogenic brain edema from tumors (both primary and metastatic), but there is limited data [18,19].

(b) *GRADE recommendations*: Corticosteroids have *no net benefit* for TBI, acute cerebral hemorrhage, and infarction. There are *trade-offs* when used for brain-tumor-related cerebral edema and presumed ICP elevation for these patients, or in the perioperative setting to help with postoperative nausea and vomiting. Side effects from corticosteroids must be considered and the inherent risk such as hyperglycemia especially in diabetic patients and gastrointenstinal bleeding or ulceration caused from such therapies. Utilization of glucose monitoring and insulin if needed for hyperglycemia and H_2 blocking medication or proton-pump inihibitor medication for gastrointestinal prophylaxis may help offset these side effects of glucocorticoids. If corticosteroids are used beyond 1–2 months for brain tumor patients, immunosuppressive risks should be considered and some prophylaxis patients for pneumocystis carinii (PCP), gastrointenstinal, and osteoporotic effects (vitamin D, calcium, or bisphosphonate agents).

Clinical question (#3): How effective is craniectomy on ICP?

Craniectomy or removal of calvarial bone is typically done after medical therapy to control ICP has failed. Decompressive hemicraniectomy (DHC) is removal of bone over one-half of the skull and is typically done for malignant MCA infarction. Bifrontal craniectomy (BFC) has been studied in one randomized controlled trial [20]. DHC has been studied in three randomized controlled trials and a meta-analysis for space-occupying malignant MCA infarction [21–23], and in one review on treatment of cerebral venous thrombosis with herniation [24]. The randomized trial data show improved survival when compared to conservative therapy that is statistically significant for malignant MCA infarction but not for TBI. For DHC for malignant MCA infarction, there is an improvement in survival but is associated with differing levels of neurological impairment due to the underlying severity of ischemic infarction [23]. For TBI with BFC, ICP was improved compared to the conservative group and had reduced ICU length of stay, but had worse functional outcomes compared to the standard therapy group [20].

(a) *GRADE level of evidence*: The quality of the evidence is *high* for craniectomy after severe TBI with elevated ICP and malignant MCA infarction when operated within 48 hours. Further studies are recommended to validate the TBI-randomized controlled trial data. For malignant MCA infarction with three randomized control trials, further studies are unlikely to demonstrate additional benefit.

(b) *GRADE level of recommendation*: There is a *net-benefit* for improved survival for patients with malignant MCA infarction who have DHC within 48 hours, but distribution of varying levels of neurological impairment related to the underlying disease. For malignant MCA infarction, the number needed to treat (NNT) = 2 for survival with a modified Rankin scale (mRS) of 4 (moderately severe disability), NNT = 4 for mRS = 3 (moderate disability), and NNT = 2 for survival regardless of functional outcome. For TBI BFC, patients did worse in terms of functional outcomes compared to standard ICU therapy, although ICP and ICU length of stay were reduced in the BFC arm of the study compared to the standard therapy group.

Clinical question (#4): Is hypothermia effective in reducing ICP?

Hypothermia has been demonstrated to be effective on reducing ICP [25], regardless of underlying type of brain injury. Hypothermia reduces ICP by reducing cerebral metabolism and cerebral blood flow in a temperature-dependent manner. However, randomized studies investigating hypothermia for TBI have failed when used for 24 hours compared to other medical therapies [25–27]. In a study by Jiang *et al.* that studied TBI patients with prolonged hypothermia up to 5 days, patients had improved outcomes compared to nonhypothermic TBI patients. This study, however, is in contrast to the National Acute Brain Injury Study: Hypothermia II (NABIS II), a randomized controlled study allocated patients to hypothermia cooled to 35°C and if they met a second set of exclusion criteria cooled to 33°C for 48 hours and then gradually rewarmed. The control group was treated with normothermia, In the NABIS II trial, there was no difference in functional outcome by 6 months.

(a) *GRADE level of evidence*: The quality of the evidence regarding hypothermia and ICP control is high, whereas the quality of evidence in TBI-related hypothermia is high for 24–48 hours, which shows no improvement in outcome. However, the studies are conflicting in the study methodology, temperature target, and duration of hypothermia (Jiang *et al.* 5 days vs. NABIS II was 48 hours).

(b) *GRADE recommendation*: There are *trade-offs* in treating patients with hypothermia including reduction in ICP, but the medical therapy needed to reduce ICP requires sedation, mechanical ventilation, and sometimes neuromuscular blockade in most studies, which limits the neurologic exam and may have complications such as bradycardia and increased risk of infection. Future studies should compare prolonged hypothermia beyond 48 hours on outcome and utilize similar methodologies and target temperature.

Summary

A variety of pathophysiologic entities can lead to raised ICP. Early recognition is critical to earlier intervention, placement of an ICP monitor in non-moribund patients or those patients who are expected to benefit from intervention, Glasgow Coma Scale is 8 or less after severe TBI, or have hydrocephalus [28]. Mannitol remains one of the most widely available and effective medical therapies for reducing ICP among a broad range of intracranial pathology, and generally safe (excluding renal failure and severe congestive heart failure). Mannitol can be given via a peripheral IV where as HTS must be given to a central line, for example, 3%, 14.6%, or 23.4%. Trials comparing equal osmolar doses of mannitol versus HTS shows similar efficacy in ICP reduction. However, HTS may be preferred in patients in which blood volume depletion with mannitol is not preferable (e.g. subarachnoid hemorrhage patients in vasospasm). Hyperventilation remains a transient effective method but can be deleterious long term or if used too aggressively ($PaCO_2$ 25 or less) [29]. Surgical DHC reduces intracranial pressure and improves survival compared to patients compared to conservative management after malignant middle cerebral artery infarction. However, surgical hemicraniectomy did not reduce mortality or underlying morbidity when craniectomy is employed for TBI patients. Hypothermia is an effective tool to reduce intracranial pressure if other medical therapies failed such as mannitol or hypertonic saline. However, hypothermia needs further study in TBI regarding the optimal duration of hypothermia (48 hours or longer), given the conflicting results of two trials, and optimal temperature target (35°C or 33°C) as well as safety of hypothermia on medical complications such as pneumonia. Therefore, hypothermia while effective on ICP does not change underlying neurological outcomes.

Disclosures

The author reports no conflict of interest or funding for this manuscript.

Acknowledgments

(Including supporting research grants): None

References

1 Wakai, A., Roberts, I. & Schierhout, G. (2007 Jan 24) Mannitol for acute traumatic brain injury. *Cochrane Database of Systematic Reviews*, (**1**), CD001049.

2 Levin, A.B., Duff, T.A. & Javid, M.J. (1979 Nov) Treatment of increased intracranial pressure: a comparison of different hyperosmotic agents and the use of thiopental. *Neurosurgery*, **5**(**5**), 570–5.

3 No authors listed (1996) The use of barbiturates in the control of intracranial hypertension. Brain Trauma Foundation. *Journal of Neurotrauma*, **13**(**11**), 711–714 Review.

4 Muizelaar, J.P., Marmarou, A., Ward, J.D. *et al.* (1991) Adverse effects of prolonged hyperventilation in patients with severe head injury: a randomized clinical trial. *Journal of Neurosurgery*, **75**, 731–739.

5 Fink, M.E. (2012) Osmotherapy for intracranial hypertension: mannitol versus hypertonic saline. *Continuum (Minneap Minn).*, **18**(**3**), 640–654.

6 No authors listed, The Brain Trauma Foundation, The American Association of Neurological Surgeons & The Joint Section on Neurotrauma and Critical Care (2000) Use of mannitol. *Journal of Neurotrauma*, **17**(**6–7**), 521–525 Review.

7 Vialet, R., Albanèse, J., Thomachot, L., Antonini, F. *et al.* (2003 Jun) Isovolume hypertonic solutes (sodium chloride or mannitol) in the treatment of refractory posttraumatic intracranial hypertension: 2 mL/kg 7.5% saline is more effective than 2 mL/kg 20% mannitol. *Critical Care Medicine*, **31**(**6**), 1683–1687.

8 Francony, G., Fauvage, B., Falcon, D. *et al.* (2008) Equimolar doses of mannitol and hypertonic saline in the treatment of increased. intracranial pressure. *Critical Care Medicine*, **36**(**3**), 795–800.

9 Mortazavi, M.M., Romeo, A.K., Deep, A. *et al.* (2012) Hypertonic saline for treating raised intracranial pressure: literature review with meta-analysis. *Journal of Neurosurgery*, **116**(**1**), 210–21.

10 Kamel, H., Navi, B.B., Nakagawa, K., Hemphill, J.C. 3rd, & Ko, N.U. (2011) Hypertonic saline versus mannitol for the treatment of elevated intracranial pressure: a meta-analysis of randomized clinical trials. *Critical Care Medicine*, **39**(**3**), 554–559 HTS may be superior to mannitol, but needs RCT validation.

11 Rasmussen, M., Tankisi, A. & Cold, G.E. (2004) The effects of indomethacin on intracranial pressure and cerebral haemodynamics in patients undergoing craniotomy: a randomised prospective study. *Anaesthesia*, **59**(**3**), 229–236.

12 Puppo, C., Lopez, L., Farina, G., Caragna, E. *et al.* (2007) Indomethacin and cerebral autoregulation in severe head injured patients: a transcranial Doppler study. *Acta Neurochirurgica (Wien)*, **149**(**2**), 139–49 discussion 149. Epub 2007 Jan 3.

13 Bauer, R.B. & Tellez, H. (1973) Dexamethasone as treatment in cerebrovascular disease. 2. A controlled study in acute cerebral infarction. *Stroke*, **4**(**4**), 547–555.

14 Tellez, H. & Bauer, R.B. (1973) Dexamethasone as treatment in cerebrovascular disease. 1. A controlled study in intracerebral hemorrhage. *Stroke*, **4**(**4**), 541–546.

15 No authors mentioned (1996) The role of glucocorticoids in the treatment of severe head injury. Brain Trauma Foundation. *Journal of Neurotrauma*, **13**(**11**), 715–718 Review.

16 Saul, T.G., Ducker, T.B., Salcman, M. & Carro, E. (1981) Steroids in severe head injury: a prospective randomized clinical trial. *Journal of Neurosurgery*, **54**(**5**), 596–600.

17 French, L.A. & Galicich, J.H. (1964) The use of steroids for control of cerebral edema. *Clinical Neurosurgery*, **10**, 212–223.

18 Ryken, T.C., McDermott, M., Robinson, P.D., Ammirati, M.A. et al. (2010) The role of steroids in the management of brain metastases: a systematic review and evidence-based clinical practice guideline. *Journal of Neuro-Oncology*, **96**(1), 103–114. doi:10.1007/s11060-009-0057-4 Epub 2009 Dec 3.

19 Bebawy, J.F. (2012) Perioperative steroids for peritumoral intracranial edema: a review of mechanisms, efficacy, and side effects. *Journal of Neurosurgical Anesthesiology*, **24**(3), 173–177. doi:10.1097/ANA.0b013e3182578bb5

20 Cooper, D.J., Rosenfeld, J.V., Murray, L. et al. (2011) Decompressive craniectomy in diffuse traumatic brain injury. *The New England Journal of Medicine*, **364**(16), 1493–502.

21 Cho, D.Y., Chen, T.C. & Lee, H.C. (2003) Ultra-early decompressive craniectomy for malignant middle cerebral artery infarction. *Surgical Neurology*, **60**(3), 227–232 discussion 232-3.

22 Jüttler, E., Bösel, J., Amiri, H. et al. (2011) DESTINY II: DEcompressive Surgery for the Treatment of malignant INfarction of the middle cerebral arterY II. *International Journal of Stroke*, **6**(1), 79–86.

23 Vahedi, K., Hofmeijer, J., Juettler, E., Vicaut, E. et al. (2007) Early decompressive surgery in malignant infarction of the middle cerebral artery: a pooled analysis of three randomised controlled trials. *Lancet Neurology*, **6**, 215–222.

24 Einhäupl, K., Stam, J., Bousser, M.G., De Bruijn, S.F. et al (2010) European Federation of Neurological Societies. EFNS guideline on the treatment of cerebral venous and sinus thrombosis in adult patients. *European Journal of Neurology*, **17**(10), 1229–1235.

25 Polderman, K. (2008) Induced hypothermia and fever control for prevention and treatment of neurological injuries. *Lancet*, **371**, 1955–1969.

26 Andrews, P.J., Sinclair, H.L., Battison, C.G. et al. (2011) Eurotherm3235Trial collaborators. European society of intensive care medicine study of therapeutic hypothermia (32-35 °C) for intracranial pressure reduction after traumatic brain injury (the Eurotherm3235Trial). *Trials*, **12**, 8. doi:10.1186/1745-6215-12-8.

27 Kramer, C., Freeman, W.D., Larson, J.S. et al. (2012) Therapeutic hypothermia for severe traumatic brain injury: a critically appraised topic. *The Neurologist*, **18**(3), 173–177.

28 Brain Trauma Foundation, American Association of Neurological Surgeons, Congress of Neurological Surgeons et al. (2007) Guidelines for the management of severe traumatic brain injury. VIII. Intracranial pressure thresholds. *Journal of Neurotrauma*, **24**(Suppl 1), S55–S58.

29 Brain Trauma Foundation, American Association of Neurological Surgeons, Congress of Neurological Surgeons et al. (2007) Guidelines for the management of severe traumatic brain injury. XIV. Hyperventilation. *Journal of Neurotrauma*, **24**(Suppl 1), S87–S90.

11

CHAPTER 11

Traumatic brain injury

Miguel Arango[1], Walter Videtta[2], and Corina Puppo[3]

[1] *The University of Western Ontario and The London Health Sciences Centre, London, Ontario, Canada.*

[2] *Intensive Care Unit, Hospital Posadas, Buenos Aires, Argentina*

[3] *Emergency Department, Clinics Hospital, University of the Repúblic School of Medicine, Montevideo, Uruguay*

Around the world, Acute Traumatic Brain Injury (TBI) continues to be an important public health problem and a leading cause of death and permanent disability. According to the National Center for Injury Prevention and Control, in the United States alone, 1,400,000 people are affected by acute head injury every year [1]. Worldwide statistics are difficult to establish its incidence because of the under-registration in developing countries. From this, 50,000 die, 230,000 require long-term hospitalization, and between 80,000 and 90,000 develop some kind of permanent neurological disability [2]. Unfortunately, most of the burden is in low- and middle-income countries [3,4].

Even though statistics are different between countries and similar within the countries, the overall mortality of acute severe head injury at high-technology centers is around 36%, with severe disability in 15%, moderate disability in 20%, and complete recovery in 25%, although these patients can remain with significant emotional and significant alterations preventing the normal reintegration into the society [2,5].

Evidence about best clinical management, monitoring, and follow-up is limited and sometimes contradictory. During the last few years, different aspects about management of acute subdural hematoma, CT scan follow-up, ICP, and antiepileptic management had been a matter of discussion.

We searched in the following databases: PubMed, Cochrane Injuries Group Specialized Register, Cochrane Central Register of Controlled Trials, MEDLINE, and LILACS.

Critical review of each question

Traumatic acute subdural hematoma in adult brain-injured patients

Nonoperative treatment
Among patients with acute traumatic brain injury with acute subdural hematoma thickness <10 mm thickness and <5 mm midline shift, how does the conservative treatment in intensive care unite with respect to immediate surgery affect the short-term, long-term mortality, the disability, and the occurrence of acute complications?

Acute subdural hematoma (ASDH), defined as a hematoma occurring within 14 days post acute trauma brain injury (TB), is a common posttraumatic clinical and radiological finding. It is diagnosed using head computed tomography scan (CTS) based on revealing extracranial, hyperdense, and dynamic collections between the dura and the brain parenchyma. Normally, all types of ASDH are managed surgically, either by craniotomy or burr holes depending on the size of the hematoma. In the past decade, there had been an increasing interest toward conservative medical therapy, although there is lack of data supporting such therapeutic strategy.

More than a decade ago, a few authors [6,7] consistently reported clinical and radiological characteristics of patients with traumatic ASDH, which might allow a nonsurgical, conservative therapeutic approach. It is important to note that because of the frequent association of ASDH with other types of parenchymal injury, nonsurgical management decisions should also take into consideration the recommendations for other types of lesions. In a recent multicenter survey [8], 729 patients with TBI and intradural mass lesion were prospectively analyzed regarding the current surgical approach: 69% of them showed that the surgical intervention remains the preferred decision taken by neurosurgeons in patients with a space occupying intradural lesion. Even though there is lack of sufficient evidence, 93% of patients with acute subdural hematoma were managed with emergency surgery. A more conservative approach is seen when treating patients with intraparenchymal brain lesions. The subset of ASDH patients who would benefit from medical management, plus indications, technique, and benefits still need to be defined, and could be the topics for future head injury research.

Objectives

To determine whether or not traumatic acute subdural hematoma could be managed conservatively. (see Table 11.1)

Criteria for considering studies for this review

Type of studies: randomized control trials (RCTs).

Type of participants: adult patients with posttraumatic ASDH.

Type of intervention: surgical versus nonsurgical treatment of ASDH.

Results

As in the first review, again we have not found any RCT comparing surgical and nonsurgical treatments of posttraumatic ASDH in adult patients (See Table 11.1).

It is important to mention that a randomized trial, where early surgery vs initial conservative treatment in spontaneous (NON – TRAUMATIC) intracerebral hematomas demonstrated no overall benefit from early surgery compared with initial conservative treatment [10].

In a prospective study [7], Servadei analyzed 65 patients with large traumatic ASDH. Of them, Glasgow Coma Scale (GCS) ≤8, 15 were initially managed conservatively based on a clinical protocol using CTS and intracranial pressure (ICP) parameters. Two CTS were performed within the first 6 hours of injury. Of the 15 cases initially treated conservatively, 7 showed improved GCS compared to admission, 4 remained in stable clinical condition, and 4 showed a decrease in the neurological status not related to the subdural hematoma itself.

Requirements for nonsurgical management were as follows: clinical improvement or stability from the scene of the accident, hematoma thickness <10 mm, midline shift (MLS) <5 mm, and ICP <20 mmHg, or 20–30 mmHg if the cerebral perfusion pressure was >75 mmHg. Two patients failed nonoperative management and as a result underwent a craniotomy after the sequential CTS was performed. When comparing the different parameters between the surgical group and the patients initially managed conservatively, hematoma thickness and shift of the midline structures were predictive of the need for surgery. Outcomes for the conservatively treated group were as follows: mortality 20% (15 patients), severe disability 13.3% (2 patients), and good recovery 66.7% (10 patients). The authors concluded that GCS scoring at the scene of the accident and in the emergency room combined with early and subsequent CT scanning is crucial when making the decision for nonoperative management for selected cases with ASDH with a thickness ≤10 mm and with a shift of the midline structures ≤5 mm.

A prospective observational study, also published by Servadei [9], reported 206 patients (all age-groups) with TBI with GCS ≥ 3 presenting with ASDH ≥5 mm thickness. The study investigates the effects of prognosis on patients with ASDH and other findings on admission CTS that could predict worsening of brain lesions and prognosis. There was no treatment protocol, and the authors conclude that hematoma thickness, MLS, status of basal cisterns, and presence of subarachnoid hemorrhage (SAH) on the initial CTS were related to poor neurological outcome.

In summary, there is insufficient information regarding the operative and nonoperative management in patients with traumatic ASDH. The prognosis of traumatic ASDH seems to be related to clinical age, pupillary status, ICP, and initial CTS variables: MLS, hematoma thickness, patency of the basal cisterns, and SAH. Sometimes surgical treatment is required for other evolving traumatic brain lesions different from the ASDH. Some subgroups of patients with traumatic acute

Table 11.1 Conservative treatment versus surgical evacuation of acute subdural haematoma in patients with acute severe TBI

Reference	Type of study	Patients	Intervention	Outcome	Results
Servadei [7]	Nonrandomized NonControlled Prospective	65 patients Severe acute TBI GCS <8	15 patients with conservative treatment CTS: hematoma <10 mm and MLS <5 mm. ICP: <20 mmHg or between 20 and 30 mmHg if CPP >75 mmHG 50 patients surgical evacuation of hematoma	GOS at 6 months post trauma	Conservative treatment: • mortality 20% • severe disability 13% • good recovery 67% Surgery: • Mortality 48% • Severe disability 6% • Good recovery 28%
Servadei [9]	Nonrandomized Observational Prospective	206 patients with TI and GCS >3 and ASDH >5 mm	Conservative treatment: Serial CT scan. First within 3h of admission, second within 12 h of admission. Subsequent according to the clinical condition	GOS at 6 months post trauma. CTS worsening	Mortality 46% Vegetative state 2% Severe disability 6% Favorable outcome 46% First CTS findings associated with poor neurological outcome

subdural hematoma would benefit from initial conservative management.

Conclusions
Implications for practice

Patients with GCS ≤8, and traumatic ASDH, with hematoma thickness <10 mm, MLS <5 mm, and patency of the basal cisterns whom are admitted to hospital, with CT scanner, 24 hours neurosurgery, and an intensive care unit with ICP monitoring, could be considered as candidates to be treated nonsurgically.

Implications for research

Prospective trials including adult patients with mild, moderate, and severe closed traumatic brain injury with MLS <5 mm, different status of the basal cisterns, SAH, and a clot thickness <10 mm must address whether or not patients with traumatic ASDH can be managed conservatively.

Serial CTSs in acute patients

Among patients with acute TBI without clinical deterioration or ICP elevation, how does the practice of serial CTSs affect the indication for surgery treatment, the short-term mortality, and the probability of acute complications?

Computed tomographic scans (CTSs) of the brain are often routinely repeated at many trauma centers for severe traumatic brain injury (TBI) patients between 12 and 48 hours after to anticipate clinical deterioration or instigate early management changes for silent lesions. CTS is the current standard imaging method for diagnosing intracranial pathology following acute traumatic head injury. It is well known that intracranial lesions after TBI are not static and develop over time. As a result of the improvements in the trauma system, emergency transport practices, and reduced times between trauma and initial CTS, the chances of finding an intracranial lesion early in its course and evolution are high. The use of sequential CTS to evaluate progression of injury is considered a common practice [11] even though the evidence of the impact in outcome is unknown. The utility of repeated head CT performed solely for routine follow-up has not yet been defined [11] (Table 11.2).

Given the conflicting results regarding the indication for a second scheduled head CT in patients with severe closed brain injury, it is disappointing that we did not find any RCTs evaluating the utility of routine repeat CTS in these patients. Only nine prospective non-RCTs for severe TBI were identified (Table 11.2).

Lobato *et al.* [12] reported a prospective study of 56 patients. The authors' intention was to determine the incidence of pathological ICP changes during the acute post-traumatic period in patients with severe acute TBI presenting with diffuse injury (DI) I-II (TCDB classification) on the admission CTS. The aim was to define the most appropriate strategy of sequential CTS and ICP monitoring for detecting new intracranial mass effect and improving the final outcome. All patients had the initial CTS less than 24 hours after injury, several control CTS within the first days of the trauma, and ICP monitoring after admission. The mean GCS was 5, and 57.1% of the patients showed CTS changes: new contusion (26.8%), growth of previous contusion (68.2%), precious extra-axial hematoma (10.7%), and generalized brain swelling (10.7%). It was found that 64.9% of the patients had favorable outcomes and 35.1% an unfavorable outcome. Overall, 27 (48.9%) patients developed clinical deterioration, 21 (37.5%) with concurrent CTS changes, and 6 (10.7%) without new pathology. The remaining 29 (51.7%) patients did not develop deterioration in spite of 11 (19.6%) showing CTS changes. The presence of contusion at the initial CTS ($P = 0.01$) and the presence of generalized brain swelling ($P = 0.003$) in posterior CTS significantly correlated with the risk of deterioration. This worsening in neurological status increased the risk of death by a factor of 10 (OR = 9.8). Eight (14.2%) patients requiring surgery showed simultaneous ICP deterioration and CTS changes, but another 11 patients in a similar condition were able to be managed without surgery. Over 50% of the patients with initial DI I-II lesions developed new CTS changes and nearly 50% showed intracranial hypertension. The discordances between ICP and CTS deterioration were seen in 30.3% of patients. Therefore, the authors recommend ICP monitoring in all patients and serial CTS at 2–4, 12, 24, 48, and 72 hours after injury with additional controls as indicated by clinical or ICP changes in all cases. Brown *et al.* [11] reported a prospective analysis of 100 patients with GSC < 14. The study was intended to examine the value of routine serial CTS after TBI in a single Level I trauma center. Repeat CTS was ordered at the discretion of the trauma team or the neurosurgical consultant with no protocol in place. Only patients who showed abnormalities subsequent to the initial CS scan were included. Patents who died within 24 hours were excluded. Patients with moderate TBI were also included. A total of 68 patients who underwent repeat CTS (Repeat Group, RG) were compared with 32 patients who had CTS only at admission (No Repeat Group, NRG) to evaluate the effect of repeat CTS on patient outcome. Primary outcome was the need for TBI-related intervention. The 68 patients in the RG underwent 90 repeat CTSs. Repeat scans were mainly done 34 ± 32 hours after admission. This group had a higher incidence of extradural hematoma (EDH), and a trend toward more SDH. Of those undergoing repeat CTS, 90% (*n* = 81) were performed on a routine basis without neurological changes. Of those routine CTS, 26%, 52%, and 22% were classified as "better," "the same," and "worse," respectively. No patient had any neurosurgical intervention after having a routine repeat CTS. In the RG, every patient (100%) with EDH, intracentricular hemorrhage (IVH) underwent sequential CTS, but only in 70%

Table 11.2 Effect on outcome and management of serial brain CTS policy

Reference	Type of study	Patients	Intervention	Outcome	Results
Lobato et al. [12]	Nonrandomized Prospective	56 patients acute severe TBI, diffuse CTS damage, ICP monitoring	Serial CTS admission 24, 48, and 72 hours	Surgery, clinical deterioration and death	CTS add information with respect to ICP monitoring alone.
Brown et al. [11]	Nonrandomized Prospective	100 patients moderate – severe acute TBI, CTS abnormality at admission	68 repeated CTS (no protocol), 32 patients only one CTS on admission	Surgery	No patient with repeated CTS had surgery
Oertel et al. [13]	Nonrandomized Prospective	142 patients acute TBI any severity, mean GCS = 8	Early repeated CTS in patients with progressive shift and brain swelling	Progression of intracranial hemorrhagic injury	50% had PHI and 25% required surgery
Servadei et al. [9]	Nonrandomized Prospective	206 patients with TI and GCS >3 and ASDH >5 mm	Conservative treatment: Serial CT scan. First within 3 hours of admission, second within 12 hours of admission. Subsequent according to the clinical condition	GOS at 6 months post trauma. CTS worsening	Mortality 46% Vegetative state 2% Severe disability 6% Favorable outcome 46% First CTS findings associated with poor neurological outcome
Lubillo et al. [14]	Nonrandomized Prospective	82 patients intracranial hematoma and surgery	CTS within 2–12 hours after surgery	Mortality and long-term outcome	CTS findings associated with final outcome
Cope et al. [15]	Nonrandomized Prospective	47 Patients acute TBI traumatic head injuries	CTS at admission, 1 month and 3 months later	Surgery	CTS allows early diagnosis of lesion requiring surgery
Roberson et al. [16]	Nonrandomized Prospective	107 patients acute TBI, coma	Serial CTS from day 1 to 12 months	Delayed intracranial lesions	18% of patients with normal CTS at admission present delayed intracranial lesion requiring surgical decompression
Ward et al. [17]	SR	Patients with traumatic acute brain injury	Repeated head CTS after admission for blunt traumatic brain injury		30 studies included. Majority retrospective

of the patients with SDH, intraparenchymal hemorrhage (IPH), contusion, MLS, or multiple injuries. Eighty-three percent of the patients with GCS <8 underwent repeat CTS scan and showed a trend toward a higher injury severely scan (ISS) and lower GCS. The authors concluded that the use of routine serial CTS in patients without neurological deterioration was not supported.

In a prospective study, Oertel et al. [13] looked at patients who underwent two CTS within 24 h after acute TBI to determine the incidence, risk factors, and clinical significance of progressive hemorrhagic injury (PHI). One single Level I Trauma center and 142 patients with mild, moderate, and severe, closed and penetrating TBI were included. The diagnosis of PHI was determined by comparing the first and second CTSs and defined as an unambiguous increase in the full film appearance of lesion size; this amounted to a 25% increase in at least one dimension of at least one lesion seen on the first postinjury CTS. The mean GCS was 8. Potential risk factors, coagulation status, temperature, ethanol, ICP, and CPP were analyzed. Increased MLS, hemispheric swelling, or progressive loss of basilar cisterns on the second CTS was defined as "progressive shift and swelling." Similarly, "progressive brain shift and swelling" was present in 23% of patients with PHI, but in only 4% of patients without PHI ($P = 0.003$). The second CTS scan was performed earlier in patients with progressive brain shift and swelling than in patients without this finding (6.4 ± 4.2 hours post injury versus 9.3 ± 3.9 post injury; $P = 0.01$). Of the 17 patients with progressive shift and swelling, 8 underwent craniotomy after the second CTS. Male sex ($P = 0.01$), older age ($P = 0.01$), time from injury to first ($P = 0.02$), and initial partial thromboplastin time ($P = 0.02$) were the best predictors of PHI. Of the 46 patients who underwent craniotomy for hematoma evacuation, 24% present hematoma after the second CTS.

Early CTS after moderate or severe TBI did not reveal the full extent of hemorrhagic injury in 45% of patients. PHI approached 50% in patients undergoing scanning within 2 hours of injury. Parenchymal lesions in the frontal and temporal lobes are the most likely to progress. Patients with PHI have a greater degree of subsequent ICP elevations, and 25% required craniotomy. The neurological outcomes at 6 months post injury were similar in both groups. The authors recommended early repeat CTS in patients with no surgically treated hemorrhage revealed on the first CTS.

In a prospective study, Servadei et al. [9] intended to establish the frequency of deterioration in CTS appearance from an admission scan to subsequent scans and the prognostic significance of such deterioration. Data have been gathered prospectively for 206 patients with moderate and severe head injury. The findings of the initial and final "worst" CTS were classified according to the Traumatic Coma Data Bank (TCDB) system, and were related to outcome using the GCS at 6 months after injury. The initial CTS findings were classified as a DI for 53% of the cohort, with 16% of these DI demonstrating deterioration on a subsequent scan. In 56 (74%) of 76 deteriorations, the change was from a DI to a mass lesion. Patients with normal CTS or with a DI I at admission showed a low rate (4%) of evolution. Patients with DI II, III, and IV showed high rates of progression to mass lesion (13–14% for DI II and III and 20% for type IV). A third CTS may be scheduled on the third day post trauma. When the initial CTS demonstrated a DI without swelling or shift, evolution to a mass lesion was associated with a significant increase in the risk of an unfavorable outcome (62% vs 38%). The authors recommended follow-up scans when admission CTS demonstrates evidence of a DI, because approximately one of six patients will demonstrate significant CT evolution of this lesion. The CRS may be repeated within 12 hours whenever the first scan is obtained, within 3 hours after injury, and within 24 hours in all other situations. A third scan was also recommended on the third day after trauma, even though the author accepted that this recommendation is empiric.

Lubillo et al. [14] prospectively studied 82 patients with isolated, severe TBI (GCS <8), all of whom had intracranial hematoma. The author analyzed the CTS appearance after evacuation of a mass lesion in relation to outcome. The CTS was performed within 2–12 hours after craniotomy; continuous monitoring of the ICP and CPP was also done after surgery. The mortality rate during the hospital stay was 37%; 50% of patients achieved a favorable outcome. The postoperative scan revealed DI III-IV in 53 patients and DI I-II in 29 patients. The percentages of the time presenting an ICP>20 mmHg and a CPP<70 mmHg were higher in the group of patients with DI III-IV ($P < 0.001$); these patients also revealed an unfavorable neurological outcome. Patients with a motor (m) GCS <3, bilateral nonreactive pupils,

associated intracranial injuries, and hypotension demonstrate high incidence of raised ICP, CPP<70 mmHg, DI III-IV, and unfavorable outcome ($P < 0.001$). The author concluded that the features on CTS obtained shortly after craniotomy constitute an independent predictor of outcome in patients with traumatic hematoma.

Cope et al. [15] reported a prospective study looking at routine serial CTS in 47 patients with TBI. This study analyzed patients who were admitted to a rehabilitation unit after initial hospitalization. Under a prospective protocol for routine scans (1- and 3-month admissions), 22% of patients required neurosurgical intervention for a variety of findings. Most patients had chronic manifestations of TBI not applicable to acutely head-injured patients. Even though there is no reference regarding exact neurological disability before routine repeat CTS, the patients who underwent neurosurgical intervention had higher disability rating score. This would imply that the clinical status of the patient, not scan findings alone, played a major role in determining the need for surgical intervention and observation. The authors concluded that routine serial scanning might allow earlier diagnosis of a progressive intracranial lesion and thereby minimize further brain injury in the rehabilitation setting.

In a prospective study, Servadei et al. [7] looked at patients with large ASDH. Of 65 comatose patients, 15 were initially managed conservatively according to a protocol based on clinical, CTS, and ICP parameters. Two patients failed nonoperative management and underwent a craniotomy after sequential scan. When comparing the different parameters between the surgical group and the patients initially managed conservative, hematoma thickness and shift of the midline structures were predictive of the need of surgery. The authors concluded that GCS scoring at the scene and in the emergency room combined with early and subsequent CTS is crucial when making the decision for nonoperative management for selected cases with ASDH with a thickness <10 mm and with a shift of the midline structures <5 mm.

Roberson et al. [16] reported a prospective study of comatose TBI patients who had routine CTS (on days 1, 3, 5, 7, 14, and at 3 and 12 months). The author compared the value of sequential scans, neurological status, and ICP in 107 patients. Thirty-eight (40%) of 95 patients had a normal CTS on admission. Seven (18%) of these 38 patients had scans demonstrating a delayed intracranial lesion requiring surgical decompression. It is important to note that all seven patients had neurological deterioration before intervention, and were not treated based on CTS results alone. They gave a confirmatory value to CTS regarding the changes in ICP monitoring and clinical examination. The authors concluded that it is useful to get a control CTS on days 3 and 7 after injury if the patient shows no clinical improvement.

In a prospective study, Brown et al [11] found that two craniotomies were performed on the basis of the results of routine CT scans in 64 patients with GCS <8. The first patient received an ICP monitor after the first scan. The second patient experienced significant change on repeat CT scan at 14 hours that was not reflected in the ICP monitor readings and underwent craniotomy.

A recent review conducted by Wang *et al.* [18] concluded that indications for repeat head CT after traumatic brain injury are unclear. The wide range of reported injury progression on CT and resulting surgical and medical treatment changes suggest that there may be a subset of patients who benefit from repeat CT. Further research should stratify by severity of traumatic brain injury, clearly define inclusion and exclusion criteria, address selection bias, quantify progression of injury on CT, determine factors predictive of injury progression and intervention, and assess risks associated with repeat CT.

In summary, there is insufficient information and conflicting data on the value of repetitive routinely head CT in adult severe closed head injury patients, some subgroups of patients with SAH, epidural hematoma, SDH, contusions, and intraparenchymal hematoma with initially conservative management would benefit from serial CTS. Patients with risk factors, such as coagulopathy and hypotension, should be scheduled for repeat CT scan. More studies are needed to address this issue. Were ever possible, uncertainty about the convenience of doing a second CTS in the absence of clinical manifestations, for example, impaired GCS and ICP elevation, must evaluate the risks/benefits of transporting patients out of the monitoring and controlled ICU environment. Further investigation is warranted into whether a repeat scan at 12 hours should unmask radiologic deterioration before clinical deterioration, and if so, whether earlier detection would change outcome. Prospective trials, including adult patients with moderate/severe blunt head injury admitted to the ICU, first CTS classified according to TCDB categories and including confounding variables, worsening GCS and/or clinical examination, elevations of ICP, hypotension, and coagulopathy, represent the next step in defining guidelines for obtaining repeat CTS.

Anticonvulsive therapy in acute traumatic brain injury patients

Among patients with acute traumatic brain injury, how does the early treatment with antiepileptic drugs affect the risk of early seizure, late seizure, and the probability of long-term death or disable condition? What are the side effects?

Trauma is an important cause of epilepsy. The incidence of posttraumatic seizures (PTS) in patients with acute traumatic brain injury is between 10% and 30%. According to some reports, between 20% and 25% of patients with severe head injury (GCS<9) might be expected to have at least one PTS during hospital stay.

Definitions

Epilepsy: Chronic disorder of the nervous system characterized by recurrent unproved seizures [19]; there should be at least two or more seizures greater than 24 hours apart [20].

Depending on the time of occurrence, the PTS can be classified as follows:

1 *Immediate seizures:* Seizures occurring within the first few hours of trauma.

2 *Early posttraumatic seizures:* Seizures that occur soon after a brain trauma. Usually, this interval is specified as 1–2 weeks after the insult. These are *provoked* seizures. The pathophysiology that underlies these provoked seizures (e.g., neuronal calcium influx, cerebral edema, intracranial blood effects, and metabolic disorders) likely differs substantially from that which contributes to the development of epilepsy.

3 *Late posttraumatic seizures:* Seizures that occur after the 1- to 2-week interval after a brain trauma. If no new CNS insult or new systemic disorder (e.g., drug withdrawal, eclampsia, and toxins) occurs during this "later" interval, these seizures are unprovoked [21].

Only recurrent late seizures make up the clinical syndrome which can be labeled as "posttraumatic epilepsy" and can be defined as a disorder characterized by *recurrent* seizures, not referable to another obvious cause ("unprovoked seizures"), in patients following traumatic brain injury. Early seizures are felt to be acute symptomatic events with a low likelihood of recurrence, whereas late seizures are likely to repeat and thus they represent epilepsy.

Antiepileptic: Prevents or reduces epileptic seizures

Neuroprotective: Prevents neuronal injury. An antiepileptic may be neuroprotective if seizures are injurious or if the compound has an additional protective activity independent of its antiepileptic activity.

Antiepileptogenic: Prevents or slows down the process of developing epilepsy. An antiepileptic might be antiepileptogenic if the seizures it blocks are themselves epileptogenic. A neuroprotective compound might be antiepileptogenic if injury leads to epilepsy. Alternatively, some compounds might have antiepileptogenic activity without either blocking seizures or preventing injury [22].

A number of human clinical trials have been conducted in preventing epilepsy development in subjects at risk for epilepsy, but only a few of these have been randomized, double-blind, placebo-controlled studies (Table 11.3).

A clinical trial by Tempkin et al [23] showed that phenytoin administration after moderate to severe TBI does not decrease the chance of unprovoked seizures after the first week of brain injury. In this well-executed blinded placebo-controlled trial, 323 patients were randomized to phenytoin or placebo within 24 hours after TBI. Half of

Table 11.3 Antiepileptic drugs for acute TBI

Trial	Participants	Outcome	No of patients	Intervention	Results
Glotzner	TBI; had one or more listed complications patients over 15 years of age	Early seizures, late seizures, overall mortality, persistent vegetative state	151	CMZ; LD 100 mg × 3 per day on day 1 and 2, 200 mg × 3 per day on day 3. MD dose adjusted according to serum concentrations. LD started immediately and given for 18 months to 2 years. If oral CMZ could not be taken, 750 mg iv PHT on day 1 and 250-500 mg on day 2, switched to CMZ when oral medication was tolerated.	Patients on carbamazepine showed a lower probability of posttraumatic seizures than those on placebo ($p < 0.05$). This difference was statistically significant with regard to early seizures within the first week and with regard to the follow-up time in total, but not regarding late seizures per se. Lost to follow up over 2 years was 20% in E and 1% in C; includes drug-related withdrawal
McQueen	TBI; no patients with early seizures; 5–65 years of age	Late seizures, overall mortality, skin rashes	164	PHT; LD 300 mg for adults; for children (<15 years), 5 mg per kg body weight; adjusted according to plasma concentrations, for 1 year.	2-year follow-up
Young, 1983	Head injured; included all penetrating injuries and for blunt injuries, had one or more listed complications	Early seizures, late seizures, overall mortality	244	PHT; LD 11 mg per kg given within 24 hours. MD adjusted according to plasma concentrations. Given for 18 months after injury. If hypersensitivity developed, switched to PB ($n=20$).	2-year follow-up Loss to follow up over 24 months was 26%
Temkin	Head injured; 16 years of age and older	Early seizures, late seizures, overall mortality, skin rashes, neurobehavioral effects, Glasgow coma outcome score [+]	586	PHT; LD 20 mg/kg of body weight given within 24 hours; adjusted according to serum concentrations, for 1 year.	Including predrug loading withdrawals 2-year follow-up. Loss to follow up over 24 m was 50% in C and 55% in E
Pechardre	TBI patients; 5–60 years of age	Early seizures, late seizures, overall mortality [+]	91	PHT; LD 11 mg/kg given within 24 hours. MD modified according to plasma concentrations. Given for 3 months or 1year	2-year follow-up. Authors report no loss to follow-up
Manaka	TBI patients with one or more listed complications; no age restrictions	Late seizures to end of year 1	169	PB; LD between 10 and 25 µg/ml started 4 weeks after head injury. Gradually reduced over 3rd year to zero	5-year follow-up. Loss to follow up at 5 years was 25%
Brackett unpublished	TBI adults	Adjusted overall seizure rates	125	PB (60 mg) and PHT (200 mg) started within 12 hours following admission. Given for 18 months.	36-month follow-up. Loss to follow up at 36 m 39%

(continued overleaf)

Table 11.3 (*continued*)

Trial	Participants	Outcome	No of patients	Intervention	Results
Brackett unpublished	TBI adults	Adjusted overall seizure rates	49	PB and PHT given for 6 months.	Study terminated early because of low accession rates. Loss to follow up at 18 months was 52%
Marshall unpublished	TBI adults	Adjusted overall seizure rates	154	PB and PHT.	Study terminated early because of drug levels unable to be kept in therapeutic range. 23% of cases lost to follow up within 48 hours
Locke unpublished	TBI adults	Adjusted overall seizure rates	303	PB or PHT or combination. Given for 6 months.	18-month follow-up. 79% of the cases died or were lost to follow up
Temkin	TBI		379	VPA versus PHT (1 week) then placebo	VPA: no benefit over short-term PHT for prevention of early seizures. Neither treatment prevents late seizures. VPA: Trend toward higher mortality. VPA should not be routinely used for the prevention of posttraumatic seizures.
Ma, C et al.	Mild, moderate, and severe TBI in adults		159	Valproate	Retrospective study Of the 87 severe TBI patients (GCS 3-8), 6 patients in the control group (6.9%) suffered from early seizures during the first week after TBI and no patient who received preventive therapy suffered from seizures.
Szaflarski	Severe TBI and SAH	GOSE and DRS at time of hospital discharge and again at 3 and 6 months after admission. Seizure frequency, any adverse events, prescribed medications, and a Resource Utilization Questionnaire were also documented at the 3- and 6-month follow-up	46 TBI and 6 SAH	(1) fosPHT LD 20 mg/kg PE IV, max 2000 mg, over 60 minutes and PHT MD (5 mg/kg per day, IV every 12 hours over 15 minutes) were days 2 and 6 adjusted by PHT levels of 10–20 μg/dl. (2) LEV LD 20 mg/kg IV, over 60 minutes MD (1000 mg, IV every 12 hours over 15 minutes) adjusted if seizures occurred to 1500 mg every 12 hours (3000 mg per day max). Both regimens maintained for 7 days. Discontinued afterward if no seizures	Patients treated with PHT vis-a'-vis LEV have the same outcomes in respect to death or seizures, but LEV results in less undesirable side effects and better long-term outcomes as measured with GOSE and DRS.

the patients continued to receive phenytoin for 1 year and the placebo group continued on placebo. The patients were observed for 2 years. There was no significant difference in late seizures in the first year (21.5% of phenytoin group and 15.7% of placebo group) or in the second year (27.5% of phenytoin group and 21.1% of control group, risk ratio 1.20, 95% CI 0.71–2.02.

Another trial performed by the same investigators [24] on TBI patients at high risk for seizures investigated 1-week phenytoin (132 p) versus 1-week valproate (120 p) versus 6-month valproate (127 p) (the first two arms received placebo until 6 months after active drug arm cessation). The cases were followed up to 2 years. This study also failed to show antiepileptogenic effects. Valproate treatment for 6 months was associated with a nonsignificant increase in late seizure rate. The mortality rates were not significantly different between treatment groups, but there was a trend toward a higher mortality rate in patients treated with valproate. The lack of additional benefit and the potentially higher mortality rate suggest that valproate should not be routinely used for the prevention of early or late posttraumatic seizures.

Other placebo-controlled trials in epilepsy prevention after traumatic brain injury (carbamazepine, phenobarbital) have also proved to be unsuccessful [25]. Non-AED interventions after TBI have also proved to be unsuccessful in blocking epileptogenesis. A trial on magnesium sulfate administration in the first 5 days after moderate to severe TBI was not associated with a significant change in late seizures over the following 6 months compared to placebo in a randomized controlled trial of 500 patients [26]. One factor that complicates trials is that the AEDs, especially the older ones, can add morbidity. Phenytoin caused significant neurobehavioral impairment months after traumatic brain injury when compared to patients receiving placebo [27].

A systematic review of the use of drugs to prevent seizures after head injury [28] identified ten randomized controlled trials, which provided data from 2036 patients. Four were unpublished studies, which turned to be unavailable. Therefore, only six trials were reviewed, which included 1218 randomized patients. Four trials randomized 890 patients in order to address prevention of early seizures (Tables 11.1 and 11.2). They found consistent evidence that the early treatment with antiepileptic drugs, most commonly phenytoin, but also carbamazepine and phenobarbitone, decreased the relative risk (RR) of early seizures (0.34 [95% CI 0.21–0.54]). For late seizures, six trials were analyzed; there was significant heterogeneity between trials, and therefore a summary relative risk could not be calculated. A reduction in late seizures was not demonstrated. Mortality data were available from five trials (1054 randomized patients), showing no beneficial effect of antiepileptics (pooled RR 1.15; 95% CI 0.89–1.51); or death and severe

neurological disability (RR 1.49, 95% CI 1.06–2.08), [29] (RR 0.96; 95% CI 0.72–1.39). Skin rashes: based on the pooled relative risk, for every 100 patients treated, 4 will develop skin rashes.

Conclusion

On the basis of these findings, antiepileptic drugs seem to control early seizures in patients with traumatic brain injury. They do not seem to prevent the subsequent development of posttraumatic epilepsy, neither change mortality nor improve disability.

As early seizures may contribute to secondary damage to the injured brain, preventive treatment with phenytoin should be initiated as the first line of choice, as soon as possible after injury among patients with severe traumatic brain injury. Anticonvulsants have not been found to reduce the incidence of developing late posttraumatic seizures, and therefore, prolonged prophylaxis with antiepileptics is not currently supported. They should not be used after the first 7 days of injury to decrease the risk of posttraumatic seizures occurring beyond that time.

The trials that have been performed to date have important drawbacks. Electroencephalography (EEG) monitoring has only been performed in one of them. It would be of great help to evaluate subclinical seizures. The trials enrolled a small number of patients; only four studies included more than 200 patients. The periods of observation after the drug was stopped were short. Few studies monitored compliance or drug concentrations. Most trials had high rates of loss to follow-up. Finally, some of them were not blinded.

Control of intracranial hypertension

Background

Controlling and preventing high ICP and aggressive treatment of ICP elevation plus avoiding cerebral ischemia maintaining the cerebral blood flow, and the cerebral perfusion pressure is in fact the standard of treatment in acute traumatic brain injury. Unfortunately, there is no consensus on the best way to achieve these therapeutic goals.

Among patients with severe acute traumatic brain injury, how does the ICP monitoring policy affect the probability of death or the severity of neurological impairment?

In 2010, a systematic review about the efficacy of routine ICP monitoring in severe acute cases in reducing the risk of all-cause mortality or severe disability was published by Forsyth R *et al.* A systematic database search approach was done in order to find all randomized controlled studies of real-time ICP monitoring by invasive or semi-invasive means in acute coma secondary to traumatic and nontraumatic events, versus no ICP monitoring or/and clinical assessment of ICP. Interesting and despite the high incidence of acute traumatic brain injury and the so-called standardized use of ICP monitoring, the authors were unable to identify any studies fulfilling the selection criteria.

Among patients with severe acute traumatic brain injury, how does ICP-lowering interventions affect the probability of death or the severity of neurological impairment?

The clinical relationship between management of increased intracranial pressure and neurological long-term outcome had been a matter of research by several investigators. Miller *et al.* [30] were among the first; Marshall *et al.* [31], Gaab and Haubitz [29], McGraw *et al.* [32], Narayan *et al.* [33], and Fearnside *et al.* [34] have demonstrated significantly worse outcomes in patients with increased ICP. Marmarou *et al.* [35] reviewed the experience of the Traumatic Coma Data Bank with regard to ICP instability and hypotension. By measuring the percentage of time that ICP was >20 mmHg, they were able to demonstrate that elevated ICP was a highly significant predictor of poor outcome. Unterberg *et al.* [5] found that patients with late (day 3–5) increases in ICP had significantly worse outcomes than patients without such an increase. The prospective analysis of 394 head injury patients obtained from the database provided by the Selfotel trial [31] showed an important decrease in neurological outcome in those patients with alterations of the ICP.

In 2008, based on the CRASH trial [36] (large cohort of international patients), a practical model for predicting outcome after traumatic brain injury was published in the BMJ [37]. The authors used a multivariable logistic regression to select variables that have an independent association with patient neurological outcome. Two models were defined: a basic model based on demographic and clinical variables and a "CT" model adding the CT finding to the basic model. The basic model includes age, GCS, presence of major extracranial trauma, and pupil reactivity. The CT model includes obliteration of the third ventricle or basal cistern, presence of petechial hemorrhages, subarachnoid bleeding, middle shift, and nonevacuated hematoma. The models demonstrated a very good discrimination (C static above 0.80), although the calibration for unfavorable outcome at 6 months in developed countries was poor in spite of having a good discrimination. That year, Roozenbeek *et al.* [38] published an external validation of the prognostic models based on the CRASH trial patient and the IMPACT patients, concluding that both models show good generalizability and they can be considered as valid tools for quantify prognosis in acute traumatic brain injury. The outcome prediction models that have evolved from these databases are undergoing further refinement and validation, and it is likely that these advances will prove valuable in education, family information, improvement in designing prospective clinical trials, and better allocation of medical resources.

An important systematic review by Roberts in 1998 [39] analyzed the effectiveness of five medical interventions routinely used in the medical management of severe acute traumatic brain injury patients. The specific interventions were hyperventilation, use of mannitol, CSF drainage, and barbiturates and corticosteroids administration. On the basis of the available randomized evidence, it was not possible to support or refute the existence of a real benefit on mortality and neurological disability from the use of these therapeutic interventions.

Hyperventilation is often associated with a rapid fall in intracranial pressure; therefore, it has been assumed to be effective in the treatment of severe head injury patients. Hyperventilation reduces raised intracranial pressure by causing cerebral vasoconstriction and a concomitant reduction in cerebral blood volume. A Cochrane systematic review was performed and published in 2000 [40] in which only one trial was found which randomized 113 patients [41]. An updated version of the systematic review was published in 2009 confirming the same results [42]. Possible disadvantages of hyperventilation include cerebral vasoconstriction to such an extent that cerebral ischemia ensues. These investigators hypothesized that the short effect of hyperventilation could be related to the CSF pH decrease, with a loss of HCO_3 buffer. The latter disadvantage might be overcome by the addition of the buffer tromethamine (THAM). Accordingly, a trial was performed with patients randomly assigned to receive normal ventilation, hyperventilation ($PaCO_2$ 25 ± 2 mmHg), or hyperventilation plus THAM ($PaCO_2$ 25 ± 2 mmHg). Stratification into subgroups of patients with motor scores of 1–3 and 4–5 took place. Outcome was assessed according to the Glasgow Outcome Scale at 3, 6, and 12 months. There were 41, 36, and 36 patients, respectively. A 100% follow-up was obtained. At 3 and 6 months after injury, the number of patients with a favorable outcome was significantly lower in the hyperventilated patients than in the other two groups. This occurred only in patients with a motor score of 4–5. At 12 months post trauma, this difference was not significant ($P = 0.13$). Biochemical data indicated that hyperventilation could not sustain alkalinization in the CSF, although THAM could. Accordingly, cerebral blood flow (CBF) was lower in the HV + THAM group than in the control and HV groups, but neither CBF nor arteriovenous difference of oxygen data indicated the occurrence of cerebral ischemia in any of the three groups. Even though mean ICP could be kept well below 25 mmHg in all three groups, the course of ICP was most stable in the HV + THAM group. It is concluded that prophylactic hyperventilation is deleterious in head-injured patients with motor scores of 4–5. Hyperventilation alone, as well as in conjunction with the buffer THAM, showed a beneficial effect on mortality at 1 year after injury, although the effect measure was imprecise ($RR = 0.73$; 95% CI 0.36–1.49 and $RR = 0.89$; 95% CI 0.47–1.72, respectively). This improvement in outcome was not supported by an improvement in neurological recovery. For hyperventilation alone, the RR for death or severe disability was 1.14 (95% CI 0.82–1.58). In the hyperventilation plus THAM group, the RR for death or severe disability was 0.87 (95% CI 0.58–1.28). The data available are inadequate to assess any potential benefit or harm that might result from hyperventilation in severe head injury. Randomized controlled trials to assess the effectiveness of hyperventilation therapy following severe head injury are needed.

Mannitol may be sometimes dramatically effective in reversing acute brain swelling, but its effectiveness in the on-going management of severe head injury remains open to question. There is evidence that, in prolonged dosage, mannitol may pass from the blood into the brain, where it might cause reverse osmotic shifts that increase intracranial pressure. A Cochrane systematic review initially published in 2003 [43] and then updated in 2007 [44] included four RCTs [45–48]. The authors concluded that there is not sufficient and reliable evidence to make any therapeutic recommendation for the use of mannitol in the management scenario of patients with TBI. Mannitol therapy for raised ICP may have a beneficial effect on mortality when compared to pentobarbital treatment. ICP-directed treatment shows a small beneficial effect compared to treatment directed by neurological signs and physiological indicators. There are insufficient data on the effectiveness of prehospital administration of mannitol to preclude either a harmful or a beneficial effect on mortality. It has to be stressed that three of these five trials did not measure ICP, because the patients were examined in the emergency room, and therefore, mannitol was administered for the treatment of clinical signs of severity.

The use of barbiturates is also relatively common in the management of patients with TBI because of the belief that reducing ICP by suppressing cerebral metabolism reduces cerebral metabolic demands and cerebral blood volume. However, barbiturates also can create brain ischemia secondary to important cerebral vasoconstriction; a reduction in blood pressure might be also present and may, therefore, adversely reduce cerebral perfusion pressure. An initial systematic review was published by Roberts I *et al.* [49], and then updated by same authors in 2009 [50]. The authors identified eight trials that met the inclusion criteria [51–54,46,17]. One article was unpublished and the other was published twice [54]. Authors conclude that there is a lack of reliable evidence in the barbiturate therapy and better neurological outcome in patients with acute TBI. It was also found that the barbiturate administration results in a fall in blood pressure in one of four treated patients.

Corticosteroids have been widely used in treating people with TBI. However, the increase in mortality with steroids demonstrated by the Cochrane Systematic Review [55] and the CRASH trial [56] suggests that steroids should no longer be routinely used in people with traumatic head injury.

References

1 Systems TJSoNaCCT. THe Brain Trauma Foundation (2000) The American Associating of Neurological Surgeons. *J Neurotrauma.*, **17**, 457–462.

2 Bruns, J.J. & Hauser, W.A. (2003) The epidemiology of traumatic brain injury: a review. *Epilepsia.*, **44(Suppl 10)**, 2–10.

3 Hofman, K., Primack, A., Keusch, G. & Hrynkow, S. (2005) Addressing the growing burden of trauma and injury in low- and middle-income countries. *Am J Public Health.*, **95**, 13–17.

4 De Silva, M.J., Roberts, I., Perel, P. *et al.* (2009) Patient outcome after traumatic brain injury in high-, middle- and low-income countries: analysis of data on 8927 patients in 46 countries. *Int J Epidemiol.*, **38**, 452–458.

5 Marshall, L.F., Gautile, T. & Klauber, M.R. (1991) The outcome of severe close head injury. *J Neurosurgery.*, **75**, s28–36.

6 Dent DL, Croce MA, Menke PG *et al.* Prognostic factors after acute subdural hematoma. *J Trauma.* 1995;**39**:36-42; discussion 42-3.

7 Servadei, F., Nasi, M.T., Cremonini, A.M., Giuliani, G., Cenni, P. & Nanni, A. (1998) Importance of a reliable admission Glasgow Coma Scale score for determining the need for evacuation of posttraumatic subdural hematomas: a prospective study of 65 patients. *J Trauma.*, **44**, 868–873.

8 Compagnone, C., Murray, G.D., Teasdale, G.M. *et al.* (2007) The management of patients with intradural post-traumatic mass lesions: a multicenter survey of current approaches to surgical management in 729 patients coordinated by the European Brain Injury Consortium. *Neurosurgery.*, **61**, 232–40 discussion 240-1.

9 Servadei, F., Nasi, M.T., Giuliani, G. *et al.* (2000) CT prognostic factors in acute subdural haematomas: the value of the 'worst' CT scan. *Br J Neurosurg.*, **14**, 110–116.

10 Pantazis, G., Tsitsopoulos, P., Mihas, C., Katsiva, V., Stavrianos, V. & Zymaris, S. (2006) Early surgical treatment vs conservative management for spontaneous supratentorial intracerebral hematomas: a prospective randomized study. *Surg Neurol.*, **66**, 492–501 discussion 501-2.

11 Brown, C.V., Weng, J., Oh, D. *et al.* (2004) Does routine serial computed tomography of the head influence management of traumatic brain injury? A prospective evaluation. *J Trauma.*, **57**, 939–943.

12 Lobato, R.D., Alen, J.F., Perez-Nunez, A. *et al.* (2005) Value of serial CT scanning and intracranial pressure monitoring for detecting new intracranial mass effect in severe head injury patients showing lesions type I-II in the initial CT scan. *Neurocirugia (Astur)*, **16**, 217–234.

13 Oertel, M., Kelly, D.F., McArthur, D. *et al.* (2002) Progressive hemorrhage after head trauma: predictors and consequences of the evolving injury. *J Neurosurg.*, **96**, 109–116.

14 Lubillo, S., Bolanos, J., Carreira, L., Cardenosa, J., Arroyo, J. & Manzano, J. (1999) Prognostic value of early computerized tomography scanning following craniotomy for traumatic hematoma. *J Neurosurg.*, **91**, 581–587.

15 Cope, D.N., Date, E.S. & Mar, E.Y. (1988) Serial computerized tomographic evaluations in traumatic head injury. *Arch Phys Med Rehabil.*, **69**, 483–486.

16 Roberson, F.C., Kishore, P.R., Miller, J.D., Lipper, M.H. & Becker, D.P. (1979) The value of serial computerized tomography in the management of severe head injury. *Surg Neurol.*, **12**, 161–167.

17 Ward, J.D., Becker, D.P., Miller, J.D. *et al.* (1985) Failure of prophylactic barbiturate coma in the treatment of severe head injury. *J Neurosurg.*, **62**, 383–388.

18 Wang, M.C., Linnau, K.F., Tirschwell, D.L. & Hollingworth, W. (2006) Utility of repeat head computed tomography after blunt head trauma: a systematic review. *J Trauma.*, **61**, 226–233.

19 Mani R, Pollard J, Dichter MA. (2011) Human clinical trials in antiepileptogenesis. *Neuroscience Letters.* **49**:251-256.

20 Hauser, W.A., Rich, S.S., Lee, J.R., Annegers, J.F. & Anderson, V.E. (1998) Risk of recurrent seizures after two unprovoked seizures. *N Engl J Med.*, **338**, 429–434.

21 Herman, S.T. (2006) Clinical trials for prevention of epileptogenesis. *Epilepsy Res.*, **68**, 35–38.

22 Dichter, M.A. & Cole, A.J. (2002) Neuroprotection and antiepileptogenesis: where are we now? *Neurology*, **59**, S36–S38.

23 Temkin, N.R., Dikmen, S.S., Wilensky, A.J., Keihm, J., Chabal, S. & Winn, H.R. (1990) A randomized, double-blind study of phenytoin for the prevention of post-traumatic seizures. *N Engl J Med.*, **323**, 497–502.

24 Temkin, N.R., Dikmen, S.S., Anderson, G.D. *et al.* (1999) Valproate therapy for prevention of posttraumatic seizures: a randomized trial. *J Neurosurg.*, **91**, 593–600.

25 Temkin, N.R. (2001) Antiepileptogenesis and seizure prevention trials with antiepileptic drugs: meta-analysis of controlled trials. *Epilepsia.*, **42**, 515–524.

26 Temkin, N.R., Anderson, G.D., Winn, H.R. *et al.* (2007) Magnesium sulfate for neuroprotection after traumatic brain injury: a randomised controlled trial. *Lancet Neurol.*, **6**, 29–38.

27 Dikmen, S.S., Temkin, N.R., Miller, B., Machamer, J. & Winn, H.R. (1991) Neurobehavioral effects of phenytoin prophylaxis of posttraumatic seizures. *JAMA.*, **265**, 1271–1277.

28 Schierhout, G. & Roberts, I. (1998) Prophylactic antiepileptic agents after head injury: a systematic review. *J Neurol Neurosurg Psychiatry*, **64**, 108–112.

29 Gaab, M.R. & Haubitz, I. (1993) Intracranial pressure, primary/secondary brain stem injury and prognosis in cerebral truam. *Intracranial Pressure*, **V**, 558–561.

30 Miller, J.D., Becker, D.P., Ward, J.D., Sullivan, H.G., Adams, W.E. & Rosner, M.J. (1977) Significance of intracranial hypertension in severe head injury. *J Neurosurg.*, **47**, 503–516.

31 Marshall, L.F., Smith, R.W. & Shapiro, H.M. (1979) The outcome with aggressive treatment in severe head injuries. Part I: the significance of intracranial pressure monitoring. *J Neurosurg*, **50**, 20–25.

32 McGraw, C.P., Howard, G. & O'Connor, C. (1983) Outcome associated with management based on ICP monitoring. In: Ishii, S., Nagai, H. & Brock, M. (eds), *Intracranial Pressure V*. Springer, Berlin, Heidelberg, pp. 558–561.

33 Narayan, R.K., Greenberg, R.P., Miller, J.D. *et al.* (1981) Improved confidence of outcome prediction in severe head injury. A comparative analysis of the clinical examination, multimodality evoked potentials, CT scanning, and intracranial pressure. *J Neurosurg*, **54**, 751–762.

34 Fearnside, M.R., Cook, R.J., McDougall, P. & McNeil, R.J. (1993) The Westmead Head Injury Project outcome in severe head injury. A comparative analysis of pre-hospital, clinical and CT variables. *Br J Neurosurg*, **7**, 267–279.

35 Marmarou, A., Anderson, R.L. & Ward, J.D. (1991) Impact of ICP instability and hypotension on outcome in patients with severe head trauma. *J Neurosurg*, **75**, S59–S66.

36 Edwards, P., Arango, M., Balica, L. *et al.* (2005) Final results of MRC CRASH, a randomised placebo-controlled trial of intravenous corticosteroid in adults with head injury-outcomes at 6 months. *Lancet.*, **365**, 1957–1959.

37 Perel, P., Arango, M., Clayton, T. *et al.* (2008) Predicting outcome after traumatic brain injury: practical prognostic models based on large cohort of international patients. *BMJ*, **336**, 425–429.

38 Roozenbeek, B., Lingsma, H.F., Lecky, F.E. *et al.* (2012) Prediction of outcome after moderate and severe traumatic brain injury: external validation of the International Mission on Prognosis and Analysis of Clinical Trials (IMPACT) and Corticoid Randomisation After Significant Head injury (CRASH) prognostic models. *Crit Care Med.*, **40**, 1609–1617.

39 Roberts, I., Schierhout, G. & Alderson, P. (1998) Absence of evidence for the effectiveness of five interventions routinely used in the intensive care management of severe head injury: a systematic review. *J Neurol Neurosurg Psychiatry.*, **65**, 729–733.

40 Schierhout, G. & Roberts, I. (2000) Hyperventilation therapy for acute traumatic brain injury. *Cochrane Database Syst Rev*, CD000566.

41 Muizelaar, J.P., Marmarou, A., Ward, J.D. *et al.* (1991) Adverse effects of prolonged hyperventilation in patients with severe head injury: a randomized clinical trial. *J Neurosurg.*, **75**, 731–739.

42 Roberts, I. (2009) *Schierhout G.* Hyperventilation therapy for acute traumatic brain injury, The Cochrane Library.

43 Roberts I, Schierhout G, Wakai A. Mannitol for acute traumatic brain injury. Cochrane Database Syst Rev. 2003;CD001049.

44 Wakai, A., Roberts, I. & Schierhout, G. (2007) Mannitol for acute traumatic brain injury. *Cochrane Database Syst Rev*, CD001049.

45 Sayre, M.R., Daily, S.W., Stern, S.A., Storer, D.L., van Loveren, H.R. & Hurst, J.M. (1996) Out-of-hospital administration of mannitol to head-injured patients does not change systolic blood pressure. *Acad Emerg Med.*, **3**, 840–848.

46 Schwartz, M.L., Tator, C.H., Rowed, D.W., Reid, S.R., Meguro, K. & Andrews, D.F. (1984) The University of Toronto head injury treatment study: a prospective, randomized comparison of pentobarbital and mannitol. *Can J Neurol Sci.*, **11**, 434–440.

47 Smith, H.P., Kelly, D.L.J., McWhorter, J.M. *et al.* (1986) Comparison of mannitol regimens in patients with severe head injury undergoing intracranial monitoring. *J Neurosurg.*, **65**, 820–824.

48 Vialet, R., Albanese, J., Thomachot, L. *et al.* (2003) Isovolume hypertonic solutes (sodium chloride or mannitol) in the treatment of refractory posttraumatic intracranial hypertension: 2 mL/kg 7.5% saline is more effective than 2 mL/kg 20% mannitol. *Crit Care Med.*, **31**, 1683–1687.

49 Roberts, I. (2000) Barbiturates for acute traumatic brain injury. *Cochrane Database Syst Rev*, CD000033.

50 Roberts, I. (2009) *Sydenham E*. Barbiturates for acute traumatic brain injury, The Cochrane Library.

51 Eisenberg, H.M., Frankowski, R.F., Contant, C.F., Marshall, L.F. & Walker, M.D. (1988) High-dose barbiturate control of elevated intracranial pressure in patients with severe head injury. *J Neurosurg.*, **69**, 15–23.

52 Levy, M.L., Aranda, M., Zelman, V. & Giannotta, S.L. (1995) Propylene glycol toxicity following continuous etomidate infusion for the control of refractory cerebral edema. *Neurosurgery.*, **37**, 363–369 discussion 369-71.

53 Perez-Barcena, J., Llompart-Pou, J.A., Homar, J. *et al.* (2008) Pentobarbital versus thiopental in the treatment of refractory intracranial hypertension in patients with traumatic brain injury: a randomized controlled trial. *Crit Care*, **12**, R112.

54 Saul, T.G. & Ducker, T.B. (1982) Effect of intracranial pressure monitoring and aggressive treatment on mortality in severe head injury. *J Neurosurg.*, **56**, 498–503.

55 Alderson, P. & Roberts, I. (2005) Corticosteroids for acute traumatic brain injury. *Cochrane Database Syst Rev*, CD000196.

56 Roberts, I., Yates, D., Sandercock, P. *et al.* (2004) Effect of intravenous corticosteroids on death within 14 days in 10008 adults with clinically significant head injury (MRC CRASH trial): randomised placebo-controlled trial. *Lancet*, **364**, 1321–1328.

12 CHAPTER 12

Myasthenia gravis

Brent P. Goodman

Department of Neurology, Mayo Clinic, Scottsdale, AZ, USA

Introduction

Myasthenia gravis (MG) is an acquired, autoimmune, neuromuscular junction disorder that results in fatigable weakness. This autoimmune disorder is characterized by a T cell-dependent, antibody-mediated process that affects the postsynaptic muscle membrane. With appropriate diagnostic testing and treatment, a normal life expectancy is expected, though many patients with MG report persistent, residual symptoms and limitations, reduction in quality of life, and the potential for treatment-related complications.

MG occurs in men and women, may develop at any age, and affect all races [1]. In a recently reported systematic review of population-based epidemiologic studies, incidence rates ranged from 1.7 to 21.3 cases per million person-years [2]. Incidence rates of MG increase with age. Historically, a bimodal pattern of incidence rates has been reported, with females more likely to be affected at younger ages, in their 20s and 30s, and men in their 60s and beyond. However, a recent meta-analysis of MG incidence rates suggested that this bimodal pattern was seen in a minority of studies. The frequency of MG seems to increase in men and women with aging in most populations [2].

The majority of patients with MG have an autoimmune disorder mediated by antibodies against acetylcholine receptors (AChR). These antibodies play a critical role not only in the immunopathogenesis of this condition, but provide confirmatory serologic evidence of MG, in the appropriate clinical context. Approximately 5% of patients with MG have antibodies against muscle-specific kinase (MuSK) [3]. MuSK plays an important role in the clustering of AChR on the postsynaptic membrane. More recently, the agrin receptor, low-density lipoprotein receptor-related protein 4 (LRP4), has been identified as an antigenic target in a small number of patients without antibodies to AChR or MuSK [4,5]. Like MuSK, agrin plays a critical role in the aggregation of AChR on the postsynaptic muscle membrane.

The diagnosis of MG is established through the demonstration of antibodies in the serum to acetylcholine receptors (AChR) or muscle-specific kinase (MuSK), and through electrodiagnostic testing, including repetitive nerve stimulation studies and single-fiber electromyography (EMG). Treatment is directed toward improving neuromuscular transmission through the use of acetylcholinesterase inhibitors, which increase the availability of acetylcholine at the neuromuscular junction and immunomodulating therapy.

The severity of the signs and symptoms of MG is quite variable as is the clinical course. This variability in symptom severity from patient to patient and across a patient population, when combined with an unpredictable clinical course that in many patients is characterized by relapses and remissions, complicates treatment decisions and certainly clinical trials in MG. For most patients with MG, disease severity peaks within 3 years [6]. However, given the predilection for impairment in bulbar and respiratory muscles in 20–30% of patients with MG, there is potential for substantial morbidity amongst patients with more severe disease.

Framing of clinical question and search strategy

The following evidence-based discussion focuses on the management of myasthenia gravis in different clinical scenarios as follows: (1) treatment of myasthenic crisis utilizing intravenous immunoglobulin and plasma exchange, (2) thymectomy in the treatment of generalized myasthenia gravis, (3) treatment of myasthenia gravis using mycophenolate mofetil as a "steroid-sparing agent," and (4) IVIg in the treatment of chronic but stable, generalized MG. The topics are presented similarly, preceded by a clinical patient scenario that provides the foundation for a clinical question, and for each topic, a subsequent critical appraisal of the literature. The general search strategy involved the use of PubMed, MEDLINE, the Cochrane Library, and the Cochrane Database of Reviews of Effectiveness utilizing the search terms "myasthenia gravis," "IVIg," "intravenous immunoglobulin," "plasma exchange," "myocophenolate mofetil," and "thymectomy."

Evidence-Based Neurology: Management of Neurological Disorders, Second Edition. Edited by Bart M. Demaerschalk and Dean M. Wingerchuk.
© 2015 John Wiley & Sons, Ltd. Published 2015 by John Wiley & Sons, Ltd.

Clinical scenario

A 62-year-old man presents to the emergency room for evaluation of dysphagia, dysarthria, and shortness of breath. He reports the onset of fatigable ptosis and diplopia before 2 months, and 2 weeks ago developed difficulties with chewing and swallowing and a fatigable, hypernasal speech. He was evaluated at that time by his primary care physician, who requested some bloodwork, and a neurological evaluation. He reports the onset of dyspnea with even minor activities about a week before. His past medical history was notable only for hypertension and hyperlipidemia, and he reported having been on a stable dose of lisinopril and statin medication for the past few years.

On neurological examination, he was afebrile and normotensive, though his heart rate was borderline elevated in the 90s in normal sinus rhythm. He was tachypneic though his oxygen saturation was normal on room air. His language and mental status examination were normal. He had a flaccid, hypernasal dysarthria, which became less intelligible the longer he spoke. His cranial nerve examination was notable for limitations with right lateral gaze, fatigable ptosis bilaterally, moderately severe weakness involving orbicularis oculi, orbicularis oris, and tongue bilaterally. He appeared to have a head drop, with at least moderate neck flexor and extensor weakness. He had mild weakness of deltoid muscles bilaterally, otherwise his manual muscle strength testing was normal in the extremities. Deep tendon reflexes, plantar responses, limb coordination, and sensory examination were all unremarkable.

Upon further communication with the patient's primary care physician, it is learned that the patient had elevated acetylcholine receptor-binding antibodies, and a chest CT had been performed and showed no evidence of thymoma or other pulmonary abnormalities. The emergency room team requests neurological recommendations on how best to treat this patient with myasthenic crisis.

Critical review of the evidence for each question

Intravenous immunoglobulin (IVIg) versus plasma exchange in myasthenic crisis

Is IVIg or plasma exchange superior in the treatment of myasthenic crisis?

MG is a T cell-dependent, antibody-mediated disorder with a number of potential immunotherapeutic options. The majority of the available immunosuppressive medications, such as corticosteroids, azathioprine, mycophenolate, cyclosporine, tacrolimus, and methotrexate, require considerable time to influence disordered immune function in MG. These medications therefore play no role in the more acute treatment necessary in a patient with myasthenic crisis.

Myasthenic crisis refers to respiratory muscle or upper airway muscle weakness in a patient with MG, and is a medical emergency. The lifetime prevalence of myasthenic crisis is 20–30%, and may occur at any point during a patient's disease course [7–9], that is, early in a patient's course before the initiation of immune-modulating therapy as in the case of the patient presented above. Myasthenic crisis may occur later in a patient's disease course, with a number of potential precipitating causes including suboptimal control of generalized myasthenia, hyperthyroidism, infection, corticosteroids, and certain medications [10]. The management of myasthenic crisis requires prompt recognition, admission to the intensive care unit for close observation and ongoing assessment to initiate intubation and mechanical ventilation with progressive symptoms. There may be some role for noninvasive ventilation as an alternative to intubation and mechanical ventilation [11]. Bedside pulmonary measurements are utilized to guide the need for respiratory support. The "20/30/40" rule has been used to determine if intubation is necessary: vital capacity <20 ml/kg; peak inspiratory pressure $\leq 30\,cmH_2O$; and peak expiratory pressure <40 cmH_2O [10].

Plasma exchange and IVIg have been the mainstays of therapy for myasthenic crisis. Plasma exchange has traditionally been administered every other day for five total treatments, while 2 g/kg of IVIg has been traditionally administered over 5 days in the treatment of myasthenic crisis. The relative efficacy of these treatments in the treatment of MG exacerbations has not been evaluated until recently.

Clinical bottom line

- Plasma exchange and IVIg have equal efficacy in the treatment of MG worsening or exacerbations.
- Because relatively few patients with myasthenic crisis have been included in clinical trials, it cannot be definitively stated whether plasma exchange or IVIg is more effective in myasthenic crisis.

Evidence

There were two clinical trials identified that examined the efficacy of IVIg versus plasma exchange in the treatment of MG exacerbation.

Study design

The first clinical trial compared the efficacy and tolerability of plasma exchange and IVIg in MG exacerbation, with the primary outcome measure being myasthenic muscle score (MMS) between randomization and on day 15 [12]. There were 41 and 46 patients in the plasma exchange and IVIg groups, respectively. The second study compared IVIg and plasma exchange in the treatment of patients with moderate to severe MG, with the primary outcome being the quantitative myasthenia gravis score in 84 total patients [13].

Summary of results

In the 1997 clinical trial comparing IVIg and plasma exchange, there was no difference between groups comparing MMS between day 0 and day 15 ($P=0.770$) [12]. In the second, 2011 clinical trial, there was no significant difference between the QMGS between the IVIg and plasma exchange treatment groups [13]. It is noteworthy that the number of patients with myasthenic crises was small, and no conclusion can therefore be made regarding the relative efficacy of IVIg versus plasma exchange in the treatment of myasthenic crisis [14].

Clinical scenario

A 28-year-old woman is referred for neurological evaluation with a 6-month history of fatigable diplopia, generalized fatigue, and extremity weakness. Her past medical history was notable only for hypothyroidism, for which she was taking thyroid replacement medication. Her general medical examination was normal aside from obesity, with body mass index of 32. On neurological examination, her speech, language, and mental status examination were normal. She had bilateral fluctuating ptosis on examination, and fatigable proximal greater than distal weakness in her extremities bilaterally. Her deep tendon reflexes, sensory examination, gait, and limb coordination were normal.

Laboratory studies were unremarkable aside from elevated AChR antibodies. Electrodiagnostic studies showed a significant decrement in her compound muscle action potential with 2-Hz repetitive stimulation of accessory and facial nerves, with unstable motor unit potentials of normal size on needle examination. A chest CT showed no evidence of thymoma.

The patient is interested in discussing options for treatment of her symptoms of MG. She has read about corticosteroids being used for MG, and is interested in avoiding those as much as possible given her obesity and the potential for weight gain with these medications. She relates that her mother was on prednisone for a number of years for the treatment of her rheumatoid arthritis and gained substantial weight. She is interested in discussing other options as well as thymectomy in the treatment of her MG.

Critical review of the evidence for each question

Thymectomy in MG

Is thymectomy effective in the treatment of myasthenia gravis?

Myasthenia gravis is a heterogenous disorder that may result in fatigable weakness, involving ocular, bulbar, trunk, and extremity muscles in isolation or in some combination. Ocular symptoms are particularly common, and are the initial manifestation of MG in approximately half of all patients

[15], ultimately develop in most MG patients, and result in diplopia, blurred vision, and ptosis. Most patients with initially ocular symptoms who go on to develop generalized MG will do so within 2 years of symptom onset. Patients with generalized MG are at risk for myasthenic crisis, and the presence of bulbar symptoms or significant limb or truncal weakness may substantially affect quality of life. For this reason, generalized MG typically requires long-term treatment with acetylcholinesterase medications and immunotherapy.

Corticosteroids are often the mainstay of generalized MG treatment, but because of their numerous side effects, other "steroid-sparing" agents such as azathioprine, mycophenolate mofetil, cyclosporine, tacrolimus, rituximab, IVIg, or cyclophosphamide are often initiated when high doses of corticosteroids are necessary to control symptoms or response with corticosteroids is suboptimal. Thymectomy has also been utilized in the long-term management of patients with generalized MG.

The thymus has long been implicated in the pathogenesis of MG, and it has been suggested that thymectomy may reduce the severity of MG by attenuating immune-mediated attack of the neuromuscular junction in patients with MG [16,17]. Approximately 70% of patients with MG have thymic follicular hyperplasia, and 10% of patients have a thymoma. All patients with thymoma require thymectomy. Cells with the medullary of the thymus contain cells that express AChR on their surface [18]; therefore, removal of the thymus may eliminate a major source of AChR antibodies in MG patients.

Clinical bottom line

- There is no definitive evidence that thymectomy is effective in the management of nonthymomatous MG.
- Despite this lack of rigorous, definitive evidence demonstrating the effectiveness of thymectomy in MG, many clinicians routinely recommend thymectomy in generalized MG, and believe in its efficacy in treating this condition.

Evidence

There are no randomized clinical trials evaluating thymectomy in the management of nonthymomatous MG.

Study design

Despite numerous retrospective studies over the past 50 years reporting the results of thymectomy in the management of nonthymomatous MG, there have not been any randomized clinical trials involving the surgical treatment of MG [19].

Summary of results

To date, no prospective, randomized clinical trial to evaluate the effectiveness of thymectomy in MG has been reported. Previously reported studies have been hampered by a number of methodological flaws, including absence of randomized treatment allocation, lack of standardized outcome measures, and the confounding difference in baseline characteristics [20].

An evidenced-based review by Gronseth and Barohn comprehensively analyzed studies evaluating the efficacy of thymectomy in MG between 1966 and 1998 [20]. Twenty-eight class II studies were analyzed in this review. There was no randomization to thymectomy or nonthymectomy. Follow-up length was not standardized and patient loss-to-follow-up was variable. There were no blinded assessment of outcomes, and nonstandard definitions of remission were used. In all but three of the studies analyzed, patients who underwent thymectomy were more likely to achieve mediation-free remission, become asymptomatic, and improve than patients who did not undergo thymectomy. A number of potentially confounding variables were identified: patients who underwent thymectomy were more likely to be female, were younger, and had more severe MG. The studies did not adequately control for confounding factors or baseline subject characteristics. Effects due to surgical timing, medical therapy, and differing surgical techniques were difficult to assess or account for. The general consensus is that thymectomy is likely beneficial in patients with myasthenia gravis. Despite the vast numbers of studies reporting benefit, methodological flaws, and particularly, lack of randomization do not permit conclusive evidence of efficacy. At the time of this writing, an international, multicenter, prospective, randomized trial, "Thymectomy in nonthymomatous MG patients receiving prednisone" is underway.

Mycophenolate mofetil in the treatment of MG

Is mycophenolate mofetil effective as a steroid-sparing agent in the treatment of generalized MG?

Mycophenolate mofetil is an inhibitor of inosine monophosphate dehydrogenase, an enzyme critical in the pathway for guanosine nucleotide synthesis. As a result, it is hypothesized that mycophenolate should inhibit the antibody response in patients with MG. There has been significant interest in and widespread use of mycophenolate mofetil in the treatment of generalized MG, particularly given its favorable side effect profile.

Clinical bottom line

• There is no definitive evidence that mycophenolate mofetil is effective as a steroid-sparing agent in generalized MG.

Evidence

There have been two clinical trials evaluating the efficacy of mycophenolate mofetil in the treatment of generalized MG.

Study design

The first was a multicenter, double-blind, placebo-controlled, parallel group trial on moderate dose prednisone in 80 patients with mild to moderate generalized MG [21]. The other study involving an international, prospective, randomized, double-blind, placebo-controlled, parallel group, 36-week trial evaluated efficacy of mycophenolate mofetil as a steroid-sparing agent in the treatment of mild to moderate, generalized, seropositive MG [22].

Summary of results

In the multicenter, double-blind, placebo-controlled, parallel group trial comparing moderate dose prednisone alone to combined mycophenolate mofetil and moderate dose prednisone, the quantitative MG score at 12 weeks was assessed and found to be similar in both. Furthermore, in an additional 24-week open-label phase, prednisone dose was tapered at a similar rate in both groups [21]. In the international, prospective, randomized, double-blind, placebo-controlled, parallel group, 36-week trial, there were no differences in primary and secondary outcomes between the treatment groups with respect to prednisone tapering [22].

These two randomized, controlled, clinical trials suggest that mycophenolate mofetil is not effective as a steroid-sparing agent in generalized MG. The results of these two rigorous clinical trials surprised many clinicians, whose anecdotal experience suggested some benefit of mycophenolate in MG patients. Furthermore, earlier, though admittedly less rigorous reports suggested clinical efficacy in patients with MG. A number of factors such as very short study duration, very small sample size, robust response of patients to prednisone, and entry of milder disease patients have been raised as potential reasons for study conclusions that appear to contradict clinical experience.

IVIg in the treatment of chronic MG

Is IVIg effective in the treatment of chronic MG?

As discussed earlier, the efficacy of IVIg in the treatment of MG exacerbations has been established. In clinical practice, IVIg has also been used to treat MG more chronically either in patients who are unable to tolerate corticosteroids, in those with relative contraindications to long-term prednisone use (patients with diabetes mellitus or severe osteoporosis), or in patients with suboptimal responses to corticosteroids. It has been suggested that IVIg is appropriate to consider in the chronic management of MG, as it affects all of the critical mediators in the pathogenesis of MG, including antibodies, T cell activation, B cells, complement, and cytokines [23,24]. However, IVIg is expensive, and has a number of potential side effects.

Clinical bottom line

• There is no definitive evidence from randomized clinical trials demonstrating efficacy in the treatment of chronic, but stable generalized MG.

Evidence

Two randomized clinical trials evaluated the efficacy of IVIg in the treatment of moderate to severe, but stable MG.

Study design

The first study compared IVIg and plasma exchange in individuals with moderate to severe, but stable MG. This was a controlled crossover study, with individuals receiving either IVIg 0.4 g/kg over 5 consecutive days and 16 weeks later with plasma exchange every other day for five treatments or plasma exchange followed by IVIg [25]. In the second study, IVIg was compared to placebo (albumin) in patients with mild to moderate generalized MG never treated with corticosteroids or other immunomodulating therapy, or in MG patients taking at least 20 mg of prednisone every other day [26]. Primary outcome in this trial was change in the QMGS from baseline to day 42.

Summary of results

In the trial comparing IVIg and plasma exchange, a significant decrease in the QMGS for both IVIg and plasma exchange was significant at 4 weeks ($P < 0.05$), but not at 8 and 16 weeks. In the second trial comparing IVIg and placebo, the change in QMGS from day 0 to day 42 was no different in the IVIg and placebo arms. These trials failed to provide any definitive evidence of the efficacy of IVIg in the treatment of chronic, but stable, generalized MG.

A recently reported retrospective study of 52 patients with generalized MG treated with chronic IVIg maintenance therapy helped to reduce symptoms of MG, but was ineffective in inducing full remission or reducing disease activity in this cohort [27]. Forty-eight of them failed to respond adequately to prednisone, azathioprine, or some combination, and nine patients did not receive prednisone due to contraindications (diabetes or osteoporosis). Thirty-seven of them were treated with IVIg for a minimum of 1 year, and there was a decrease in their Myasthenia Gravis Foundation of America (MGFA) of at least one class. Six of them were able to stop prednisone therapy and another 24 were able to reduce their prednisone dose. In 15 patients, there was no improvement after a loading dose and two additional doses, and treatment was discontinued. None of the patients achieved complete stable or pharmacologic remission.

A need for further clinical trials utilizing IVIg maintenance therapy in the treatment of chronic, but stable MG has been suggested [14].

Conclusions

MG is a relatively rare, heterogenous, autoimmune disorder with the potential to result in substantial morbidity, adversely affecting quality of life. There is very little definitive evidence regarding the roles of various immunotherapies and surgical therapies in the treatment of MG. Both plasma exchange and IVIg are unequivocally effective in the treatment of MG exacerbations. There are no definitive randomized, controlled clinical trials demonstrating efficacy in the chronic treatment of generalized but stable MG with various immunotherapies or thymectomy.

References

1 Kurtzke, J.F. (1978) Epidemiology of myasthenia gravis. *Advances in Neurology*, **19**, 55–566.

2 Carr, A.S., Cardwell, C.R., McCarron, P.O. & McConville, J. (2010) A systematic review of population based epidemiologic studies in myasthenia gravis. *BMC Neurology*, **10**, 46.

3 Hoch, W., McConville, J., Helms, S., Newsom-Davis, J. *et al.* (2001) Auto-antibodies to the receptor tyrosine kinase MuSK in patients with myasthenia gravis without acetylcholine receptor antibodies. *Nature Medicine*, **7**, 365–368.

4 Higuchi, O., Hamuro, J., Motomura, M. & Yamanashi, Y. (2011) Autoantibodies to lowdensity lipoprotein receptor-related protein 4 in myasthenia gravis. *Annals of Neurology*, **69**, 418–22.

5 Pevzner, A., Schoser, B., Peters, K. *et al.* (2012) Anti-LRP4 autoantibodies in AChR- and MuSK-antibody-negative myastheniagravis. *Journal of Neurology*, **259**, 427–35.

6 Grob, D., Brunner, N.G. & Namba, T. (1981) The natural course of myasthenia gravis and effect of therapeutic measures. *Annals of the New York Academy of Sciences*, **377**, 652–669.

7 Lacomis, D. (2005) Myasthenic crisis. *Neurocritical Care*, **3**, 189–194.

8 Mayer, S.A. (1997) Intensive care of the myasthenic patient. *Neurology*, **48**, S70–5.

9 Juel, V.C. (2004) Myasthenia gravis: management of myasthenic crisis and perioperative care. *Seminars in Neurology*, **24**, 75–81.

10 Chaudhuri, A. & Behan, P.O. (2009) Myasthenic crisis. *QJM*, **102(2)**, 97–107.

11 Agarwal, R., Reddy, C. & Gupta, D. (2006) Noninvasive ventilation in acute neuromuscular respiratory failure due to myasthenic crisis: case report and review of literature. *Emergency Medicine Journal*, **23**, 6–7.

12 Gajdos, P., Chevret, S., Clair, B. *et al.* (1997) Clinical trial of plasma exchange and high-dose intravenous immunoglobulin in myasthenia gravis. Myasthenia Gravis Clinical Study Group. *Annals of Neurology*, **41(6)**, 789–796.

13 Barth, D., Nouri, N.N., Ng, E. *et al.* (2011) Comparison of IVIg and PLEX in patients with myasthenia gravis. *Neurology*, **76(23)**, 2017–2023.

14 Gajdos, P., Chevret, S. & Tokya, K.V. (2012) Intravenous immunoglobulin for myasthenia gravis (Review). *Cochrane Database of Systematic Reviews*, **12**, 1–38.

15 Bever, C.T., Aquino, A.V., Penn, A.S. *et al.* (1983) Prognosis of ocular myasthenia. *Annals of Neurology*, **14(5)**, 516–519.

16 Penn, A.S. (1994) Thymectomy for myasthenia gravis. In: Lisak, R.P. (ed), *Handbook of Myasthenia Gravis and Myasthenic Syndrome*. Marcel Dekker, New York, pp. 321–339.

17 Kaminsi, H.J. (2003) *Myasthenia Gravis and Related Disorders.* Humana Press, Totowa, NJ.

18 Schluep, M., Wilcox, N., Vincent, A. *et al.* (1987) Acetylcholine receptors in human thymic myoid cells in situ:an immunohistological study. *Annals of Neurology,* **22**(**2**), 212–222.

19 Cea, G., Benatar, M., Verdugo, R.J. & Salinas, R.A. (2013) Thymectomy for non-thymomatous myasthenia gravis (Review). *Cochrane Database of Systematic Reviews,* **10**, 1–19.

20 Gronseth, G.S. & Barohn, R.J. (2000) Practice parameter: thymectomy for autoimmune myasthenia gravis (an evidence-based review). Report of the quality standards subcommittee of the American Academy of Neurology. *Neurology,* **55**, 7–15.

21 Muscle Study Group (2008) A trial of mycophenolate mofetil with prednisone as initial immunotherapy in myasthenia gravis. *Neurology,* **71**, 394–399.

22 Sanders, D.B., Hart, I.K., Mantegazza, R. *et al.* (2008) An international phase II randomized trial of mycophenolate mofetil in myasthenia gravis. *Neurology,* **71**, 400–406.

23 Dalakas, M.C. (2013) Novel future therapeutic options in myasthenia gravis. *Autoimmunity Reviews,* **12**, 936–941.

24 Dalakas, M.C. (2010) Evidence-based efficacy of intravenous immunoglobulin in human myasthenia gravis and mechanisms of action. In: Premkumar, C. (ed), *Myasthenia Gravis: Mechanisms of Disease and Immune Intervention.* Linus Publication, Inc, New York, pp. 89–102.

25 Ronager, J., Ravnborg, M., Hermansen, J. *et al.* (2001) Immunoglobulin treatment versus plasma exchange in patients with chronic moderate to severe myasthenia gravis. *Artificial Organs,* **25**(**12**), 967–973.

26 Wolfe, G.I., Barohn, R.J., Foster, B.M. *et al.* (2002) Randomized, controlled trial of intravenous immunoglobulin in myasthenia gravis. *Muscle and Nerve,* **26**(**4**), 549–552.

27 Hellman, M.A., Mosberg-Gallili, R., Lotan, I. & Steiner, I. (2014) Maintenance IVIg therapy in myasthenia gravis does not affect disease activity. *Journal of Neurological Sciences,* **338**(**1–2**), 39–42.

13 CHAPTER 13
Acute visual loss

Byron Roderick Spencer

Blue Sky Neurology(Division of Carepoint), Denver, CO, USA

Acute vision loss can be a challenging and potentially devastating condition that can be the result of various unique conditions. In the outpatient setting, ophthalmologists and neuro-ophthalmologists are often the first to see these patients; however, in the hospital setting, often they are first seen by the emergency room physician or internist who then subsequently relies on the neurologist to aid with diagnosis and management recommendations. This chapter will review some of the most common neuro-ophthalmic conditions seen in the hospital setting that may be associated with acute vision loss.

Non-arteritic ischemic optic neuropathy

Background

Non-arteritic anterior ischemic optic neuropathy (NA-AION) is one of the most common causes of sudden painless vision loss in middle-aged or elder adults. This disease is thought to occur due to optic nerve head infarction secondary to local vascular impairment [1,2]. Patients who develop NA-AION tend to have underlying vascular risk factors such as diabetes, hyperlipidemia, hypertension, and obstructive sleep apnea. NA-AION has also been associated with hematologic disorders, systemic vasculitis, and vasculopathies [3]. Vision loss is usually realized upon wakening, and tends to be painless. Clinical evaluation often reveals hyperemic optic nerve swelling often in a segmental pattern, flame hemorrhages, relative afferent papillary defect, and decreased visual acuity. Visual field testing frequently shows an altitudinal field defect.

Treatment

Biousse and Hayreh, along with several others, have published numerous studies analyzing various treatment modalities including optic nerve sheath decompression (possibly harmful) [2]; unfortunately, there are currently no acute treatment options for non-arteritic ischemic optic neuropathy. Because patients with NA-AION often have a "disk at risk" in the unaffected eye, preventive measures often include treatment of systemic risk factors, including trying to reduce the chance of nocturnal hypotension [4].

Arteritic anterior ischemic optic neuropathy or giant cell arteritis

Background

Giant cell arteritis (GCA) is a systemic vasculitis that most commonly affects the elderly population. GCA is an autoimmune-mediated disorder in which T-cells attack the internal elastic lamina of medium- and large-sized blood vessels, causing occlusion of the lumen [5]. Classically, GCA presents with the combination of headache, scalp tenderness, and vision loss. Other symptoms can include arthralgias, fever, jaw or tongue claudication, myalgias, and weight loss. Laboratory studies often reveal elevated serum inflammatory markers such as C-reactive protein (CRP), erythrocyte sedimentation rate (ESR), and platelet count, since this condition can exist in the presence of both a normal ESR and CRP.

Unlike non-arteritic ischemic optic neuropathy funduscopic evaluation of patients with giant cell arteritis tends to show a pale or "chalky" white edematous optic nerve and, occasionally, cotton wool spots indicating retinal ischemia. Neuro-ophthalmic complications can include amaurosis fugax, central retinal artery occlusion (cilioretinal artery occlusion), diplopia, eye pain, ocular hypotony, ptosis, and visual hallucinations [5,6]. Systemic complications of GCA include aortic aneurysm, aortic dissection, and large artery stenosis. Visual field testing can reveal central defects, peripheral constriction and sector defects [6]. To make a definitive diagnosis of giant cell arteritis, temporal artery biopsy is required. In some cases, the unilateral biopsy may be negative; thus, it may require contralateral artery biopsy.

Evidence-Based Neurology: Management of Neurological Disorders, Second Edition. Edited by Bart M. Demaerschalk and Dean M. Wingerchuk.
© 2015 John Wiley & Sons, Ltd. Published 2015 by John Wiley & Sons, Ltd.

Treatment

Vision loss associated with GCA can be shattering if not identified early. Bilateral eye involvement can often occur, with the second eye affected within 2 weeks of the first eye [5]. Once profound vision loss has occurred, even with rapid treatment, chance of marked visual improvement is low. The mainstay of treatment is the combination of intravenous and oral corticosteroids. Currently there is no evidence supporting the use of other immunosuppressants [6].

Retinal vascular occlusion syndromes

Branch and central retinal artery occlusion

Background

Central retinal artery occlusion (CRAO) can be a destructive disorder that causes ischemia and necrosis of the inner retina, ultimately causing permanent vision loss [1]. Patients often present with abrupt, painless, and extensive vision loss in the affected eye. The clinical examination may show attenuated retinal arteries, retinal edema, a relative afferent papillary defect, and severe visual impairment. The distinct characteristic of central retinal artery occlusion is the cherry-red spot. This red spot indicates edema of the retina and it occurs as a result of the choroidal blood supply beneath the fovea being unaffected.

The most common cause of a central retinal artery occlusion is embolism. Retinal emboli may be glistening or non-glistening cholesterol with associated, platelet-fibrin composition from sources such as the heart (aortic arch disease, atrial fibrillation, and valvular disease), carotid artery, and optic disc, respectively. Emboli may also be calcific in etiology [1,7]. Arteritic CRAO has been affiliated with vasculitic conditions, such as giant cell arteritis, Henoch–Schonlein purpura, Kawasaki disease, polyarteritis, nodosum, systemic lupus, and Wegner's granulomatosis [1,8].

Evaluation of a central retinal artery occlusion requires a comprehensive search for a cause, including carotid artery imaging via carotid ultrasound, computed tomography (CT) angiography or magnetic resonance (MR) angiography. Echocardiogram (transthoracic or transesophageal) is also necessary. Pertinent laboratory studies, such as ESR, C-reactive protein, C- and P-ANCA, should also be checked based on constitutional symptoms.

Treatment

The first problem with instituting treatment is recognition by the patient that vision loss has occurred. Secondly, the promptness with which an implemented treatment method can affect outcome. The longer the retina is ischemic, the less likely it is to recover. The ischemic retina has been known to survive up to 4 hours [7]. Hayreh [9] demonstrated that

without arterial blood flow, the retina in the rhesus monkey can survive up to 100 min, and between 180 and 240 min when collateral circulation is present [7,9]. Several authors have published articles on the management of central retinal artery occlusion ranging from conservative to aggressive; however, no premier treatment has come to the forefront. Conservative management options include acetazolamide, aspirin, anterior chamber paracentesis, a combination of 5% carbon and 95% oxygen inhalation and ocular massage [1,7,8].

A meta-analysis of all of the trials for IA thrombolysis for CRAO showed that IA may provide better outcomes for CRAO than conservative and conventional treatments [10]. Aldrich *et al.* reported a prospective non-randomized case series of intra-arterial tPA use in CRAO up to 15 hours from the onset of CRAO and 75% of tPA patients had VA improvement [11] European Assessment Group for Lysis in the Eye (EAGLE) is a multicentered trial initiated in 2006 by 16 centers located in Austria, Germany, and Switzerland [12]. To date, the centers involved in this study have the most experience with IA thrombolysis. This study includes patients up to 20 hours out from CRAO. Patients were treated with a maximum dose of 50 mg of tissue plasminogen activator [7,13]. EAGLE did not show an improvement in VA after thrombolysis, but did suggests that a delay in treatment after the onset of symptom renders thrombolysis ineffective and that if thrombolytics are administered earlier, then there is an increased chance of better visual outcomes.

Chen *et al.* are recently held the first prospective randomized, placebo-controlled multicentered trial comparing the efficacy of intravenous tPA and placebo in acute CRAO. Their work revealed early improvement in visual acuity of three lines or more in two of eight tPA subjects but in none of the placebo subjects. This improvement was prudent during the first week after tPA, but was not sustained over a 6-month period; therefore, the primary outcome measure was not achieved. Both subjects received tPA within 6 hours of symptom onset. Visual deterioration in the two subjects was mainly due to artery reocclusion that was confirmed via fluorescein angiography.

The most dreaded adverse effect of intravenous thrombolytic administration is either intracerebral or systemic hemorrhage. The expected risk of hemorrhage should be comparable to that faced in coronary artery or peripheral vascular thrombolysis given that brain tissue is assumed to be normal. Thus, the risk of intracerebral hemorrhage is 0.3% (95% CI 0.2–0.4) based on the more than 6000 patients in the GISSI-2 trial who received systemic tPA in myocardial infarction [11]. In Chen *et al.*'s recent study, they had one patient who sustained intracerebral hemorrhage post tPA administration.

Terson's syndrome

Background

Some patients who sustain intracranial hemorrhage, in particular a subarachnoid hemorrhage, can acutely develop increased intracranial pressure, which can impede ocular venous outflow and subsequently cause vitreous hemorrhage. This phenomenon is known as Terson's syndrome [14]. The pathophysiology of this syndrome is hotly debated. Theories include blood arising from a ruptured capillary or vein causes hydro-dissection of the retinal inner limiting membrane [15]. As well as that vitreous hemorrhage happens because of a sharp elevation of intracranial pressure transmitted throughout the venous channels into the orbital veins and that pressure is not adequately spread down the sheath space [14].

Terson's syndrome occurs in 8–14.5% of patients with subarachnoid hemorrhage [14,16]. A common complication of this syndrome is the accumulation of blood in the area of the macula, which can contribute to the patient's decreased visual acuity secondary to vitreous hemorrhage. Other clinical findings may include altered level of consciousness secondary to intracranial bleeding and headache [16]. Studies have revealed that approximately 89% of patients who developed intraocular hemorrhage had a history of coma compared to patients who did not have intraocular hemorrhage [14,16,17]. Therefore, it is extremely important that these individuals have a thorough ocular examination.

Treatment

Terson's syndrome often goes unrecognized. In one study, approximately half the patients with a subarachnoid or sub-dural hemorrhage did not receive funduscopic evaluation [14]. Despite the clinical implications of this patient population, ophthalmologists are rarely consulted. In addition to the clinical examination, detailed evaluation of the globe on a CT scan may show Terson's hemorrhage and alert clinicians that a careful ophthalmoscopic examination is required [18].

Even though most Terson's hemorrhages resolve spontaneously, vitrectomy can be a viable option. Many studies have shown this procedure to be a low surgical risk that often produces excellent outcomes and allow for quick rehabilitation [14–18]. Complications associated with vitrectomy include, cataract, endophthalmitis, macular hole, retinal detachment, and retinal tear [14].

Stroke

Even though it is beyond the scope of this chapter to discuss the in-depth details and management of stroke, it would be remiss not acknowledge that stroke is often a cause of acute vision loss. More than three out of four stroke sufferers report some form of disability, of which visual impairment is becoming more recognized. Approximately 16% of these have a homonymous visual field defect post-stroke [19].

Zhang *et al.* looked at 880 brain lesion locations and determined that homonymous field defects due to occipital lobe lesions were found in 45% of cases, followed by optic radiation (33%), optic tract (10.2%), multiple sites (11.4%), and lateral geniculate body (1%) [20]. Townsend *et al.* looked at 61 consecutive stroke admissions who were then subsequently assessed with formal perimetric visual field testing 9 months post-stroke and found that 16% of patients had homonymous field defects. Of these patients, none were aware of their vision loss. This study also looked at visual field testing using the confrontational method utilized in The National Institutes of Health Stroke Scale (NIHSS). Only two patients had visual field defects on using this method. Their data revealed that NIHSS confrontational visual field testing had a sensitivity of 20% (95% CI=4–56%) for post-stroke homonymous visual field loss and a specificity of 98% (95% CI=88–99%) when compared to objective perimetry. Their conclusion was that the prevalence of post-stroke homonymous visual field loss is relatively high and is underestimated by confrontational testing, and that these patients are commonly unaware of their defects.

Treatment

Management of vision loss due to stroke is focused on addressing the corresponding symptoms caused by the visual defect. The first step in treatment is to accurately determine what the true defect is. Having the patient undergo formal perimetry testing does this. In cases of homonymous hemianopia, treatment can be directed based on the patients' ability to deal with their surrounding environment, driving, and reading.

Navigating one's environment with a visual field defect can be quite challenging, but can sometimes be achieved by directing the eyes toward the hemianopic field using large eye movements into the blind field, then letting the eyes return to the object. Prism placed in glasses can also be used to help a person compensate for the visual field loss. Prism or glasses attempt to shift or move the visual field toward the defect to attract attention to objects. A prism deviates the light emerging from an object toward its base, causing the object to appear displaced toward the apex of the prism [21]. When this occurs, a stationary object seen through a prism with its base facing the left will look as though it has been shifted to the right and into the right half of the visual field. In case of left-sided homonymous hemianopia, the prism is placed in the left sector of each lens (the patient's left) with the base facing the left. If the patient needs information from the left half of the visual field, he/she must make an eye movement to the left to access the prism. The prism will then move the user's visual world about 10° into the "seeing half" of the field. This process requires the ability to generate saccadic movement. Because saccadic eye movements are often affected by strokes, a patient may benefit from saccadic training [21]. Visual rehabilitation in the past has also included visual restorative therapy (VRT); however, this strategy is expensive and has not been proved to be very effective. Spitznya *et al.* found a strategy that has been found to be very helpful in improving saccades in patients with hemianopic alexia is *read right*. This study showed a significant improvement in patients using a simple moving text stimulus. This improvement was dependent on the specific intervention and not because of generation of random saccades, placebo or visual stimulation [22,23]. This protocol can be accessed free of cost at http://www.readright.ucl.ac.uk [23].

Optic nerve disorders

Optic neuritis

Background

Optic neuritis (ON) is often a painful acute inflammatory disorder affecting the optic nerve, and is the most common cause of unilateral vision loss in those below the age of 50 with an incidence of 1–5 in 100 000 per year [1,24]. Even though the most common cause of optic neuritis is demyelinating disease, the differential diagnosis is very broad – including: acute glaucoma, B12 deficiency, infection (HIV, histoplasmosis, syphilis, varicella, west Nile virus), multiple sclerosis, neuromyelitis optica, recurrent idiopathic optic neuritis, retinal artery occlusion, retinal detachment, rheumatologic disease (antiphospholipid antibody syndrome, Behcet's disease, SLE, Sjogren's syndrome), and sarcoidosis [1,25].

One of the distinct characteristics of optic neuritis is eye pain or tenderness with eye movement or touch. Clinical evaluation may reveal decreased visual acuity, red desaturation, and reduced contrast sensitivity. A relative afferent pupillary defect is a distinguishing component and should almost always be present. In about two-thirds of cases of optic neuritis, the optic disc may appear normal whereas the other one-third may have a swollen optic nerve [1,25,26]. The appearance of a macular star and optic neuritis suggests an infectious cause. Perimetry testing may show a central scotoma, but can also show altitudinal, arcuate defects or peripheral constriction.

Neuroimaging is critical in the work-up of optic neuritis. Magnetic resonance imaging with and without gadolinium will often show optic nerve enhancement. MRI may also show lesion suggestive of demyelinating diseases such as acute disseminated encephalomyelitis (ADEM), multiple sclerosis or neuromyelitis optica. The most predictive factor for the development of multiple sclerosis after optic neuritis is the presence of asymptomatic demyelinating lesions in the central nervous system [24].

Treatment

Intravenous (IV) methylprednisolone has become the standard in management of acute optic neuritis. Doses may vary from 500 to 1000 mg daily over a 3- to 5-day course. The use of IV steroids within 2–3 weeks of initial symptom onset can hasten visual recovery, but has no influence on long-term visual outcome[24–29]. The Optic Neuritis Treatment Trial (ONTT) [27–29] has been considered the major study which established the guidelines for optic neuritis management. In the ONTT, almost 80% of patients showed improvement by week 3 and about 93% at week 5. Improvement may continue to occur up to 1 year; however, 5–10% of patients fail to have any meaningful recovery.

Neuromyelitis optica

Background

Devic's disease or neuromyelitis optica (NMO) can be a devastating, immune-mediated, inflammatory demyelinating disease which targets the brain, optic nerve, and spinal cord (1). Lennon *et al.* determined that the NMO-Ig specifically targets aquaporin 4 water channels located in the blood–brain barrier of the central nervous system [30,31]. MRI brain lesions can be found in the area postrema, peri-fourth ventricle, nucleus tractus solitaries, and the subependymal regions [30].

NMO can present with features of optic neuritis or transverse myelitis separately over time or simultaneously.

Apart from symptoms associated with optic neuritis (pain, vision loss) or transverse myelitis (sensory, motor impairment) if the brainstem is involved, examination findings can consist of varying degrees of diplopia, facial weakness, hearing loss, intractable hiccups, nausea, nystagmus, ptosis, trigeminal neuralgia, respiratory failure, vertigo, and vomiting [1,30,32].

The 5-year survival rate for those with a monophasic course is 90%, whereas for those with a relapsing course it is lower at 68%. Respiratory failure and subsequent death due to cervical spinal cord involvement occurs in approximately 32% of people [31].

Treatment

The mainstay of therapy for neuromyelitis optica is a combination of steroids (intravenous methylprednisolone or oral prednisone) and azathioprine. There have also been several studies confirming disease response to agents such as immunomodulators, mitoxantrone, mycophenolate mofetil, plasmapheresis, and rituximab [1].

Idiopathic intracranial hypertension

Background

Idiopathic intracranial hypertension (IIH) is a condition that most commonly affects obese young women between the ages of 15 and 45. In more than 90% of patients, the most common presenting symptom of idiopathic intracranial hypertension is headache [1]. The distinct clinical exam finding of IIH is papilledema. A prospective study of 50 patients diagnosed with IIH found that 94% of them had transient visual obscuration, 58% described intracranial noises, 54% had photopsias and 44% complained of retrobulbar pain (Wall and George) [34]. In some cases, IIH can be associated with a sixth nerve palsy; however, if other focal neurologic deficits are found, strongly consider a different diagnosis. In the beginning stages of IIH-associated papilledema, visual acuity may be normal; however, if the intracranial pressure persistently remains elevated, papilledema can worsen, and vision can rapidly deteriorate leading to complete vision loss [1].

Neuroimaging, including CT, computer tomography venography (CTV), MRI or magnetic resonance venography (MRV) of the brain to exclude intracranial pathology (e.g., tumor and venous sinus thrombosis), a lumbar puncture to accurately record normal CSF constituents, and an elevated opening CSF pressure ($>25 \, cmH_2O$) are the three vital components needed for the diagnosis of IIH [1,34,35]. Mimickers of papilledema include anomalous or tilted disks and optic nerve head drusen. Neuroimaging, such as MRI, can sometimes reveal tilting of the optic nerve, and CT may reveal optic nerve calcification. Fluorescein angiography (FA) can be performed in the outpatient setting, and can also be used to distinguish anomalous optic nerves from true papilledema. True papilledema generally shows both elevation of the optic nerves and obscuration of the vessels around the nerve [1].

Treatment

Because of the scarceness of evidence-based clinical treatment trials, there are no precise treatment recommendations for IIH. Management of IIH must focus on protecting visual function as well as symptom relief [34]. Some patients with headache and minimal visual signs are often managed conservatively provided they are monitored regularly with frequent visual fields to make sure there are no signs of visual deterioration. Intractable headache and evidence of vision loss are the primary indicators to initiate treatment [1]. Treatment modalities include diuretics and weight loss, serial lumbar punctures, optic nerve sheath fenestration, ventricular-peritoneal or lumbar peritoneal shunts, and stenting [1]. Headache can be best treated with a combination of a diuretic such as acetazolamide and anti-migraine drugs [1,4]. Topiramate can also be an effective alternative as it is FDA approved for migraine prophylaxis, has weak diuretic properties and has a known side effect of weight loss [1].

Non-physiologic vision loss

Functional vision loss is an important entity to keep in the differential diagnosis for acute vision loss, especially in the setting of a normal ocular and neurologic examination. One of the key points to understand is that non-physiologic vision loss is a diagnosis of exclusion. It is imperative that true pathology is ruled out via the detailed history of physical neuroimaging. Because it can be quite difficult to distinguish physiologic and non-physiologic vision loss in the hospital setting, ancillary neuro-ophthalmic evaluation needs to be performed in the outpatient setting. Testing as in the clinical setting can include use of an OKN drum, mirror, perimetry testing (Goldman and automated), prism dissociation test and fogging with a phoropter or trial lens fogging. One test that can be performed in either the hospital or outpatient setting is the fingertip touching test. In this test, a person who is truly blind can readily touch his/her fingertips together because of intact proprioception, whereas the patient in non-physiologic vision loss will be unable to touch the fingertips together. Once the diagnosis of non-organic vision loss is made, it must be determined whether the condition is due to malingering, Munchausen's syndrome or psychogenic disturbance. If the latter two are the cause, it is important that the patient be referred to appropriate psychologic/psychiatric services.

References

1 Spencer, B. & Digre, K. (2010) Treatments for Neurophthalmic Conditions. *Neurologic Clinics*, **28**(4), 1005–1035.

2 Guyer, D.R., Miller, N.R., Auer, C.L. & Fine, S.L. (1985) The risk of cerebrovascular and cardiovascular disease in patients with anterior ischemic optic neuropathy. *Archives of Ophthalmology*, **103**, 1136–1142.

3 Purvin, V. & Kawasaki, A. (2005) Neuro-ophthalmic emergencies for the neurologist. *The Neurologist*, **11**, 195–233.

4 Hayreh, S.S. (2009) Ischemic optic neuropathy. *Progress in Retinal and Eye Research*, **28**(1), 34–62.

5 Schwedt, T.J., Dodick, D.W. & Caselli, R.J. (2006) Giant cell arteritis. *Current Pain and Headache Reports*, **10**, 415–420.

6 Phillips, P.H. (2007) Treatment of diplopia. *Seminars in Neurology*, **27**, 288–298.

7 Biousse, V., Calvetti, O., Bruce, B.B. & Newman, N.J. (2007) Thrombolysis for central retinal artery occlusion. *Journal of Neuro-Ophthalmology*, **27**, 215–230.

8 Hazin, R., Dixon, J.A. & Bhatti, T. (2009) Thrombolytic therapy in central retinal artery occlusion: cutting edge therapy, standard of care therapy, or impractical therapy. *Current Opinion in Ophthalmology*, **20**, 210–218.

9 Hayreh, S.S., Kolder, H.E. & Weingeist, T.A. (1980) Central retinal artery occlusion and retinal tolerance time. *Ophthalmology*, **87**, 75–78.

10 Noble, J., Weizblit, N., Baerlocher, M.O. Intra-arterial thrombolysis for central retinal artery occlusion: a systematic review. *Br J Ophthalmol.* 2008;**92**(**5**):588-593. doi: 10.1136/bjo.2007.133488.

11 Chen, C.S., Lee, A.W., Campbell, B. *et al.* (2011) Efficacy of intravenous tissue-type plasminogen activator in central retinal artery occlusion. *Stroke*, **42**, 2229–2234.

12 Feltgen, N., Neubauer, A., Jurklies, B. *et al.* (2006) Mutlicenter study of the European assessment group for lysis in the eye

(EAGLE) for the treatment of central retinal artery occlusio: design issues and implications. EAGLE study report no. 1. *Graefe's Archive for Clinical and Experimental Ophthalmology*, **244**, 950–956.

13 Klein, R., Klein, B.E., Moss, S.E. *et al.* (2000) The epidemiology of retinal vein occlusion: the Beaver Dam Eye Study. *Transactions of the American Ophthalmological Society*, **98**, 133–141.

14 Ogawa, T., Kitaoka, T., Dake, Y. & Amemiya, T. (2001) Terson syndrome, a case report suggesting the mechanism of vitreous hemorrhage. *Ophthalmology*, **108**, 1654–1656.

15 Garweg, J.G. & Koerner, F. (2009) Outcome indicators for vitrectomy in Terson syndrome. *Acta Ophthalmologica*, **87**, 222–226.

16 Roux, F.X., Panthier, J.N., Tanghe, Y.M. *et al.* (1991) Terson's syndrome and intraocular complications in meningeal hemorrhages. *Neurochirurgie*, **37**, 106–110.

17 Swallo, C.E., Tsuruda, J.S., Digre, K.B., Glaser, M.J., Davidson, H.C. & Harnsberger, H.R. (1998 Apr) Terson syndrome: CT evaluation in 12 patients. *AJNR American Journal of Neuroradiology*, **19**(**4**), 743–747.

18 Rinker, J.R. & Cross, A.H. (2007) Diagnosis and dfferential diagnosis of Multiple Sclerosis. *Contiunuum Lifelong Learning in Neurology*, **13**(**5**), 13–34.

19 Townsend, B.S., Sturm, J.W., Petsoglou, C., O'leary, B., Whyte, S. & Crimmins, D. (2007) Perimetric homonymous visual field loss Post-Stroke. *Journal of Clinical Neuroscience*, **14**, 754–756.

20 Zhang, X., kedar, S., Lynn, M.J., Newman, N.J. & Biousse, V. (2006) Homonymous Hemianopias: Clinical-anatomic correlation in 904 cases. *Neurology*, **66**, 906–910.

21 Khan, S., Leung, E. & Joy, W. (2008) Stroke and Visual Reahbilitation. *Topics in Stroke Rehabilitation*, **15**(**1**), 27–36.

22 Spitznya, G.A., Wise, R.J., McDonald, S.A., Plant, G.T., Crewes, H. & Leff, A.P. (2007) Optikokinetic therapy improves text reading in patients with hemianopic alexia: a controlled trial. *Neurology*, **68**(**22**), 1922–1930.

23 Glisson, C.C. & Galetta, S.L. (2007) Visual Rehabilitation: now you see it; now you don't. *Neurology*, **68**(**22**), 1881–1882.

24 Voss, E., Raab, P., Trebst, C. & Stangel, M. (2011) Clinical approach to optic neuritis: pitfalls, red flags and differential diagnosis. *Therapeutic Advances in Neurological Disorders*, **4**(**2**), 123–34.

25 Chu, E.R. & Chen, C.S. (2000) Optic neuritis more than a loss of vision. *Australian Family Physician*, **30**(**10**), 789–793.

26 Keltner, J.L., Johnson, C.A., Spur, J.O. *et al.* (1993) Baseline visual field profile of optic neuritis. The experience of the optic neuritis treatment trial. Optic Neuritis Study Group. *Archives of Ophthalmology*, **111**, 231–234.

27 Beck, R.W. (1992) The optic neuritis treatment trial. Implications for clinical practice. Optic Neuritis Study Group [Editorial]. *Archives of Ophthalmology*, **110**, 331–332.

28 Beck, R.W., Cleary, P.A. & Backlund, J.C. (1994) The course of visual recovery after optic neuritis. Experience of the Optic Neuritis Treatment Trial. *Ophthalmology*, **101**, 1771–1778.

29 Peixoto, M.A. (2008) Devic's neuromyelitis optica. *Arq Neuropsiquiatr*, **66**(**1**), 120–138.

30 Wingerchuk, D.M., Hogancamp, W.F., Obrien, P.C. & Weinshenker, B.G. (1999) The clinical course of neuromyelitis optica (Devic's syndrome). *Neurology*, **53**, 1107–1114.

31 Lennon, V.A., Wingerchuk, D.M., Kryser, T.J. *et al.* (2004) A serum autoantibody marker of neuromyelitis optica: distinction from multiple sclerosis. *Lancet*, **364**, 2106–2112.

32 Vernant, J.C., Cabre, P., Smadja, D. *et al.* (1997) Recurrent optic neuromyelitis with endocrinopathies: a new syndrome. *Neurology*, **45**, 58–64.

33 Miller, N.L., Walsh, F.B., Newman, N.J., Biousse, V. & Kerrison, J.B. (2007) *Walsh and Hoyt's Clinical Neuro-Ophthalmology: The Essentials*. Lippincott Williams & Wilkins, Philadelphia, PA, pp. 122–146.

34 Wall, M. & George, D. (1991) Idiopathic intracranial hypertension(pseudotumor cerebri), a prospective study of 54 patients. *Brain*, **114**, 155–180.

35 Mathew, N.T., Ravishankar, K. & Sanin, L.C. (1996) Coexistence of migraine and idiopathic intracranial hypertension without papilledema. *Neurology*, **46**, 1226–1230.

CHAPTER 14
Secondary prevention of stroke

Gord Gubitz

Dalhousie University, Division of Neurology, Department of Medicine, Halifax, Nova Scotia, Canada

What can be done to prevent further strokes in stroke survivors?

Quite simply put, prevention of further strokes in stroke survivors involves a detailed assessment and management plan for each stroke survivor's vascular risk factors. It should be emphasized that managing risk factors for stroke has added the benefit of helping to manage other vascular diseases, including coronary artery disease and peripheral vascular disease. In addition, all of this information applies equally to persons who have experienced a transient ischemic attack (TIA), as the risk of subsequent stroke is the same as for a completed stroke, regardless of the stroke severity.

There are a number of publicly available national guideline statements that contain specific evidence-based approaches to the secondary prevention of stroke. Most of these are complementary (i.e., they arrive at the same general conclusions for a given topic), but there may be some variation, depending on when the guideline was last updated – this should be relatively easy to determine. *Caveat emptor.*

Examples of national stroke prevention initiatives include the following:

http://stroke.ahajournals.org/content/42/1/227.full.pdf
(American Stroke Association)

www.strokebestpractices.ca (Canadian Stroke Best Practice Recommendations)

http://www.rcplondon.ac.uk/resources/stroke-guidelines
(UK National Stroke Guidelines)

http://www.sign.ac.uk/guidelines/published/index.html
(Scottish Intercollegiate Guidelines)

http://strokefoundation.com.au/health-professionals/
clinical-guidelines (Australian Guidelines)

The reader is also invited to explore the National Guideline Clearinghouse for a more comprehensive list of stroke prevention guidelines, documents, and other resources:

http://www.guideline.gov/search/search.aspx?term=
stroke+prevention

Vascular risk factor modification for secondary stroke prevention

Vascular risk factor modification for the prevention of recurrent stroke can be divided into two categories: non-modifiable vascular risk factors and modifiable vascular risk factors.

Non-Modifiable Vascular Risk Factors cannot be treated, and include: age, sex, a history of previous stroke or other vascular disease, and a strong family history of stroke or other vascular disease.

Modifiable Vascular Risk Factors can be measured and treated, and include the following:

1 Hypertension management
2 Dyslipidemia management
3 Diabetes management
4 Smoking cessation
5 Antithrombotic agents in stroke survivors with atrial fibrillation
6 Antiplatelet agents in stroke survivors without atrial fibrillation
7 Endarterectomy for symptomatic carotid disease
8 Obstructive sleep apnea management
9 Lifestyle management (eating a balanced diet, limiting salt intake, moderating alcohol consumption, increasing physical activity, and optimizing weight).

Hypertension
General statement

It is generally accepted that hypertension is the most important modifiable risk factor for stroke, and that as blood pressure increases, so does the risk of stroke. This was demonstrated in the INTERSTROKE study [1], an international observational study, which shows that hypertension contributed to 34.6% of the population-attributed risk (PAR) for stroke (and 52% when blood pressures were

Evidence-Based Neurology: Management of Neurological Disorders, Second Edition. Edited by Bart M. Demaerschalk and Dean M. Wingerchuk.
© 2015 John Wiley & Sons, Ltd. Published 2015 by John Wiley & Sons, Ltd.

greater than 160/90 mmHg). Healthcare practitioners should be trained in the proper technique for measuring blood pressure, and blood pressure must be treated to current standards. In general, a target blood pressure of less than 140/80 mmHg (and less than 130/70 mmHg for diabetics) is a reasonable goal for stroke survivors. The preferred agents for secondary stroke prevention include a combination of a diuretic and an ACE Inhibitor.

Brief evidence summary

A systematic review [2] assessed the effectiveness of lowering BP in preventing recurrent vascular events in patients with previous stroke (ischemic or hemorrhagic) or TIA. Seven randomized controlled trials, with eight comparison groups, were included. The results of the meta-analysis indicated that lowering BP or treating hypertension with a variety of antihypertensive agents reduced a number of outcome events, including stroke (OR 0.76, 95% CI 0.63–0.92), non-fatal stroke (OR 0.79, 95% CI 0.65–0.95), myocardial infarction (MI) (OR 0.79, 95% CI 0.63–0.98), and total vascular events (OR 0.79, 95% CI 0.66–0.95). Importantly, heterogeneity was present for several outcomes and was partly related to the class of antihypertensive drugs used. **The meta-analysis indicated that ACE inhibitors and diuretics separately,** *and especially together,* **reduced vascular events**, while beta-receptor antagonists had no discernable effect. The reduction in stroke was related to the difference in systolic BP between treatment and control groups ($P < 0.002$). In addition, vascular prevention was associated positively with the magnitude by which BP is reduced. The authors of the systematic review indicated that the trial evidence supported the use of antihypertensive agents in lowering BP for the prevention of vascular events in patients with previous stroke or TIA.

In order to address the question about BP lowering in the elderly, the *HYVET study* [3] randomly assigned 3845 patients who were > 80 years of age to receive either antihypertensive therapy or matching placebo. The results showed that lowering mean blood pressure by 15.0/6.1 mmHg associated with a 30% reduction in the rate of fatal or non-fatal stroke (95% CI 1% to 51%, $p = 0.06$), a 21% reduction in the rate of death from all causes (95% CI 4% to 35%, $p = 0.02$), and a 39% reduction in the rate of death from stroke (95% CI 1% to 62%, $p = 0.05$). Fewer serious adverse events were reported in the active treatment group (358 vs 448 in the placebo group, $p = 0.001$). The authors concluded that antihypertensive treatment in patients of ≥80 years of age was beneficial. This finding was confirmed in an open-label active treatment extension of the HYVET study including 1682 patients from both the original treatment and placebo group [4].

Dyslipidemia

General statement

There is abundant evidence that elevated blood LDL levels are associated with a higher risk of stroke and myocardial infarction. It is recommended that a statin drug should be prescribed as secondary prevention to most patients who have had an ischemic stroke or transient ischemic attack in order to achieve an LDL cholesterol of <2.0 mmol/L, or a 50% reduction in LDL cholesterol from baseline. In addition to statin use, stroke survivors should be counseled regarding lifestyle changes, including dietary modification and regular exercise as part of a comprehensive plan to help reduce LDL values.

Brief evidence summary

The *Heart Protection Study* (*HPS*) [5] randomized 20 536 patients, 40–80 years, at elevated risk of coronary heart disease death because of past history of MI or other coronary heart disease, occlusive disease of non-coronary arteries, diabetes mellitus or treated hypertension or had baseline blood total cholesterol of ≥ 3.5 mmol/L. They were randomized to simvastatin 40 mg versus placebo. The trial demonstrated benefit in patients with prior stroke and TIA, even if their LDL cholesterol level was not significantly elevated. Simvastatin significantly reduced the first event rate of stroke versus placebo. There was no significant difference in strokes attributed to hemorrhage (51 vs 53, $P < 0.8$). Simvastatin also reduced the number of patients having transient cerebral ischemic attacks alone (2.0% vs 2.4%, $P < 0.02$) or requiring carotid endarterectomy or angioplasty (0.4% vs 0.8%, $P < 0.0003$). The benefits were evident in every subgroup tested, and were independent of the baseline cholesterol level.

The *Stroke Prevention by Aggressive Reduction in Cholesterol Levels* (*SPARCLs*) [6] trial randomized 4731 patients with stroke or TIA in the past 6 months, and LDL levels of 2.6–4.9 mmol/L and no known coronary artery disease to atorvastatin 80 mg once daily or placebo. The 5-year absolute reduction in risk of any stroke was 2.2%, relative risk reduction was 16%, and adjusted hazard ratio (HR) was 0.84 (95% CI 0.71–0.99, $p = 0.03$). The reduction in ischemic stroke (HR 0.78, 95% CI 0.66–0.94) should be weighed against the statistically significant increase in hemorrhagic stroke (HR 1.66, 95% CI 1.08–2.55). The 5-year absolute reduction in risk of major cardiovascular events was 3.5% (HR 0.80, 95% CI 0.69–0.92, $p = 0.002$). The statistically significant increase in hemorrhagic stroke, not seen in other statin trials, remains unexplained.

Diabetes

General statement

Diabetes is a major risk factor for all vascular disease and is known to be an independent risk factor for ischemic stroke, but the interaction between diabetes and other conventional risk factors is complex. The Framingham Study found a 2.5-fold incidence of ischemic stroke in diabetic men and a 3.6-fold incidence in diabetic women [7]. For secondary prevention in stroke survivors with type 1 or type 2 diabetes, there is general agreement that efforts should be made to achieve a glycated hemoglobin (Hb_{A1C}) level of $\leq 7.0\%$, using a combination of diet, oral hypoglycemic agents, and insulin if necessary. Close control of other vascular risk factors (treating BP to <130/80, statin use, initiation of antithrombotic therapy, advice regarding diet, exercise, and smoking cessation) should also be undertaken unless specifically contraindicated, as many diabetics have components of the metabolic syndrome; these risk factors compound the stroke risk for diabetic stroke survivors.

Brief evidence summary

The *ACCORD Study* [8] enrolled 10 251 patients, mean age 62 years, A1c at entry 8.1%, with a combination of Type II DM and cardiovascular disease. Patients were randomized to intensive control (A1C < 6%) versus conventional care (A1C 7.0–7.9%). The primary outcome (a composite of non-fatal myocardial infarction, non-fatal stroke or death from cardiovascular causes) showed a non-statistically significant difference between the intensive group (6.86%) and the conventional group (7.23%, HR 0.90, 95% CI 0.78–1.04, $p = 0.16$). There was a non-significant decrease in non-fatal stroke, but a significant increase in all-cause mortality in the intensively treated group (HR 1.22, 95% CI 1.01–1.46, $P = 0.04$). This finding led to a discontinuation of intensive therapy after a mean of 3.5 years of follow-up. The study identified a previously unrecognized harm of *intensive* glucose lowering in high-risk patients with type 2 diabetes.

The *ADVANCE Study* [9] enrolled 11 140 patients, mean age 66 years, A1C at entry 7.5%, with a combination of type II DM, cardiovascular disease, and stroke (9%). Patients were randomized to intensive control (A1C < 6.5%) versus conventional care (AIC ~ 7%). The primary vascular outcome showed a non-statistically significant decrease in macrovascular outcomes, and non-fatal stroke, with a decrease in nephropathy in the intensively treated group.

The *PROACTIVE Study* [10] enrolled 5238 patients, mean age 61 years, A1C at entry 7.8%, with a combination of Type II DM, cardiovascular disease, and stroke (19%). Patients were randomized to routine care plus Pioglitazone or placebo. The primary outcome was not statistically significant. However, the subgroup with a history of previous stroke demonstrated a decrease in cardiovascular events in the pioglitazone group.

Smoking cessation

General statement

The INTERSTROKE study [1] reported that current smokers had an increased risk of stroke, and that the risk increased with the number of cigarettes smoked per day; the impact of smoking on stroke was second only to hypertension. As smoking is now recognized as an addiction and not a 'habit', every stroke survivor who is a smoker should be offered unambiguous, non-judgmental advice about smoking cessation, either directly or through referral to a local addictions specialist. A combination of behavioral therapy

and patient-specific pharmacological therapy (with either nicotine replacement therapy, bupropion or varenicline) should be offered.

Brief evidence summary

In a Cochrane Collaboration systematic review [11], smoking cessation interventions that used behavioral therapy strategies, either solely or in combination with pharmacotherapy, produced a significant effect in favor of the intervention (RR 1.43, 95% CI 1.03–1.98, $p = 0.032$).

A systematic review and meta-analysis of pharmacological smoking cessation therapies [12] found that Bupropion trials were superior to controls at one year (12 RCTs, OR 1.56, 95% CI 1.10–2.21, $p = 0.01$). Two RCTs provided evidence to support bupropion over nicotine replacement therapy (NRT) at one year (OR 1.14, 95% CI 0.20–6.42, $p \leq 0.0001$). Three RCTs evaluated the effectiveness of varenicline versus bupropion at one year (OR 1.58, 95% CI 1.22–2.05). Using indirect comparisons, varenicline was superior to NRT when compared to placebo (OR 1.66, 95% CI 1.17–2.36, $p = 0.004$) or to all controls at one year (OR 1.73, 95% CI 1.22–2.45, $p = 0.001$). Adverse events were not systematically different across studies.

Antithrombotic agents in stroke survivors with atrial fibrillation

General statement

Atrial fibrillation (AF) is an important modifiable risk factor for stroke. Epidemiological evidence demonstrates that about one in six patients with ischemic stroke will have AF. Strokes caused by atrial fibrillation tend to be larger, and often result in worse clinical outcomes. If AF can be detected, strokes caused by AF can be prevented. It is now generally held that most patients with acute ischemic stroke and AF should receive oral anticoagulant therapy with the new oral anticoagulants (NOACs: apixaban, dabigatran, rivaroxaban), in preference to warfarin. Antiplatelets should only be used in that small minority of patients who are genuinely not able to tolerate an anticoagulant, as antiplatelet agents offer inferior protection against stroke. Anticoagulant therapy should be started as soon as it is thought to be safe for the patient. For stroke prevention, the NOACs have advantages in safety, efficacy or both when compared with warfarin.

Brief evidence summary
Warfarin versus placebo in patients with atrial fibrillation and stroke

One Cochrane systematic review sought to assess the effect of anticoagulants (warfarin) for secondary prevention, after a stroke or TIA, in patients with NRAF [13]. Two trials involving 485 people were included. Follow-up time was 1.7 years in one trial and 2.3 years in the other. Warfarin reduced the odds of recurrent stroke by two-thirds (OR 0.36, 95% CI 0.22–0.58). The odds of all vascular events were almost halved by treatment (OR 0.55, 95% CI 0.37–0.82).

The odds of major extracranial hemorrhage were increased (OR 4.32, 95% CI 1.55–12.10). No intracranial bleeds were reported among people given anticoagulants. The authors concluded that warfarin was beneficial, without serious adverse effects, for people with NRAF and recent cerebral ischemia.

Warfarin versus antiplatelet agents in patients with atrial fibrillation and stroke

One Cochrane systematic review compared the effect of warfarin with antiplatelet agents, for secondary prevention, in people with NRAF and previous cerebral ischemia [14]. Two trials were identified; The European Atrial Fibrillation Trial (EAFT) involving 455 patients, who received either warfarin (International Normalized Ratio (INR) 2.5–4.0) or aspirin (300 mg/day). Patients joined the trial within 3 months of TIA or minor stroke. The mean follow-up time was 2.3 years. In the Studio Italiano Fibrillazione Atriale (SIFA) trial, 916 patients with NRAF and a TIA or minor stroke within the previous 15 days were randomized to open-label warfarin (INR 2.0–3.5) or indobufen (a reversible platelet cyclooxygenase inhibitor, 100 or 200 mg bid). The follow-up time was 1 year. The combined results show that warfarin was significantly more effective than antiplatelet therapy both for all vascular events (Peto odds ratio (Peto OR) 0.67, 95% CI 0.50–0.91) and for recurrent stroke (Peto OR 0.49, 95% CI 0.33–0.72). Major extracranial bleeding complications occurred more often in patients with warfarin (Peto OR 5.16, 95% CI 2.08–12.83), but the absolute difference was small (2.8% per year vs 0.9% per year in EAFT and 0.9% per year vs 0% in SIFA). Warfarin did not cause any significant increase in intracranial bleeds. The authors concluded that the evidence from two trials suggests that anticoagulant therapy is superior to antiplatelet therapy for the prevention of stroke in people with NRAF and recent non-disabling stroke or TIA. The risk of extracranial bleeding was higher with anticoagulant therapy than with antiplatelet therapy.

Warfarin versus the novel anticoagulants (NOACs) in patients with atrial fibrillation

At present, there are three NOACs that have been studied against warfarin (the gold standard), in properly conducted randomized controlled clinical trials.

Dabigatran

The **RE-LY (Randomized Evaluation of Long-term Anticoagulant Therapy) trial** [15] compared two doses of dabigatran (a direct thrombin inhibitor) to warfarin in 18 130 patients with atrial fibrillation at increased risk of stroke (mean $CHADS_2 = 2.1$) in a non-inferiority trial with a prospective, randomized, open-label (warfarin only) design. Patients were randomized to dabigatran 110 mg ($n = 6015$) or 150 mg ($n = 6076$) twice daily, or warfarin adjusted to an INR of 2.0–3.0 ($n = 6022$), and followed for a median of 2 years. The primary outcome was a composite of stroke or systemic embolism. Warfarin patients in the RE-LY trial had a therapeutic INR about 64% of the time. The primary end point rates were 1.69% per year in the warfarin group, 1.53% per year in the dabigatran 110 mg arm (relative risk [RR] for dabigatran, 0.91; 95% confidence interval [CI] 0.74–1.11; $p < 0.001$ for non-inferiority), and 1.11% per year in the 150 mg dabigatran arm (RR 0.66; 95% CI 0.53–0.82, $p < 0.001$ for superiority). There was no statistically significant change in mortality rates when warfarin and dabigatran were compared. The rate of hemorrhagic stroke was 0.38% per year in the warfarin group, 0.12% per year in the dabigatran 110 mg arm ($p < 0.001$), and 0.10% per year in the dabigatran 150 mg arm ($p < 0.001$). The rates of major bleeding were 3.36% per year in the warfarin group, 2.71% per year in the dabigatran 10 mg arm ($p = 0.003$), and 3.11% per year in the dabigatran 150 mg arm ($p = 0.31$). The rates of intracranial bleeding were significantly lower in the dabigatran 110 mg arm (0.23% vs 0.76%, $p < 0.001$) and in the dabigatran 150 mg arm (0.32% vs 0.76%, $p < 0.001$). Dyspepsia occurred in 5.8% of the warfarin arm, 11.8% of the dabigatran 110 mg arm, and 11.3% of the dabigatran 150 mg arm ($p < 0.001$ for both comparisons).

In a subgroup analysis of the RE-LY data published separately [16], Eikelboom *et al.* further assessed bleeding risk in the RE-LY population. It was determined that both doses of dabigatran compared with warfarin were associated with an increasing relative risk of major bleeding with increasing age categories (<65 years, 65–74 years, > 75 years) (p for interaction <0.001 for each analysis). Furthermore, in patients with atrial fibrillation at risk for stroke, both doses of dabigatran compared with warfarin were found to have lower risks of both intracranial and extracranial bleeding in patients aged <75 years. In those aged > 75 years, intracranial bleeding risk was lower, but extracranial bleeding risk is similar or higher with both doses of dabigatran compared with warfarin.

Rivaroxaban

The *ROCKET-AF trial* [17] compared rivaroxaban (a factor Xa inhibitor) to warfarin in 14 624 patients with non-valvular AF who were at increased risk of stroke (mean $CHADS_2$ approximately 3.4). Patients were randomized to either fixed-dose rivaroxaban (20 mg daily or 15 mg daily in patients with a creatinine clearance of 30–49 ml per minute) or adjusted-dose warfarin (target INR 2.0–3.0). The primary end point was a composite of stroke (ischemic or hemorrhagic) and systemic embolism. Warfarin-assigned patients in the ROCKET-AF had a therapeutic INR about 55% of the time. The primary end point occurred at a rate of 1.7% per year in the rivaroxaban group, and at a rate of 2.2% per year in the warfarin group (HR 0.79, 95% confidence interval [CI], 0.66–0.96, $p < 0.001$ for non-inferiority). Major and non-major clinically relevant bleeding occurred at a rate of 14.9% per year in the rivaroxaban group, and at a rate of 14.5% per year in the warfarin group (HR 1.03, 95% CI 0.96–1.11, $p = 0.44$), with statistically significant reductions in intracranial hemorrhage (0.5% per year vs 0.7% per year, $p = 0.02$) and fatal bleeding (0.2% per year vs 0.5% per year, $p = 0.003$) in the rivaroxaban group.

Apixaban

The *ARISTOTLE trial* [18] compared apixaban (a factor Xa inhibitor) to warfarin in 18 210 patients in a double-blind, double-dummy RCT. Patients with atrial fibrillation and at least one additional risk factor for stroke (mean $CHADS_2$ score = 2.1) were randomized to either apixaban (5 mg twice daily) or adjusted-dose warfarin (target INR = 2.0–3.0). The primary outcome was ischemic or hemorrhagic stroke or systemic embolism. Warfarin-assigned patients in the ROCKET-AF had a therapeutic INR about 62% of the time. The rate of the primary outcome was 1.27% per year in the apixaban arm, and 1.60% per year in the warfarin arm (HR with apixaban = 0.79, 95% confidence interval [CI], 0.66–0.95, $p < 0.001$ for non-inferiority, $p = 0.01$ for superiority). The rates of death from any cause were 3.52% and 3.94%, respectively (HR 0.89, 95% CI 0.80–0.99, $p = 0.047$). The rate of hemorrhagic stroke was 0.24% per year in the apixaban arm and 0.47% per year in the warfarin arm (HR 0.51, 95% CI 0.35 to 0.75, $p < 0.001$). The rate of major bleeding was 2.13% per year in the apixaban arm and 3.09% per year in the warfarin arm (HR 0.69, 95% CI 0.60–0.80, $p < 0.001$). There was a statistically significant decrease in intracranial hemorrhage in the apixaban arm (0.33% per year vs 0.80% per year, $p < 0.0001$).

General comments about the NOACs.

1 The NOACs have each been compared to warfarin in properly designed RCTs, but have *not been directly compared to each other*. Therefore, it is not possible to make *any* statement about whether any one of the NOACs is 'superior', as indirect comparisons are fraught with error and bias, and should be avoided. Each of the NOACs does offer certain advantages, depending on the characteristics of the individual patient being treated. Such characteristics may include age, concerns regarding compliance, once daily versus bid dosing, diminished renal function as measured by creatinine clearance, gastrointestinal upset, and cost.

2 Unlike warfarin, the NOACs do not require routine blood monitoring. However, every effort must be made to educate patients to ensure compliance with the drug (as the half-lives of the NOACs are very short when compared with warfarin). In addition, routine monitoring of creatinine clearance is undertaken (i.e., at least annually, or if there is a change in the health status of the patient) in order to ensure that the patient's kidney function is sufficient to continue NOAC use. Patients with inadequate creatinine clearance

should be switched to warfarin, with appropriate education and monitoring.

3 None of the NOACs have been approved for use in patients with prosthetic cardiac valves.

Anticoagulants for patients with non-cardiac stroke

One Cochrane systematic review sought to determine the effect of prolonged warfarin therapy (compared with placebo or open control) following presumed non-cardioembolic ischemic stroke or TIA [19]. Eleven trials involving 2487 patients were included. The quality of the nine trials, which predated routine computerized tomography scanning and the use of the INR to monitor anticoagulation, was poor. There was no evidence of an effect of warfarin therapy on either the odds of death or dependency (two trials, OR 0.83, 95% CI 0.52–1.34) or of 'non-fatal stroke, MI or vascular death' (four trials, OR 0.96, 95% CI 0.68–1.37). Death from any cause (OR 0.95, 95% CI 0.73–1.24) and death from vascular causes (OR 0.86, 95% CI 0.66–1.13) were not significantly different between treatment and control groups. The inclusion of two recent completed trials did not alter these conclusions. There was no evidence of an effect of warfarin therapy on the risk of recurrent ischemic stroke (OR 0.85, 95% CI 0.66–1.09). However, warfarin increased fatal ICH (OR 2.54, 95% CI 1.19–5.45) and major extracranial hemorrhage (OR 3.43, 95% CI 1.94–6.08). This is equivalent to warfarin therapy causing about 11 additional fatal ICH and 25 additional major extracranial hemorrhages per year for every 1000 patients treated. The authors concluded that, compared with control, there was no evidence of benefit from long-term warfarin therapy in people with presumed non-cardioembolic ischemic stroke or TIA, but there was a significant bleeding risk.

Antiplatelet agents in stroke survivors without atrial fibrillation

Antiplatelet agents other than aspirin

The most widely studied and prescribed antiplatelet agent for the prevention of stroke and other serious vascular events among high vascular risk patients is aspirin [20]. One Cochrane systematic review sought to determine the effectiveness and safety of thienopyridine derivatives (ticlopidine and clopidogrel) versus aspirin for the prevention of serious vascular events (stroke, MI or vascular death) in patients at high risk of such events, and specifically in patients with a previous TIA or ischemic stroke [21]. Four trials involving a total of 22 656 high vascular risk patients were included. The trials were of high quality and comparable. Aspirin was compared with ticlopidine in three trials (3471 patients) and with clopidogrel in one trial (19 185 patients). Allocation to a thienopyridine was associated with a modest, yet statistically significant, reduction in the odds of a serious vascular event

(12.0% vs 13.0%, OR 0.91, 95% CI 0.84–0.98, $2P = 0.01$), corresponding to the avoidance of 11 (95% CI 2–19) serious vascular events per 1000 patients treated for about 2 years. There was also a reduction in stroke (5.7% vs 6.4%, OR 0.88, 95% CI 0.79–0.98, 7 (95% CI 1–13) strokes avoided per 1000 patients treated for 2 years). Compared with aspirin, thienopyridines produced a significant reduction in the odds of gastrointestinal haemorrhage and other upper gastrointestinal upset, but a significant increase in the odds of skin rash and of diarrhea. However, the increased odds of skin rash and diarrhea were greater for ticlopidine than for clopidogrel. Allocation to ticlopidine, but not clopidogrel, was associated with a significant increase in the odds of neutropenia (2.3% vs 0.8%, OR 2.7, 95% CI 1.5–4.8). In the subset of patients with TIA/ischemic stroke, the results were similar to those for all patients combined. However, since these patients are at particularly high risk of stroke, allocation to a thienopyridine was associated with a larger absolute reduction in stroke (10.4% vs 12.0%, OR 0.86, 95% CI 0.75–0.97, 16 (95% CI 3–28) strokes avoided per 1000 patients treated for 2 years). The authors concluded that the thienopyridine derivatives are modestly but significantly more effective than aspirin in preventing serious vascular events in patients at high risk (and specifically in TIA/ischemic stroke patients), but there is uncertainty about the size of the additional benefit. The thienopyridines are also associated with less gastrointestinal hemorrhage and other upper gastrointestinal upset than aspirin, but an excess of skin rash and diarrhea. The risk of skin rash and diarrhea is greater with ticlopidine than with clopidogrel. Ticlopidine, but not clopidogrel, is associated with excess neutropenia and of thrombotic thrombocytopenic purpura.

Combinations of antiplatelet agents (in the non-acute phase)

The combination of ASA and clopidogrel for secondary stroke prevention has been studied in two randomized controlled trials. The MATCH trial determined that adding aspirin to clopidogrel in high-risk patients with recent ischemic stroke or TIA was associated with an increased risk of bleeding and a non-significant reduction in major ischemic vascular events [22]. The combination of ASA and clopidogrel for the secondary prevention of stroke was further studied in the CHARISMA study, which investigated clopidogrel and aspirin versus aspirin alone in lower and higher risk patients [23]. In this trial, there was a suggestion of benefit with clopidogrel treatment in patients with symptomatic atherothrombosis and a suggestion of harm in patients with multiple risk factors but no vascular symptoms. Overall, clopidogrel plus aspirin was not significantly more effective than aspirin alone in reducing the rate of MI, stroke or death from cardiovascular causes.

Endarterectomy for symptomatic carotid disease

General statement

The current standard of care indicates that stroke survivors with ipsilateral 50–99% internal carotid artery stenosis (measured by two concordant non-invasive imaging modalities such as Dopplers, CTA or MRA) should be evaluated by an individual with stroke expertise (neurosurgeon/vascular surgeon) and that *selected* patients should be offered carotid endarterectomy as soon as possible within *2 weeks* of the stroke event, once the patient is clinically stable. Further to this, it is also agreed that carotid endarterectomy should be performed by a surgeon with a known perioperative morbidity and mortality of less than 6%.

Evidence summary

It has been well established that carotid endarterectomy is beneficial for stroke prevention in appropriate patients. A pooled analysis of three large trials of endarterectomy for symptomatic stenosis [24] (the North American Symptomatic Carotid Endarterectomy Trial (NASCET), the European Carotid Surgery Trial (ECST) and the Veterans Affairs Trial) demonstrated that endarterectomy is highly beneficial in symptomatic patients with severe (70–99%) angiographic stenosis (NNT = 6 to prevent one stroke over 5 years), moderately beneficial for symptomatic patients with moderate (50–69%) stenosis (NNT = 22 to prevent one stroke over 5 years) and not beneficial for mild (< 50%) stenosis.

The Carotid Endarterectomy Trialists' Collaboration analyzed pooled data (5893 patients with 33 000 patient-years of follow-up) from the European Carotid Surgery Trial and North American Symptomatic Carotid Endarterectomy Trial [25]. The findings indicated that the benefit from endarterectomy depends not only on the degree of carotid stenosis but also on several other clinical characteristics, including the timing of surgery after the presenting event. In patients with severe stenosis (70–99%), surgery was most effective when performed within 2 weeks of the index transient ischemic attack or stroke (NNT = 3 to prevent one stroke in 5 years), and this benefit declined quickly over time (NNT = 125 for patients who undergo surgery more than 12 weeks after the symptomatic event). This time-dependent decline in benefit was even more pronounced in patients with moderate stenosis (50–69%); endarterectomy performed within the first 2 weeks of the ischemic event was beneficial, but the benefit was lost (and there was net harm) when surgery was delayed more than 3 months. The summary recommendation is that carotid endarterectomy should be done within 2 weeks of the patient's last symptoms.

Endovascular treatment (angioplasty and stenting) for carotid stenosis

An updated Cochrane systematic review [26] included 16 trials involving 7572 patients. The reviewers found that in patients with symptomatic carotid stenosis at standard surgical risk, endovascular treatment was associated with a higher risk of the following outcome measures occurring between randomization and 30 days after treatment than endarterectomy: death or any stroke (the primary safety outcome) (OR 1.72, 95% CI 1.29–2.31, $p = 0.0003$, $I^2 = 27\%$), death or any stroke or myocardial infarction (OR 1.44, 95% CI 1.15–1.80, $p = 0.002$, $I^2 = 7\%$), and any stroke (OR 1.81, 95% CI 1.40–2.34, $p < 0.00001$, $I^2 = 12\%$). The OR for the primary safety outcome was 1.16 (95% CI 0.80–1.67) in patients with age <70 years and 2.20 (95% CI 1.47–3.29) in patients with age ≥ 70 years (interaction $p = 0.02$).

The rate of death or major or disabling stroke did not differ significantly between treatments (OR 1.28, 95% CI 0.93–1.77, $p = 0.13$, $I^2 = 0\%$). Endovascular treatment was associated with lower risks of myocardial infarction (OR 0.44, 95% CI 0.23–0.87, $p = 0.02$, $I^2 = 0\%$), cranial nerve palsy (OR 0.08, 95% CI 0.05–0.14, $p < 0.00001$, $I^2 = 0\%$), and access site hematomas (OR 0.37, 95% CI 0.18–0.77, $p = 0.008$, $I^2 = 27\%$).

The combination of death or any stroke up to 30 days after treatment or ipsilateral stroke during follow-up (the primary combined safety and efficacy outcome) favored endarterectomy (OR 1.39, 95% CI 1.10–1.75, $p = 0.005$, $I^2 = 0\%$), but the rate of ipsilateral stroke after the peri-procedural period did not differ between treatments (OR 0.93, 95% CI 0.60–1.45, $p = 0.76$, $I^2 = 0\%$).

Restenosis during follow-up was more common in patients receiving endovascular treatment than in patients assigned surgery (OR 2.41, 95% CI 1.28–4.53, $p = 0.007$, $I^2 = 55\%$). In patients with asymptomatic carotid stenosis, treatment effects on the primary safety (OR 1.71, 95% CI 0.78–3.76, $p = 0.18$, $I^2 = 0\%$) and combined safety and efficacy outcomes (OR 1.75, 95% CI 0.92–3.33, $p = 0.09$, $I^2 = 0\%$) were similar to symptomatic patients, but differences between treatments were not statistically significant. Among patients who are not suitable for surgery, the rate of death or any stroke between randomization and end of follow-up did not differ significantly between endovascular treatment and medical care (OR 0.22, 95% CI 0.01–7.92, $p = 0.41$, $I^2 = 79\%$).

The reviewers concluded by stating that carotid stenting may be considered for patients who are not operative candidates for technical, anatomic or medical reasons. Interventionalists should have expertise in carotid procedures and an expected risk of peri-procedural morbidity and mortality rate of less than 5%. It should be noted that carotid endarterectomy is more appropriate than carotid stenting for patients over 70 years of age who are otherwise fit for surgery because stenting carries a higher short-term risk of stroke and death.

Obstructive sleep apnea management

General statement

Sleep apnea is now recognized as a modifiable risk factor for stroke. Observational studies have demonstrated that people with obstructive sleep apnea are 1.6–2.7 times more likely to experience a stroke [27]. Therefore, it is increasingly recommended that specific targeted management strategies should be initiated for stroke survivors with confirmed sleep apnea following an objective clinical assessment. Even though there is a lack of well-powered randomized controlled trials, treatments for sleep apnea may include avoidance of sedative medications and alcohol, advice to avoid sleeping on their back, weight loss, use of continuous positive airway pressure (CPAP) devices, and appropriately fitted dental appliances.

Evidence summary

One study [28] demonstrated that patients with moderate to severe obstructive sleep apnea who could not tolerate CPAP showed an increased adjusted incidence of new ischemic strokes (HR 2.87, 95% CI 1.11–7.71, $p = 0.03$), compared to patients with moderate to severe obstructive sleep apnea who were able to tolerate CPAP.

Lifestyle management (eating a balanced diet, limiting salt intake, moderating alcohol consumption, increasing physical activity, and optimizing weight)

General statement

Stroke survivors should be assessed for lifestyle management issues that are known to impact on the other major vascular risk factors. Stroke survivors should receive patient-specific information and counseling about possible strategies to modify their lifestyles appropriately.

• *Eating a balanced diet*: Unless contraindicated for other reasons, stroke survivors should consume a diet rich in fruits and vegetables (fresh, frozen or canned), low-fat dairy products, dietary and soluble fiber, whole grains and protein from plant sources. The diet should be low in saturated fat and cholesterol.

• *Limiting salt intake:* For persons of 9–50 years of age, total daily sodium intake from all sources should not exceed 1500 mg. This decreases to 1300 mg for persons of 51–70 years of age and to 1200 mg for persons over 70 years of age. Patients should be counseled not to add salt to food, not to cook with salt, and to learn more about the sodium content of packaged foods.

• *Moderating alcohol consumption:* Limit consumption to two or fewer standard drinks per day for men and one drink per day for women who are not pregnant.

• *Increasing physical activity:* After being assessed by a healthcare provider, stroke survivors should be encouraged to gradually establish a moderate exercise program such as walking, jogging, cycling, swimming or other dynamic exercise 4–7 days every week, in addition to routine activities of daily living.

• *Optimizing weight:* Through the use of the aforementioned suggested strategies, stroke survivors should be encouraged to maintain a body mass index (BMI) of 18.5–24.9 kg/m².

Evidence summary
Diet

A meta-analysis of studies evaluating fruit and vegetable consumption and stroke risk [29] (257 551 individuals over a 13-year follow-up time) showed that consumption of five or more servings of fruits and vegetables per day is associated with a lower risk of stroke. Compared with individuals who had fewer than three servings of fruit and vegetables per day, the pooled relative risk of stroke was 0.89 (95% CI 0.83–0.97) for those with three to five servings per day, and 0.74 (95% CI 0.69–0.79) for those with more than five servings per day. A more broadly designed study compared four diet regimes and their impact on stroke risk [30]. These diets included the Healthy Eating Index 2005 (HEI-2005), the Dietary Approaches to Stop Hypertension (DASH), the Greek Mediterranean Index or the Italian Mediterranean Index. The study found that all four diets had an inverse relationship to stroke occurrence, and that the Italian Mediterranean Index showed the best overall results [HR 0.37 (95% CI 0.19–0.70) and was the only one of the four diets to show an association with hemorrhagic stroke as well [HR 0.51(95% CI 0.22–1.20), $p = 0.07$)] [10].

Sodium

It is well documented that a chronically high dietary sodium intake is associated with elevated blood pressure [31]. Furthermore, the available evidence suggests that lowering sodium consumption to adequate intake levels could reduce the incidence of stroke and heart disease by as much as 30%, and has a significant impact on lowering blood pressure [32].

Alcohol

A meta-analysis of 35 observational studies examining the effects of alcohol consumption on stroke risk revealed a significant ($p = 0.004$) J-shaped relationship between the amounts of alcohol consumed per day and the risk of ischemic stroke [33]. In the analysis, it was found that individuals who consumed one to two drinks per day had the least risk for ischemic stroke (RR = 0.72), while those

having more than five drinks per day had the most risk (RR = 1.69) when compared with a group of abstainers. The analysis also confirmed that alcohol consumption has a linear, dose-dependent effect on risk of hemorrhagic stroke. Heavy drinking (more than five drinks per day) was associated with a relative risk of hemorrhagic stroke of 2.18. Irregular and binge drinking (more than five drinks at one sitting) has also been associated with an increase in risk for hemorrhagic stroke.

Physical activity

A meta-analysis derived from 33 prospective cohort studies and 10 case–control studies that addressed the potential effect of physical activity on stroke showed physical activity reduced the risk of all stroke types (RR = 0.32) for men and women combined [34].

Weight reduction

Observational studies have examined the relationship between body mass index (BMI) and stroke risk. One study [35] compared high BMIs of 27.0–29.9 kg/m² and BMI of ≥ 30.0 kg/m² to a 'healthy' BMI between 23.0 and 24.9 kg/m², and reported hazard ratios for increased stroke risk as 1.09 and 1.25 for men, and 1.29 and 2.16 for women. In addition, in women, an increase in weight of greater than 10% over the last 5 years was also associated with increased stroke risk. Other studies have looked at measurements of waist circumference; a case-controlled observational study of independent risk factors for stroke reported an odds ratio of 4.0 for persons with increased waist to hip ratios [36].

Disclosure

G. Gubitz is a member of the Steering Committee for the Canadian Best Practice Recommendations for Stroke Care (www.strokebestpractices.ca), and has borrowed extensively from and paraphrased this evidence base in the preparation of this chapter.

References

1 O'Donnell, M.J., Denis, X., Liu, L. *et al.* (2010) Risk factors for ischemic and intracerebral hemorrhagic stroke in 22 countries (the INTERSTROKE study): A case-control study. *The Lancet,* **376**, 112–123.

2 Rashid, P. *et al.* (2003) Blood pressure reduction and secondary prevention of stroke and other vascular events. A systematic review. *Stroke,* **34**, 2741–9.

3 Beckett, N.S., Peters, R., Fletcher, A.E. *et al.* (2008) Treatment of hypertension in patients 80 years of age and older. *New England Journal of Medicine,* **358**, 1887–98.

4 Beckett, N., Peters, R., Tuomilehto, J. *et al.* & for the HYVET Study Group (2012) Immediate and late benefits of treating very

elderly people with hypertension: results from active treatment extension to hypertension in the very elderly randomized controlled trial. *BMJ*, **344**, d7541.4.

5 Heart Protection Study Collaborative Group (2004) Effects of cholesterol lowering with simvastatin on stroke and other major vascular events in 20,536 people with cerebrovascular disease or other high risk conditions. *Lancet*, **363**, 757–67.

6 Amarenco, P., Bogousslavsky, J., Callahan, A. 3rd, *et al.* (2006) Stroke Prevention by Aggressive Reduction in Cholesterol Levels (SPARCL) Investigators. High-dose atorvastatin after stroke or transient ischemic attack. *New England Journal of Medicine*, **355**, 549–59.

7 Karapanayiotides, T., Piechowski-Jozwiak, B., van Melle, G. *et al.* (2004) Stroke patterns, etiology, and prognosis in patients with diabetes mellitus. *Neurology*, **62**, 1558–1562.

8 The Action to Control Cardiovascular Risk in Diabetes (ACCORD) Study Group (2008) Effects of Intensive Glucose Lowering in Type 2 Diabetes. *New England Journal of Medicine*, **358**, 2545–2559.

9 ADVANCE Collaborative Group (2008) Intensive blood glucose control and vascular outcomes in patients with type 2 diabetes. *New England Journal of Medicine*, **358**, 2560–2572.

10 Dormand, J.A. *et al.* (2005) Secondary prevention of macrovascular events in patients with type 2 diabetes in the PROactive Study (PROspective pioglitAzone Clinical Trial In macroVascular Events): a randomized controlled trial. *Lancet*, **366**, 1279–1289.

11 Ussher, M.H., Taylor, A. & Faulkner, G. (2012) Exercise interventions for smoking cessation. *Cochrane Database of Systematic Reviews*, (**1**). Art. No.: CD002295.

12 Wu, P., Wilson, K., Dimoulas, P. & Mills, E.J. (2006) Effectiveness of smoking cessation therapies: a systematic review and meta-analysis. *BMC Public Health*, **6**.: article number 300.

13 Saxena, R. & Koudstaal, P.J. (2004) Anticoagulants for preventing stroke in patients with nonrheumatic atrial fibrillation and a history of stroke or transient ischaemic attack. *Cochrane Database of Systematic Reviews*, (**2**. Art. No.: CD000185.). doi:10.1002/14651858.CD000185.pub2.

14 Saxena, R. & Koudstaal, P.J. (2004) Anticoagulants versus antiplatelet therapy for preventing stroke in patients with non-rheumatic atrial fibrillation and a history of stroke or transient ischemic attack. *Cochrane Database of Systematic Reviews*, (**4**. Art. No.: CD000187). doi:10.1002/14651858.CD000187.pub2.

15 Connolly, S.J., Ezekowitz, M.D., Yusuf, S. *et al.* (2009) And the RE-LY Steering Committee and Invcstigators. Dabigatran versus Warfarin in patients with atrial fibrillation. *NEJM*, **361**, 1139–1151.

16 Eikelboom, J.W., Wallentin, L., Connolly, S.J. *et al.* (2011) Risk of bleeding with 2 doses of dabigatran compared with warfarin in older and younger patients with atrial fibrillation: an analysis of the randomized evaluation of long-term anticoagulant therapy (RE-LY) trial. *Circulation*, **123**, 2363–2372.

17 Patel, M.D. *et al* (2011) Rivaroxaban versus Warfarin in Nonvalvular Atrial Fibrillation. *NEJM*, **365**, 883–891.

18 Granger, C. *et al.* (2011) Apixaban versus Warfarin in Patients with Atrial Fibrillation. *NEJM*, **365**, 981–992.

19 Sandercock, P.A.G., Gibson, L.M. & Liu, M. (2009) Anticoagulants for preventing recurrence following presumed non-cardioembolic ischaemic stroke or transient ischaemic attack. *Cochrane Database of Systematic Reviews*, (**2**. Art. No.: CD000248.). doi:10.1002/14651858.CD000248.pub2.

20 Antithrombotic Trialists' Collaboration (2002) Collaborative meta-analysis of randomized trials of antiplatelet therapy for prevention of death, myocardial infarction, and stroke in high-risk patients. *BMJ*, **324**, 71–86.

21 Sudlow, C.L.M., Mason, G., Maurice, J.B., Wedderburn, C.J. & Hankey, G.J. (2009) Thienopyridine derivatives versus aspirin for preventing stroke and other serious vascular events in high vascular risk patients. *Cochrane Database of Systematic Reviews*, (**4**. Art. No.: CD001246.). doi:10.1002/14651858.CD001246.pub2

22 Diener, H., Bogousslavsky, J., Brass, L. & for the MATCH Investigators (2004) Aspirin and clopidogrel compared with clopidogrel alone after recent ischemic stroke or transient ischaemic attack in high-risk patients (MATCH): randomized, double-blind, placebo-controlled trial. *Lancet*, **364**, 331–337.

23 Bhatt, D., Fox, K., Hacke, W. *et al.* & for the Charisma Investigators (2006) Clopidogrel and aspirin versus aspirin alone for the prevention of atherothrombotic events. *New England Journal of Medicine*, **354**, 1706–1717.

24 Rerkasem, K. & Rothwell, P.M. (2011) Carotid endarterectomy for symptomatic carotid stenosis. *Cochrane Database of Systematic Reviews*, (**4**. Art. No.: CD001081.). doi:10.1002/14651858.CD001081.pub2

25 Rothwell, P.M., Eliasziw, M., Gutnikov, S.A. *et al.* & Carotid Endarterectomy Trialists' Collaboration (2003) Analysis of pooled data from the randomized controlled trials of endarterectomy for symptomatic carotid stenosis. *Lancet*, **361**, 107–116.

26 Bonati, L.H. *et al.* (2012) Percutaneous transluminal balloon angioplasty and stenting for carotid artery stenosis. *Cochrane Database of Systematic Reviews*, (**9**. Art. No.: CD000515.). doi:10.1002/14651858.CD000515.pub4

27 Bassetti, C., Aldrich, M.S., Chervin, R.D. & Quint, D. (1996) Sleep apnea in patients with transient ischemic attack and stroke: a prospective study of 59 patients. *Neurology*, **47**, 116–117.

28 Martinez-Garcia, M.A., Galiano-Blancar, R., Roman-Sanchez, P., Soler-Cataluna, J.J., Cabero-Salt, L. & Salcedo-Maiques, E. (2005) Continuous positive airway pressure treatment in sleep apnea prevents new vascular events after ischemic stroke. *Chest*, **128(4)**, 2123–2129.

29 He, F.J., Nowson, C.A. & MacGregor, G.A. (2006) Fruit and vegetable consumption and stroke: meta-analysis of cohort studies. *Lancet*, **367**, 320–326.

30 Agnoli, C., Krogh, V., Grioni, S. *et al.* (2011) A priori-defined dietary patterns are associated with reduced risk of stroke in a large Italian cohort. *Journal of Nutrition*, **141**, 1552–1558.

31 He, F.J. & MacGregor, G.A. (2011) Salt reduction lowers cardiovascular risk: meta-analysis of outcome trials. *Lancet*, **378**, 380–381.

32 Saito, I., Iso, H., Kokubo, Y., Inoue, M. & Tsugane, S. (2011) Body mass index, weight change and risk of stroke and stroke

subtypes: the Japan public health center-based prospective (JPHC) study. *International Journal of Obesity*, **35**, 283–229.

33 Mazzaglia, G., Britton, A.R., Altmann, D.R. *et al.* (2001) Exploring the relationship between alcohol consumption and non-fatal or fatal stroke: a systematic review. *Addiction*, **96**, 1743–1756.

34 Lee, C.D., Folsom, A.R. & Blair, S.N. (2003) Physical activity and stroke risk: a meta-analysis. *Stroke*, **34**, 2475–2481.

35 Dalton, M., Cameron, A.J., Zimmet, P.Z. *et al.* (2003) on behalf of the AUSDIAB Steering Committee. Waist circumference, waist-hip ration and body mass index and their correlation with cardiovascular disease risk factors in Australian adults. *Journal of Internal Medicine*, **254**, 555–563.

36 Janssen, I., Katzmarzyk, P.T. & Ross, R. (2004) Waist circumference and not body mass index explains obesity-related health risk. *American Journal of Clinical Nutrition*, **79**, 379–384.

PART 3

Evidence-based neurology in the clinic

CHAPTER 15

Central nervous system infections

Gloria von Geldern and Avindra Nath
Section of Infections of the Nervous System, NINDS, National Institutes of Health, Bldg 10/ 7C-103, 10 Center Drive, Bethesda, MD, 20892 USA

Bacterial meningitis

Vaccines have changed the epidemiology and predominant pathogens in many countries, but bacterial meningitis continues to be an important neurological disease worldwide. It is associated with high mortality and frequent neurological sequelae and requires expeditious management.

Timing of antibiotics

The 2008 guidelines of the European Federation of Neurological Societies (EFNS) recommend that patients with suspected bacterial meningitis should be hospitalized as soon as possible [1]. The importance of prompt initiation of antibiotics has been demonstrated in several studies. A French prospective multicenter study of 156 patients admitted to an intensive care unit for pneumococcal meningitis found that a delay in antibiotic treatment of more than 3 h after hospitalization was a strong and independent risk factor for 3-month mortality (OR 14.1, 95% CI 3.93–50.9). Delayed therapy was a stronger predictor of mortality than penicillin-resistance (OR 6.83, 95% CI 2.94–20.8) or clinical examination at presentation (OR 1.12, 95% CI 1.072–1.153) [2]. Similarly, retrospective single-center studies from Croatia and Canada found decreased mortality and morbidity in patients with community-acquired bacterial meningitis who received antibiotics early in their disease course [3,4]. A retrospective Danish multicenter study found that the odds for unfavorable outcome increased up to 30% per hour of treatment delay [5]. Empiric antibiotics should therefore be started as soon as possible after obtaining blood cultures and CSF (if lumbar puncture is deemed safe and can be done quickly). Blood and CSF culture data remain important in confirming the diagnosis and identifying the organism and its susceptibility, which enables a more targeted antibiotic regimen. The EFNS recommends initiation of empiric antibiotic treatment within 60 minutes of hospitalization, and no longer than 3 h after initial contact with a healthcare provider [1].

The benefit of pre-hospital administration of antibiotics for suspected bacterial meningitis is unclear. There are no randomized controlled trials (RCTs) or prospective case–control studies of the potential benefit of pre-hospital antibiotic treatment. In a retrospective case–control study of 158 children with suspected meningococcal disease, pre-hospital treatment with parenteral penicillin was associated with an increase in mortality (OR 7.4, 95% CI 1.5–37.7), which may be due to more severe disease in these cases [6]. EFNS guidelines still recommend pre-hospital administration of antibiotics in patients with expected delay in hospital transfer or in those with a high suspicion for meningococcal disease given the risk of early cardiovascular decompensation in these patients [1].

Empiric antibiotic therapy

Empiric therapeutic regimens for bacterial meningitis depend on the patient's age. This chapter focuses on treatment of older children and adults and does not cover special considerations in neonates and infants. Standard empiric treatment of community-acquired acute bacterial meningitis in adults and older children consist of parenteral penicillin or third-generation cephalosporins (cefotaxime or ceftriaxone). High-dose vancomycin should be used in combination with a third-generation cephalosporin in areas with penicillin-resistant pneumococcus. On the basis of data from a rabbit meningitis model, cephalosporins should be continued to treat even strains with intermediate susceptibility or resistance to ceftriaxone as the combination with vancomycin is synergistic [7]. Vancomycin plus chloramphenicol is generally recommended in patients with severe beta-lactam allergy. A Cochrane review of the efficacy and safety of third-generation cephalosporins (ceftriaxone or cefotaxime) versus chloramphenicol analyzed the results of 19 RCTs with a total of 1496 patients (adults and children). None of the studies found a difference in mortality or deafness between the different antibiotics [8]. Cephalosporins were associated with a higher risk of diarrhea. However, as most of the studies in this review were conducted in the 1980s or early 1990s, these findings need to be viewed with some caution because of an increasing development of antibiotic resistance.

Patients with more than 50 years of age or with a compromised immune system (including diabetics and alcoholics) are at higher risk for listeria meningitis, although it can also occur in immune-competent individuals. Empiric therapy for listeria may be necessary in patients with subacute onset of basilar or brain stem encephalitis since the organism is intracellular and may be difficult to isolate. No controlled trials have been conducted to establish a drug of choice or optimal duration of therapy for CNS listeriosis, and treatment recommendations are based on data obtained from in-vitro susceptibility testing, animal models, and reported clinical experience with small numbers of patients. On the basis of these data, intravenous ampicillin is found to be the most widely used antibiotic to treat listerial infection and should be given in addition to the aforementioned antibiotics [9]. The combination of ampicillin or other beta-lactam antibiotics with aminoglycosides such as gentamicin has been shown in vitro and in animal models to have a synergistic effect against listeria [10,11]. In patients with severe penicillin allergy, trimethoprim-sulfamethoxazole is generally recommended [12]. Moxifloxacin is another alternative based on in vitro and animal studies [13].

No studies address how to best treat nosocomial meningitis, for example, after neurosurgical interventions. However, antibiotic treatment recommendations in these settings differ from community-acquired meningitis as organisms found in neurosurgical patients in large prospective surveillance studies were significantly different from those seen in community-acquired meningitis [14]. On the basis of such observations, empiric therapy must cover both Gram-positive and Gram-negative bacteria such as *Pseudomonas aeruginosa*. Most authors recommend vancomycin to cover methicillin-resistant *Staphylococcus aureus* plus ceftazidime, cefepime or meropenem [15]. Ceftazidime is a cephalosporin with good anti-pseudomonal activity, but the fourth-generation cephalosporin cefepime may be the better choice as it has a better coverage of penicillin-resistant pneumococci [16]. Meropenem also has some Gram-negative coverage and is helpful in treatment of extended-spectrum B-lactamase producing enterobacter. More detailed coverage of nosocomial meningitis, particularly in patients with indwelling devices such as ventriculo-peritoneal shunts is beyond the scope of this chapter.

There is insufficient evidence to establish the optimal duration of antibiotic treatment. A meta-analysis of five open-label RCTs involving 426 children found no difference in morbidity or mortality between intravenous ceftriaxone given over 4–7 days versus longer treatment duration of 7–14 days [17]. However, as pointed out in a commentary by van de Beek and Brower, these findings may not apply to patients with severe illness, with drug-resistant pneumococcal meningitis or in patients receiving concomitant dexamethasone [18] and further investigation of optimal treatment duration seems warranted.

Corticosteroids

While more than 20 randomized trials have sought to address whether adjunctive treatment with the glucocorticosteroids such as dexamethasone improves mortality or morbidity, there remains an ongoing debate about its use in different patient populations. A Cochrane review based on 18 RCT published until the end of 2003 concluded that the use of dexamethasone was associated with overall reduction in mortality, hearing loss and neurological sequelae in children in high-income countries and in adults worldwide [19]. A meta-analysis of individual patient data of five trials published since 2001 including 2029 patients found no significant reduction in mortality and only a slight reduction in hearing loss. The authors therefore concluded that adjunctive dexamethasone is not justified [15]. However, these findings may at least in part be influenced by a subset of patients from resource-poor settings such as Malawi, where delayed presentation and untreated HIV infection are common [20,21]. Since the entry of vancomycin into the CSF may be reduced by the decrease in inflammation with dexamethasone, rifampin or daptomycin have been suggested as alternatives for vancomycin during steroid use based on animal model data [22].

Supportive care

Supportive therapy includes careful management of fluid and electrolyte balance. A Cochrane review assessing the optimal approach to intravenous fluids identified three randomized controlled trials [23]. There was no statistical difference in mortality or overall neurological sequelae between patients receiving maintenance fluids and those receiving restricted fluids in the first 48 h after admission. However, fluid restriction was correlated with higher rates of spasticity and seizures as well as severe neurological sequelae at 3 months in patients presenting later in their disease course. Whether these findings can guide treatment in other patients remains unclear. A prospective Dutch multicenter observational study of 671 patients showed that hypernatremia was an independent predictor of unfavourable outcome and death [18]. It is, however, not clear whether hypernatremia is a manifestation of severe disease or directly contributes to the outcome, and the impact this finding should have on fluid management needs to be further studied.

In comatose patients, monitoring intracranial pressure (ICP) may be helpful for management, though no randomized controlled trials have investigated the utility of ICP monitoring [24]. Most data regarding treatment of increased

ICP are in traumatic brain injury and whether the findings in those patients can be applied in bacterial meningitis is doubtful. Hyperosmolar glycerol has been studied in a randomized trial in adults with bacterial meningitis in Malawi, but this trial was stopped early as the interim analysis demonstrated increased mortality in the glycerol group [25]. The reason for this finding is unclear, but might relate to an increased incidence of seizures in patients who received glycerol or may be related to rebound increase in ICP. Some studies using glycerol in children with bacterial meningitis show a more favorable tendency, though more data are needed to assess this [26].

Prevention

To avoid spread of the disease, the Centers for Disease Control and Prevention (CDC) recommends droplet precautions for the first 24 h after hospitalization for patients with known or suspected meningitis caused by *Hemophilus influenzae* or *Neisseria meningitides* [27]. A 2011 Cochrane review assessed the efficacy of chemoprophylaxis for those in close contact with patients with meningococcal disease [28]. In 24 RCTs with 6885 patients, no meningococcal disease occurred after administration of antibiotics for 1 week. Ciprofloxacin, minocycline, penicillin and rifampin were all found to be effective, but the use of rifampin was associated with development of resistant isolates. There was only limited direct comparison between the efficacies of these agents.

Vaccines have been implemented to help reduce the incidence of bacterial meningitis. Meningitis due to *H. influenzae* decreased after widespread use of *H. influenzae* type b conjugate vaccines for children of least 18 months old in 1987 and infants of least 2 months old in 1990 [29]. The effect of meningococcal vaccine on the epidemiology of bacterial meningitis is somewhat less clear as its use is typically limited to high-risk groups such as military recruits since the 1980s and college freshmen since 2000 [30]. After implementation of routine vaccination of young children with pneumococcal vaccine in the US in 2000, pneumococcal meningitis hospitalization rates decreased by 33.0% overall and by 66.0% in children under 2 years [30]. These findings stress the importance of preventative measures in containing infectious diseases.

CNS tuberculosis

Tuberculosis (TB) caused by *Mycobacterium tuberculosis* is a global epidemic with highest prevalence in sub-Saharan Africa, India, China, and Southeast Asia and intermediate rates in Central and South America, Eastern Europe, and northern Africa, though it also occurs in the US, Western Europe, Canada, Japan, and Australia. CNS TB occurs in 1% of patients with tuberculosis. Meningitis is the most common form of CNS TB, but cerebral abscesses or a tuberculoma and

spinal arachnoiditis can also occur. Infection of the vertebrae can lead to collapse of the vertebral bodies resulting in Pott's disease with possible neurological deficits.

First-line therapies

Antibiotic treatment should be initiated when CNS TB is suspected rather than after confirmation by PCR, which does not have a high sensitivity [31], or by culture, which usually requires several weeks and also has limited sensitivity [32]. Since there are no sufficient data from RCTs to establish the optimal medication regimen for CNS tuberculosis, most treatment recommendations are based on data from pulmonary TB. The American and British Thoracic Societies, the Infectious Disease Society of America and the Centers for Disease Control and Prevention recommend an initial 2-month intensive therapy with four drugs, followed by a prolonged continuation phase lasting 7–10 months, depending on clinical response and antibiotic sensitivity [33,34].

During the initial 2 months of intensive therapy, a four-drug regimen is used, typically consisting of the three bactericidal first-line drugs: isoniazid (INH), rifampin (RIF), and pyrazinamide (PZA), combined with either ethambutol (EMB) or streptomycin (STM). INH, RIF, and PZA are bactericidal, and INH and PZA both have excellent CNS penetration with CSF levels equivalent to serum levels in the setting of inflamed meninges [35]. INH is more active against rapid dividing than semi-dormant mycobacterium. Dosing for INH is typically 10 mg/kg per day and should be administered with 50–100 mg pyridoxine (vitamin B6) a day to minimize the risk of peripheral neuropathy. PZA adds efficacy to the regimen without significantly increasing hepatotoxicity. Dosing ranges from 15 to 30 mg/kg per day. CNS penetration of RIF is less than that of INH, and PZA and CSF levels rarely exceed the minimal inhibitory concentration [35]. RIF, however, is active against both rapidly dividing organisms and semi-dormant organisms and is thought to be important in aiding elimination of mycobacterium from the body. The recommended dose is 10–15 mg/kg per day. EMB has poor penetration with normal meninges but reaches adequate CSF levels in inflamed meninges. At high doses, EMB can lead to optic neuritis but ocular toxicity is rare at the recommended dose of 15 mg/kg per day [36]. While the aforementioned drugs can be given orally, STM requires intramuscular application. CSF penetration is poor, and the use of STM is generally limited to regions with a high prevalence of INH resistance. Dosage is typically 15 mg/kg per day to a maximum of 1 g per day in adults and 20–40 mg/kg per day in children [37]. The continuation phase usually consists of 7–10 months of INH and RIF alone if the organism is susceptible (for drug-resistant TB, see below). If patients have tuberculoma, treatment is usually extended to 18 months [38], though no studies have been undertaken to support this practice.

Drug resistance

Mycobacterium strains resistant to antituberculosis drugs are becoming increasingly prevalent. The World Health Organization (WHO) defines multidrug-resistant TB (MDR-TB) as caused by bacteria resistant to at least isoniazid and rifampicin. Extensively drug-resistant TB (XDR-TB) is caused by strains that are additionally resistant to fluoroquinolone and second-line injectable antituberculosis drugs (amikacin, kanamycin or capreomycin). In 2008, about 440,000 cases of MDR-TB occurred, which constitutes about 3.6% of all incident TB. In some countries of Eastern Europe or Central Asia, 6% or more of new TB cases are MDR-TB and 50% or more among previously treated cases [39]. The impact of resistance on treatment outcome appears to vary depending on which drug is ineffective. A prospective study from Vietnam of 180 adults with TB meningitis found resistance to at least one antituberculosis drug in 40% of the isolates and resistance to at least INH and rifampin in 5.6%. While resistance to INH and STM was significantly associated with slower clearance of mycobacterium from CSF, clinical outcome was not significantly impacted, whereas combined INH and RIF resistance was strongly predictive of death (RR 11.6, 95% CI 5.2–26.3) [40].

Second-line therapies that have been used for treatment of drug-resistant strains include the aforementioned fluoroquinolones and the parenteral agents amikacin, kanamycin and capreomycin. Oral bacteriostatic second-line drugs include ethionamide, prothionamide, cycloserine, terizidone, and p-aminosalicylic acid (PAS). Clofazimine, linezolid, amoxicillin/clavulanate, thioacetazone, clarithromycin, and imipenem are also considered second-line antituberculosis drugs. While there are no data from controlled trials to guide treatment in MDR-TB, the WHO recommends using four second-line antituberculosis drugs likely to be effective as well as pyrazinamide [41]. A fluoroquinolone, a parenteral agent, ethionamide or prothionamide, and cycloserine (or PAS if cycloserine cannot be used) should be included in the regimen. There are also no data from clinical trials regarding the optimal duration of therapy in patients with multidrug-resistant mycobacterium strains. Extending the treatment duration to 18–24 months is often recommended. Several new antituberculosis medications are currently under development, and bedaquiline and delamanid are currently in phase III clinical trials [42].

HIV-infected patients

Co-infection with HIV is common in patients with TB meningitis and is associated with higher mortality [43]. The antibiotic regimen in HIV-positive patients does not differ significantly from treatment of patients without HIV. Rifampicin significantly reduces levels of protease inhibitors and some non-nucleoside reverse transcriptase inhibitors, so rifabutin may be used as an alternative [44]. Drug resistance

appears to be more prevalent in HIV-co-infected patients, which should be considered in choosing an empiric antibiotic regimen [45].

Optimal timing of initiating HIV-therapy in antiretroviral-naïve patients with TB meningitis is not clear. After initiation of antiretrovirals, clinical worsening can occur due to immune reconstitution inflammatory syndrome (IRIS). A recent randomized controlled trial compared starting antiretrovirals immediately at the time of diagnosis of TB meningitis versus after 2 months on TB therapy [46]. Immediate antiretroviral therapy was associated with significantly more serious adverse events, although mortality was not significantly different. The CDC recommends for patients with a CD4+ count <100 cells/µL initiating antiretrovirals after 2 weeks of TB treatment [47]. For patients with a CD4+ count of 100–200 cells/µL, they recommend a delay until after 2 months of TB treatment.

Glucocorticosteroids

Adjunctive corticosteroid may attenuate the inflammatory response in mycobacterial meningitis and thus lead to improve outcome. A 2008 Cochrane review assessed seven trials with 1140 patients and found that overall corticosteroids reduced mortality (RR 0.78, 95% CI 0.67–0.91) [48]. Three trials with 720 patients assessed disabling residual neurological deficit and showed that corticosteroids reduce the risk of death or neurological sequelae (RR 0.82, 95% CI 0.70–0.97). Adverse events in these trials included gastrointestinal bleeding, bacterial and fungal infections, and hyperglycemia, but they were mild and treatable. The largest randomized controlled trial assessing corticosteroid use is a trial of 545 Vietnamese patients, which compared a dexamethasone taper for the first 6–8 weeks of treatment with placebo and found a significantly reduced mortality (32% vs 41%) [49]. The reduced mortality seemed to be in part due to a reduction in side effects like hepatitis (9.5 versus 16.6%), leading to the need for a change in the antituberculous regimen. Dexamethasone did not lead to improved survival in the 98 HIV-infected patients included in the trial, and overall there is not enough evidence to support or refute addition of corticosteroids in HIV-positive patients. A randomized trial in South African children found that addition of prednisone (4 mg/kg per day) during the first month of treatment was associated with a significantly reduced mortality (4% vs 17%) and higher IQs. In addition, tuberculomas resolved faster with additional prednisone [50].

Surgical interventions

Hydrocephalus is a frequent complication, especially in children. Surgical decompression may be required and has been associated with decreased mortality in retrospective studies especially when done early [51,52]. Unlike other CNS mass lesions, medical management is preferred for clinical tuberculomas, as surgical removal has often been complicated by severe fatal meningitis, unless the lesion produces obstructive hydrocephalus or compression of the brainstem or spinal cord [38]. If the diagnosis is unclear, a biopsy may be preferable over resection [53].

Additional management considerations

Patients with tuberculous meningitis can develop a syndrome of inappropriate antidiuretic hormone release (SIADH). The resulting hyponatremia may worsen cerebral edema. While water restriction is typically the main treatment for SIADH, hypovolemia may lead to decreased cerebral perfusion [54], making fluid management in these patients challenging, and more studies assessing optimal fluid management in patients with TB meningitis are necessary.

Given the high prevalence of ischemic strokes as a complication of tuberculous meningitis, especially in children, a randomized controlled South African study recently assessed whether addition of aspirin would improve outcome in children with tuberculous meningitis. Motor and cognitive outcomes were unchanged whether patients received low-dose aspirin (75 mg), high-dose aspirin (100 mg/kg per day) or placebo, though assessment of stroke incidence could not be accurately assessed as only CT but not MRI was available [55].

HSV encephalitis

Herpes simplex virus 1 (HSV-1) is the most common cause of encephalitis in adults worldwide and the most common cause of fatal sporadic encephalitis in the US. Untreated HSV-1 encephalitis has a mortality of up to 70% and most survivors have significant neurological sequelae [56]. Therefore early empiric therapy is crucial.

Acyclovir

The most important medication in the treatment of HSV-1 encephalitis to date is acyclovir, a purine nucleoside analogue. The first report describing the effectiveness of acyclovir in herpes encephalitis was published in 1977 [57]. Until then vidarabine had been the standard of care, this medication was found to reduce mortality in two small studies of patients with biopsy-proven HSV encephalitis [58,59]. The pivotal trials confirming the importance of acyclovir were done in the mid-1980s. In a Swedish study, 51 patients with HSV encephalitis (confirmed by brain biopsy or antibody responses in serum and CSF) were randomized to receive acyclovir or vidarabine. Mortality was reduced from 50% in the vidarabine to 19% in the acyclovir-treated group [60]. The second study comparing vidarabine and acyclovir [61] looked at 69 patients with biopsy-proven HSV encephalitis. Mortality was 54% in the vidarabine-treated

patients and 28% in patients on acyclovir, a difference that remained significant even when adjusted for differences in age between the two groups. Both studies also showed better functional outcome after 6 months in the patients treated with acyclovir: The Swedish study showed that 56% of patients on acyclovir had returned to normal life compared to 13% of vidarabine-treated patients; in the second study, 38% of acyclovir-treated patients versus only 14% of patients in the vidarabine group returned to normal function.

In the initial trials, acyclovir was given at a dose of 10 mg/kg IV every 8 h. The drug needs to be diluted to a concentration of 7 mg/ml or less and given by intravenous infusion over an hour to prevent phlebitis and renal toxicity. A recent prospective observational study in France showed that a higher dose of acyclovir did not lead to better outcome [62]. The dose needs to be adjusted in patients with renal insufficiency. Acyclovir should be accompanied with sufficient intravenous hydration to prevent crystalluria and renal failure. Because acyclovir is only effective in halting viral replication, and HSV encephalitis is associated with significant morbidity and mortality, early acyclovir administration is generally recommended. This practice is supported by a retrospective multicenter study of 93 adults assessing the risk of death or disability at 6 months. Initiation of acyclovir more than 2 days after admission or poor clinical status at presentation was found to be the only independent risk factor for poor outcome [63].

Duration of treatment

While the treatment duration in the initial trials documenting the efficacy of acyclovir was 10 days, a longer treatment course of 14–21 days is generally recommended since case reports of recurrence in patients receiving shorter antiviral courses have been reported, in particular in infants [64] but also less frequently in adults [65].

Whether empirically started, acyclovir can be safely discontinued once the HSV PCR in CSF is found to be negative, depends on the clinical constellation. In patients with a low pre-test probability of HSV encephalitis, a negative test essentially excludes the diagnosis; but in patients with a high pre-test probability of HSV encephalitis, a negative test, although significantly decreasing the likelihood of HSV encephalitis, does not entirely exclude it. As part of the California Encephalitis Project, 11 of 291 patients were found to have HSV1 encephalitis and 3 of these 11 patients had a negative HSV PCR on presentation but positive PCR results at day 4, 7 and 14 [66]. A smaller prospective study and retrospective case series described similar cases of negative HSV PCR early in the course of infection [67–70]. Depending on the clinical presentation, repeated CSF sampling may therefore be necessary to confirm the diagnosis of HSE, especially if brain imaging and EEG are consistent with the diagnosis of HSV encephalitis.

Acyclovir resistance

While acyclovir has been used extensively for the past 30 years, drug resistance is still relatively uncommon. Resistance has mainly been described in immunocompromised patients, who had received repeated acyclovir treatments. Up to 10% of transplant patients and HIV-positive individuals carry acyclovir-resistant HSV strains [71,72]. In immunocompetent patients, large population-based studies found only up to 0.7% acyclovir resistance [73,74], and only one case of acyclovir-resistant HSV encephalitis has been described to date in an immunocompetent adult. Acyclovir resistance should be suspected if the clinical condition deteriorates and CSF viral load increases despite acyclovir treatment, especially in immunocompromised patients.

Foscarnet is typically used in cases of acyclovir resistance, and the EFNS guidelines recommend treatment with 60 mg/kg intravenously infused over 1 h every 8 h for 3 weeks [75]. The use of Foscarnet appears reasonable in cases of acyclovir resistance despite the lack of RCTs in HSV encephalitis. Foscarnet does not require phosphorylation by viral kinases, and acyclovir resistance is usually caused by viral mutations leading to thymidine kinase deficiency. A small randomized control trial showed better efficacy of foscarnet compared with vidarabine in treatment of acyclovir-resistant mucocutaneous HSV infection [76]. Foscarnet possesses antiviral activity against all herpesviruses and penetrates well into the CNS. Case reports show efficacy in HHV6 and CMV encephalitis [77,78] as well as acyclovir-resistant HSV encephalitis [71].

Oral antiviral therapy

While the initial studies used intravenous (IV) acyclovir for treatment of encephalitis, IV medications are expensive and often not available in developing countries. There is currently no randomized trial assessing the clinical efficacy of oral options. However, there is a very small case series from Vietnam, looking at CSF data of patients treated with oral valacyclovir (1 g three times a day). The four patients with confirmed HSV-1 encephalitis in this study achieved higher CSF peak concentrations than the 50% inhibitory concentration for HSV-1 and HSV-2. After 10 days of treatment, these patients had a negative HSV PCR in CSF. Since this trial did not address the effect of oral valacyclovir on morbidity and mortality, intravenous acyclovir remains the standard of care but oral valacyclovir may be considered, if IV acyclovir is not available. Randomized trials to assess the clinical efficacy of oral treatments would be necessary to better address this question.

Steroids

There is currently not sufficient evidence to answer the question whether steroids are beneficial or harmful in patients with HSV encephalitis. Before acyclovir was available, there were some case reports in the 1970s that showed good outcome in patients with HSV encephalitis who were treated with steroids [79,80]. A more recent Japanese non-randomized retrospective study of 45 patients showed that the 22 patients who received steroids in conjunction with acyclovir had better outcome at 3 months ($R = 0.594$, $p = 0.0001$) than the patients who only received acyclovir [81]. However, this was not a randomized trial, and the dosage and duration of steroid administration varied between patients. Animal models seem to support the usefulness of steroids in HSV encephalitis: In mouse models of HSV-1 encephalitis, additive application of methylprednisolone has been shown to lead to fewer abnormalities on brain MRI than acyclovir alone [82] and can have a neuroprotective effect when given 3 days after acyclovir [83].

A prospective randomized placebo-controlled trial is currently ongoing. The "German trial of Acyclovir and corticosteroids in Herpes-simplex-virus-encephalitis" (GACHE) is a multicenter trial studying adult patients with HSV encephalitis in Germany, Austria, and the Netherlands [84]. In this trial, all patients receive acyclovir intravenously and are randomized to receive adjunctive therapy with dexamethasone 40 mg IV Q24 hours for 4 days versus placebo. The study will assess functional outcome at 6 months, mortality and development of seizures and will hopefully help to answer this question.

Supportive treatments

Seizures are common in the acute stage of HSV encephalitis and are estimated to occur in about 60% of patients [85], whereas status epilepticus is much less common [86]. There is no clear consensus about the use of prophylactic antiepileptics in HSV encephalitis, but most guidelines do not support treatment unless seizures occur [87].

Increased ICP is common in patients with HSV encephalitis and may eventually lead to death [88]. No sufficient evidence exists to evaluate the use of osmotherapy, hyperventilation, barbiturates, normothermia or similar measures in reducing ICP in viral encephalitis [24]. Case reports advocate the use of craniectomy in cases of encephalitis associated with severely elevated ICP [89,90].

Finally, rehabilitation is an important addition in the treatment of patients after the acute phase of their disease. Many survivors of HSV encephalitis are left with neurocognitive deficits, underscoring the importance of neuropsychological rehabilitation [91].

Cryptococcal meningitis

Fungal infections of the CNS occur primarily in immunocompromised individuals and have gained importance with the increased number of patients with immune deficits. *Cryptococcus neoformans* is the most common cause of meningitis in patients with HIV infection [92] and is frequently seen in transplant patients [93].

Antifungals in HIV-infected patients
Induction therapy

Treatment of cryptococcal meningitis consists of three phases: an induction, a consolidation and a maintenance phase. A randomized multicenter trial assessed induction therapy with intravenous amphotericin B (AmB) at 0.5 mg/kg per day compared to oral fluconazole (200 mg per day) and found the same efficacy in achieving negative CSF cultures at 10 weeks [94]. However, CSF sterilization was faster with AmB. There was no difference in mortality, although at 2 weeks it was higher in the fluconazole group. A subsequent large randomized study in HIV-positive patients used a higher dose of AmB (0.7 mg/kg per day) with or without flucytosine (100 mg/kg per day) as induction therapy for 2 weeks [95]. The addition of flucytosine was associated with an increased rate of CSF sterilization but no difference in mortality, though the mortality at 2 weeks in this study was decreased when compared with the lower dose AmB regimens used in previous studies. A randomized trial involving HIV-infected patients from Thailand evaluated 64 patients receiving AmB alone (0.7 mg/kg per day), AmB plus flucytosine (100 mg/kg per day), AmB plus fluconazole (400 mg per day) or triple drug therapy. The combination of AmB plus flucytosine cleared the cryptococci from CSF most rapidly [96]. An observational cohort study of HIV-positive and HIV-negative patients showed significantly higher treatment failure (cryptococcus in CSF or death) at 2 weeks and at 3 months in patients who were treated with antifungals other than AmB plus flucytosine or who received less than 14 days of the induction regimen [97]. Higher doses of AmB (0.7 vs 1.0 mg/kg per day) plus flucytosine were used in a more recent study. The higher dosage was more fungicidal, although no difference in 2- and 10-week mortality was observed [98]. A Cochrane review updated in 2011 states that the optimal dosing of AmB remains unclear.

AmB therapy is often limited by significant renal toxicity. A lipid-associated preparation can reduce toxicity and is equally effective in several older trials [99,100]. A trial randomized HIV-positive patients to treatment with conventional AmB (at 0.7 mg/kg per day) or with liposomal AmB at two different doses (3 or 6 mg/kg per day). The liposomal formulation at 3 mg/kg per day had significantly less renal toxicity and other side effects, and mortality was the same in all three treatment arms. The use of intrathecal AmB has been reported in individual patients but its benefit is unclear [101,102]. The 2010 guidelines of the Infectious Diseases Society of America (IDSA) recommend for HIV-positive patients induction therapy with conventional AmB at 0.7–1.0 mg/kg per day (or liposomal AmB at 3–4 mg/kg per day) plus 100 mg/kg per day flucytosine for at least 2 weeks. The CDC guidelines recommend a higher liposomal AmB dose of 4–6 kmg/kg per day [47].

Adjuvant subcutaneous interferon gamma-1b may be beneficial during induction therapy. In a small randomized trial, more patients had negative CSF cultures at 2 weeks with interferon gamma at 100 or 200 mcg three times per week compared to placebo [103]. A randomized trial added interferon gamma-1b (100 mcg every other day) to an induction treatment with high dose AmB plus flucytosine and found faster CSF clearance at 2 weeks in patients receiving additional interferon gamma (both with two and six doses). Mortality was not different between groups.

Since access to flucytosine is limited in many areas of the world, recent studies have assessed the efficacy of AmB in combination with fluconazole as induction therapy. A randomized open-label trial in the US and Thailand compared 2 weeks of AmB (0.7 mg/kg per day) to induction therapy with AmB plus fluconazole at two doses (400 or 800 mg per day). A higher frequency of survival, neurologic stability and negative CSF culture was seen in patients with additional fluconazole at the higher dose (800 mg per day) [104]. A recent trial assessed higher doses of fluconazole and randomized patients to either AmB (0.7–1 mg/kg) plus flucytosine, AmB plus fluconazole (800 mg daily), AmB plus fluconazole (600 mg twice daily) or AmB plus voriconazole (300 mg twice daily). There were no statistically significant differences in the rate of clearance from CSF samples among the four treatment groups, suggesting that AmB plus fluconazole at higher doses (800–1200 mg per day) represents an alternative to the standard regimen of AmB plus fucytosine [105]. Voriconazole showed promising results, though more data evaluating this medication are necessary. Induction therapy using solely the fungistatic (and in contrast to AmB not fungicidal) fluconazole had been shown to be inferior at lower fluconazole doses of 200–400 mg per day [106,94]. Higher doses of fluconazole (800, 1200, 1600 and 2000 mg per day) were used for 10 weeks without prior AmB induction and survival and time to negative CSF cultures improved with increasing doses [107]. At higher daily doses of fluconazole, divided doses are recommended to minimize gastrointestinal toxicity. Fluconazole resistance leading to relapses and high mortality may occur with monotherapy as seen in a prospective observational study [108].

Consolidation and maintenance therapy

Following induction treatment, patients should receive consolidation therapy with fluconazole (200–400 mg a day) for eight weeks. A large randomized trial compared fluconazole with itraconazole (both at 400 mg per day) for 8 weeks, followed by a maintenance therapy with the same agent at 200 mg per day. Fluconazole was associated with a higher rate of CSF sterilization, but clinical outcome was the same with itraconazole [95].

Maintenance therapy or secondary prophylaxis is recommended for at least 1 year but also depends on the immune status. A large multicenter study randomized patients to continue or discontinue secondary prophylaxis when the CD4 count had increased to >100 cells/μL and an undetectable HIV RNA level had been sustained for 3 months. No recurrent cryptococcal meningitis was seen in the subsequent 48 weeks in either group [109]. A small observational cohort study showed no relapses in patients whose maintenance therapy was discontinued with CD4 count >100 or 200 cells [110]. However, a larger retrospective study showed four relapses when secondary prophylaxis was stopped after obtaining CD4 count >100 cells [111]. Overall, discontinuation of secondary prophylaxis can be considered once CD4 count is >100 cells but reinstitution of maintenance therapy should be considered if the CD4 count decreases to <100 cells/mL.

Immune reconstitution syndrome

Limited data exist to determine the optimal timing of initiation or reinstitution of antiretroviral therapy for treatment of HIV infection in patients with cryptococcal meningitis. A South African study showed that initiation of antiretrovirals within 14 days of treatment of opportunistic infections was associated with lower mortality [112]. However, earlier antiretroviral treatment may be associated with greater risk of immune reconstitution syndrome (IRIS) [113]. Limited evidence also exists in determining best management of IRIS. A few small randomized trials have shown that corticosteroid addition to continued antiretrovirals and antifungal treatments is safe and could be beneficial [114,115].

HIV-negative patients

Less evidence exists for optimal treatment of HIV-negative patients. In organ transplant recipients with cryptococcal meningitis, antifungal therapy should generally be accompanied by an adjustment in their immunosuppressive regimen. Because of a high rate of reduced renal function in transplant recipients and increased risk of nephrotoxicity from concomitant calcineurin use, conventional AmB is not a first-line therapy in this population. In a prospective cohort study of solid organ transplant recipients, the lipid formulation of AmB was associated with a lower 90-day mortality than conventional AmB [116]. This study did not show a difference in mortality when flucytosine was added, though the numbers may have been too small for meaningful results. Bone marrow toxicity due to flucytosine is a concern in transplant patients, especially since a decreased renal function can lead to elevated flucytosine levels; hence close monitoring of laboratory values is important in these patients. The IDSA recommends the same first-line treatment in transplant patients as in HIV-positive patients consisting of induction with AmB plus flucytosine followed by fluconazole consolidation and maintenance (Perfect, 2010). Data in non-HIV-infected and non-transplant patients are very limited. This population

is very heterogeneous and includes hematological malignancies, severe liver disease, idiopathic CD4-deficiency and those with an apparently normal immune system. The optimal duration of induction treatment in these patients is debated (Perfect, 2010).

Increased intracranial pressure

Elevated ICP is common in cryptococcal meningitis and is associated with increased morbidity and mortality [117] and should therefore be managed aggressively. Medical treatment with acetazolamide has not been shown to be effective [118]. While there are no data from randomized trials, daily lumbar punctures are recommended to reduce the opening pressure to <20 cmH$_2$O or by 50% of the initial value. Lumbar drains can be placed in patients who require frequent spinal taps. A patient who continues to require serial lumbar punctures after 4 weeks of appropriate therapy likely needs a ventricular shunt [117].

References

1 Chaudhuria, A., Martinb, P.M., Kennedyc, P.G.E. *et al.* (2008) EFNS guideline on the management of community-acquired bacterial meningitis: report of an EFNS Task Force on acute bacterial meningitis in older children and adults. *European Journal of Neurology*, **15**, 649–659.

2 Auburtin, M., Wolff, M., Charpentier, J. *et al.* (2006) Detrimental role of delayed antibiotic administration and penicillin-nonsusceptible strains in adult intensive care unit patients with pneumococcal meningitis: the PNEUMOREA prospective multicenter study. *Critical Care Medicine*, **34**(**11**), 2758.

3 Lepur, D. & Barsić, B. (2007) Community-acquired bacterial meningitis in adults: antibiotic timing in disease course and outcome. *Infection*, **35**(**4**), 225.

4 Proulx, N., Fréchette, D., Toye, B., Chan, J. & Kravcik, S. (2005) Delays in the administration of antibiotics are associated with mortality from adult acute bacterial meningitis. *QJM*, **98**(**4**), 291.

5 Køster-Rasmussen, R., Korshin, A. & Meyer, C.N. (2008) Antibiotic treatment delay and outcome in acute bacterial meningitis. *Journal of Infection*, **57**, 449–454.

6 Harnden, A., Ninis, N., Thompson, M. *et al.* (2006) Parenteral penicillin for children with meningococcal disease before hospital admission: case–control study. *British Medical Journal*, **332**, 1295–1298.

7 Friedland, I.R., Paris, M., Ehrett, S., Hickey, S., Olsen, K. & McCracken, G.H. Jr. (1993) Evaluation of antimicrobial regimens for treatment of experimental penicillin- and cephalosporin-resistant pneumococcal meningitis. *Antimicrobial Agents and Chemotherapy*, **37**(**8**), 1630.

8 Prasad, K., Kumar, A., Singhal, T. & Gupta, P.K. (2007) Third generation cephalosporins versus conventional antibiotics for treating acute bacterial meningitis. *Cochrane*

Database of Systematic Reviews, (**4**), CD001832 DOI: 10.1002/14651858.CD001832.pub3.

9 Clauss, H.E. & Lorber, B. (2008) Central nervous system infection with Listeria monocytogenes. *Current Infectious Disease Reports*, **10**(**4**), 300.

10 Scheld, W.M., Fletcher, D.D., Fink, F.N. *et al.* (1979) Response to therapy in an experimental rabbit model of meningitis due to Listeria monocytogenes. *Journal of Infectious Diseases*, **140**, 287–94.

11 Azimi, P.H., Koranyi, K. & Lindsey, K.D. (1979) Listeria monocytogenes: synergistic effects of ampicillin and gentamicin. *American Journal of Clinical Pathology*, **72**, 974–977.

12 Boisivon, A., Guiomar, C. & Carbon, C. (1990) In-vitro bactericidal activity of amoxicillin, gentamicin, rifampicin, ciprofloxacin and trimethoprim-sulfamethoxazole alone or in combination against Listeria monocytogenes. *European Journal of Clinical Microbiology and Infectious Diseases*, **9**, 206–209.

13 Sipahi, O.R., Turhan, T., Pullukcu, H., Calik, S. *et al.* (2008) Moxifloxacin versus ampicillin 1 gentamicin in the therapy of experimental Listeria monocytogenes meningitis. *Journal of Antimicrobial Chemotherapy*, **61**, 670–673.

14 Korinek, A.M., Baugnon, T., Golmard, J.L., van Effenterre, R., Coriat, P. & Puybasset, L. (2006) Risk factors for adult nosocomial meningitis after craniotomy: role of antibiotic prophylaxis. *Neurosurgery*, **59**(**1**), 126.

15 van de Beek, D., Drake, J.M. & Tunkel, A.R. (2010) Nosocomial bacterial meningitis. *The New England Journal of Medicine*, **362**, 146–54.

16 Sáez-Llorens, X. & O'Ryan, M. (2001) Cefepime in the empiric treatment of meningitis in children. *Pediatric Infectious Disease Journal*, **20**(**3**), 356.

17 Karageorgopoulos, D.E., Valkimadi, P.E., Kapaskelis, A. *et al.* (2009) Short versus long duration of antibiotic therapy for bacterial meningitis: a meta-analysis of randomised controlled trials in children. *Archives of Disease in Childhood*, **94**, 607–14.

18 van de Beek, D., Brouwer, M. & de Gans, J. (2007b) Hypernatremia in bacterial meningitis. *Journal of Infection*, **55**(**4**), 381–2.

19 van de Beek, D., de Gans, J., McIntyre, P. & Prasad, K. (2007a) Corticosteroids for acute bacterial meningitis. *Cochrane Database of Systematic Reviews*, (**1**), CD004405 DOI: 10.1002/14651858.CD004405.pub2.

20 McIntyre, P. (2010) Adjunctive dexamethasone in meningitis: does value depend on clinical setting? *The Lancet Neurology*, **9**, 229–231.

21 Scarborough, M., Gordon, S.B., Whitty, C.J. *et al.* (2007) Corticosteroids for bacterial meningitis in adults in sub-Saharan Africa. *The New England Journal of Medicine*, **357**, 2441–50.

22 Egermann, U., Stanga, Z., Ramin, A., Acosta, F. *et al.* (2009) Combination of daptomycin plus ceftriaxone is more active than vancomycin plus ceftriaxone in experimental meningitis after addition of dexamethasone. *Antimicrobial Agents and Chemotherapy*, **53**(**7**), 3030–3033.

23 Maconochie, I.K. & Baumer, J.H. (2008) Fluid therapy for acute bacterial meningitis. *Cochrane Database of Systematic*

Reviews, (**1**), CD004786 DOI: 10.1002/14651858.CD004786.pub3.

24 Kramer, A.H. & Bleck, T.P. (2007) Neurocritical care of patients with central nervous system infections. *Current Infectious Disease Reports*, **9**(**4**), 308.

25 Ajdukiewicz, K.M., Cartwright, K.E., Scarborough, M. *et al.* (2011) Glycerol adjuvant therapy in adults with bacterial meningitis in a high HIV seroprevalence setting in Malawi: a double-blind, randomised controlled trial. *Lancet Infectious Diseases*, **11**(**4**), 293.

26 Peltola, H., Roine, I., Fernández, J. *et al.* (2007) Adjuvant glycerol and/or dexamethasone to improve the outcomes of childhood bacterial meningitis: a prospective, randomized, double-blind, placebo-controlled trial. *Clinical Infectious Diseases*, **45**(**10**), 1277.

27 Siegel, J.D., Rhinehart, E., Jackson, M., Chiarello, L., and Healthcare Infection Control Practices Advisory Committee. (2007) *Guideline for isolation precautions: preventing transmission of infectious agents in healthcare settings.*

28 Zalmanovici Trestioreanu, A., Fraser, A., Gafter-Gvili, A., Paul, M. & Leibovici, L. (2011) Antibiotics for preventing meningococcal infections. *Cochrane Database of Systematic Reviews*, (**8**), CD004785 DOI: 10.1002/14651858.CD004785.pub4.

29 Adams, W.G., Deaver, K.A., Cochi, S.L. *et al.* (1993) Decline of childhood Haemophilus influenzae type b (Hib) disease in the Hib vaccine era. *JAMA*, **269**, 221–226.

30 Tsai, C.J., Griffin, M.R., Nuorti, J.P. & Grijalva, C.G. (2008) Changing epidemiology of pneumococcal meningitis after the introduction of pneumococcal conjugate vaccine in the United States. *Clinical Infectious Diseases*, **46**, 1664–1672.

31 Pai, M., Flores, L.L., Pai, N., Hubbard, A., Riley, L.W. & Colford, J.M. Jr. (2003) Diagnostic accuracy of nucleic acid amplification tests for tuberculous meningitis: a systematic review and meta-analysis. *Lancet Infectious Diseases*, **3**(**10**), 633.

32 Zunt, J.R. & Marra, C.M. (1999) Cerebrospinal fluid testing for the diagnosis of central nervous system infection. *Neurologic Clinics*, **17**, 675–689.

33 Blumberg, H.M., Burman, W.J., Chaisson, R.E. *et al.* (2003) American Thoracic Society/Centers for Disease Control and Prevention/Infectious Diseases Society of America: treatment of tuberculosis. *American Journal of Respiratory and Critical Care Medicine*, **167**(**4**), 603.

34 Thwaites, G., Fisher, M., Hemingway, C., Scott, G., Solomon, T. & Innes, J. (2009) British Infection Society guidelines for the diagnosis and treatment of tuberculosis of the central nervous system in adults and children. *Journal of Infection*, **59**(**3**), 167–187.

35 Donald, P.R. (2010) Cerebrospinal fluid concentrations of anti-tuberculosis agents in adults and children. *Tuberculosis*, **90**(**5**), 279–292.

36 Griffith, D.E., Brown-Elliott, B.A., Shepherd, S., McLarty, J., Griffith, L. & Wallace, R.J. Jr. (2005) Ethambutol ocular toxicity in treatment regimens for Mycobacterium avium complex lung

disease. *American Journal of Respiratory and Critical Care Medicine*, **172**(2), 250.

37 Rock, R.B., Olin, M., Baker, C.A., Molitor, T.W. & Peterson, P.K. (2008) Central nervous system tuberculosis: pathogenesis and clinical aspects. *Clinical Microbiology Reviews*, **21**(2), 243–61.

38 Li, H., Liu, W. & You, C. (2012) Central nervous system tuberculoma. *Journal of Clinical Neuroscience*, **19**(5), 691–695.

39 World Health Organization. (2010) *Multidrug and extensively drug-resistant TB (M/XDR-TB): 2010 global report on surveillance and response.* WHO Library Cataloguing-in-Publication Data.

40 Thwaites, G.E., Lan, N.T., Dung, N.H. *et al.* (2005) Effect of anti-tuberculosis drug resistance on response to treatment and outcome in adults with tuberculous meningitis. *Journal of Infectious Diseases*, **192**(1), 79.

41 World Health Organization. (2011) *Guidelines for the programmatic management of drug-resistant tuberculosis 2011 update.* First edition, 2006; Emergency update, 2008; WHO Library Cataloguing-in-Publication Data.

42 Ginsberg, A.M. (2010) Drugs in development for tuberculosis. *Drugs*, **70**(17), 2201–2214.

43 Marx, G.E. & Chan, E.D. (2011Article ID 798764) TuberculousMeningitis: diagnosis and treatment overview. *Tuberculosis Research and Treatment*, 9 doi:10.1155/2011/798764.

44 Vinnard, C. & Macgregor, R.R. (2009) Tuberculous meningitis in HIV-infected individuals. *Current HIV/AIDS Reports*, **6**(3), 139–145.

45 Cecchini, D., Ambrosioni, J., Brezzo, C. *et al.* (2007) Tuberculous meningitis in HIV-infected patients: drug susceptibility and clinical outcome. *AIDS*, **21**(3), 373–374.

46 Torok, M.E., Yen, N.T.B. & Chau, T.T.H. (2011) Timing of initiation of antiretroviral therapy in human immunodeficiency virus (HIV)-associated tuberculousmeningitis. *Clinical Infectious Diseases*, **52**(11), 1374–1383.

47 Kaplan, J.E., Benson, C., Holmes, K.H., Brooks, J.T., Pau, A. & Masur, H. (2009) Guidelines for prevention and treatment of opportunistic infections in HIV-infected adults and adolescents: recommendations from CDC, the National Institutes of Health, and the HIV Medicine Association of the Infectious Diseases Society of America. *Morbidity and Mortality Weekly Report. Recommendations and Reports*, **58**(**RR-4**), 1–207.

48 Prasad, K. & Singh, M.B. (2008) Corticosteroids for managing tuberculous meningitis. *Cochrane Database of Systematic Reviews*, (1), CD002244 DOI: 10.1002/14651858.CD002244.pub3.

49 Thwaites, G.E., Nguyen, D.B., Nguyen, H.D. *et al.* (2004) Dexamethasone for the treatment of tuberculous meningitis in adolescents and adults. *New England Journal of Medicine*, **351**(17), 1741–51.

50 Patel, V.B., Padayatchi, N., Bhigjee, A.I. *et al.* (2004) Multidrug-resistant tuberculous meningitis in KwaZulu-Natal, South Africa. *Clinical Infectious Diseases*, **38**, 851–856.

51 Kemaloglu, S., Özkan, Ü., Bukte, Y., Ceviz, A. & Özates, M. (2002) Timing of Shunt surgery in childhood tuberculous meningitis with hydrocephalus. *Pediatric Neurosurgery*, **37**, 194–198.

52 Srikantha, U., Morab, J.V., Sastry, S. *et al.* (2009) Outcome of ventriculoperitoneal shunt placement in Grade IV tubercular meningitis with hydrocephalus: a retrospective analysis in 95 patients. *Journal of Neurosurgery: Pediatrics*, **4**(2), 176–183.

53 Bayindir, C., Mete, Ő. & Bilgic, B. (2006) Retrospective study of 23 pathologically proven cases of central nervous system tuberculomas. *Clinical Neurology and Neurosurgery*, **108**(4), 353–357.

54 Møller, K., Larsen, F.S., Bie, P. & Skinhøj, P. (2001) The syndrome of inappropriate secretion of antidiuretic hormone and fluid restriction in meningitis—how strong is the evidence? *Scandinavian Journal of Infectious Diseases*, **33**(1), 13–26.

55 Schoeman, J.F., van Rensburg, A.J., Laubscher, J.A. & Springer, P. (2011) The role of aspirin in childhood tuberculous meningitis. *Journal of Child Neurology*, **26**, 956.

56 Kimberlin, D.W. (2007) Management of HSV encephalitis in adults and neonates: diagnosis, prognosis and treatment. *Herpes*, **14**, 11–16.

57 Elion, G.B., Furman, P.A., Fyfe, J.A. *et al.* (1977) Selectivity of action of an antiherpetic agent 9-(2-hydroxyethoxymethyl) guanine. *PNAS*, **74**, 5716–5720.

58 Whitley, R.J., Soong, S.-J., Dolin, R. *et al.* (1977) Adenine arabinoside therapy of biopsy-proved herpes simplex encephalitis. *The New England Journal of Medicine*, **297**, 289–294.

59 Whitley, R.J., Soong, S.J., Hirsch, M.S. *et al.* (1981) Herpes simplex encephalitis. Vidarabine therapy and diagnostic problems. *The New England Journal of Medicine*, **304**, 313–318.

60 Sköldenberg, B., Forsgren, M., Alestig, K. *et al.* (1984) Acyclovir versus vidarabine in herpes simplex encephalitis. Randomized multicentre study in consecutive Swedish patients. *Lancet*, **2**, 707.

61 Whitley, R.J., Alford, C.A., Hirsch, M.S. *et al.* (1986) Vidarabine versus acyclovir therapy in herpes simplex encephalitis. *The New England Journal of Medicine*, **314**, 144.

62 Stahl, J.P., Mailles, A. *et al* (2011) Herpes simplex encephalitis and management of acyclovir in encephalitis patients in France. *Epidemiology and Infection*, 1–10.

63 Raschilas, F., Wolff, M., Delatour, F. *et al.* (2002) Outcome of and prognostic factors for herpes simplex encephalitis in adult patients: results of a multicenter study. *Clinical Infectious Diseases*, **35**, 254–260.

64 Valencia, I., Miles, D.K., Melvin, J. *et al.* (2004) Relapse of herpes encephalitis after acyclovir therapy: report of two new cases and review of the literature. *Neuropediatrics*, **35**(6), 371.

65 Sköldenberg, B. *et al.* (2006) Incidence and pathogenesis of clinical relapse after herpes simplex encephalitis in adults. *Journal of Neurology*, **253**, 163–170.

66 Weil, A.A., Glaser, C.A., Amad, Z. & Forghani, B. (2002) Patients with suspected herpes simplex encephalitis: rethinking an initial negative polymerase chain reaction result. *Clinical Infectious Diseases*, **34**(8), 1154–1157.

67 Studahl, M., Bergstrom, T. & Hagsberg, L. (1998) Acute viral encephalitis in adults—a prospective study. *Scandinavian Journal of Infectious Diseases*, **30**, 215–220.

68 Guffond, T., Dewilde, A., Lobert, P.E., Caparros-Lefebvre, D., Hober, D. & Wattre, P. (1994) Significance and clinical relevance of the detection of herpes simplex virus DNA by the polymerase chain reaction in cerebrospinal fluid from patients with presumed encephalitis. *Clinical Infectious Diseases*, **18**, 744–749.

69 Koskiniemi, M., Piiparinen, H., Mannonen, L., Rantalaiho, T. & Vaheri, A. (1996) Herpes encephalitis is a disease of middle aged and elderly people: polymerase chain reaction for detection of herpes simplex virus in the CSF of 516 patients with encephalitis. *Journal of Neurology, Neurosurgery, and Psychiatry*, **60**, 174–178.

70 Aurelius, E., Johansson, B., Skoldenberg, B., Staland, A. & Forsgren, M. (1991) Rapid diagnosis of herpes simplex encephalitis by nested polymerase chain reaction assay of cerebrospinal fluid. *Lancet*, **337**, 189–192.

71 Chen, Y., Scieux, C., Garrait, V. *et al.* (2000) Resistant herpes simplex virus type 1 infection: an emerging concern after allogeneic stem cell transplantation. *Clinical Infectious Diseases*, **31**, 927–935.

72 Ziyaeyan, M. *et al.* (2007) Frequency of acyclovir-resistant herpes simplex viruses isolated from the general immunocompetent population and patients with acquired immunodeficiency syndrome. *International Journal of Dermatology*, **46**, 1263–1266.

73 Piret, J. & Boivin, G. (2011) Resistance of herpes simplex viruses to nucleoside analogues: mechanisms, prevalence, and management. *Antimicrobial Agents and Chemotherapy*, **55**(2), 459–472.

74 Bacon, T.H., Levin, M.J., Leary, J.J. *et al.* (2003) Herpes simplex virus resistance to acyclovir and penciclovir after two decades of antiviral therapy. *Clinical Microbiology Reviews*, **16**, 114–128.

75 Steiner, I., Budka, H., Chaudhuri, A. *et al.* (2010) Viral meningoencephalitis: a review of diagnostic methods and guidelines for management. *European Journal of Neurology*, **17**, 999–1009.

76 Safrin, S., Crumpacker, C., Chatis, P. *et al.* (1991) A controlled trial comparing foscarnet with vidarabine for acyclovir-resistant mucocutaneous herpes simplex in the acquired immunodeficiency syndrome. *The New England Journal of Medicine*, **325**, 551–555.

77 Pöhlmann, C., Schetelig, J., Reuner, U. *et al.* (2007) Cidofovir and foscarnet for treatment of human herpesvirus 6 encephalitis in a neutropenic stem cell transplant recipient. *Clinical Infectious Diseases*, **44**, e118–e120.

78 Hubacek, P., Keslova, P., Formankova, R. *et al.* (2009) Staryl J, Sedlacek1 P: Cytomegalovirus encephalitis/retinitis in allogeneic haematopoietic stem cell transplant recipient treated successfully with combination of cidofovir and Foscarnet. *Pediatric Transplantation*, **13**(7), 919–922.

79 Habel, A.H. & Brown, J.K. (1972) Dexamethasone in herpes-simplex encephalitis. *Lancet*, **1**, 695.

80 Upton, A.R., Foster, J.B. & Barwick, D.D. (1971) Dexamethasone treatment in herpes-simplex encephalitis. *Lancet*, **1**, 861.

81 Kamei, S., Sekizawa, T., Shiota, H. *et al.* (2005) Evaluation of combination therapy using aciclovir and corticosteroid in adult patients with herpes simplex virus encephalitis. *Journal of Neurology, Neurosurgery, and Psychiatry*, **76**, 1544–1549.

82 Meyding-Lamadé, U.K., Oberlinner, C., Rau, P.R. *et al.* (2003) Experimental herpes simplex virus encephalitis: a combination therapy of acyclovir and glucocorticoids reduces long-term magnetic resonance imaging abnormalities. *Journal of Neurovirology*, **9**(1), 118–125.

83 Sergerie, Y. *et al.* (2007) Delayed but not early glucocorticoid treatment protects the host during experimental herpes simplex virus encephalitis in mice. *Journal of Infectious Diseases*, **195**, 817–825.

84 Martinez-Torres, F., Menon, S., Pritsch, M. *et al.* (2008) Protocol for German trial of Acyclovir and corticosteroids in Herpes-simplex-virus-encephalitis (GACHE): a multicenter, multinational, randomized, double-blind, placebo-controlled German, Austrian and Dutch trial. *BMC Neurology*, **8**, 40.

85 McGrath, N., Anderson, N.D., Crixson, M.C. & Powell, K.F. (1997) Herpes simplex encephalitis treated with acyclovir: diagnosis and longterm outcome. *Journal of Neurology, Neurosurgery, and Psychiatry*, **63**, 321–326.

86 Gunduz, A., Beskardes, A.F., Kutlu, A., Ozkara, C., Karaagae, N. & Yeni, S.N. (2006) Herpes simplex encephalitis as a cause of nonconvulsive status epilepticus. *Epileptic Disorders*, **8**, 57–60.

87 Liu, K.C. & Bhardwaj, A.A. (2007) Use of Prophylactic Anticonvulsants in Neurologic Critical Care: A Critical Appraisal. *Neurocritical Care*, **7**, 175–184.

88 Barnett, G.H., Ropper, A.H. & Romeo, J. (1988) Intracranial pressure and outcome in adult encephalitis. *Journal of Neurosurgery*, **68**, 585–588.

89 Schwab, S., Jünger, E., Spranger, M. *et al.* (1997) Craniectomy: an aggressive treatment approach in severe encephalitis. *Neurology*, **48**, 412–417.

90 Taferner, E. & Pfausler, B. (2001) Craniectomy in severe, life-threatening encephalitis: a report on outcome and long-term prognosis of four cases. *Intensive Care Medicine*, **27**(8), 1426–1428.

91 Arciniegas, D.B. & Anderson, C.A. (2004) Viral encephalitis: neuropsychiatric and neurobehavioral aspects. *Current Psychiatry Reports*, **6**(5), 372.

92 Price, R.W. (1996) Neurological complications of HIV infection. *Lancet*, **348**(9025), 445–452.

93 Wu, G., Vilchez, R.A., Eidelman, B., Fung, J., Kormos, R. & Kusne, S. (2002) Cryptococcal meningitis: an analysis among 5521 consecutive organ transplant recipients. *Transplant Infectious Disease*, **4**(4), 183–188.

94 Saag, M.S., Powderly, W.G., Cloud, G.A. *et al.* (1992) Comparison of amphotericin B with fluconazole in the treatment of acute AIDS-associated cryptococcal meningitis. The NIAID Mycoses Study Group and the AIDS Clinical Trials Group. *The New England Journal of Medicine*, **326**, 83.

95 van der Horst, C.M., Saag, M.S., Cloud, G.A. *et al.* (1997) Treatment of cryptococcal meningitis associated with the acquired immunodeficiency syndrome. National Institute of Allergy and Infectious Diseases Mycoses Study Group and

AIDS Clinical Trials Group. *The New England Journal of Medicine*, **337**, 15–21.

96 Brouwer, A.E., Rajanuwong, A., Chierakul, W. *et al.* (2004) Combination antifungal therapies for HIV-associated cryptococcal meningitis: a randomized trial. *Lancet*, **363**, 1764–1767.

97 Dromer, F., Bernede-Bauduin, C., Guillemot, D. *et al.* (2008) Major role for amphotericin B- flucytosine combination in severe cryptococcosis. *PLoS One*, **3**, e2870.

98 Bicanic, T., Wood, R., Meintjes, G. *et al.* (2008) High-dose amphotericin B with flucytosine for the treatment of cryptococcal meningitis in HIV-infected patients: a randomized trial. *Clinical Infectious Diseases*, **47**, 123–130.

99 Leenders, A.C., Reiss, P., Portegies, P. *et al.* (1997) Liposomal amphotericin B (AmBisome) compared with amphotericin B both followed by oral fluconazole in the treatment of AIDS-associated cryptococcal meningitis. *AIDS*, **11**(12), 1463.

100 Sharkey, P.K., Graybill, J.R., Johnson, E.S. *et al.* (1996) Amphotericin B lipid complex compared with amphotericin B in the treatment of cryptococcal meningitis in patients with AIDS. *Clinical Infectious Diseases*, **22**(2), 315.

101 Diamond, R.D. & Bennett, J.E. (1973) A subcutaneous reservoir for intrathecal therapy of fungal meningitis. *The New England Journal of Medicine*, **288**(4), 186.

102 Yuchong, C., Jianghan, C., Hai, W. & Julin, G. (2011) Lumbar puncture drainage with intrathecal injection of amphotericin B for control of cryptococcal meningitis. *Mycoses*, **54**(4), e248–e251.

103 Pappas, P.G., Bustamante, B., Ticona, E. *et al.* (2004) Recombinant interferon- gamma 1b as adjunctive therapy for AIDS-related acute cryptococcal meningitis. *Journal of Infectious Diseases*, **189**(12), 2185.

104 Pappas, P.G., Chetchotisakd, P., Larsen, R.A. *et al.* (2009) A phase II randomized trial of amphotericin B alone or combined with fluconazole in the treatment of HIV-associated cryptococcal meningitis. *Clinical Infectious Diseases*, **48**(12), 1775–1783.

105 Loyse, A., Wilson, D., Meintjes, G. *et al.* (2012) Comparison of the Early Fungicidal Activity of High-Dose Fluconazole, Voriconazole, and Flucytosine as Second-Line Drugs Given in Combination With amphotericin B for the Treatment of HIV-Associated Cryptococcal Meningitis. *Clinical Infectious Diseases*, **54**(1), 121–128.

106 Larsen, R.A., Leal, M.A. & Chan, L.S. (1990) Fluconazole compared with amphotericin B plus flucytosine for cryptococcal meningitis in AIDS. A randomized trial. *Annals of Internal Medicine*, **113**(3), 183–187.

107 Milefchik, E., Leal, M.A., Haubrich, R. *et al.* (2008) Fluconazole alone or combined with flucytosine for the treatment of AIDS-associated cryptococcal meningitis. *Medical Mycology*, **46**, 393–395.

108 Bicanic, T., Harrison, T., Niepieklo, A., Dyakopu, N. & Meintjes, G. (2006) Symptomatic relapse of HIV-associated cryptococcal meningitis after initial fluconazole monotherapy: the role of fluconazole resistance and immune reconstitution. *Clinical Infectious Diseases*, **43**(8), 1069.

109 Vibhagool, A., Sungkanuparph, S., Mootsikapun, P. *et al.* (2003) Discontinuation of secondary prophylaxis for cryptococcal meningitis in human immunodeficiency virus-infected patients treated with highly active antiretroviral therapy: a prospective, multicenter, randomized study. *Clinical Infectious Diseases*, **36**(10), 1329.

110 Kirk, O., Reiss, P., Uberti-Foppa, C. *et al.* (2002) Cohorts. Safe interruption of maintenance therapy against previous infection with four common HIV-associated opportunistic pathogens during potent antiretroviral therapy. *Annals of Internal Medicine*, **137**(4), 239.

111 Mussini, C., Pezzotti, P., Miró, J.M. *et al.* (2004) Discontinuation of maintenance therapy for cryptococcal meningitis in patients with AIDS treated with highly active antiretroviral therapy: an international observational study. *Clinical Infectious Diseases*, **38**(4), 565.

112 Zolopa, A., Andersen, J., Powderly, W. *et al.* (2009) Early antiretroviral therapy reduces AIDS progression/death in individuals with acute opportunistic infections: a multicenter randomized strategy trial. *PLoS One*, **4**(5), e5575.

113 Bicanic, T., Meintjes, G., Rebe, K. *et al.* (2009) Immune reconstitution inflammatory syndrome in HIV-associated cryptococcal meningitis: a prospective study. *Journal of Acquired Immune Deficiency Syndromes*, **51**(2), 130.

114 Shelburne, S.A. 3rd, Darcourt, J., White, A.C. Jr. *et al.* (2005) The role of immune reconstitution inflammatory syndrome in AIDS-related Cryptococcus neoformans disease in the era of highly active antiretroviral therapy. *Clinical Infectious Diseases*, **40**, 1049–1052.

115 Lesho, E. (2006) Evidence base for using corticosteroids to treat HIV-associated immune reconstitution syndrome. *Expert Review of Anti-Infective Therapy*, **4**, 469–478.

116 Sun, H.Y., Alexander, B.D., Lortholary, O. *et al.* (2009) Lipid formulations of amphotericin B significantly improve outcome in solid organ transplant recipients with central nervous system cryptococcosis. *Clinical Infectious Diseases*, **49**(11), 1721.

117 Graybill, J.R., Sobel, J., Saag, M. *et al.* (2000) Diagnosis and management of increased intracranial pressure in patients with AIDS and cryptococcal meningitis. The NIAID Mycoses Study Group and AIDS Cooperative Treatment Groups. *Clinical Infectious Diseases*, **30**(1), 47.

118 Newton, P.N., Thai le, H., Tip, N.Q. *et al.* (2002) A randomized, double-blind, placebo-controlled trial of acetazolamide for the treatment of elevated intracranial pressure in cryptococcal meningitis. *Clinical Infectious Diseases*, **35**(6), 769.

16

CHAPTER 16
Evidence-based neuro-oncology

Michael G Hart[1] and Robin Grant[2]
[1]*Department of neurosurgery, Addenbrooke's Hospital, Cambridge, UK*
[2]*Division of Clinical Neurosciences, Western General Hospital, Edinburgh, UK*

Introduction

Epidemiology, prognostic factors and molecular markers

Primary brain tumours account for only 2% of all cancers and are the most common solid malignancy of childhood, the fourth most common in the under 45 age group, and the eighth most common in the under 65 age group [1]. Overall, brain tumours are the second most common cause of death from neurological disease, after stroke. Management depends on important pre-operative prognostic factors: age, disability (performance status), site, suspected imaging diagnosis and presence of co-morbid diseases (Table 16.1). Important molecular diagnostic and prognostic markers are chromosome 1p and 19q for oligodendroglial tumours, methyl-guanine methyl transferase (MGMT) for glioblastoma multiforme (GBM) and isocitrate dehydrogenase (IDH-1), which helps differentiate glioblastomas that have arisen from low-grade glioma (secondary GBM) from more aggressive de-novo GBM (primary GBM).

Trial outcome criteria and defining response to therapy

At least one-third of patients treated with radiotherapy with concomitant and then adjuvant Temozolomide (chemo-radiation) will develop apparent tumour 'progression' on magnetic resonance imaging (MRI) within the first 3 months of completion of radiotherapy [3] (Figure 16.1). Approximately 50% of them will have true progression and the other 50% will have 'pseudo-progression' [4]. Pseudo-progression corresponds to the 'early delayed radiation reaction' that mimics tumour progression. There seems no simple structural or metabolic imaging way of distinguishing the two conditions, although methionine positron emission tomography (PET) may help distinguish to some extent.

Pseudo-progression, paradoxically, is associated with a better survival than those that do not have a stable response.

This finding of pseudo-progression has huge implications for all previous studies of experimental therapies where treatment was started within the first 3 months of completion of radiotherapy because of presumed tumour progression as they may overstate response rate to the experimental treatment.

A further potential problem has been identified using contrast enhanced T1-weighted MRI to measure the dimensions of the tumour in trials of anti-angiogenic agents, for example, bevacizumab. There can be reduction of size of the lesion on T1-weighted imaging and co-existent progression of imaging on T2-weighted images: this has been termed 'pseudo-response'.

Finally, MRI tumour volume measurements (rather than product of maximum perpendicular diameters used in McDonald criteria) are being increasingly used in trials [5]. Volumetric measurements will overestimate the extent of reduction in tumour size, compared with previous studies using McDonald criteria, thereby reporting a higher response rate.

Because of all the aforementioned problems, new response criteria have been developed (RANO criteria). These include guidance on imaging and how to manage suspected tumour progression within the first 3 months of completion of radiation therapy [6].

Best pre-operative medical management

Steroids

Most malignant brain tumours are associated with the surrounding vasogenic oedema that can cause headache or progressive focal neurological deficit. Dexamethasone has a widely accepted role in providing control of oedema and producing symptomatic improvement [7,8]. There is no indication to start steroids in the absence of raised intracranial pressure or focal neurological deficit. Even though there is limited RCT evidence for the use of corticosteroids,

Table 16.1 Recursive partitioning analysis for high-grade glioma

Category	Median survival in months (95% confidence intervals)	2-year survival (%)
Group 1: low risk (age < 40 years, frontal tumour)	132 (110–226)	65
Group 2: low to moderate risk (age < 40 years, other tumour sites)	71 (60–97)	35
Group 3: moderate- to high-risk group (age 40–65 years, KPS > 70, STR or GTR)	63 (58–69)	17
Group 4: high risk (age > 65 years or age 40–65 years and KPS < 80 or age 40–65 years and KPS > 70 and biopsy only)	37 (32–42)	4

STR = sub-total resection; GTR = gross total resection; KPS = Karnofsky Performance Score.
Source: Lamborn et al. 2004 [2]. Reproduced with permission of Oxford University Press.

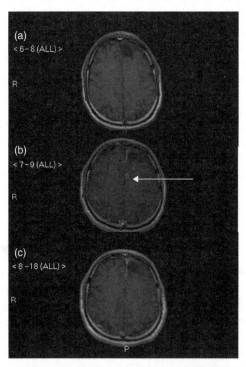

Figure 16.1 MRI 'pseudo-progression'. (a) Serial MRI scans demonstrating Gadolinium enhanced T1 weighted image after concomitant chemo-radiation. (b) Development of new focus of enhancement during adjuvant chemotherapy with Temozolomide ? Tumour progression. (c) Enhancement resolves on follow-up without changing treatment plan of completion of adjuvant Temozolomide.

clinical experience and data from retrospective studies have established their role beyond reasonable doubt. Side effects are common and a balance needs to be reached between the dose and duration of treatment.

A low oral dose of 4 mg dexamethasone for 28 days is as effective as an 8 mg or 16 mg daily in producing symptomatic improvement and results in fewer side effects [9]. The mean improvement in Karnofsky Performance Score (KPS) – a standard measure of neurological impairment [10] – for 4 mg dexamethasone was 6.7 points (SD 11.3). Up to 50% of patients will show an improvement of 10 points in Karnofsky Performance Status (KPS) and 17% had an improvement of over 20 points. Low-dose dexamethasone (4 mg) has significantly lower rates of proximal myopathy (14% vs 38%) and Cushingoid facies (32% vs 69%). The specific side effects with low-dose dexamethasone (4 mg) at day 28 were gastric upset (18%), mental changes (14%), infection (9%) and hypertension (45%).

Seizures

Seizures are the presenting feature of tumours in about one-fourth of patients with single intracerebral tumours [11]. Prophylactic anti-epileptic drugs (AEDs) should not be prescribed in the absence of seizures pre-operatively, as they can be associated with serious side effects and show no significant benefit [12,13]. Following a single seizure, there is a very high likelihood of further seizures (>80%), and hence AEDs should be commenced. There is debate over which is the most appropriate AED [14]. There are specific evidence-based guidelines for status epilepticus and these should be followed [15]. Enzyme-inducing AEDs (Table 16.2) may reduce the serum concentration of dexamethasone and certain chemotherapy agents (e.g. vorinostat and irinotecan) that also utilise cytochrome P450 enzymatic metabolism, thereby potentially reducing the effectiveness of these agents. Enzyme inhibitors (e.g. valproate) may reduce

Table 16.2 Cytochrome P450 enzyme inducers and inhibitors

Enzyme inducers	Non-inducers
Phenytoin	Valproic acid or sodium valproate (enzyme inhibitor)
Phenobarbital	
Oxcarbazepine	Lamotrigine
Carbamazepine	Ethosuximide
Primidone	Gabapentin
Topiramate	Pregabalin
	Levetiracetam
	Tiagabine
	Rufinamide
	Lacosamide
	Zonisamide
	Vigabatrin
	Clobazam/midazolam

excretion of Temozolomide through the kidneys potentially increasing the effectiveness or toxicity of chemotherapy. The clinical effect of these interactions on response, and survival remains uncertain. There is one small randomised controlled trial in patients with brain tumours, demonstrating that it is feasible to switch from phenytoin to levetiracetam without deleterious effects in the post-operative period [16].

Best surgical treatment in primary brain tumours

Introduction

Imaging is accurate for the diagnosis of an intra-cranial tumour, but not for the specific type or grade [17,18]. Histological diagnosis is usually required before treatment of intra-cranial tumours. Surgery may take the form of biopsy or resectional surgery. Biopsy may be 'open' (through a craniotomy) or via a burr hole. Samples may be obtained 'freehand' (based on macroscopic vision) or using neuro-navigation (with or without a stereotactic frame). A retrospective analysis of 7471 biopsies suggests morbidity of 3.5% and mortality < 0.7% [19]. Sampling error may occur with biopsy due to the heterogenous nature of many brain tumours. The accuracy of identifying tumour in a stereotactic biopsy in two prospective series is 98.5% [20,21]. Stereotactic biopsy agreed with the diagnosis and grade at subsequent craniotomy (a mean of 3 weeks later) in 74% and correctly guided therapy in 91% [22]. Biopsy may under-grade tumours, due to sampling error, and consequently, some of those in the biopsy arm of low-grade glioma trials may have an unexpectedly poor survival.

Biopsy versus resection for high-grade glioma

Benefits of resection include larger tissue sample to allow molecular analysis (e.g. MGMT), avoidance of sampling error, possibility of intra-operative therapies (e.g. Gliadel®), relief from symptoms of mass effect, improved symptom control during radiotherapy, reduced steroid requirements and possibly longer progression free and overall survival. Some benefit may also be conferred by the greater effect of adjuvant therapies in patients with limited post-operative tumour burden. A Cochrane review of biopsy versus resection for high-grade glioma [23] identified only one small RCT including patients aged over 65 from a single centre in Finland [24]. Thirty elderly patients were randomised, but due to errors in diagnosis and missing data only 18 patients were assessable. Resection was reported as being associated with improved survival, but this trial was grossly under-powered and at high risk of bias, making conclusions unreliable.

Intra-operative imaging to maximise extent of resection

Surgical research has focussed on the extent of resection as a significant prognostic factor. Intra-operative imaging

techniques have developed to assist increasing the extent of resection. Analyses from non-randomised studies are fraught with bias and, because of the infiltrative nature of many glial cell tumours, increasing the extent of resection predisposes to the development of post-operative neurological deficits.

Gliolan® (5-aminolevulinic acid or 5-ALA) administered orally pre-operatively results in the accumulation of fluorescent porphyrins within tumour tissue to identify infiltrative margins. An RCT of 322 patients evaluated resection performed with 5-ALA under UV light versus standard microscopic resection under white light. This found that 5-ALA was associated with an increase in the likelihood of obtaining a complete resection (65% vs 36%) as assessed by post-operative MR imaging and improved progression free survival at 6 months (41% vs 21%) but did not affect overall survival [25]. A subsequent analysis revealed greater morbidity according to the NIH-SS score in those treated with 5-ALA, although early deficits commonly improved later [26] (Stummer 2011). Analysis of this trial found that patients who achieved a complete tumour resection (regardless of the use of 5-ALA) had an improved median survival of 16.7 vs 11.8 months [27], supporting the value of extent of resection. An RCT of neuro-navigation did not find that this improved outcome, but neuro-navigation, has become well established in planning surgery and minimising morbidity related to the surgical approach [28]. An unblinded RCT of 58 patients found that complete resection rate was improved with the use of intra-operative MRI compared to microscopic resection (96% vs 68%) and that no new neurological deficits were detected: survival outcomes were not reported [29]. There is currently an ongoing RCT investigating the diagnostic properties of three-dimensional ultrasound (Sonowand®). A Cochrane review has compared all of the above methods of intra-operative imaging [30]. The most compelling evidence was for 5-ALA and intra-operative MRI increasing extent of resection. Trials directly comparing interventions will potentially be available in the future.

Techniques to make surgery safer

Complimentary to the techniques aiming to maximise resection is research on improving the safety of brain tumour surgery in eloquent areas of the brain. Motor tract identification using diffusion tensor MRI was assessed in an RCT of 238 patients [31]. Motor deterioration occurred in 15% of those treated with tractography versus 33% of the control arm: extent of resection and overall survival were also improved. Awake craniotomy has been evaluated in a small randomised study of 53 patients with intrinsic lesions in eloquent areas [32]. Paradoxically, there was a trend for those undergoing awake craniotomy to have more deficits and greater residual tumour volume. Reasons for this could have been a lack of intra-operative cortical mapping, the learning curve of the technique and variations in intra-operative assessment.

Best oncological treatment in primary brain tumours

Chemotherapy can be given locally or systemically, alone or in combination with radiotherapy and as part of primary treatment or at relapse after initial treatment.

Local chemotherapy

A RCT of 240 patients randomised to either carmustine-impregnated wafers (Gliadel®) or placebo wafers, placed in the resection cavity of patients with presumed high-grade glioma, demonstrated a 2.2-month survival advantage (13.8 months vs 11.6 months) with chemotherapy [33]. A Cochrane review found three RCTs in total and supported the survival advantage for primary therapy (hazard ratio 0.65 or 35% reduction in risk of death) but not for recurrent disease [34]. However, only 20% of patients with malignant brain tumours are eligible for treatment, based on study entry criteria [35].

Systemic chemotherapy

Multi-agent adjuvant chemotherapy with nitrosoureas, procarbazine and platinum derivatives has been used for many years. Young patients are more likely to respond to chemotherapy (<40 years (40%), 40–60 years (17%), >60 years (<5%)) [36]. Patients with WHO grade 3 tumours and oligodendroglial histology are more likely to have an imaging response. A Cochrane review has been conducted on the use of chemotherapy for adult high-grade glioma [37]. Individual patient data meta-analysis from 12 randomised controlled trials of chemotherapy showed a 2-month survival advantage from 10 months to 12 months in high-grade glioma, which equates to an increase in 1-year survival from 40% to 46% and in 2-year survival from 10% to 15%. The hazard ratio (HR) was 0.85 (95% CI 0.78–0.92), equating to a 15% risk reduction of death for each patient randomised. However, reanalysis of cases aged >70 years showed a non-significant deleterious effect of chemotherapy (personal communication with L Stewart).

A trial of 573 patients aged <70 years, with glioblastoma (GBM), randomised to concomitant Temozolomide chemotherapy with standard radiotherapy (60 Gy in 30 fractions), followed by adjuvant courses of Temozolomide on days 1–5, repeated every 4 weeks, for six courses versus standard radiotherapy also found a 2.5-month survival advantage with chemotherapy, but more importantly demonstrated an improvement in 2-year survival from 10.4% to 26.5% [38]. As a result of this study concomitant and adjuvant Temozolomide chemotherapy are recommended in fit patients with GBM, <70 years of age. Subgroup analysis demonstrated that biopsy and poor performance status patients did not do significantly differently from given radiotherapy alone (and later 'salvage' chemotherapy or other treatments at relapse). An RCT that compared standard chemo-radiation with intensified Temozolomide chemotherapy ('dose-dense') in 833 patients showed a median survival of 16.6 months in standard Temozolomide versus 14.9 months with dose-dense t (P = 0.63; hazard ratio 0.87), and toxicity was worse with dose dense [39].

The value of treatment in the elderly is more controversial. Sixty per cent of all malignant glioma occurs in people aged >65 years. A French study randomised 85 selected patients with GBM aged >70 years to either radiotherapy (50 Gy over 6 weeks) or supportive care alone [40]. This study closed early after an interim analysis showed a statistically significant improvement in overall survival (OS) in the radiotherapy group (median OS; 29.1 weeks vs 16.9 weeks; HR for death in the RT group was 0.47 (95% CI, 0.29–0.76; P = 0.002). There did not appear to be a difference in quality of life between the groups in this study, but patients were highly selected at entry. Two trials have examined the role of chemotherapy in the elderly in comparison with radiotherapy. The German NOA-8 trial randomized 373 good prognosis malignant glioma patients (glioblastoma and anaplastic glioma), aged >65 years to radiotherapy or "dose-dense" temozolomide (ref). Overall, median survival was not different (9.8 (RT) vs 8.6 (Tem)). Event Free Survival was better with temozolomide in methylated GBM (8.4 months vs 4.6 months) and the reverse was true for unmethylated GBM (3.3 months vs 4.6 months). There was a high frequency of bone marrow toxicity with temozolomide [41]. A Nordic Trial included 342 good prognosis GBM patients aged >60 years, 291 of whom were randomised either to: 60 Gy in 30 fractions radiotherapy; hypo-fractionated radio-herapy (34 Gy in 10 fractions) or standard-dose schedule of Temozolomide (5 out of 28 days). Median survival was 6.0 months vs 7.5 months vs 8.3 months, respectively. There was an unexpected poor outcome with standard radiotherapy but they concluded that chemotherapy might be an alternative to short course radio-therapy [42]. The best management in the elderly therefore remains contentious. It seems that hypo-fractionated radio-therapy is at least as good as standard radiotherapy and takes less patient time and may be the option of choice especially in unmethylated GBM. Chemotherapy, alone, may be an alternative, and maybe option of choice in methylated GBM. In patients with newly diagnosed GBM, the use of anti-angiogenic therapy does not improve survival, despite evidence of improved progression-free survival" [43–45].

A randomised controlled trial of over 400 chemo-naive patients with recurrent malignant glioma, following standard radiotherapy, compared PCV chemotherapy (procarbazine, lomustine and vincristine) against Temozolomide given either as standard regime (5/28) or a 21-day regime [46]. There was no survival difference between Temozolomide and PCV chemotherapy (hazard ratio [HR] 0.91, 95% CI, 0.74–1.11, P = 0.350). Standard-dose Temozolomide demonstrated better progression free survival (HR 1.38, 95% CI, 1.05–1.82, P = 0.023), overall survival (HR 1.32, 95% CI, 0.99–1.75, P = 0.056) and global quality of life than the 21-day regimen.

Best treatment of brain metastasis?

Introduction

Brain metastases are usually multiple and occur most often in the setting of active extra-cranial disease; in this instance, management is palliative and prognosis is very poor. A small subgroup of those with a single brain metastasis may enjoy longer survival, particularly if the brain is the only site of metastatic disease ('solitary' metastasis), or extra-cranial disease is well controlled [47]. Treatment options for brain metastases can involve surgical resection or radiotherapy. The latter can be in the form of whole brain radiation therapy (WBRT) or as a focal technique (e.g. stereotactic radiosurgery (SRS) or stereotactic radiotherapy (SRT)). Chemotherapy is seldom used as primary therapy alone [48].

Historical series of patients with good prognostic features suggests that WBRT is associated with an improved life expectancy from 3 months with steroids alone to 7 months with steroids and WBRT [49]. Even though WBRT has not been thoroughly assessed in RCTs, it has become the standard palliative treatment, associated with late side effects characterised by dementia, ataxia and incontinence. Adverse events occurred in < 11% of longer term survivors treated by high doses of WBRT in one study [50].

Role of surgical resection

Three RCTs from the 1990s have compared surgery followed by WBRT versus WBRT alone (standard palliative treatment at the time) [51–53]. Two of the three trials suggested a benefit from surgery. Meta-analysis is invaluable in this situation of small conflicting studies and has recently been analysed in a Cochrane review [54]. This did not demonstrate a significant survival advantage from surgery or in reducing the number of deaths from neurological cause. Only one of the three trials provided information on functionally independent survival for the complete sample population, and although this did suggest an improvement with surgery, the small sample size makes firm conclusions difficult. It should be noted that all the trials recruited a highly selected cohort of patients and the findings are not necessarily generalisable to all clinical scenarios. For instance, patients with cerebellar metastases, hydrocephalus, or significant mass effect were not randomised as the indications or surgery are better understood. Nevertheless, it may be that the benefits of surgery for increasing survival for even highly selected patients with single brain metastases may be more tenuous than previously appreciated. It is important to consider each case individually, use prognostic factors judiciously, and consider other outcomes than survival (Table 16.3).

Role of SRS

Focal radiotherapy techniques (SRS or stereotactic radiotherapy) have received increased attention in recent years as a means of selectively delivering a high dose of radiation. Numerous phase II studies have suggested benefit. Three RCTs have been performed to assess whether the addition of SRS to WBRT confers any advantage over WBRT alone, for patients with one to four brain metastases and analysed in a Cochrane review [55]. Two of the three studies have such serious methodological shortcomings as to render them un-interpretable [56,57]. The single RCT of satisfactory methodological quality included 333 patients and found that those with a single brain metastasis had a statistically significant increase in median survival from 4.9 to 6.5 months, but there was no difference for those with more than one brain metastasis [58]. Local control was better in the SRS and WBRT arm. From these studies it appears that for those with a single un-resectable brain metastasis, SRS and WBRT should be the standard treatment.

Table 16.3 Current randomised controlled trials of concomitant and adjuvant chemotherapy with Temozolomide and control groups in primary disease and Temozolomide alone at recurrence

	Intervention arm	Control arm			
		Radiotherapy only	Chemotherapy		
			Temozolomide 'dose dense'	PCV/nitrosourea	Other
Primary disease	Temozolomide	Stupp 2005 & 2009 & Taphoorn 2005 Athanassiou 2005 Kocker 2008	Clarke 2009	Qian 2009 (CCNU) Wick 2009 (NOA-04)*	
Recurrent disease treatment	Temozolomide			Yung 2000 (CCNU) Osama 2000a (QOL)* Brada et al. [46]* (BR-12 'dose dense')	van den Bent 2009 (erlotinib) Bogdahn 2011 (CED)*

PCV = procarbazine, CCNU and vincristine; CCNU = *N*-(2-chloroethyl)-*N*'-cyclohexyl-*N*-nitrosourea (lomustine); QOL = quality of life.
*WHO Grade 3 tumours (+/− grade 4).

Role of non-focal therapy (WBRT) after focal therapy (SRS or surgery)

Modern imaging more accurately detects very small metastases, and the value of WBRT to treat undetected micro-metastasis is uncertain. Theoretically, a single metastasis should be able to be definitively treated with either surgery or SRS, and if there are subsequent metastases, salvage whole brain radiotherapy therapy can then be given. Only one RCT of 95 patients has demonstrated an advantage with post-operative WBRT in the setting of surgically resected single brain metastasis [59]. This found a decrease in the number of deaths from neurological disease (44–14%) and reduced recurrence rates both locally (46–10%) and throughout the brain (37–14%), but overall survival was not increased. Four RCTs have examined the addition of WBRT after focal therapy (surgery or SRS). The addition of WBRT does not improve survival, but does improve intra-cranial disease control and reduces the need for later therapy [60–63]. Potential benefits of SRS over WBRT in reducing cognitive decline were investigated in a single study but unfortunately data analysis issues, including low statistical power and questionable methodological techniques, render this still an open question. A meta-analysis of this area is needed to accurately stratify the risks and benefits of WBRT to allow accurate counselling of patients before treatment.

Surgery versus SRS (+/− WBRT)

Focal radiotherapy with SRS has generated debate regarding whether it may be a simpler and more effective focal treatment than surgery. RCTs treating single brain metastases with SRS (with or without WBRT) have been found to have shorter survival times than RCTs involving surgery. This is mainly due to selection bias. Two RCTs have attempted to answer this question [64,65]. Both were stopped early due to poor recruitment and included only 85 patients. No statistically significant differences were found (Table 16.4).

Summary

The evidence base in neuro-oncology is improving, but there will remain areas where evidence is patchy and a clinical decision must be taken based on clinical experience, ideally through a multi-disciplinary team model. Results from RCTs are only robust, when the individual patient falls within the inclusion and exclusion criteria of the appropriate trial. The fact that a study is randomised and controlled not by itself is an indication of quality, and statistical significance must not be confused with clinical significance. With these caveats in mind, however we are much better placed than previously to advise patients about the relative value of treatments.

In high-grade glioma, morbidity and mortality are lower with stereotactic biopsy than surgery. These features tend to make biopsy the more realistic surgical option for those with poor performance status, advanced age, or certain types of lesions (e.g. those that are diffuse, deep, or in eloquent areas), if indeed surgery is contemplated. In other selected groups of patients with lobar tumours, there may be a greater likelihood for benefit with resection. The balance of evidence supports a relationship between better resection and delayed tumour progression. Intra-operative imaging in its various forms is becoming increasingly utilised, and chemo-radiation is now the standard of care for younger patients with high-grade glioma who are

Table 16.4 Current randomised controlled trials of surgery, whole brain radiotherapy and focal radiation for brain metastases

Intervention arm		Control arm		
Focal therapy	Additional radiotherapy	WBRT & SRS	WBRT & surgery	WBRT alone
Surgery	WBRT	Roos *et al.* [65]		Patchell *et al.* [51] Vecht *et al.* [52] Mintz *et al.* [53]
	Nil		Patchell *et al.* [59] Roos *et al.* [60] Kocher *et al.* [63]	
SRS	WBRT			Kondziolka *et al.* [56] Chougule *et al.* [57] Andrews *et al.* [58]
	Nil	Aoyama *et al.* [61] Roos *et al.* [60] Chang *et al.* [62] Kocher *et al.* [63]	Muacevic *et al.* [64]	

SRS = stereotactic radiosurgery; WBRT = whole brain radiation therapy.

otherwise fit. Attention to prognostic factors and thorough multi-disciplinary consultation and discussion with the patient over risks and side effects of chemotherapy are necessary to make the best decision for each patient. Much has been learnt from research about how to influence tumour cell biology and the challenges of measuring response and clinical trial end points. However, the effectiveness of molecular 'targeted' therapies (including gene, stem cell or vaccine) for gliomas remains to be proved.

In patients with brain metastasis, there is increasing understanding of the complexities of focal brain therapies and whole brain radiotherapy. In those with multiple metastases, the addition of SRS to WBRT is potentially unnecessary. Treatment with SRS or surgery alone initially may have benefits in terms of later cognitive impairment but at the risk of reduced local disease control and need for further treatment. Despite all these trials in therapy for brain metastases the main cause of death is systemic rather than neurological disease. The main cause of death in patients with brain metastases is the activity of extra-cranial disease. Benefits of other treatments including systemic and local chemotherapy are more uncertain. It is likely that the benefits of these therapies will only be confirmed in trials of individual tumour types (e.g. melanoma, renal, lung, and breast) as all metastases are not similarly responsive to treatment.

References

1 Counsell, C.E. & Grant, R. (1998) Incidence studies of primary and secondary intracranial tumors: a systematic review of their methodology and results. *Journal of Neuro-Oncology*, **37**(**3**), 241–250.

2 Lamborn, K.R., Chang, S.M. & Prados, M.D. (2004) Prognostic factors for survival of patients with glioblastoma: Recursive partitioning analysis. *Neuro-Oncology*, **6**, 227–235.

3 de Wit, M.C., de Bruin, H.G., Eijkenboom, W., Sillevis Smitt, P.A. & van den Bent, M.J. (2004) Immediate post-radiotherapy changes in malignant glioma can mimic tumor progression. *Neurology*, **63**, 535–553.

4 Taal, W., Brandsma, D., de Bruin, H. *et al.* (2008) Incidence of early pseudo-progression in a cohort of malignant glioma patients treated with chemoirradiation with remozolomide. *Cancer*, **113**, 405–410.

5 Macdonald, D.R., Cascino, T.L., Schold, S.C. Jr., & Cairncross, J.G. (1990) Response criteria for phase II studies of supratentorial malignant glioma. *Journal of Clinical Oncology*, **8**, 1277–1280.

6 van den Bent, M.J., Wefel, J.S., Schiff, D. *et al.* (2011) Response assessment in neuro-oncology (a report of the RANO group): assessment of outcome in trials of diffuse low-grade gliomas. *Lancet Oncology*, **12**(**6**), 583–593.

7 French, L.A. & Galicich, J.H. (1962) The use of steroids for control of cerebral oedema. *Cinical Neurosurgery*, **10**, 212–223.

8 Kaal, E.C.A. & Vecht, C.J. (2004) The management of brain edema in brain tumours. *Current Opinion in Oncology*, **16**, 593–600.

9 Vecht, C.J., Hoverstadt, A., Verbiest, H.B. *et al.* (1994) Dose-effect relationship of dexamethasone on Karnofsky performance in metastatic brain tumors; a randomized controlled study of 4, 8 and 16mg per day. *Neurology*, **44**, 675–680.

10 Karnofsky, D.A., Abelmann, W.H., Craver, L.H. *et al.* (1948) The use of nitrogen mustards in the palliative treatment of cancer. *Cancer*, **1**, 634–656.

11 Grant, R. (2004) Overview: brain tumour diagnosis and management/Royal College of Physicians guidelines. *Journal of Neurology, Neurosurgery, and Psychiatry*, **75**, 18–23.

12 Tremont-Lukats, I.W., Ratilal, B.O., Armstrong, T. & Gilbert, M.R. (2008) Antiepileptic drugs for preventing seizures in people with brain tumors. *Cochrane Database of Systematic Reviews*, (**2**. Art. No.: CD004424.). doi:10.1002/14651858.CD004424.pub2.

13 Perry, J., Zinman, L., Chambers, A. *et al.* (2006) The use of prophylactic anticonvulsants in patients with brain tumours — a systematic review. *Current Oncology*, **13**(**6**), 222–229.

14 Kerrigan, S. & Grant, R. (2011) Antiepileptic drugs for treating seizures in adults with brain tumours. *Cochrane Database of Systematic Reviews*, (**8**CD008586).

15 Meierkord, H., Boon, P., Engelsen, B. *et al.* (2006) EFNS guideline on the management of status epilepticus. *European Journal of Neurology*, **13**, 445–450.

16 Lim, D.A., Tarapore, P., Chang, E. *et al.* (2009) Safety and feasibility of switching from phenytoin to levetiracetam monotherapy for glioma-related seizure control following craniotomy: a randomized phase II pilot study. *Journal of Neuro-Oncology*, **93**(**3**), 349–354.

17 Kondziolka, D., Lunsford, L.D. & Martinez, A.J. (1993) Unreliability of contemporary neurodiagnostic imaging in evaluating suspected adult supratentorial (low-grade) astrocytoma. *Journal of Neurosurgery*, **79**(**4**), 533–536.

18 Murphy, M., Loosemore, A., Clifton, A.G. *et al.* (2002) The contribution of proton magnetic resonance spectroscopy (1HMRS) to clinical brain tumour diagnosis. *British Journal of Neurosurgery*, **16**(**4**), 329–334.

19 Hall, W.A. (1998) The safety and efficacy of stereotactic biopsy for intracranial lesions. *Cancer*, **82**(**9**), 1749–1755.

20 Fadul, C., Wood, J., Thaler, H., Galicich, J., Patterson, R.H. Jr., & Posner, J.B. (1988) Morbidity and mortality of craniotomy for excision of supratentorial gliomas. *Neurology*, **38**(**9**), 1374–1379.

21 Sawaya, R., Hammoud, M., Schoppa, D. *et al.* (1998) Neurosurgical outcomes in a modern series of 400 craniotomies for treatment of parenchymal tumors. *Neurosurgery*, **42**(**5**), 1044–1055.

22 Woodworth, G., McGirt, M.J., Samdani, A., Garonzik, I. *et al.* (2005) Accuracy of frameless and frame-based image-guided stereotactic brain biopsy in the diagnosis of glioma: comparison of biopsy and open specimen. *Neurological Research*, **27**, 358–362.

23 Hart, M.G., Grant, R. & Metcalfe, S.E. (2000) Biopsy versus resection for high grade glioma. *Cochrane Database of Systematic Reviews*, (**2**. Art. No.: CD002034.). doi:10.1002/14651858.CD002034.

24 Vuorinen, V., Hinkka, S., Farkkila, M. & Jaaskelainen, J. (2003) Debulking or biopsy of malignant glioma in elderly people - a randomised study. *Acta Neurochirurgica*, **145**(**1**), 5–10.

25 Stummer, W., Pichlmeier, U., Meinel, T. *et al.* (2006) Fluorescence-guided surgery with 5-aminolevulinic acid for resection of malignant glioma: a randomised controlled multicentre phase III trial. *Lancet Oncology,* **7**, 392–401.

26 Stummer, W., Tonn, J.-C., Mehdorn, H.M. *et al.* (2011) Counterbalancing risks and gains from extended resections in malignant glioma surgery: A supplemental analysis from the randomized 5-aminolevulinic acid glioma resection study. *Journal of Neurosurgery,* **114**(3), 613–623.

27 Pichlmeier, U., Bink, A., Schackert, G. & Stummer, W. (2008) Resection and survival in glioblastoma multiforme: An RTOG recursive partitioning analysis of ALA study patients and the ALA Glioma Study Group. *Neuro-Oncology,* **10**, 1025–1034.

28 Willems, P.W.A., Taphoorn, M.J.B., Burger, H. *et al.* (2006) Effectiveness of neuronavigation in resecting solitary intracerebral contrast-enhancing tumors: A randomized controlled trial. *Journal of Neurosurgery,* **104**(3), 360–368.

29 Senft, C., Bink, A., Franz, K. *et al.* (2011) Intraoperative MRI guidance and extent of resection in glioma surgery: A randomised, controlled trial. *Lancet Oncology,* **12**(11), 997–1003.

30 Barone, D.G., Lawrie, T.A., Hart, M.G. (2014) Image guided surgery for the resection of brain tumours. *Cochrane Database of Systematic Reviews,* (**1**).

31 Wu, J.-S., Zhou, L.-F., Tang, W.-J. *et al.* (2007) Clinical evaluation and follow-up outcome of diffusion tensor imaging-based functional neuronavigation: A prospective, controlled study in patients with gliomas involving pyramidal tracts. *Neurosurgery,* **61**(5), 935–948.

32 Gupta, D.K., Chandra, P.S., Ojha, B.K., Sharma, B.S., Mahapatra, A.K. & Mehta, V.S. (2007) Awake craniotomy versus surgery under general anesthesia for resection of intrinsic lesions of eloquent cortex--a prospective randomised study. *Clinical Neurology and Neurosurgery,* **109**(4), 335–343.

33 Westphal, M., Hilt, D.C., Bortey, E. *et al.* (2003) A phase 3 trial of local chemotherapy with biodegradable carmustine (BCNU) wafers (Gliadel wafers) in patients with primary malignant glioma. *Neuro-Oncology,* **5**(2), 79–88.

34 Hart, M.G., Grant, R., Garside, R. *et al.* (2011) Chemotherapy wafers for high grade glioma. *Cochrane Database of Systematic Reviews,* (**3**. Art. No.: CD007294.). doi:10.1002/14651858. CD007294.pub2.

35 Whittle, I.R., Lyles, S. & Walker, M. (2003) Gliadel therapy given for first resection of malignant glioma: a single centre study of the potential use of Gliadel. *Journal of Neurosurgery,* **17**(4), 352–354.

36 Grant, R., Liang, B.C., Page, M.A., Crane, D.L., Greenberg, H.S. & Junck, L. (1995) Age influences chemotherapy response in astrocytomas. *Neurology,* **45**(5), 929–933.

37 Glioma Meta-Analysts Trialists (GMT) Group (2002) Chemotherapy for High Grade Glioma. *Cochrane Database of Systematic Reviews.*; CD003913(3).

38 Stupp, R., Mason, W.P., van den Bent, M.J. *et al.* (2005) Radiotherapy plus concomitant and adjuvant temozolomide for glioblastoma. *New England Journal of Medicine,* **352**(10), 987–996.

39 Gilbert, M.R., Wang, M., Aldape, A.D. *et al.* (2006) RTOG 0525: A randomized phase III trial comparing standard adjuvant temozolomide (TMZ) with a dose-dense (dd) schedule in newly diagnosed glioblastoma (GBM). *Journal of Clinical Oncology,* **29**, 2011.

40 Keime-Guibert, F., Chinot, O., Taillandier, L. *et al.* (2007) Radiotherapy for glioblastoma in the elderly. *New England Journal of Medicine,* **356**, 1527–1535.

41 Wick, W., Platten, M., Meisner, C. *et al.* (2012) Temozolomide chemotherapy alone versus radiotherapy alone for malignant astrocytoma in the elderly: the NOA-08 randomised, phase 3 trial. *Lancet Oncol,* **13**(7), 707–715.

42 Malmstrom, A., Gronberg, B.H., Marosi, C. *et al.* (2012) Temozolomide versus standard 6-week radiotherapy versus hypofractionated radiotherapy in patients older than 60 years with glioblastoma: the Nordic randomised, phase 3 trial. *Lancet Oncol,* **13**(9), 916–926.

43 Khasraw, M., Ameratunga, M.S., Grant, R. *et al.* (2014) Antiangiogenic therapy for high-grade glioma. *Cochrane Database of Systematic Reviews,* **9**, CD008218.

44 Chinot, O.L., Wick, W., Mason, W. *et al.* (2014) Bevacizumab plus radiotherapy-temozolomide for newly diagnosed glioblastoma. *New England Journal of Medicine,* **370**, 709–722.

45 Gilbert, M.R., Dignam, J.J., Armstrong, T.S. *et al.* (2014) A randomized trial of bevacizumab for newly diagnosed glioblastoma. *New England Journal of Medicine,* **370**, 699–670.

46 Brada, M., Stenning, S., Gabe, R. *et al.* (2010) Temozolomide versus procarbazine, lomustine, and vincristine in recurrent high-grade glioma. *Journal of Clinical Oncology,* **28**(30), 4601–4608.

47 Gaspar, L., Scott, C., Rotman, M. *et al.* (1997) Recursive partitioning analysis (RPA) of prognostic factors in three radiation therapy oncology group (RTOG) brain metastases trials. *International Journal of Radiation Oncology Biology Physics,* **37**(4), 745–751.

48 Patchell, R.A. (2003) The management of brain metastases. *Cancer Treatment Reviews,* **29**(6), 533–540.

49 Diener-West, M., Dobbins, T.W., Phillips, T.L. & Nelson, D.F. (1989) Identification of an optimal subgroup for treatment evaluation of patients with brain metastases using RTOG study 7916. *International Journal of Radiation Oncology Biology Physics,* **16**(3), 669–673.

50 DeAngelis, L.M., Delattre, J.Y. & Posner, J.B. (1989) Radiation-induced dementia in patients cured of brain metastases. *Neurology,* **39**(6), 789–796.

51 Patchell, R.A., Tibbs, P.A., Walsh, J.W. *et al.* (1990) A randomized trial of surgery in the treatment of single metastases to the brain. *New England Journal of Medicine,* **322**(8), 494–500.

52 Vecht, C.J., Haaxma-Reiche, H., Noordijik, E.M. *et al.* (1993) Treatment of single brain metastasis: radiotherapy alone or combined with neurosurgery? *Annals of Neurology,* **33**(6), 583–590.

53 Mintz, A.H., Kestle, J., Rathbone, M.P. *et al.* (1996) A randomized trial to assess the efficacy of surgery in addition to radiotherapy in patients with a single cerebral metastasis. *Cancer,* **78**(7), 1470–1476.

54 Hart, M.G., Grant, R., Walker, M. & Dickinson, H. (2005) Surgical resection and whole brain radiation therapy versus whole brain radiation therapy alone for single brain metastases. *Cochrane Database of Systematic Reviews.*; CD003292.

55 Patil, C.G., Pricola, K., Garg, S.K., Bryant, A. & Black, K.L. (2010) Whole brain radiation therapy (WBRT) alone versus WBRT and radiosurgery for the treatment of brain metastases. *Cochrane Database of Systematic Reviews*, (**6**. Art. No.: CD006121.). doi:10.1002/14651858.CD006121.pub2.

56 Kondziolka, D., Patel, A., Lunsford, L.D., Kassam, A. & Flickinger, J.C. (1999) Stereotactic radiosurgery plus whole brain radiotherapy versus radiotherapy alone for patients with multiple brain metastases. *International Journal of Radiation Oncology Biology Physics*, **45**, 427–434.

57 Chougule, P.B., Burton-Williams, M., Saris, S. *et al.* (2000) Randomized treatment of brain metastasis with gamma knife radiosurgery, whole brain radiotherapy or both. *International Journal of Radiation Oncology Biology Physics*, **48(3)**, 114.

58 Andrews, D.W., Scott, C.B., Sperduto, P.W. *et al.* (2004) Whole brain radiation therapy with or without stereotactic radiosurgery boost for patients with one to three brain metastases: phase III results of the RTOG 9508 randomised trial. *Lancet*, **363(9422)**, 1665–1672.

59 Patchell, R.A., Tibbs, P.A., Regine, W.F. *et al.* (1998) Postoperative radiotherapy in the treatment of single metastases to the brain: a randomized trial. *JAMA*, **280(17)**, 1485–1489.

60 Roos, D.E., Wirth, A., Burmeister, B.H. *et al.* (2006) Whole brain irradiation following surgery or radiosurgery for solitary brain metastases: Mature results of a prematurely closed randomized Trans-Tasman Radiation Oncology Group trial (TROG 98.05). *Radiotherapy Oncology*, **80(3)**, 318–322.

61 Aoyama, H., Shirato, H. & Tago, M. (2006) Stereotactic radiosurgery plus whole-brain radiation therapy vs stereotactic radiosurgery alone for treatment of brain metastases. *JAMA*, **295(21)**, 2483–2491.

62 Chang, E.L., Wefel, J.S., Hess, K.R. *et al.* (2009) Neurocognition in patients with brain metastases treated with radiosurgery or radiosurgery plus whole-brain irradiation: a randomised controlled trial. *Lancet Oncology*, **10**, 1037–1044.

63 Kocher, M., Soffietti, R., Abacioglu, U. *et al.* (2011) Adjuvant whole-brain radiotherapy versus observation after radiosurgery or surgical resection of one to three cerebral metastases: results of the EORTC 22952-26001 study. *Journal of Clinical Oncology*, **29(2)**, 134–141.

64 Muacevic, A., Wowra, B., Siefert, A., Tonn, J.C., Steiger, H.J. & Kreth, F.W. (2008) Microsurgery plus whole brain irradiation versus Gamma Knife surgery alone for treatment of single metastases to the brain: a randomized controlled multicentre phase III trial. *Journal of Neuro-Oncology*, **87**, 299–307.

65 Roos, D.E., Smith, J.G. & Stephens, S.W. (2011) Radiosurgery versus surgery, both with adjuvant whole brain radiotherapy, for solitary brain metastases: A randomised controlled trial. *Clinical Oncology*, **23**, 646–651.

17 CHAPTER 17
Epilepsy

Sridharan Ramaratnam[1] and Anthony G. Marson[2]
[1]*Department of Neurology, SIMS Hospitals, Chennai, Tamil Nadu, India*
[2]*Department of Molecular and Clinical Pharmacology, Institute of Translational Medicine, University of Liverpool, Liverpool, Merseyside, UK*

Background

Definition

An epileptic seizure is a transient occurrence of signs and/or symptoms due to abnormal excessive or synchronous neuronal activity in the brain. Epilepsy is a disorder of the brain characterised by an enduring predisposition to generate epileptic seizures and by the neurobiological, cognitive, psychological and social consequences of this condition. A person is considered to have epilepsy if he/she had had two or more unprovoked seizures or at least one epileptic seizure with a strong likelihood of recurrence [1]. Seizures can be classified by type as focal (earlier called as partial) and generalised (categorised as generalised tonic clonic, absence, myoclonic, tonic and atonic seizures) [2]. Generalised seizure types are thought to occur within and result from rapid engagement of bilaterally distributed systems. Focal epileptic seizures are conceptualised as originating within networks limited to one hemisphere. Focal seizures may occur without impairment of consciousness or awareness (earlier called as simple partial) or with alteration of cognition (earlier called as complex partial or dyscognitive) or evolve to bilateral, convulsive seizure (earlier called as secondary generalised).

Incidence/prevalence

Epilepsy (generalised or partial) is common, with an estimated average prevalence in the developed world of 5–10/1000 and an annual incidence of approximately 50/100 000. The prevalence and incidence rates in the developing world are reported to be higher. About 3% of people will be diagnosed with epilepsy at some time in their lives [3].

Aetiology/risk factors

Epilepsy may be caused by various disorders involving the brain. The causes/risk factors include birth/neonatal injuries, congenital or metabolic disorders, head injuries, tumours, infections of the brain or meninges, genetic defects, degenerative disease of the brain or cerebrovascular disease.

Classification

Classification of epilepsy is in effect an organisation by consensus, as we cannot classify according to the biology of this disorder in a scientific way. Epilepsy can be classified by aetiology as follows [2]: genetic (previously called idiopathic), structural-metabolic (previously called symptomatic – wherein there is a distinct structural or metabolic condition such as tuberous sclerosis or tumour congenital defect) or unknown (previously called cryptogenic). Genetic epilepsy is the direct result of a known or inferred genetic defect(s) and seizures are the core symptom of the disorder, for example, juvenile myoclonic epilepsy or childhood absence epilepsy.

Prognosis

About 60% of untreated people have no further seizures in the 2 years after their first seizure [4]. A diagnosis of epilepsy is usually made following two or more unprovoked seizures, and for most people with epilepsy the prognosis is good. About 70% go into remission, defined as being seizure-free for 5 years on or off treatment. This leaves 20–30% of people who develop chronic epilepsy, which is often treated with multiple antiepileptic drugs (AEDs) [5].

Interventions

People with epilepsy of various types are treated with one or more of the following interventions, namely antiepileptic drugs used alone or in combination, non-drug treatments such as psychological treatments, complementary alternative treatments, surgery such as temporal lobectomy, lesionectomy, hemispherectomy and corpus callosotomy or vagus nerve stimulation

Evidence-Based Neurology: Management of Neurological Disorders, Second Edition. Edited by Bart M. Demaerschalk and Dean M. Wingerchuk.
© 2015 John Wiley & Sons, Ltd. Published 2015 by John Wiley & Sons, Ltd.

Aims of the intervention

- Seizure freedom/seizure control without adverse effects.
- To withdraw AEDs without causing seizure recurrence, for people in remission.
- To improve quality of life.

Outcomes investigated

- For treatment after a single seizure: Time to recurrence; proportion of people having recurrence of seizure 1, 2 or 5 years after the first seizure; time to achieve a 12-month or 2-year remission; proportion of people achieving a 1-year or 2-year remission 2 or 5 years after their first seizure; quality of life (QOL) and adverse effects.
- For treatment of newly diagnosed epilepsy: Retention on allocated treatment or time to withdrawal of allocated treatment, time to 12-month remission, time to first seizure after treatment, recurrence rates, QOL and adverse effects.
- For treatment of drug-resistant epilepsy: Percentage reduction in seizure frequency, proportion of responders (response defined as 50% or greater reduction in seizure frequency), withdrawal from treatment, QOL and side effects.
- For drug withdrawal: Time to seizure recurrence, improvement in QOL and side effects.
- For epilepsy surgery: Seizure freedom 1 or 2 years after surgery, mortality/morbidity, QOL and adverse effects.

Methodology

We searched the Cochrane Epilepsy Group Trial Register, Cochrane Systematic Reviews (Cochrane Library July 2014) and Medline in October 2011. The authors were also contributors to the BMJ Clinical Evidence Chapter on Epilepsy and had access to the Clinical Evidence Team Searches. An additional search within the Cochrane Library was carried out for the Database of Abstracts of Reviews of Effects (DARE) and Health Technology Assessment (HTA). We included published systematic reviews of RCTs and RCTs in any language, single- or double-blinded for drug trials and containing more than 20 individuals of whom more than 80% were followed up for at least 3 months. We included systematic reviews of RCTs and RCTs where harms of an included intervention were studied.

AED Treatment After First Seizure

In persons with the first unprovoked seizure (single seizure), does AED treatment, started immediately, affect the probability of seizure recurrence and long-term prognosis?

We found no systematic review. We found five randomised controlled trials (RCTs).

The Multicentre Study of Early Epilepsy and Single Seizures (MESS study) [6] was an unmasked, multicentre study of 1443 patients (children and adults) with single seizures (56%) or early epilepsy (44%) randomised to immediate ($n = 722$) and deferred AED treatment ($n = 721$). Outcomes comprised time to first, second and fifth seizures; time to 2-year remission; no seizures between years 1 and 3 and between years 3 and 5 after randomisation and quality of life. Immediate treatment increased time to first, second, and fifth tonic clonic seizures. It also reduced the time to achieve 2-year remission of seizures ($P = 0.023$). At 5-year follow-up, 76% of patients in the immediate-treatment group and 77% of those in the deferred treatment group were seizure-free between 3 and 5 years after randomisation (difference – 0.2% [95% CI (confidence interval) – 5.8–5.5%]). The two policies did not differ with respect to quality of life outcomes or serious complications. It found that carbamazepine monotherapy significantly increased time to first seizure, but that the effects of sodium valproate were inconclusive. Thirty-nine per cent of people in the immediate-treatment group reported at least one adverse event, including depression, dizziness and gastrointestinal symptoms, compared to 31% of people with deferred treatment.

The FIRST Group [7] randomised 419 people (42% women, 28% aged <16 years, 66% aged 16–60 years, 6% aged >60 years) presenting within 7 days of their first unprovoked tonic clonic seizure to immediate treatment or no immediate treatment. Longer term follow-up of the RCT [8] found that there were half as many second seizures with immediate treatment compared with no immediate treatment at 2 years (hazard ratio (HR) 0.4, 95% CI 0.2–0.5). However, no significant difference was found in the proportion of people achieving a 2-year remission in seizures (absolute risk (AR) 60% with immediate treatment versus 68% with no treatment; relative risk (RR) 0.82, 95% CI 0.64–1.03; RR adjusted for time of starting treatment 0.96, 95% CI 0.77–1.22). Forty-one patients discontinued AEDs of whom 14 cited adverse effects.

Gilad [9] randomised 91 adult patients aged 18–50 years, presenting to the hospital within 24 hours of the first unprovoked seizure to treatment with carbamazepine (CBZ) [$n = 46$] or no medication ($n = 45$) and followed up for 36 months. Nine subjects, who did not tolerate CBZ, were changed over to treatment with sodium valproate (VPA). Seizures recurred in 29 of the untreated and 10 in the treatment group. The number of patients having seizure recurrences in the treatment and control groups were 6 versus 24 at the end of 1 year, 9 versus 28 at the end of 2 years and 10 versus 29 at the end of 3 years. The risk rates for relapse (AR) at the end of 1, 2 and 3 years in the treatment group were 0.1, 0.2 and 0.4, respectively compared to 0.33, 0.62 and 0.77 in untreated $P < 0.001$; 95% CI not given.

Chandra [10] performed a double-blind RCT of 228 adult patients (aged 16–79 years) presenting within 2 weeks after the first seizure to treatment with sodium valproate or placebo. They were followed up for 12 months. Five of the

115 patients treated with VPA and 63 of the 113 on placebo had recurrence of seizures. Side effects were noted in 10 on VPA and 2 on placebo but were not considered serious.

Camfield [11] randomised 31 children with first afebrile seizure to treatment with CBZ or no immediate treatment. At the end of 1 year, afebrile seizures recurred in 2 of the 14 randomised to CBZ and 9 of 17 with no medication. Four discontinued CBZ due to side effects and two on CBZ had febrile recurrences. One year after their initial seizure, 6 of the 14 taking CBZ and 7 of 17 on no medication were seizure-free and without adverse effects.

Summary

RCTs found that AED treatment following a single seizure reduces seizure recurrence at 1–3 years compared with no treatment. However, we found no evidence that treatment alters long-term prognosis or increases the proportion of people who achieve remission at 2–5 years. Quality of life outcomes from the MESS study indicate that the benefits of preventing seizure are balanced by the adverse effects and stigma of taking AEDs. Antiepileptic drug treatment may be associated with harmful effects such as idiosyncratic reactions, teratogenesis, adverse effects on bone mineral density, suicidality [12] and cognitive effects.

AED monotherapy for partial epilepsy

In patients with partial epilepsy, which AED is most effective and safe?

carbamazepine monotherapy for partial epilepsy
Carbamazepine versus placebo

We found no placebo-controlled RCTs of CBZ used as monotherapy in people with partial epilepsy, but widespread consensus holds that it is effective. Placebo-controlled trials of carbamazepine would now be considered unethical.

We found the following systematic reviews comparing carbamazepine with VPA, phenobarbital (PHB), phenytoin (PHT), lamotrigine (LTG) and RCTs; comparing CBZ with oxcarbazepine (OXC), gabapentin (GBP), topiramate (TOP) and levetiracetam (LEV). The results of the systematic reviews are given in Table 17.1.

Carbamazepine versus sodium valproate

A systematic review (5 RCTs, 1265 people, of whom 830 had partial epilepsy and 395 had generalised epilepsy, aged 3–83 years, follow-up time<5 years) compared VPA and CBZ and included a meta-analysis of the subgroup of people with partial epilepsy [14]. Carbamazepine significantly decreased time to 12-month remission and reduced the risk of first seizure compared with VPA. There was no significant difference for treatment withdrawal between VPA and CBZ. The meta-analysis provides weak evidence in support of the

consensus view to use CBZ as the drug of choice in people with partial epilepsy (Table 17.1).

Carbamazepine versus phenobarbital

A systematic review (4 RCTs, 680 people aged between 2 and 68 years, of whom 523 (77%) had partial epilepsy) compared CBZ and PHB [13]. For people with partial epilepsy, it found no significant difference in remission during the next 12 months. The review found that PHB significantly increased time to first seizure compared with CBZ, but was significantly more likely to be withdrawn compared with CBZ (Table 17.1).

Carbamazepine versus phenytoin

A systematic review (3 RCTs, 552 adults and children, of whom 431 (78%) had partial epilepsy) compared CBZ and PHT [18]. The review did not present results separately for people with partial and generalised epilepsy. Overall, however, it found no significant difference between CBZ and PHT for treatment withdrawal, first seizure or 12-month remission (Table 17.1).

Carbamazepine versus lamotrigine:

We found one systematic review (search date 2007), comparing CBZ and LTG monotherapy [15]. This systematic review (5 RCTs, 1384 people, of whom 1108 (80%) had partial epilepsy, 51% men) included a meta-analysis of the subgroup of people with partial epilepsy. Carbamazepine significantly increased the proportion of seizure-free people after 6 months (48% with CBZ vs 41% with LTG). There was no significant difference in time to first seizure between LTG and CBZ. The review found that LTG significantly increased time to treatment withdrawal compared with CBZ.

We also found three subsequent RCTs. The first RCT [20] compared CBZ (standard release) with LTG in elderly people with newly diagnosed epilepsy. It included 593 older people (mean age 72 years) with new-onset epilepsy (75% with partial-onset seizures and 25% with generalised tonic clonic seizures only). This was a three-arm trial comparing CBZ (198 people), LTG (200 people) and gabapentin (GBP) (195 people). The RCT found no significant difference among the three treatment groups in the proportion of people who remained in the study at 3 months and who were seizure-free after the start of treatment (seizure-free rates at 3 months: 64% with CBZ vs 63% with LTG vs 62% with GBP, $P=0.09$). The RCT found that, at 12 months, CBZ was significantly more likely to lead to treatment withdrawal compared with LTG ($P<0.0001$) and significantly increased the number of people who withdrew from treatment because of adverse effects ($P<0.0001$). The RCT found that CBZ significantly increased hypersensitivity reactions (rash of any degree) compared with LTG ($P=0.007$) [20].

The second RCT (186 elder people aged at least 65 years with newly diagnosed epilepsy, 55% male, at least

Table 17.1 Comparisons of antiepileptic drug monotherapy in partial and generalised epilepsy (results of systematic reviews)

SR (reference number)	Outcome (time to event)	Partial hazard ratio (95% CI)	Generalised hazard ratio (95% CI)	Both hazard ratio (95% CI)	Remarks
CBZ versus PHB [13]	12-month remission	1.03 (0.72–1.49)	0.61 (0.36–1.03)	0.87 (0.65–1.17)	Search date 2006, 4 RCTs, 680 people including 157 with generalised epilepsy; Advantage to PHB in partial seizures; more withdrawals with PHB; statistically significant difference for partial onset but with significant heterogeneity
	First seizure	0.71 (0.55–0.91) PHB better	1.50 (0.95–2.35)	0.85 (0.68–1.05)	
	Withdrawal	1.60 (1.18–2.17) PHB Worse	1.78 (0.87–3.62)	1.63 (1.23–2.15) PHB Worse	
CBZ versus VPA [14]	12-month remission	0.82 (0.67–1.00) VPA Worse	0.96 (0.75–1.24)	0.87 (0.74–1.02)	5 RCTs, search date 2007, Advantage for CBZ, for partial seizures
	First seizure	1.22 (1.04–1.44) VPA worse	0.86 (0.68–1.09)	1.09 (0.96–1.25)	
	Withdrawal	1.0 (0.79–1.26)	0.89 (0.62–1.29)	0.97 (0.79–1.18)	
CBZ versus LTG [15]	6-month remission	0.72 (0.54–0.97) CBZ better	1.37 (0.74–2.56)	0.92 (0.81–1.04)	5 RCTs, search date 2007; 1384 people; 80% partial epilepsy
	First seizure	1.28 (0.98–1.66)	0.96 (0.62–1.47)	1.14 (0.92–1.43)	
	Withdrawal	0.62 (0.45–0.86) LTG Better	0.48 (0.26–0.89) LTG Better	0.55 (0.35–0.84) LTG Better	
PHT versus VPA [16]	12-month remission	0.90 (0.63–1.29), 244 pts, 4 studies	1.04 (0.77–1.40), 270 pts, 4 studies	0.98 (0.78–1.23), 514 pts, 4 studies	5 RCTS, search date 2013, 669 people including 395 with generalised epilepsy; Differences not statistically significant
	First seizure	0.83 (0.62–1.11), 244 pts, 4 studies	1.03 (0.77–1.39), 395 pts, 5 studies	0.93 (0.75–1.14), 639 pts, 5 studies	
	Withdrawal	1.20 (0.74–1.95), 187 pts, 4 studies	0.98 (0.59–1.64), 341 pts, 5 studies	1.09 (0.76–1.55), 528 pts, 5 studies	
PHT versus PHB [17]	12-month remission	0.96 (0.70–1.33), 468 pts, 4 studies	0.77 (0.46–1.28), 131 pts, 3 studies	0.90 (0.69–1.19), 599 pts 4 studies	HR >1 event more with PHB
	First Seizure	0.78 (0.61–1.01), 461 pts, 4 studies	1.14 (0.73–1.78), 131 pts, 3 studies	0.86 (0.69–1.08), 592 pts, 4 studies	Advantage for PHT;
	Withdrawal	1.48 (1.10–1.98), 404 pts, 3 studies	4.04 (1.61–10.14), 95 pts, 2 studies	1.62 (1.22–2.14), 499 pts, 3 studies	Statistically significant
PHT versus CBZ [18]	12-month remission			1.0 (0.78–1.29)	HR >1 event more with PHT. Data for partial and generalised seizures not available.
	First seizure			0.91 (0.74–1.12)	
	Withdrawal			0.97 (0.74–1.28)	
PHT versus OXC [19]	12-month remission	0.92 (0.64–1.33), 326 pts, 2 studies	1.01 (0.59–1.73), 142 pts, 2 studies	0.95 (0.70–1.29), 468 pts, 2 studies	search date 2013, 2 RCTs, 480 people, in which 69% had partial epilepsy
	First seizure	1.08 (0.80–1.47), 326 pts, 2 studies	0.94 (0.56–1.56), 142 pts, 2 studies	1.04 (0.80–1.35), 468 pts, 2 studies	Less withdrawals with OXC
	Withdrawal	1.95 (1.15–3.33), 333 pts, 2 studies OXC Better	1.16 (0.54–2.46), 143 pts, 2 studies	1.64 (1.06–2.54), 476 pts, 2 studies OXC Better	

2 partial-onset or generalised tonic clonic seizure in the previous 6 months) compared LTG at a flexible dosing range 25–400 mg daily with CBZ controlled release (CR) at a flexible dosing range of 100–800 mg over 40 weeks [21]. The RCT did not report subgroup analyses according to seizure type or epilepsy type and did not specify how many people had partial epilepsy. The RCT found no significant difference in time to withdrawal between LTG and CBZ-CR (HR (LTG vs CBZ) 0.77, 95% CI 0.45–1.31, P = 0.33, ITT) [21]. The RCT found similar rates of treatment-emergent adverse effects in both groups (88% with LTG vs 86% with CBZ-CR). Central nervous system effects were the most

common adverse effect for both LTG (47%) and CBZ (49%). The RCT found no significant difference in withdrawals due to adverse effects between groups (14% with LTG vs 25% with CBZ-CR, $P = 0.078$) [21].

The third RCT (SANAD study – 1721 people, 88% partial epilepsy, 10% unclassified) had a pragmatic design comparing the effectiveness of CBZ versus newer antiepileptics – GBP, LTG, OXC and TPM in the treatment of partial epilepsy [22]. This open-label RCT allowed clinicians to determine what they considered the optimum rate of titration and dosing regime. The RCT found that CBZ was associated with a significantly higher risk of treatment failure (defined as unacceptable adverse effects after randomisation and inadequate seizure control) compared with LTG (HR >1 indicates that failure occurs more rapidly with LTG; HR 0.78, 95% CI 0.63–0.97). LTG has mild advantage over CBZ and is probably better tolerated

Carbamazepine versus topiramate

We found two RCTs. The first RCT (621 people, 19% children, 53% male, 63% partial epilepsy) compared TPM (210 patients taking 100 mg and 199 patients taking 200 mg), CBZ (126 people) and VPA (78 people) [23]. The RCT combined efficacy data for TPM 100 and 200 mg doses and compared with CBZ and VPA. The study found no significant difference in time to exit for any reason ($P = 0.53$), in time to first seizure ($P = 0.35$) or in the proportion of people without seizures during the last 6 months of the study between TPM and CBZ (49% with TPM 100 mg vs 44% with TPM 200 mg vs 44% with CBZ). The follow-up time of the study is not clear and only 45% of people randomised completed the study [23].

The second RCT [22] (SANAD study) found no significant difference in time to treatment failure between CBZ and TPM [intention-to-treat analysis (ITT) HR 1.22, 95% CI 0.99–1.49]. However, there was no significant difference in 12-month remission between CBZ and TPM (HR 0.86, 95% CI 0.72–1.03).

Carbamazepine versus gabapentin

We found one RCT (593 older people, mean age 72 years) with new-onset epilepsy (75% with partial-onset seizures and 25% with generalised tonic clonic seizures only), which was a three-arm trial comparing CBZ (198 people), LTG (200 people) and GBP (195 people) [20]. The RCT found no significant difference among treatment groups in the proportion of people who remained in the study at 3 months and were seizure-free after start of treatment (seizure-free rates at 3 months: 64% with CBZ vs 63% with LTG vs 62% with GBP, $P = 0.09$). The RCT found that, at 12 months, CBZ was significantly more likely to lead to treatment withdrawal compared with GBP ($P = 0.008$). After 12 months of treatment, weight gain was significantly more among people

treated with GBP ($P = 0.002$), while hyponatraemia (sodium <130 mmol/L) occurred more frequently with CBZ [20].

SANAD study [22]: there was no significant difference in time to treatment failure between CBZ and GBP (ITT – HR >1 indicates that failure occurs more rapidly with GBP; HR 1.21, 95% CI 0.99–1.48). The RCT found that CBZ was significantly more effective at achieving 12-month remission compared with GBP (HR >1 indicates that failure occurs more rapidly on GBP; HR 0.75, 95% CI 0.63–0.90).

Carbamazepine versus oxcarbazepine

SANAD [22]: There was no significant difference in time to treatment failure between CBZ and OXC (ITT – HR 1.04, 95% CI 0.78–1.39). There was no significant difference in 12-month remission between CBZ and OXC (ITT – HR 0.92, 95% CI 0.73–1.18).

Carbamazepine versus levetiracetam

We found one RCT (579 people, mean age 39 years, 55% male, at least two partial or generalised tonic clonic seizures in the previous year, 80% with partial epilepsy) comparing LEV (1000–3000 mg per day) with CBZ (controlled release, 400–1200 mg per day) in people with newly diagnosed epilepsy [24]. The RCT did not report subgroup analyses for seizure types or epilepsy type. The RCT found no significant difference in the proportion of people seizure-free for at least 6 months at 26 weeks (ITT – 67% with both drugs). The RCT also found no significant difference in the proportion seizure-free for at least 1 year at 52 weeks (ITT – 50% with LEV vs 53% with CBZ). The RCT found that the majority of people achieving at least 6 months' seizure freedom were taking either LEV at a dose of 1000 mg daily or CBZ-CR at a dose of 400 mg daily. Similar rates of any adverse effect were reported in both groups (80% with LEV vs 81% with CBZ). Depression and insomnia were reported significantly more often with LEV compared with CBZ-CR (depression: 6% with LEV vs 2% with CBZ, RR 3.06, 95% CI 1.23–7.61; insomnia: 6% with LEV vs 2% with CBZ, RR 2.48, 95% CI 1.04–5.89) while back pain was reported significantly more often with CBZ-CR (3% with LEV vs 7% with CBZ, RR 0.41, 95% CI 0.18–0.91).

Phenobarbitone Monotherapy for Partial Epilepsy
Phenobarbitone versus Placebo

We found no placebo-controlled RCTs of PHB used as monotherapy in people with partial epilepsy, but widespread consensus holds that it is effective. Placebo-controlled trials of PHB would now be considered unethical.

We found two systematic reviews comparing PHB, CBZ and PHT.

Phenobarbital versus phenytoin

The first systematic review (3 RCTs, 599 people with partial or generalised epilepsy, aged 3–77 years) compared PHB and PHT [17], found no significant difference in 12-month remission or first seizure, but the treatment withdrawal was greater with PHB than with PHT, presumably because it was less well tolerated (Table 17.1).

Phenobarbital versus carbamazepine
The second systematic review (4 RCTs, 680 people, of whom 523 had partial epilepsy) compared CBZ and PHB [13]. For people with partial epilepsy, it found no significant difference in remission during the next 12 months. However, it found that PHB significantly increased time to first seizure compared with CBZ but was significantly more likely to be withdrawn (Table 17.1).

Phenytoin monotherapy for partial epilepsy
Phenytoin versus placebo:
We found no placebo-controlled RCTs of phenytoin used as monotherapy in people with partial epilepsy, but widespread consensus holds that it is effective. Placebo-controlled trials of PHT would now be considered unethical.

We found four systematic reviews comparing phenytoin with VPA, PHB, CBZ and OXC.

Phenytoin versus sodium valproate
The first systematic review (5 RCTs, 250 people with partial epilepsy and 395 with generalised epilepsy, aged 3–95 years, follow-up time < 5 years) compared VPA and PHT [16]. It included a meta-analysis of people with partial epilepsy. It found no significant difference in 12-month remission, or first seizure or in treatment withdrawal between PHT and VPA (Table 17.1).

Phenytoin versus phenobarbitone
The second systematic review (3 RCTs, 599 people with partial or generalised epilepsy, aged 3–77 years) compared PHB and PHT [17]. Overall, it found no significant difference in 12-month remission or first seizure. The review found that treatment withdrawal was greater with PHB than with PHT, presumably because it was less well tolerated (Table 17.1).

Phenytoin versus carbamazepine
The third systematic review (3 RCTs, 552 adults and children, of whom 431 had partial epilepsy) compared CBZ and PHT [18]. The review did not present results separately for people with generalised epilepsy and people with partial epilepsy. Overall, however, it found no significant difference between CBZ and PHT for treatment withdrawal, first seizure or 12-month remission (Table 17.1).

Phenytoin versus oxcarbazepine
The fourth systematic review (search date 2008, 2 RCTs, 480 people, of whom 333 (69%) had partial epilepsy) comparing OXC with PHT [19]. The review carried out a subgroup analysis in people with partial epilepsy. It found no significant difference between OXC and PHT in time to first seizure or in achieving 6-month or 12-month remission. The review found a significantly lower risk of treatment withdrawal with OXC compared with PHT. However, a test for statistical interaction between partial and generalised epilepsy was not significant. These subgroup analyses must therefore be treated with caution (Table 17.1).

Sodium valproate monotherapy for partial epilepsy
Sodium valproate versus placebo:
We found no placebo-controlled RCTs of VPA used as monotherapy in people with partial epilepsy, but widespread consensus holds that it is effective. Placebo-controlled trials of VPA would now be considered unethical.

We found two systematic reviews comparing VPA with CBZ and PHT.

Sodium valproate versus carbamazepine
The first systematic review (5 RCTs, 1265 people, of whom 830 had partial epilepsy and 395 had generalised epilepsy, aged 3–83 years, follow-up time <5 years) compared VPA and CBZ [14]. For details, see 2.1.1 (CBZ Vs VPA).

Sodium valproate versus phenytoin
The second systematic review (5 RCTs, 250 people with partial epilepsy and 395 with generalised epilepsy, aged 3–95 years, follow-up time <5 years) compared VPA and PHT [16]. It included a meta-analysis in people with partial epilepsy. It found no significant difference in 12-month remission or first seizure or in treatment withdrawal between VPA and PHT (Table 17.1).

Sodium valproate versus topiramate
We found one RCT (621 people, 19% children, 53% male, 63% partial epilepsy) comparing TPM (210 people taking 100 mg and 199 people taking 200 mg), CBZ (126 people) and VPA (78 people) [23]. The RCT did not undertake subgroup analyses for people with partial or generalised epilepsy. No statistically significant differences were observed in time to exit, time to first seizure and the proportion of seizure-free patients during the last 6 months of treatment between VPA and TPM.

Lamotrigine monotherapy for partial epilepsy
Lamotrigine versus placebo
We found no placebo-controlled RCTs of LTG used as monotherapy in people with partial epilepsy. Placebo-controlled trials of LTG would now be considered unethical.

Lamotrigine versus carbamazepine
See CBZ versus LTG (carbamazepine versus lamotrigine).

Lamotrigine versus Gabapentin

We found no systematic review, but three RCTs. The first RCT (described in CBZ), 593 elder people with new-onset epilepsy, was a three-arm trial comparing CBZ (198 people), LTG (200 people) and GBP (195 people) [20]. The RCT found no significant difference among the three treatment groups in the proportion of people who remained in the study at 3 months and who were seizure-free after start of treatment. Withdrawal from study due to adverse effects was significantly less likely with LTG compared with GBP (P = 0.015). Weight gain was significantly more with GBP compared with LTG (P = 0.001).

The second RCT (291 patients aged 13–78 years, 80% with partial seizures, 52% male, >2 seizures/12 months) compared GBP (1200–3600 mg per day) and LTG (100–300 mg per day) in people with newly diagnosed epilepsy [25]. The RCT found no significant difference in time to exit, between GBP and LTG at 24 weeks for all subjects (HR 1.04, 95% CI 0.60–1.8) as well as for people with partial seizures (exit events 12% with GBP vs 16% with LTG). The study found no significant difference in the proportion of people withdrawing due to adverse events between GBP (11%) and LTG (15%). The most frequent adverse effects in both treatment groups were dizziness, asthenia and headache.

The SANAD study [22] found that LTG was associated with a significantly lower risk of treatment failure compared with GBP (HR >1 indicates that failure occurs more rapidly with LTG; HR 0.65, 95% CI 0.52–0.80). The RCT found that LTG was significantly less effective at achieving 12-month remission compared with GBP (HR >1 indicates that failure occurs more rapidly with LTG; HR 1.21, 95% CI 1.01–1.46).

Lamotrigine versus topiramate

The SANAD study [22] found that LTG was associated with a significantly lower risk of treatment failure compared with TPM (HR >1 indicates that failure occurs more rapidly with TPM; HR 1.56, 95% CI 1.26–1.93). However, there were no significant differences in time to achieve 12-month remission between LTG and TPM (HR >1 indicates that failure occurs more rapidly with topiramate; HR 0.94, 95% CI 0.78–1.113).

Lamotrigine versus oxcarbazepine

SANAD study [22] found no significant differences in time to treatment failure (HR 1.15, 95% CI 0.86–1.54) or in time to achieve 12-month remission between LTG and OXC (HR >1 indicates that remission occurs more rapidly with OXC; HR 1.15, 95% CI 0.89–1.47).

Topiramate monotherapy for partial epilepsy
Topiramate versus placebo

We found no placebo-controlled RCTs of TPM used as monotherapy in people with partial epilepsy. Placebo-controlled trials of TPM would now be considered unethical.

Topiramate versus carbamazepine

Described in CBZ versus TPM (carbamazepine versus topiramate).

Topiramate versus sodium valproate

We found one RCT [23] described in VPA versus TPM (Sodium valproate versus topiramate).

Harms of TPM versus CBZ versus VPA: The RCT [23] reported that the most common adverse effects were paraesthesia (25% with TPM 100 mg vs 33% with TPM 200 mg vs 4% with CBZ vs 3% with VPA), fatigue (20% with TPM 100 mg vs 23% with TPM 200 mg vs 29% with CBZ vs 18% with VPA), headache (25% with TPM 100 mg vs 18% with TPM 200 mg vs 29% with CBZ vs 18% with VPA), dizziness (13% with TPM 100 mg vs 12% with TPM 200 mg vs 16% with CBZ vs 10% with VPA) and upper respiratory tract infections (18% with TPM 100 mg vs 17% with TPM 200 mg vs 15% with CBZ vs 12% with VPA).

Topiramate versus lamotrigine

See LTG versus TPM (lamotrigine versus topiramate)

Topiramate versus gabapentin

The SANAD study [22] found no significant differences in time to treatment failure (HR 1.01, 95% CI 0.83–1.23) or in achieving12-month remission between TPM and GBP (HR >1 indicates that failure occurs more rapidly with TPM; HR 1.14, 95% CI 0.95–1.37).

Topiramate versus oxcarbazepine

The SANAD [22] study found no significant differences in time to treatment failure, or in achieving12-month remission between TPM and OXC (HR 1.10, 95% CI 0.86–1.42).

Levetiracetam monotherapy for partial epilepsy
Levetiracetam versus placebo

We found no systematic review or RCTs. Placebo-controlled trials of LEV will now be considered unethical.

Levetiracetam versus carbamazepine

See CBZ versus LEV (carbamazepine versus levetiracetam)

Gabapentin monotherapy for partial epilepsy
Gabapentin versus placebo

We found no systematic review or RCTs. Placebo-controlled trials of GBP will now be considered unethical.

Gabapentin versus Lamotrigine

See LTG versus GBP (lamotrigine versus gabapentin)

Gabapentin versus Topiramate:

See TOP versus GBP (topiramate versus gabapentin)

Gabapentin versus carbamazepine
See CBZ versus GBP (carbamazepine versus gabapentin)

Oxcarbazepine monotherapy for partial epilepsy
Oxcarbazepine versus placebo:
We found no systematic review or RCTs. Placebo-controlled trials of GBP will now be considered unethical.

Oxcarbazepine versus carbamazepine:
See CBZ (Carbamazepine versus oxcarbazepine)

Oxcarbazepine versus phenytoin
See PHT (phenytoin versus oxcarbazepine).

Oxcarbazepine versus lamotrigine
See LTG (lamotrigine versus oxcarbazepine).

Oxcarbazepine versus topiramate
See TPM (topiramate versus oxcarbazepine).

Addition of second-line AEDs

What are the effects of adding newer AED versus placebo in people with partial epilepsy not responding to the first-line AED?

We found 13 systematic reviews that compared the addition of second-line drugs (clobazam, eslicarbazepine, gabapentin, lacosamide, lamotrigine, levetiracetam, losigamone, pregabalin, oxcarbazepine, tiagabine, topiramate, vigabatrin or zonisamide) and placebo in people who had not responded to usual drug treatment (26, 27, 28, 29, 30, 31, 32, 33, 34, 35, 36, 37, 38, 39)

Clobazam versus placebo
One systematic review [26] (search date 2011, 4 crossover RCTs, 196 people) concluded that adding clobazam may be an effective add-on therapy in people with refractory partial-onset or generalised-onset seizures, compared to adding a placebo. The review did not pool data because of methodological differences between studies, methodological deficiencies and differences in outcome measures. One RCT included in the review found higher rates of adverse effects with adding clobazam (36%) than with adding placebo (12%). Drowsiness (71% with clobazam vs 16% with placebo) and dizziness (26% with clobazam vs 6% with placebo) were the most common adverse effects reported with clobazam [26].

Eslicarbazepine acetate versus placebo
We found one systematic review (search date 2011, 4 RCTs, 1146 people) [27]. Eslicarbazepine (ESL) was found superior to placebo for 50% or greater reduction in seizure frequency outcome. Dose regression analysis showed evidence that ESL

reduced seizure frequency with an increase in efficacy with increasing doses of ESL. ESL was significantly associated with seizure freedom (RR 3.04, 95% CI 1.44–6.42). Participants were more likely to have ESL withdrawn for adverse effects. Dizziness, nausea and diplopia were significantly associated with ESL (see Table 17.2).

Gabapentin versus placebo
One systematic review [28] (search date July 2013, meta-analysis of 6 RCTs, 1206 people) found that adding GBP to usual treatment significantly reduced seizure frequency compared with adding placebo, and that efficacy increased with increasing dose. Adverse effects (dizziness, fatigue and somnolence) were reported significantly more with GBP than with placebo (see Table 17.2) [28].

Lacosamide versus placebo
A systematic review (3 RCTs, 1092 people, search date 2009) found that 50% or higher seizure reduction was significantly more likely in patients treated with lacosamide, but were significantly more likely to withdraw from study compared to placebo treatment [29]. Ataxia, dizziness and nausea were significantly more with lacosamide (see Table 17.2).

Lamotrigine versus placebo:
One systematic review [30] (search date 2012, 14 RCTs, 1806 people) found that adding LTG to usual treatment significantly reduced seizure frequency compared with adding placebo. Lamotrigine is associated with a rash, which may be avoided by slower titration of the drug. The review found that adverse effects (ataxia, dizziness, diplopia, nausea and somnolence) were reported significantly more frequently with adding lamotrigine than with placebo (see Table 17.2) [30].

Levetiracetam versus placebo:
One systematic review [31] (search date 2012; 11 RCTs, 1861 people) found that adding LEV to usual treatment significantly reduced seizure frequency compared with adding placebo. The review found that adverse effects (somnolence and infection) were reported significantly more frequently with adding LEV (see Table 17.2) [31].

Losigamone versus placebo
One systematic review (search date 2012, 2 RCTS, 467 people) assessed the effects of losigamone 1200 or 1500 mg per day as an add-on therapy for partial epilepsy. One trial was assessed as being of good methodological quality while the other was of uncertain quality. Patients taking losigamone were significantly more likely to achieve a 50% or greater reduction in seizure frequency, but with a significant increase of treatment withdrawal when compared to those taking placebo [32]. Dizziness was the only adverse event

Table 17.2 Effects of additional drug treatment and dose-response in people not responding to usual treatment: results of systematic reviews

Drug	Daily dose (mg)	Percentage responding or RR (95% CI)*	RR treatment withdrawal (95% CI) Any Reason	RR adverse effects with CI (99% unless otherwise stated)	Comment
Eslicarbazepine [27]	400–1200 400 800 1200	1.86 (1.46–2.36) 1.22 (0.80–1.85) 2.00 (1.49–2.68) 2.13 (1.59–2.84)	Any reason: 1.07 (0.73–1.57) Adverse Effects: 2.26 (0.98–5.21)	Dizziness: 3.09 (1.76–5.43) Nausea: 3.06 (1.07–8.74) Diplopia: 3.73 (1.19–11.64)	4 RCTs 1146 people, search date 2011; Dose regression analysis showed evidence that ESL reduced seizure frequency with an increase in efficacy with increasing doses. RR for seizure freedom 3.04 (1.44–6.42)
Gabapentin [28]	Placebo 600 900 1200 1800 600–1800	9.7 (7.26–12.9) 13.6 (11.4–16.1) 16.0 (13.7–18.6) 18.7 (15.8–22.1) 25.3 (19.3–32.3) RR 1.89 (1.4–2.55)	1.05 (0.74–1.49)	Dizziness: 2.43 (1.44–4.2) Fatigue: 1.95 (0.99–3.82) Somnolence: 1.93 (1.22–3.06) Ataxia: 2.01 (0.98–4.11)	11 RCTs 2125 patients; (6 RCTs, 1206 patients in meta-analysis); search date July 2013; Efficacy increased with increasing dose. No plateauing of response; So doses tested may not have been optimal
Lacosamide [29]	Up to 600	OR 2.06 (1.54–2.75)	OR 1.8 (1.26–2.56)	Ataxia: 3.45 (1.44–8.26) Dizziness: 3.82 (2.31–6.33) Nausea: 2.34 (1.11–4.93)	3 RCTs 1092 people; search date 2009; non-Cochrane Review
Lamotrigine [30]	200–600	1.80 (1.45–2.23)	1.11 (0.90–1.36)	Ataxia: 3.34; (2.01–5.55) Diplopia: 3.79; (2.15–6.68) Dizziness: 2.00; (1.51–2.64) Nausea: 1.81; (1.22–2.68) Somnolence: 1.39; (0.96–2.00)	14 RCTs; search date 2012; 1806 people
Levetiracetam [31] Children	60 mg/Kg per day	52%; 1.91 (1.38–2.63)	0.80; (0.43–1.46)	Behaviour changes: 1.90; (1.16–3.11)	Search date August 2012; 2 RCTs, 296 children; NNT=4 (95% CI 3–7)
Levetiracetam [31] adults	1000 2000 3000 All doses	33%; 2.49 (1.78–3.5) 37%; 4.91 (2.75–8.77) 44%; 2.59 (2.01–3.33) 39%; 2.43 (2.04–2.9)	0.98; (0.73–1.32)	Somnolence: 1.51; (1.06–2.17) Infection: 1.76; (1.03–3.02) Accidental injury 0.60; (0.39–0.92) More with placebo	Search date 2012; 9 RCTs, 1565 adults. NNT = 5 (95% CI 4–6) Significant heterogeneity between trials
Losigamone [32]	1200–1500 1500 1200	1.75 (1.14–2.72) 1.94 (1.25–3.01) 1.47 (0.70–3.08) NS	2.16; (1.28–3.67)	Dizziness: 3.82; (1.69–8.64)	2 RCTs 467 adults; search date May 2012
Oxcarbazepine [33] adults and children	600–2400	2.51 (1.88–3.33)	1.72 (1.35–2.18)	Ataxia: 3.54; (1.75–7.13) Dizziness: 2.87; (1.82–4.52) Fatigue: 1.81; (1.00–3.29) Nausea: 3.09; (1.74–5.49) Somnolence: 2.36; (1.54–3.62) Diplopia: 7.25; (3.12–16.80)	2 RCTs 961 persons, search date 2006

(continued overleaf)

Table 17.2 (continued)

Drug	Daily dose (mg)	Percentage responding or RR (95% CI)*	RR treatment withdrawal (95% CI) Any Reason	RR adverse effects with CI (99% unless otherwise stated)	Comment
Pregabalin [34]	50–600 50 150 300 600 Titrated 150–600	2.61 (1.70–4.01) 1.06 (0.52–2.12) 2.22 (1.36–3.63) 2.86 (1.65–4.94) 2.86 (2.32–3.54) 2.86 (1.42–5.76)	1.39 (1.13–1.72)	Ataxia: 3.90; (2.05–7.42) Dizziness: 3.06; (2.16–4.34) Somnolence: 2.08; (1.45–2.99) Weight gain: 4.92 (2.41–10.03)	6 RCTs, 2009 patients; search date March 2014. RR for seizure freedom 2.59 (1.05–6.36)
Tiagabine [35]	16–56	3.16 (1.97–5.07)	1.81 (1.25–2.62)	Dizziness: 1.69; (1.13–2.51) Tremor: 4.56; (1.00–20.94)	4 RCTs+ 2 crossover trials, 900 people, search date 2011; Regression models do not provide accurate estimates for response to individual doses
Topiramate [36]	Placebo 200 200–1000	14.9 (12.1–18.2) 39.5 (36.7–42.3) 2.97 (2.38–3.72)	2.44 (1.64–3.62)	Ataxia: 2.29; (1.1–4.77) Concentration difficulty: 7.81; (2.08–29.29) Dizziness: 1.54; (1.07–2.22) Fatigue: 2.19; (1.42–3.4) Paraesthesia: 3.91; (1.51–10.12) Somnolence: 2.29; (1.49–3.51) 'Thinking abnormally': 5.70; (2.26–14.38) Weight loss: 3.47; (1.55–7.79)	11 RCTs, 1401 people, search date 2007; Dose regression analysis shows increasing effect with increasing dose, but found no advantage for doses over 300 or 400 mg per day. RR for seizure freedom 3.41 (1.37–8.51)
Vigabatrin [37] adults	1000–6000	2.58 (1.87–3.57)	2.49 (1.05–5.88)	Dizziness: 1.60; (0.98–2.59) Fatigue or drowsiness: 1.76; (1.25–2.47) 40% develop concentric visual-field abnormalities	11 RCTs, 747 people, search date December 2012
Zonisamide [39]	100–500	1.92 (1.52–2.42)	1.47 (1.07–2.01)	Ataxia: 3.77; (1.28–11.11) Somnolence: 1.83; (99% CI 1.08–3.11) Agitation: 2.35; (1.05–5.27) Anorexia: 2.71; (1.29–5.69)	5 RCTs, 949 people, search date 2013
LTG versus PGB [34]	LTG 300–600 PGB 300–600	1.47 (1.03–2.12) PGB Better	1.07 (0.75–1.52)	Dizziness: 2.94; (1.32–6.52) More with PGB	1 RCT, 434 adults; search date March 2014; seizure freedom RR 1.39 (0.40–4.83)
LTG versus GBP [29]		OR 1.34 (0.78–2.28)	OR 1.26 (0.76–2.08)		3 RCTs, no significant difference
LTG versus TPM [29]		OR 0.51 (0.29–0.91) TPM better	OR 0.55 (0.37–0.81) LTG better		1 RCT
LTG versus LEV [29]		OR 1.01 (0.56–1.83)	OR 0.91 (0.55–1.52)		1 RCT, no significant difference

Results show percentage responding at particular daily doses, but results for treatment withdrawal and adverse effects are calculated for all doses.

significantly associated with losigamone. Higher dose of losigamone (1500 mg per day) is associated with a greater reduction in seizure frequency than lower doses, but is also associated with more dropouts due to adverse events (see Table 17.2).

Oxcarbazepine versus placebo:
One systematic review [33] (search date 2006, 2 RCTs, 961 adults and children) found that adding OXC to usual treatment significantly reduced seizure frequency compared with adding placebo. Withdrawal from treatment was also more among those treated with OXC. The review found that adverse effects (ataxia, dizziness, fatigue, nausea, somnolence and diplopia) were reported significantly more frequently with adding OXC than with placebo (see Table 17.2).

Pregabalin versus placebo
Systematic review (search date 2012, 6 RCTs, 2009 people with treatment-resistant partial epilepsy, aged 12–82 years, about 50% male) found that adding pregabalin to usual treatment (1–4 antiepileptic drugs) significantly reduced seizure frequency compared with adding placebo [34]. Trials tested doses of pregabalin ranging from 50 mg per day to 600 mg per day. The primary outcome, 50% or higher seizure reduction was significantly more likely in patients randomised to pregabalin than to placebo. A dose–response analysis suggested increasing effect with increasing dose. Pregabalin was significantly associated with seizure freedom (RR 2.59; 95% CI 1.05–6.36). Withdrawal from allocated treatment was more likely with pregabalin than with placebo. Ataxia, dizziness, somnolence and weight gain were significantly associated with pregabalin. The odds of response doubled with an increase in dose from 300 to 600 mg per day (see Table 17.2).

Tiagabine versus placebo
One systematic review [35] (search date 2011; 4 parallel and 2 crossover RCTs, 900 people) found that adding tiagabine to usual treatment significantly reduced seizure frequency, but was associated with higher withdrawal from study compared with adding placebo. Dizziness and tremors were reported significantly more frequently with adding tiagabine than with placebo (see Table 17.2) [35].

Topiramate versus placebo
One systematic review [36] (search date 2007; 10 RCTs, 1312 people) found that adding TPM to usual treatment significantly reduced seizure frequency compared with adding placebo. Adverse effects (ataxia, concentration difficulty, dizziness, fatigue, paraesthesia, somnolence, thinking abnormally and weight loss) were reported significantly more frequently with adding TPM (see Table 17.2).

Vigabatrin versus placebo
One systematic review [37] (search date 2012, 11 RCTs, 747 people) found that adding vigabatrin to usual treatment significantly reduced seizure frequency compared with adding placebo. Adverse effects (dizziness, fatigue/ drowsiness) were reported significantly more frequently with adding vigabatrin (see Table 17.2). Vigabatrin causes concentric visual-field abnormalities in about 40% of people, which are probably irreversible [38]. Because of this, the consensus view among neurologists is not to recommend vigabatrin.

Zonisamide versus placebo
One systematic review [39] (search date 2013, 5 RCTs, 949 people) found that adding zonisamide to usual treatment significantly reduced seizure frequency compared with adding placebo. Adverse effects and treatment withdrawal were more frequent with zonisamide than with placebo. Adverse effects (ataxia, somnolence, agitation/irritability and anorexia) were reported significantly more frequently with adding zonisamide (see Table 17.2). A drug safety alert has been issued on the risk of metabolic acidosis associated with zonisamide (http://www.fda.gov).

Head-to-head comparisons of newer AEDs (add-on treatment)
We found the following comparisons.

Lamotrigine versus pregabalin
We found one systematic review [34] (1 RCT, 434 people). The review found that participants allocated to pregabaline were significantly more likely to achieve a 50% or greater reduction in seizure frequency than those allocated to LTG. No significant differences were found between pregabalin and LTG for seizure freedom (RR 1.39; 95% CI 0.40–4.83); withdrawal from the study due to any reason (RR 1.07; 95% CI 0.75–1.52) or for withdrawal from the study due to adverse events (RR 0.96; 95% CI 0.57–1.60). Patients allocated to pregabalin were significantly more likely to experience dizziness (RR 2.94; 99% CI 1.32–6.52) than those allocated to lamotrigine. No significant differences were found between pregabalin and lamotrigine for other adverse events such as ataxia, fatigue, somnolence, weight gain or headache (see Table 17.2)

Lamotrigine versus gabapentin
We found one systematic review (search date 2009, 3 RCTs, 408 people) [29]. The review reported no differences in responder rate, withdrawal rate or seizure-free rate between LTG and GBP (see Table 17.2).

Lamotrigine versus topiramate
We found one systematic review (search date 2009, 1 RCT, 192 people) [29]. The RCT found that TPM had

better responder rate and seizure-free rate compared to lamotrigine. LTG was superior to TPM for withdrawal rate (see Table 17.2).

Lamotrigine versus levetiracetam
We found one systematic review (search date 2009, 1 RCT, 268 people) [29]. There was no significant differences in responder rate, seizure-free rate or withdrawal rate between LTG and LEV (see Table 17.2).

The results of these systematic reviews are presented in Table 17.2.

Indirect comparisons of antiepileptic drugs
Indirect comparison of newer AEDs
We found one systematic review [29] (search date 2009, 62 placebo-controlled RCTs with 12 902 patients and 8 head-to-head RCTs 1370 patients) were included. Indirect comparisons of responder rates (ORs) revealed that TPM was more effective, while GBP and lacosamide were less effective, without significant heterogeneity. When analyses were based on absolute estimates (NNTs), TPM and LEV were more effective, while GBP and tiagabine were less effective. Withdrawal rates were higher with OXC (OR 1.60; 1.12–2.29) and TPM (OR 1.68; 1.07–2.63) and lower with GBP (OR 0.65; 0.42–1.00) and LEV (OR 0.62; 0.43–0.89). The frequency of the most common side effects is comparable between the new AEDs. The differences found are of relatively small magnitude to allow any definitive conclusion about which new AED(s) has superior effectiveness, based on indirect evidence. Caution must be exercised with this meta-analysis as the results are only valid for the drug doses used within the trials. The reviews did not present separate results for adults and children.

Indirect comparison of 'older' and 'newer' AEDs
We found one review using multiple treatment comparisons of eight AEDs [40]. Individual patient data from epilepsy 20 monotherapy RCTs of 8 AEDs (6418 patients, 4628 with partial-onset epilepsy) were synthesised in a single stratified Cox regression model adjusted for treatment by epilepsy-type interactions and making use of direct and indirect evidence. Outcomes studied were time to treatment failure, time to 12-month remission from seizures and time to first seizure (secondary outcome). For partial-onset seizures, LTG, CBZ and OXC provide the best combination of seizure control and treatment failure. Lamotrigine is clinically superior to all other drugs for treatment failure, but estimates suggest a disadvantage compared to CBZ for time to 12-month remission (hazard ratio (95% confidence interval) = 0.87 (0.73–1.04)) and time to first seizure (1.29 (1.13–1.48)). Phenobarbitone may delay time to first seizure (0.77 (0.61–0.96)) but at the expense of increased treatment failure (1.60 (1.22–2.10)).

Summary

Systematic reviews in people with drug-resistant partial epilepsy found that adding clobazam, eslicarbazepine, gabapentin, levetiracetam, lacosamide, lamotrigine, losigamone, oxcarbazepine, pregabaline, tiagabine, topiramate, vigabatrin or zonisamide to existing treatment reduced seizure frequency in the short term compared with adding placebo. The reviews found that adding any of the drugs increased the frequency of adverse effects compared with adding placebo. Little information is available from RCTs regarding longer term outcomes or safety with long-term usage. We found no good evidence from RCTs on which to base a choice of drug therapy in people with drug-resistant partial epilepsy.

AED withdrawal for people in remission

How does the withdrawal of AEDs in persons with epilepsy who are seizure-free with medication affect the probability of seizure recurrence?

Withdrawal versus continued treatment
One large RCT (1013 people, 49% men who had been seizure-free for >2 years) compared continued antiepileptic treatment with slow AED withdrawal [41,42]. At 2 years, 78% of people who continued treatment remained seizure-free compared with 59% in the withdrawal group. There were no significant differences in psychosocial outcomes between groups.

Risk reductions with 95% CI for the main factors predicting recurrence of seizures are tabulated (Table 17.3). A total of 16 people died during the trial, 10 in the continued treatment group and 6 in the withdrawal group. Only two deaths (in people randomised to continued treatment) were attributed to epilepsy. People with a seizure recurrence were less likely to be in paid employment at 2 years.

The second RCT [43] (160 adults, seizure-free for at least 2 years on monotherapy, 76% partial epilepsy) compared continued AED treatment (CBZ, VPA, PHT, PHB and LTG) and drug withdrawal at a rate of 20% dose reduction every 6 weeks. One year after AED withdrawal, 7% of people with continued treatment and 15% of people with AED withdrawal had seizure relapse (RR 2.46, 95% CI 0.85–7.08, $P = 0.095$). It found no significant difference between groups in health-related quality of life after 1 year. People with normal neurological examination and those receiving CBZ before withdrawal were more likely to remain seizure-free 1 year after AED withdrawal (Table 17.3). The RCT reported in further follow-up (median 47 months, and 41 months for people off medication) that four people died, two from apparently sudden unexpected death in epilepsy (one a few weeks after withdrawal, and one 4 years after withdrawal) [43].

Table 17.3 Risk of seizure recurrence after AED withdrawal

Study (reference number)	Prognostic variable	RR (95% CI)	Remarks
MRC [41,42]	Age <16 years:	1.8 (1.3–2.4)	Risk at 2 years
	Tonic clonic seizure:	1.6 (1.1–2.2)	
	Myoclonus:	1.8 (1.1–3.0)	
	Receiving more than one AED:	1.9 (1.4–2.4)	
	Seizures after starting AEDs:	1.6 (1.2–2.1)	
	Any EEG abnormality:	1.3 (1.0–1.8)	
Lossius [43]	Normal neurological examination	OR 2.77 (1.18–142.86)	1 year after withdrawal
	Use of CBZ before withdrawal	OR 2.86 (1.31–6.26)	
Sirven [44]	<2 years seizure freedom (SF) before taper	1.32 (1.02–1.70)	Follow-up time 2–5 years
	<2 years SF + partial seizures	1.52 (0.95–2.41)	
	<2 years SF + abnormal EEG	1.67 (0.93–3.00)	
Ranganathan [45]	Mental Retardation	3.1 (1.5–6.2)	Follow-up time 11–105 months (mean 39)
	Spikes in EEG	1.9 (1.0–3.4)	

One systematic review of observational studies [46] found that, at 2 years, 29% (95% CI 24–34%) of people in remission from all types of epilepsy would relapse if AEDs were withdrawn.

Early versus late discontinuation

One systematic review (7 RCTs, 924 randomised children) [44] investigated seizure relapse risk after early (<2 seizure-free years) versus late (>2 seizure-free years) AED withdrawal in epilepsy patients. No eligible trials evaluating seizure-free adults were found. The pooled RR for seizure relapse in early versus late AED withdrawal was 1.32 (95% CI 1.02–1.70, NNH = 10). Early discontinuation was associated with greater relapse rates in people with partial seizures or an abnormal electroencephalograph (EEG) (see Table 17.3).

Rapid versus slow withdrawal of AED

One systematic review [45] (one quasi-randomised trial, 149 children, mean age 11 years, 53% boys, majority on one or two AEDs, 16 lost to follow-up before taper) to either a 6-week or a 9-month period of drug tapering, after which therapy was discontinued. Each group was composed of patients who had been seizure-free for either 2 or 4 years before drug tapering was begun. Seizures recurred in 53 patients (40%). The mean duration of follow-up was 39

months (range 11–105) for the patients who did not have a recurrence of seizures. Neither the length of the taper period nor the length of time the patients were seizure-free before the taper period was begun significantly influenced the risk of seizure recurrence. The presence of mental retardation or spikes in the EEG at the time of tapering increased the risk of seizure recurrence (Table 17.3). This small open-label quasi-randomised study with four arms may not have had the power to detect important differences in the effects of treatment policies.

Summary

Two RCTs in people who had been seizure-free for at least 2 years found that recurrence of seizures was more likely in people who had their AEDs stopped compared to those continued on antiepileptic medication. Clinical predictors of relapse after drug withdrawal included age, seizure type, number of AEDs being taken, whether seizures had occurred since AEDs were started and the period of remission before drug withdrawal. Abnormalities in neurological examination and EEG may also be predictors for recurrence after AED withdrawal. There is a need to trade off between benefits and harms (potential adverse effects) while attempting to withdraw AEDs in seizure-free individuals. There is evidence to support waiting for at least two or more seizure-free years before discontinuing AEDs in children, particularly if individuals have an abnormal EEG and partial seizures. There is insufficient evidence regarding withdrawal of AEDs in children with generalised seizures, timing of withdrawal of AEDs in seizure-free adults or the rate at which the drugs should be withdrawn.

Surgery

For people with drug-resistant temporal lobe epilepsy, what is the probability that temporal lobe surgery will render them seizure-free after 1 year? Is surgical treatment safe?

Temporal lobectomy
One RCT [47] (80 adults with poorly controlled temporal lobe epilepsy) compared temporal lobectomy and medical treatment for 1 year.

Benefits
• Temporal lobectomy significantly increased the proportion of people who were completely free of seizures and the proportion who were seizure-free with or without auras compared with medical treatment at the end of 1 year. (seizure-free: 38.0% with surgery versus 2.5% with control; number needed to treat (NNT) 3, 95% CI 2−5; seizure-free with or without auras: 58.0% with surgery versus 7.5% with control; NNT 2, 95% CI 2−3).
• The quality of life improved at 1 year in the surgical group compared with medical treatment (QOLIE 89 scores: 73.8 with surgery versus 64.3 with medical treatment; $P < 0.001$ after adjusting for baseline differences).
• More people who underwent surgery were employed or attending school (56.4%) at 1 year compared with medical treatment (38.5%), but the increase was not significant ($P = 0.11$).

Harms
• There were no deaths at 1 year among those who underwent surgery and one death, of unknown cause, in the control group.
• Neurological adverse effects were more common with surgery (4/40 with surgery (one small thalamic infarct causing thigh dysaesthesia, one infected wound, two people with decline in verbal memory affecting occupation for 1 year) versus 0/40 with medical treatment). Fifty-five per cent of people had asymptomatic superior sub-quadrantic visual-field defects after surgery. Depression was detected almost equally with surgical (18%) and medical treatment (20%). Transient psychosis occurred in one person in each group.
• We found two systematic reviews of non-randomised studies reporting long-term outcomes after resectional epilepsy surgery [48,49]. The first review found that, in

the long term (>5 years), seizure freedom after temporal lobectomy was 66% (19 studies, 1803 people, 95% CI 64−69) using Engel's classification of seizure freedom [48]. On average, 14% (95% CI 11−17) of people were able to discontinue their antiepileptic drug treatment, 50% (95% CI 45−55) achieved antiepileptic monotherapy and 33% remained on polytherapy (95% CI 29−38) [49]. Even though non-controlled studies consistently reported an improvement in the long-term psychosocial outcomes (such as driving status, quality of life, educational and employment status, interpersonal relationships and social behaviour), the effect was less clear in studies that included a medically treated control group. Mortality was lower in people who become seizure-free after epilepsy surgery, but was still higher compared with the general population. Five studies found no worsening in intelligence scores. Three studies found conflicting information on long-term memory outcomes, depending on factors such as side of surgery and seizure freedom [49]

Amygdalohippocampectomy
We found no systematic review and no RCTs that examined the effect of amygdalohippocampectomy in people with drug-resistant temporal lobe epilepsy.

Lesionectomy
We found one systematic review of observational studies (no RCTs) that examined the effects of lesionectomy in people with drug-resistant epilepsy secondary to a known cerebral lesion. The systematic review of observational studies [50] (8 studies, 131 people with lesions) found that between 1 and 4 years, 63% of the 131 people who had lesionectomy were free of disabling seizures.

Summary

One RCT found that temporal lobectomy improved seizure control and quality of life after 1 year compared with continued medical treatment in people with poorly controlled temporal lobe epilepsy. There is consensus that temporal lobectomy is beneficial for people with drug-resistant temporal lobe epilepsy.

Though no RCTs are available, there is consensus that amygdalohippocampectomy is probably beneficial for people with drug-resistant temporal lobe epilepsy.

The effect of lesionectomy for seizure control is not known, though surgical removal of tumours and vascular lesions may be indicated to prevent haemorrhage, herniation or paralysis.

Vagus nerve stimulation for drug-resistant epilepsy
What are the effects of high-level vagus nerve stimulation and low-level (control) stimulation?

We found one systematic review (search date 2007, 2 parallel RCTs, 312 adults) [51] comparing high-level vagus nerve stimulation (VNS) and low-level VNS (control) over 12–16 weeks in people with medication-resistant partial seizures. All participants were implanted with a stimulator, but the control group received less-frequent and lower-intensity stimulation. In addition, the control group did not receive any electrical current when the device was manually activated by the participant. Twenty-six per cent of people on high-level VNS had 50% or greater reduction in seizure frequency compared to 15% with low-level VNS.

The review found no significant difference in treatment withdrawal between high-level VNS and low-level VNS. One participant had an infection at the site of device implantation and was not randomised. Hoarseness and dyspnoea were significantly more frequent in the high-level than in the low-level stimulation group, and may be attributable to stimulation. Hoarseness, cough and paraesthesia were significantly more frequent in the low-level stimulation group compared with baseline, and may be attributable to device implantation. Hoarseness, cough, dyspnoea, pain and paraesthesia were more frequent in the high-level stimulation group compared with baseline, and may be attributable to implantation plus stimulation. The results are given in Table 17.4.

What are the effects of different stimulation cycles?

An RCT (61 people) compared three distinctive stimulation cycles: 7 seconds on and 18 seconds off (rapid cycle) versus 30 seconds on and 30 seconds off (medium cycle) versus 30 seconds on and 3 minutes off (slow cycle) [52]. The proportion of 50% responders was similar among the groups (31.6 % for rapid cycle; 31.7% for medium cycle and 26.1% for slow cycle). Cough and voice alteration were more common with rapid-cycle stimulation compared with less-rapid cycles of stimulation (26% with rapid cycle vs 5% with medium cycle vs 9% for slow cycle).Three participants withdrew from the study: one did not tolerate rapid-cycle stimulation, one due to infection and the third was not followed up [52].

Summary

High-level vagus nerve stimulation may be more effective than low-level vagus nerve stimulation in reducing the frequency of seizures at 12–16 weeks in people with medication-resistant partial seizures (low-quality evidence). The adverse effects include hoarseness, cough and paraesthesia (attributable to device implantation); hoarseness and dyspnoea (attributable to stimulation); hoarseness, cough, dyspnoea, pain and paraesthesia (probably attributable to implantation plus stimulation) [51]. It is possible that investigators and participants were not adequately blinded to the treatment groups, in these short-duration studies. We do not know which stimulation cycle (7 seconds on/18 seconds off; 30 seconds on/30 seconds off; 30 seconds on/3 minutes off) is more effective at reducing seizure frequency.

Generalised epilepsy

In patients with generalised epilepsy (absence seizures), which AED is most effective and safe?

One systematic review (search date 2009) [53] found five small trials, four of which were of poor methodological quality. One trial (29 participants) compared LTG with placebo using a response conditional design. Individuals taking LTG were significantly more likely to be seizure-free than participants taking placebo during this short trial. Three

Table 17.4 Effects of vagus nerve stimulation

Comparison	Outcome	RR (95% CI)	Comments
High-level VNS versus low-level VNS	50% responders	1.71 (1.08–2.70)	Probably beneficial
	Treatment withdrawal	1.08 (0.07–17.09)	
High-level VNS versus low-level VNS	Hoarseness	2.36, 99% CI 1.62–3.45	Adverse effects of stimulation
	Dyspnoea	2.25, 99% CI 1.09–4.67	
Low-level stimulation compared to baseline	Hoarseness	4.37, 99% CI 1.83–10.44	Attributable to device implantation
	Cough	2.15, 99% CI 1.29–3.61	
	Paraesthesia	7.00, 99% CI 2.27–21.63	
High-level stimulation versus baseline	Hoarseness	14.08, 99% CI 5.20–38.11	Attribun to implantation and stimulation
	Cough	1.81, 99% CI 1.12–2.92	
	Dyspnoea	4.39, 99% CI 1.48–13.03	
	Pain	2.87, 99% CI 1.46–5.64	
	Paraesthesia	12.02, 99% CI 1.85–77.94	

studies compared ethosuximide and VPA, but because of diverse study designs and populations studied, the results could not be pooled. None of these studies found a difference between VPA and ethosuximide with respect to seizure control. A subsequent RCT [54] comparing ethosuximide, VPA or LTG in children with newly diagnosed childhood absence epilepsy found that LTG was significantly less effective than ethosuximide or VPA at reducing treatment failure. Even though ethosuximide, LTG and VPA are commonly used to treat people with absence seizures, there is insufficient evidence to inform clinical practice, since the available trials are of poor quality.

Carbamazepine for generalised epilepsy

What are the effects of monotherapy in generalised epilepsy (tonic clonic type)?

Carbamazepine versus placebo
We found no systematic review or RCTs.

Carbamazepine versus sodium valproate
We found one systematic review comparing carbamazepine and sodium valproate (search date 2007, 5 RCTs, 4 of the RCTs included 395 people with generalised epilepsy, aged 3–79 years). A meta-analysis of the generalised epilepsy subgroup found no significant difference between VPA and CBZ for 12-month remission or time to first seizure or for treatment withdrawal (Table 17.1). Even though the systematic review found no significant difference between sodium valproate and carbamazepine, the confidence interval is wide and this result does not establish equivalence of sodium valproate and carbamazepine. The age distribution of people classified as having generalised epilepsy suggests errors in the classification of epilepsy type. Failure of the RCTs to document generalised seizures other than tonic clonic seizures is an important limitation. The review did not present results separately for adults and children [14].

Carbamazepine versus phenobarbital
We found one systematic review (search date 2006, 4 RCTs, 680 people aged 2–68 years, 157 with generalised epilepsy) comparing CBZ and PHB [13]. Meta-analysis of the subgroup of people with generalised epilepsy found no significant difference between CBZ and PHB in time to first seizure or in 12-month remission or for treatment withdrawal (see Table 17.1). The review did not present results separately for adults and children.

Carbamazepine versus phenytoin
We found one systematic review (search date 2009, 10 RCTs, 903 people aged 4–82 years with partial-onset epilepsy or generalised-onset tonic clonic seizures) [18]. The review carried out a meta-analysis using individual patient data;

however, it did not present a separate analysis in people with generalised-onset epilepsy and the majority of people (78%) had partial-onset epilepsy.

Carbamazepine versus lamotrigine
See Lamotrigine.

Carbamazepine versus other antiepileptic drugs
We found no systematic review or RCTs.

Phenobarbital for generalised epilepsy
Phenobarbital versus placebo
We found no systematic review or RCTs.

Phenobarbital versus carbamazepine
See Carbamazepine.

Phenobarbital versus phenytoin
We found one systematic review [17] comparing PHT and PHB monotherapy in patients with generalised epilepsy (3 RCTs, 131 patients). There was no significant difference achieving 12-month remission or in time to first seizure, but significantly more people randomised to PHB withdrew from the study compared to those on PHT (Table 17.1).

Phenobarbital versus other antiepileptic drugs
We found no systematic review or RCTs.

Phenytoin for generalised epilepsy
Phenytoin versus placebo
We found no systematic review or RCTs.

Phenytoin versus sodium valproate:
We found one systematic review (search date 2013, 5 RCTs, 395 people aged 3–95 years had generalised epilepsy) [16]. A meta-analysis of the generalised epilepsy subgroup found no significant difference between sodium valproate and phenytoin in 12-month remission or in time to first seizure or in time to treatment withdrawal in people with generalised epilepsy [16].

Phenytoin versus carbamazepine:
See Carbamazepine.

Phenytoin versus oxcarbazepine
We found one systematic review (search date 2013, 2 RCTs, 147 with generalised epilepsy) comparing OXC and PHT [19]. The subgroup analysis of people with generalised epilepsy, revealed no significant difference between OXC and PHT for time to first seizure in people with generalised epilepsy or in achieving 6-month or 12-month remission or for time to treatment withdrawal in people with generalised epilepsy.

Phenytoin versus phenobarbitone:
See phenobarbitone.

Phenytoin versus other antiepileptic drugs

We found no systematic review or RCTs.

Sodium valproate for generalised epilepsy
Sodium valproate versus placebo

We found no systematic review or RCTs.

Sodium valproate versus carbamazepine

See section on carbamazepine.

Sodium valproate versus phenytoin

See section on phenytoin.

Sodium valproate versus other antiepileptic drugs

We found one large RCT [55] SANAD study, 716 people, 63% idiopathic generalised epilepsy, 27% unclassified epilepsy) of a pragmatic design that compared VPA, LTG and TPM in people with generalised epilepsy [55]. The RCT was open label and allowed clinicians to determine the rate of titration and dosing regimen they thought best for each person. The RCT found no significant differences in time to treatment failure (due to unacceptable adverse effects or inadequate seizure control) between VPA and LTG (HR >1 indicates that failure occurs more rapidly with lamotrigine; HR 1.25, 95% CI 0.94–1.68). However, VPA was associated with a lower risk of treatment failure compared with TPM (HR >1 indicates that failure occurs more rapidly with TPM; HR 1.57, 95% CI 1.19–2.08). The RCT found that VPA significantly increased the proportion of people who achieved 12-month remission compared with LTG (HR >1 indicates that 12-month remission occurs more rapidly with LTG; HR 0.76, 95% CI 0.62–0.94) but there was no significant difference compared with TPM (HR >1 indicates that 12-month remission occurs more rapidly with TPM; HR 1.93, 95% CI 0.76–1.15).

Lamotrigine for generalised epilepsy
Lamotrigine versus placebo

We found no systematic review or RCTs.

Lamotrigine versus carbamazepine

We found one systematic review [15] (5 RCTs, search date 2007; 1384 people; 20% generalised epilepsy) had subgroup analysis (with individual patient data) for people with generalised epilepsy. The review found no significant difference between LTG and CBZ for achieving 6-month remission or for time to first seizure. LTG was better than CBZ for time to treatment withdrawal.

Lamotrigine versus other antiepileptic drugs

We found one systematic review (search date 2009) comparing ethosuximide, VPA, LTG or placebo in children or adolescents with absence seizures [53] and a subsequent RCT [54] comparing ethosuximide, VPA or LTG in children with newly diagnosed childhood absence epilepsy. For details, see section on absence epilepsy. See SANAD study in section on sodium valproate for comparison of LTG with VPA and TPM.

Topiramate for generalised epilepsy
Topiramate versus placebo:

We found no systematic review or RCTs.

Topiramate versus other antiepileptic drugs

The SANAD study compared the effectiveness of VPA, LTG and TPM in the treatment of people with generalised epilepsy [21]. For details, see section on VPA.

Levetiracetam for generalised epilepsy
Levetiracetam versus placebo:

We found no systematic review or RCTs.

Levetiracetam versus other antiepileptic drugs

We found no systematic review or RCTs.

Gabapentin for generalised epilepsy
Gabapentin versus placebo

We found no systematic review or RCTs.

Gabapentin versus other antiepileptic drugs

We found no systematic review or RCTs.

Conclusion

Carbamazepine, gabapentin, lamotrigine, levetiracetam, phenobarbital, phenytoin, sodium valproate and topiramate are widely considered effective in controlling seizures in newly diagnosed generalised (tonic clonic) epilepsy, but we found no RCTs comparing them with placebo, and a placebo-controlled trial would now be considered unethical. Systematic reviews found no reliable evidence on which to base a choice among antiepileptic drugs; we do not know if any one antiepileptic drug is more likely to reduce seizures compared with the others.

Additional treatments

What are the effects of additional treatments in people with drug-resistant generalised epilepsy?

Lamotrigine add-on versus adding placebo

We found one systematic review [56] and one subsequent RCT [57] comparing addition of LTG and addition of placebo in people with generalised tonic clonic seizures with or without other generalised seizure types (e.g. absence or myoclonic seizures) who had not responded to usual drug treatment. The systematic review (search date 2010, 1 crossover and 1 parallel RCTs, 143 people, aged 2–55 years) did not pool the data due to differences in study design between the two RCTs [56].

The crossover design RCT included in the systematic review [58] enrolled 26 people with absence, myoclonic or generalised tonic clonic seizures or a combination of these [excluding Lennox–Gastaut epilepsy]. It found that adding LTG 75–150 mg daily (compared to adding placebo) significantly increased the responder rates for generalised seizures and absence seizures but not for myoclonic seizures. Seven patients on LTG developed drug rash with two withdrawals compared to none on placebo.

The second RCT (parallel design, 121 people with primary generalised tonic clonic seizures, aged 2–55 years) compared adding LTG (maximum 200–400 mg per day) and adding placebo to usual drug treatment [59]. The RCT found that adding LTG significantly increased the proportion of people with a 50% or greater reduction in primary generalised tonic clonic seizures (over both dose-escalation and maintenance phases: 64% with LTG vs 39% with placebo, $P < 0.05$; over maintenance phase only: 72% with LTG vs 49% with placebo, $P < 0.05$, ITT). Twenty-eight per cent of people in the RCT did not complete the study. The RCT found higher rates of dizziness (LTG 5% vs placebo 2%), nausea (LTG 5% vs placebo 3%) and somnolence (LTG 5% vs placebo 2%).

The subsequent RCT (153 people with primary generalised tonic clonic seizures with or without other generalised seizure types, three or more seizures during 8-week baseline period, aged at least 13 years) found that adding extended-release LTG (200–500 mg per day) significantly decreased frequency of primary generalised tonic clonic seizures compared with placebo (70% on LTG had 50% or greater reduction in seizure frequency vs 32% with placebo; $P < 0.0001$) [57]. Withdrawal from the study due to adverse effects and side effects were not significantly higher in the LTG extended-release group.

Levetiracetam add-on versus placebo

We found two RCTs comparing addition of levetiracetam versus addition of placebo in people who had not responded to usual drug treatment [60,61].

The first RCT [60] (164 people, aged 4–65 years, at least three generalised tonic clonic seizures/8-week baseline period) found that adding LEV (1000–3000 mg per day in adults, 20–60 mg/kg per day in children) significantly reduced seizure frequency and increased the proportion of responders, compared with placebo at 24 weeks (generalised tonic clonic seizures: 72% with LEV vs 45% with placebo for generalised tonic clonic seizures; $P < 0.001$; all seizures: 60% with LEV vs 30% with placebo; $P < 0.001$). The RCT found similar rates of adverse effects between the two groups.

The second RCT (122 people, aged 12–65 years) found that adding LEV 3000 mg daily to usual care significantly increased the proportion of 50% responders (at least a 50% reduction from baseline) compared with adding placebo

(myoclonic seizure days per week: 58% with LEV vs 23% with placebo; OR 4.77, 95% CI 2.12–10.77; $P < 0.001$; All seizure days per week: 57% with LEV vs 22% with placebo; OR 5.90, 95% CI 2.48–14.04; $P < 0.001$). LEV also increased the proportion of people seizure-free compared with placebo (13% with LEV vs 0% with placebo; $P = 0.006$) [61]. The adverse effects did not differ significantly in both groups.

Summary

Adding lamotrigine or levetiracetam seems more effective at decreasing the frequency of generalised tonic clonic seizures compared to adding placebo. Few RCTs have compared second-line drugs directly against each other. The RCTs did not report outcomes separately for adults and children.

Abbreviations

PHB Phenobarbital or phenobarbitone
PHT Phenytoin
CBZ Carbamazepine
VPA Sodium Valproate
LTG Lamotrigine
GBP Gabapentin
TPM Topiramate
LEV Levetiracetam
OXC Oxcarbazepine
ESL Eslicarbazepine
ITT Intention to treat analysis
OR Odds ratio
CI Confidence intervals

References

1 Fisher, R.S., Boas, W.M., Blume, W. *et al.* (2005) Epileptic seizures and epilepsy: definitions proposed by the International League Against Epilepsy (ILAE) and the International Bureau for Epilepsy (IBE). *Epilepsia*, **46**, 470–472.

2 Berg, A.T. & Scheffer, I.E. (2011) New concepts in classification of the epilepsies: entering the 21st century. *Epilepsia*, **52(6)**, 1058–1062.

3 Hauser, A.W., Annegers, J.F. & Kurland, L.T. (1993) Incidence of epilepsy and unprovoked seizures in Rochester, Minnesota 1935–84. *Epilepsia*, **34**, 453–468.

4 Berg, A.T. & Shinnar, S. (1991) The risk of seizure recurrence following a first unprovoked seizure: a quantitative review. *Neurology*, **41**, 965–972.

5 Cockerell, O.C., Johnson, A.L., Sander, J.W. *et al.* (1995) Remission of epilepsy: results from the national general practice study of epilepsy. *Lancet*, **346**, 140–144.

6 Marson, A., Jacoby, A., Johnson, A. *et al.* & On behalf of the Medical Research Council MESS study Group (2005) Immediate

versus deferred antiepileptic drug treatment for early epilepsy and single seizures: a randomized controlled trial. *Lancet*, **365**, 2007–2013.

7 First Seizure Trial Group (FIRST Group) (1993) Randomized clinical trial on the efficacy of antiepileptic drugs in reducing the risk of relapse after a first unprovoked tonic clonic seizure. *Neurology*, **43**, 478–483.

8 Musicco, M., Beghi, E., Solari, A. *et al.* & for the FIRST Group (1997) Treatment of first tonic clonic seizure does not improve the prognosis of epilepsy. *Neurology*, **49**, 991–998.

9 Gilad, R., Lampl, Y., Gabbay, U., Eshel, Y. & Sarova-Pinhas, I. (1996) Early treatment of a single generalized tonic-clonic seizure to prevent recurrence. *Archives of Neurology*, **53**, 1149–1152.

10 Chandra, B. (1992) First seizure in adults: to treat or not to treat. *Clinical Neurology and Neurosurgery*, **94**(**Suppl**), S61–S63.

11 Camfield, P., Camfield, C., Dooley, J., Smith, E. & Garner, B. (1989) A randomized study of carbamazepine versus no medication after a first unprovoked seizure in childhood. *Neurology*, **39**, 851–852.

12 U.S Food and Drug Administration. (2008) *Information for Healthcare Professionals: Suicidal Behavior and Ideation and Antiepileptic Drugs.* Available at http://www.fda.gov/Drugs/DrugSafety/PostmarketDrugSafetyInformationforPatientsandProviders/ucm100192.htm (Accessed 15 October 2012). FDA.

13 Tudur Smith C, Marson AG, Williamson PR. Carbamazepine versus phenobarbitone monotherapy for epilepsy. *Cochrane Database of Systematic Reviews* 2003, **1**: CD001904. 10.1002/14651858. CD001904.

14 Marson AG, Williamson PR, Hutton JL, Clough HE, Chadwick DW. Carbamazepine versus valproate monotherapy for epilepsy. *Cochrane Database of Systematic Reviews* 2000, **3**: CD001030. 10.1002/14651858.CD001030.

15 Gamble CL, Williamson PR, Marson AG. Lamotrigine versus carbamazepine monotherapy for epilepsy. *Cochrane Database of Systematic Reviews* 2006, **1**: CD001031. 10.1002/14651858. CD001031.pub2.

16 Nolan SJ, Marson AG, Pulman J, Tudur Smith C. Phenytoin versus valproate monotherapy for partial onset seizures and generalised onset tonic-clonic seizures. *Cochrane Database of Systematic Reviews* 2013, **8**: CD001769. 10.1002/14651858. CD001769.pub2.

17 Nolan SJ, Tudur Smith C, Pulman J, Marson AG. Phenobarbitone versus phenytoin monotherapy for partial onset seizures and generalised onset tonic-clonic seizures. *Cochrane Database of Systematic Reviews* 2013, **1**. CD002217. 10.1002/14651858.CD002217.pub2.

18 Tudur Smith C, Marson AG, Clough HE, Williamson PR. Carbamazepine versus phenytoin monotherapy for epilepsy. *Cochrane Database of Systematic Reviews* 2002, **2**: CD001911. 10.1002/14651858.CD001911.

19 Nolan SJ, Muller M, Tudur Smith C, Marson AG. Oxcarbazepine versus phenytoin monotherapy for epilepsy. *Cochrane Database of Systematic Reviews* 2013, **5**: CD003615. 10.1002/14651858.CD003615.pub3.

20 Rowan, A.J., Ramsay, R.E., Collins, J.F. *et al.* (2005) New onset geriatric epilepsy: a randomized study of gabapentin, lamotrigine, and carbamazepine. [see comment]. *Neurology*, **64**, 1868–1873.

21 Saetre E, Perucca E, Isojarvi J, *et al.* An international multicenter randomized double-blind controlled trial of lamotrigine and sustained-release carbamazepine in the treatment of newly diagnosed epilepsy in the elderly. *Epilepsia* 2007 **48**: 1292–1302.

22 Marson, A.G., Al-Kharusi, A.M., Alwaidh, M. *et al.* (2007) The SANAD study of effectiveness of carbamazepine, gabapentin, lamotrigine, oxcarbazepine, or topiramate for treatment of partial epilepsy: an unblinded randomised controlled trial. [see comment]. *Lancet*, **369**, 1000–1015.

23 Privitera, M.D., Brodie, M.J., Mattson, R.H. *et al.* (2003) Topiramate, carbamazepine and valproate monotherapy: double-blind comparison in newly diagnosed epilepsy. *Acta Neurologica Scandinavica*, **107**, 165–175.

24 Brodie, M.J., Perucca, E., Ryvlin, P. *et al.* (2007) Comparison of levetiracetam and controlled release carbamazepine in newly diagnosed epilepsy. *Neurology*, **68**, 402–408.

25 Brodie MJ, Chadwick DW, Anhut H, *et al.* Gabapentin versus lamotrigine monotherapy: a double-blind comparison in newly diagnosed epilepsy. *Epilepsia* 2002;**43**:993–1000.

26 Michael B, Marson AG. Clobazam as an add-on in the management of refractory epilepsy. *Cochrane Database of Systematic Reviews* 2008, **2**: CD004154. 10.1002/14651858. CD004154.pub4.

27 Chang XC, Yuan H, Wang Y, Xu HQ, Zheng RY. Eslicarbazepine acetate add-on for drug-resistant partial epilepsy. *Cochrane Database of Systematic Reviews* 2011, **12**: CD008907. 10.1002/14651858.CD008907.pub2.

28 Al-Bachari S, Pulman J, Hutton JL, Marson AG. Gabapentin add-on for drug-resistant partial epilepsy. *Cochrane Database of Systematic Reviews* 2013, **7**: CD001415. 10.1002/14651858.CD001415.pub2.

29 Costa J, Fareleira F, Ascencao R, Borges M, Sampaio C, Vaz-Carneiro A. Clinical comparability of the new antiepileptic drugs in refractory partial epilepsy: a systematic review and meta-analysis. *Epilepsia*, **52**(7):1280–1291, 2011. 10.1111/j.1528-1167.2011.03047.x.

30 Ramaratnam S, Marson AG, Baker GA. Lamotrigine add-on for drug-resistant partial epilepsy. *Cochrane Database of Systematic Reviews* 2001, **3**: CD001909. 10.1002/14651858.CD001909. (Update under Publication).

31 Mbizvo GK, Dixon P, Hutton JL, Marson AG. Levetiracetam add-on for drug-resistant focal epilepsy: an updated Cochrane Review. *Cochrane Database of Systematic Reviews* 2012, **9**: CD001901. 10.1002/14651858.CD001901.pub2.

32 Xiao Y, Luo M, Wang J, Luo H. Losigamone add-on therapy for partial epilepsy. *Cochrane Database of Systematic Reviews* 2012, **6**: CD009324. 10.1002/14651858.CD009324.pub2.

33 Castillo SM, Schmidt DB, White S, Shukralla A. Oxcarbazepine add-on for drug-resistant partial epilepsy. *Cochrane Database of Systematic Reviews* 2000, **3**: CD002028. 10.1002/14651858. CD002028.

34 Pulman J, Hemming K, Marson AG. Pregabalin add-on for drug-resistant partial epilepsy. *Cochrane Database of Systematic Reviews* 2014, **3**: CD005612. 10.1002/14651858. CD005612.pub3.

35 Pulman J, Marson AG, Hutton JL. Tiagabine add-on for drug-resistant partial epilepsy. *Cochrane Database of Systematic Reviews* 2012, **5**: CD001908. 10.1002/14651858. CD001908.pub2.

36 Pulman J, Jette N, Dykeman J, Hemming K, Hutton JL, Marson AG. Topiramate add-on for drug-resistant partial epilepsy. *Cochrane Database of Systematic Reviews* 2014, **2**: CD001417. 10.1002/14651858.CD001417.pub3.

37 Hemming K, Maguire MJ, Hutton JL, Marson AG. Vigabatrin for refractory partial epilepsy. *Cochrane Database of Systematic Reviews* 2013, **1**: CD007302. 10.1002/14651858. CD007302.pub2.

38 Kalviainen, R., Nousiainen, I., Mantyjarvi, M. *et al.* (1999) Vigabatrin, a gabaergic antiepileptic drug, causes concentric visual field defects. *Neurology,* **53**, 922–926.

39 Carmichael K, Pulman J, Lakhan SE, Parikh P, Marson AG. Zonisamide add-on for drug-resistant partial epilepsy. *Cochrane Database of Systematic Reviews* 2013 **12**: CD001416. 10.1002/ 14651858.CD001416.pub3.

40 Smith CT, Marson AG, Chadwick DW, Williamson PR. Multiple treatment comparisons in epilepsy monotherapy trials. *Trials.* 2007; **8**: 34. Published online Nov 5, 2007 10.1186/1745-6215-8-34.

41 Medical Research Council Antiepileptic Drug Withdrawal Study Group (1991) Randomised study of antiepileptic drug withdrawal in patients in remission. *Lancet,* **337**, 1175–1180.

42 Medical Research Council Antiepileptic Drug Withdrawal Study Group (1993) Prognostic index for recurrence of seizures after remission of epilepsy. *BMJ,* **306**, 1374–1378.

43 Lossius MI, Hessen E, Mowinckel P, *et al.* Consequences of antiepileptic drug withdrawal: a randomized, double-blind study (Akershus Study). *Epilepsia* 2008;49:455–463.

44 Sirven, J.I., Sperling, M. & Wingerchuk, D.M. (2006) Early versus late antiepileptic drug withdrawal for people with epilepsy in remission (Cochrane Review). In: *The Cochrane Library.* John Wiley & Sons, Ltd., Chichester, UK.

45 Ranganathan, L.N. & Ramaratnam, S. (2006) Rapid versus slow withdrawal of antiepileptic drugs (Cochrane Review). In: *The Cochrane Library.* John Wiley & Sons, Ltd., Chichester, UK.

46 Berg, A.T. & Shinnar, S. (1994) Relapse following discontinuation of antiepileptic drugs: a meta-analysis. *Neurology,* **44**, 601–608.

47 Wiebe, S., Blume, W.T., Girvin, J.P. *et al.* (2001) A randomized, controlled trial of surgery for temporal lobe epilepsy. *The New England Journal of Medicine,* **345**, 311–318.

48 Tellez-Zenteno, J.F., Dhar, R., Wiebe, S. *et al.* (2005) Long-term seizure outcomes following epilepsy surgery: a systematic review and meta-analysis. *Brain,* **128**, 1188–1198.

49 Téllez-Zenteno, J.F., Dhar, R., Hernandez-Ronquillo, L. *et al.* (2007) Long-term outcomes in epilepsy surgery: antiepileptic drugs, mortality, cognitive and psychosocial aspects. *Brain,* **130**, 334–345.

50 Engel, J. Jr.,, Wiebe, S., French, J. *et al.* (2003) Practice parameter: temporal lobe and localized neocortical resections for epilepsy: report of the Quality Standards Subcommittee of the American Academy of Neurology, in association with the American Epilepsy Society and the American Association of Neurological Surgeons. *Neurology,* **60**, 538–547 [Erratum in: Neurology 2003;60:1396].

51 Privitera, M.D., Welty, T.E., Ficker, D.M. & Welge, J. (2009) Vagus nerve stimulation for partial seizures (Cochrane Review). In: *The Cochrane Library.* John Wiley & Sons, Ltd., Chichester, UK Search date 2007.

52 DeGiorgio, C., Heck, C., Bunch, S. *et al.* (2005) Vagus nerve stimulation for epilepsy: randomized comparison of three stimulation paradigms. *Neurology,* **65**, 317–319.

53 Posner EB, Mohamed KK, Marson AG. Ethosuximide, sodium valproate or lamotrigine for absence seizures in children and adolescents. *Cochrane Database of Systematic Reviews* 2005 **4**: CD003032. 10.1002/14651858.CD003032.pub2.

54 Glauser, T.A., Cnaan, A., Shinnar, S. *et al.* (2010) Ethosuximide, valproic acid, and lamotrigine in childhood absence epilepsy. *The New England Journal of Medicine,* **362**, 790–799.

55 Marson, A.G., Al-Kharusi, A.M., Alwaidh, M. *et al.* (2007) The SANAD study of effectiveness of valproate, lamotrigine, or topiramate for generalised and unclassifiable epilepsy: an unblinded randomised controlled trial. *Lancet,* **369**, 1016–1026.

56 Tjia-Leong E, Leong K, Marson AG. Lamotrigine adjunctive therapy for refractory generalized tonic-clonic seizures. *Cochrane Database of Systematic Reviews* 2010 **12**: CD007783 10.1002/14651858.CD007783.pub2.

57 Biton V, Di Memmo J, Shukla R, *et al.* Adjunctive lamotrigine XR for primary generalized tonic-clonic seizures in a randomized, placebo-controlled study. *Epilepsy and Behavior* 2010;19: 352–358.

58 Beran RG, Berkovic SF, Dunagan FM, *et al.* Double-blind, placebo-controlled, crossover study of lamotrigine in treatment-resistant generalised epilepsy. *Epilepsia* 1998;39: 1329–1333.

59 Biton, V., Sackellares, J.C., Vuong, A. *et al.* (2005) Double-blind, placebo-controlled study of lamotrigine in primary generalized tonic-clonic seizures. *Neurology,* **65**, 1737–1743.

60 Berkovic SF, Knowlton RC, Leroy RF, *et al.* Placebo-controlled study of levetiracetam in idiopathic generalized epilepsy. *Neurology* 2007;69:1751–1760.

61 Noachtar S, Andermann E, Meyvisch P, *et al.* Levetiracetam for the treatment of idiopathic generalized epilepsy with myoclonic seizures. *Neurology* 2008;70:607–616.

18 CHAPTER 18

Cognitive disorders: mild cognitive impairment and Alzheimer's disease

Charlene H. Snyder, Bryan K. Woodruff, and Richard J. Caselli

Department of Neurology, Mayo College of Medicine, Mayo Clinic, Scottsdale, AZ, USA

Introduction

Alzheimer's disease (AD) is a degenerative brain disease that is the most common cause of dementia. Incidence and prevalence increase exponentially with age through at least the ninth decade, with little evidence of a plateau at higher ages. The prevalence of severe dementia in all persons above age 60 is estimated to be 5%, and, in those above age 85, it is estimated to be 20–50%. The lifetime risk of AD is estimated at 12–17% [1]. With more people living longer, the prevalence of AD is increasing. Since 1980, the number of Americans with AD has doubled to 4.5 million and may triple by 2050 [2]. Prevalence estimates of the co-occurrence of dementia and Parkinsonism vary widely among studies, but average 20–30%; annual incidence rates of dementia in established Parkinsonism also vary, but average 5–6% [3]. Statistics for other forms of dementia are less precise, but frontotemporal dementia is probably about one-tenth as common as AD. Vascular changes are common in dementia patients, but the frequency of mixed vascular-degenerative dementia – especially AD – is much more common than "pure" vascular dementia (VaD).

Even though most cases of AD occur after age 60, about 5% are early-onset familial cases related to one of three autosomal dominant mutations. Early-onset familial AD typically strikes young people ranging in age from the mid-30s to the mid-50s. To date, three separate genetic mutations have been identified that may cause early-onset familial AD, and all three are inherited in an autosomal dominant pattern. The most common mutation thought to account for most of the autosomal dominant kindred is presenilin-1 [4], and it is the only one of the three for which there is currently a commercially available genetic test. The other two include the amyloid precursor protein gene on chromosome 21 [5] and presenilin-2 on chromosome 1 [6]. All result in increased concentrations of Abeta amyloid, which underscores the pathogenic importance of Abeta amyloid in the evolution of AD [7]. The genetic risk factor that accounts for more cases of AD than any other, however, is the apolipoprotein E e4 allele located on chromosome 19. The apolipoprotein E e4 allele is associated with late-onset familial and "sporadic" AD, not autosomal dominant early-onset familial AD [8]. The prevalence of the apolipoprotein E e4 allele varies worldwide, but is about 20% in North America [9].

Dementia imposes an immense burden on families because 70% of these patients are cared for at home [10]. The cost of care averages $42,000 annually [11], so reducing the financial as well as the medical burden of AD is a major goal of medical diagnosis and management. Parkinsonism further adds to the cost of care. These statistics primarily reflect that most AD patients are retirees and do not account for the few patients who lose years of work productivity because of early-onset AD. The statistics also do not account for potentially reversible conditions mistaken for AD or for the increased medical burden of stress-related illness in caregivers.

Treatment of AD and other forms of dementia primarily focuses on symptoms. Nearly all therapeutic trials have been conducted in patients with AD, with results extrapolated, correctly or not, to other etiologic categories. There is little evidence-based support for any putative prevention therapy; approaches that have shown disappointing results in controlled clinical trials include estrogen replacement [12], nonsteroidal anti-inflammatory drugs [13], vitamin E [14], high-dose B vitamins [15]. and ginkgo biloba [16]. Intellectual impairment benefits modestly from cholinesterase inhibitor therapy [17] in mild to moderate AD and memantine hydrochloride therapy in moderate to severe AD [18]. Behavioral management includes the control of psychosis and agitation. Even though atypical antipsychotic drugs have

Evidence-Based Neurology: Management of Neurological Disorders, Second Edition. Edited by Bart M. Demaerschalk and Dean M. Wingerchuk.
© 2015 John Wiley & Sons, Ltd. Published 2015 by John Wiley & Sons, Ltd.

gained widespread use in this regard, they lack approval from the US Food and Drug Administration for this specific use. The Food and Drug Administration in 2005 required a black box warning label on atypical antipsychotics used to treat elderly patients with dementia because of unpublished data suggesting an increased risk of mortality (http://www.fda. gov/cder/drug/advisory/antipsychotics.htm). Other important aspects of management are lifestyle changes (e.g., driving restrictions [19]), caregiver burnout [20], and assisted living, legal guardianship, and related interventions.

Many controversies and uncertainties about the pathogenesis, diagnosis, and treatment of AD confront the clinicians and scientists, and will continue to do so until mechanistic insights translate into more effective clinical therapeutics. Evidence will always be an important cornerstone of therapy, but it is especially vital as long as therapeutic inefficacy fosters the proliferation of witch doctors and snake-oil purveyors.

Framing the clinical questions

This chapter on evidence-based management of Alzheimer's disease addresses four main clinical topics: (1) treatment of mild cognitive impairment for delaying progression to AD, (2) treatment of mild to moderate dementia due to AD, (3) treatment of moderate to severe dementia due to AD, and (4) treatment of agitation in dementia. The topics are similarly structured, with a clinical patient scenario that has been converted into a focused answerable patient or problem, intervention, comparison intervention, and outcomes (PICO) model question. For each question, a critically appraised topic review is presented. The review outlines the clinical bottom line or take-home summary message and then delves into the evidence itself, a short summary of the results, and a commentary.

Search strategy

Given that all four main clinical topics concern therapy, the general search strategy was to look first for the highest level of evidence, systematic reviews, and meta-analyses of randomized-controlled trials in the Cochrane Library, the Cochrane Database of Reviews of Effectiveness, and MEDLINE from 2003 to 2011. This strategy updates the available research originally presented in the first edition chapter. When necessary, individual randomized-controlled trials in the Cochrane Registry and MEDLINE were sought next.

Clinical questions

Treatment of mild cognitive impairment
The term mild cognitive impairment (MCI) has evolved from when it was first introduced to define an intermediate state of cognitive function between the cognitive changes seen in aging and those with all the findings of dementia or Alzheimer's disease to the present classification scheme for mild or early-stage nondisabling cognitive syndromes [20]. There are major categories of MCI: amnestic MCI and non-amnestic MCI that are further sub-classified by involvement of either single or multiple cognitive domains. Amnestic MCI (single and multiple domains) is the most common prodrome of AD, whereas the non-amnestic forms can be associated with other degenerative diseases such as dementia with Lewy bodies, frontotemporal lobar degeneration and vascular cognitive impairment. The defining feature shared by all MCI subtypes is that of an acquired cognitive abnormality, that has not yet progressed to the point of causing functional impairment. As the cognitive skills decline, the ability to manage normal daily affairs falters, and "conversion" to AD becomes apparent defined by this progression to disability. It is thought that a combination of causal factors interrelate in MCI, including cholinergic dysfunction, white-matter lesions and cerebral infarctions, extracellular amyloid deposition, and intracellular neurofibrillary tangle formation.

Longitudinal studies of patients with MCI have shown a conversion to dementia at about 10–15% per year [21]. This pattern of decline over time has sparked interest in using ChEIs as a treatment strategy to preserve cognitive skills and delay conversion to dementia. To date, there are no FDA-approved pharmacological treatments for persons with MCI. However, given the known frequent association of MCI and AD, many clinicians entertain a discussion with individual patients to determine if they would like to consider AD treatment at the MCI stage. In order to facilitate this discussion, the following critical appraisal of the topic is offered for clinicians interested in an evidence-based practice approach.

Clinical scenario
A 75-year-old woman presents with a 1-year history of short-term memory complaints, without any reduction in her ability to function fully; this is corroborated by her spouse. Her mother died at the age of 92 from presumed AD and she is anxious to prevent conversion to AD. She asks about starting on pharmacological treatment.

Focused clinical question: *Is pharmacological treatment effective in treating Mild Cognitive impairment to delay progression of AD?*

Cholinesterase inhibitors
Evidence
In the past decade, there have been several meta-analyses performed on individual ChEI agents or as a drug class but only the most recent found a small, but positive effect on long-term conversion to AD [22–26]. The most recent meta-analysis was selected, because it used progression to AD as an outcome, which best answered our clinical

question and was supported by appropriate inclusion criteria. The meta-analysis was conducted on four randomized control trials (RCTs) (one published study on donepezil (5 or 10 mg), two unpublished trials on galantamine (16–24 mg), and one published trial on rivastigmine (5.67 ± 3 mg) to assess whether pooled analysis could show the benefit of these drugs in delaying the progression of MCI to AD [26]. All enrolled participants in the two meta-analyses were determined to have MCI for inclusion, having scored 24 or more on a mini-mental state examination (MMSE) and a Clinical Dementia Rating (CDR) score of 0.5 [26].

Summary of results

The meta-analysis includes a total of 3574 subjects (1784 in the ChEI-treated group and 1790 in the placebo group) from four RCTs [26]. Sixty percent of treated group completed the study compared to 71% in placebo group. A total of 275 subjects (15.4%) progressed to AD/dementia in the ChEI-treated group, and 366 subjects (20.4%) progressed to AD/dementia in the placebo group, the relative risk (RR) for progression to AD/dementia in the ChEI-treated group was 0.75 (95% CI 0.6–0.9). Of the 1784 subjects in the ChEI-treated group, 60% completed the trial compared to 70% of the 1790 subjects in the placebo group. The rate of serious adverse events in the ChEI-treated group was NNH 5 (−4–5). (Table 18.1) Death rate in the ChEI-treated group was reported as 1.7% (31/1784) and 1.6% (30/1790) in the placebo group.

Commentary

Trials were suitably pooled for meta-analysis, and heterogeneity was assessed using the Jadad quality scale [27]. That analysis found beneficial reduction in conversion rates favoring ChEIs. While there was no significant difference in adverse events reported between the two groups, there was a higher withdrawal rate amongst the ChEI-treated group compared with placebo, which could underestimate the adverse events due to treatment.

Clinical bottom line

Long-term use of cholinesterase inhibitors may modestly reduce the risk of conversion to dementia, NNT 19 (95% CI 13–40). There was no significant difference between cholinesterase inhibitors and placebo in serious adverse events of NNH 96 (95% CI −53 to 25). However, withdrawal rates were high in the ChEI group and caution should be exercised in interpreting side effect results [26].

Other agents

A nutraceutical, homotaurine, also known as Alzhemed is being marketed for brain protection. It is the identical agent tramiprosate that was suspended during phase III trials in 2007 due to methodology problems. Because of the need to clearly define the clinical efficacy and safety of this agent, an active protocol in the Cochrane Database of Systematic Reviews has been published [28].

Clinical implications

MCI continues to be a heterogeneous clinical condition that makes it difficult for researchers to design studies that assess treatment outcomes for conversion to AD. Because the trial populations and the outcome assessment tools used have not been homogenous, the clinical usefulness of pooled analysis remains uncertain. Additional prospective studies are warranted to determine the clinical and neurobiological factors that predict conversion to dementia. Future research will hopefully clarify which group(s) of MCI patients will benefit from treatment without exposing a large population to possible side effects.

Table 18.1 Efficacy and harm of cholinesterase inhibitors for mild to moderate AD

Intervention/ dosage	Outcome	Follow-up time	Treatment number/ total (%)	Placebo number/ total (%)	WMD (95% CI)	Odds ratio (%)	Relative risk (95% CI)	Absolute risk reduction (95% CI)	NNT or NNH (95% CI)	Comment
ChEIs (donepezil 10 mg per day, galantamine 24 mg per day, rivastigmine 5.67 ± 3.00)	Progression to AD or dementia*	2–4 years	275/1784 (15)	366/1790 (20)			0.75 (0.66–0.87)		19 (13–40)	Favors ChEIs
	One or more adverse events		333/1531 (22)	349/1531 (23)			0.95 (0.83–1.09)		96 (−53–25)	Mostly gastrointestinal

CI, confidence interval; WMD, weighted mean difference; NNH, number needed to harm; NNT, number needed to treat;
*Progression to AD or dementia as defined by psychological tests or CDR >1.
Source: Data from Diniz *et al.* [26].

Treatment of mild to moderate Alzheimer's disease

Currently, five drugs in two drug classes have US Food and Drug Administration (FDA) approval for the management of AD. Cholinesterase inhibitors (ChEIs) were the first group to receive approval (donepezil hydrochloride, rivastigmine tartrate, and galantamine hydrobromide). They degrade acetylcholinesterase, which increases the availability of acetylcholine, facilitating cholinergic transmission [29]. Since their introduction, new formulations of these medications have emerged, including rivastigmine transdermal patch, extended release galantamine, and generic formulations. The second class approved for AD was the *N*-methyl-*D*-aspartic acid (NMDA) receptor antagonist (memantine), preventing excess stimulation of the glutamate system, which improves cognition in moderate to severe AD. Memantine received FDA approval for treatment of moderate to severe AD; however, a few studies do address its use in mild to moderate AD [30].

Clinical problem

A 69-year-old woman presents with her daughter for evaluation of progressive memory loss identified during the past year. She has forgotten several social engagements and appointments and frequently repeats herself, according to her daughter. She is also bothered by word-finding difficulties. Her daughter also notes that she has made several errors managing her household finances. She is having increasing difficulty finding her way around her community when driving. Her neurologic examination is unremarkable aside from memory and orientation difficulties on an office mental status assessment. Magnetic resonance imaging of the brain shows mild generalized cerebral atrophy, and routine laboratory studies are unrevealing. Formal neuropsychological assessment shows severe deficits with learning and recall of verbal and nonverbal material. She also demonstrates moderate anomia and deficits in cognitive flexibility consistent with early dementia. You diagnose her with dementia, likely due to underlying AD. She and her daughter ask what treatments are available.

Focused clinical question: *Is pharmacological treatment effective for mild to moderate AD?*

Cholinesterase inhibitors

A Cochrane systematic review identified 13 studies for inclusion. All examined the cognitive, functional and global effects of a CHEI on patients with dementia due to AD [31]. All the 13 were multicenter, randomized, double-blind parallel-group studies designed to evaluate the efficacy and safety of one of the three ChEIs (donepezil, galantamine or rivastigmine) at the manufactured recommended dose over 6 months compared to patients receiving placebo. A meta-analysis was performed on the intention to treat

ITT population. One study was a crossover study. Primary outcomes were changes in global clinical state, cognition or ADL. Secondary outcomes were adverse events.

Summary of results

The pooled results of 10 trials demonstrated a dose-related beneficial effect of ChEIs versus placebo on cognitive function, on average −2.7 points (95% CI −3 to 2.3), and measures of global clinical state at 24 weeks (Table 18.2). A benefit of treatment was found on activities of daily living (ADL). However, none of the treatment effects was large. On average, 70% of the treatment group completed the trial compared to 82% in the placebo group, with dropouts due to adverse events. The ChEI groups had more adverse events compared to placebo with gastrointestinal symptoms predominating.

Only one double-blind RCT study has been done comparing two ChEIs, donepezil and rivastigmine. There was no significant difference between the two agents as measured on cognitive function, activities of daily living, behavioral disturbances and global assessment at 16 weeks. There were fewer adverse events reported with donepezil than rivastigmine. The newer formulation of the rivastigmine daily patch was studied only comparing dosing strengths [31]. There was no difference between 20 cm² patch and 10 cm² patches at 24 weeks as shown by one study, assessing cognition, ADL, behavioral disturbance and withdrawals before end of treatment. There was a significant difference between the larger and smaller patches in favor of the smaller patch for the total number of patients who had at least one adverse event, 200/303 compared with 147/291, odds ratio (OR) 1.90, (95% CI 1.37–2.65), NNH 19, but no difference for serious adverse events, withdrawals due to adverse events and deaths. Overall, there is evidence that the lower dose smaller patch is associated with fewer side effects than the capsules or the higher dose larger patch and has comparable efficacy to both [30].

Commentary

This meta-analysis allowed for a large pooling of trial data on the efficacy and side effects of ChEIs. Even with the strength of pooled data, the improvement in outcome measures was not large. The studies were relatively brief (24 weeks) for a disease that affects the individual and caregiver for up to two decades. The validity of the study may be called into question when one considers together the high withdrawal and adverse event rates.

Clinical bottom line

All three ChEIs improved cognitive function compared to placebo at 6 months as shown in the Alzheimer's Disease Assessment Scale-Cognitive Subscale (ADAS-Cog), effect size −2.37 (95% CI −2.73 to −2.02). Each of the three ChEIs

Table 18.2 Efficacy and harm of ChEIs and NMDA for mild to moderate AD

Intervention/ dosage	Number of trials	Outcome	Follow-up time	Treatment number/ total (%)	Placebo number/ total (%)	WMD (95% CI)	Odds ratio (%)	Relative risk (95% CI)	Absolute risk reduction (95% CI)	NNT or NNH (95% CI)	Comment
ChEIs (donepezil 10 mg per day galantamine 24 mg per day rivastigmine 5.67 ± 3.00)	3	Global rating*	24 weeks	428/1755 (24)	277/1647 (17)	–	1.56 (1.32–1.85)	–	0.10 (13–8)	10 (8–13)	Favors ChEIs
	10	ADAS-COG†	24 weeks	–	–	–2.66 (–3.02 to –2.31)	–	–	–	–	Favors ChEIs
	5	ADL Score‡	24 weeks	–	–	2.40 (1.55–3.37)	–	–	–	–	Favors ChEIs
	10	One or more adverse events	24 weeks	1326/2309 (57)	1802/2515 (72)	-	2.51 (2.14–2.95)	–	0.27 (0.29–25)	4 (3–4)	Mostly gastrointestinal
	10	Nausea	24 weeks	833/1815	222/2219	–	4.7 (4.13–5.14)	–	0.22 (–0.24 to –0.20)	5 (4 to 5)	Favors placebo
Memantine 20 mg per day	3	Global rating*	24 weeks	720	561	0.13 (0.01–0.25)	–	–	–	–	No significant difference
	3	ADAS-COG†	24 weeks	718	561	0.99 (0.21–1.78)	–	–	–	–	No significant difference
	3	ADL Score‡	24 weeks	714	557	0.20 (–0.87 to 21.27)	–	–	–	–	No significant difference
	3	One or more adverse events	24 weeks	493/736	397/570	–	1.04 (0.81–1.33)	–	0.52 (0.001–0.10)	19 (0–1034)	No significant difference

CI, confidence interval; WMD, weighted mean difference; NNT, number needed to treat; NNH, number needed to harm;

*Global rating an assessment of those showing improvement or no change or improvement on Clinician's Interview-Based Impression of Change, plus caregiver input (CIBIC-Plus);

†ADAS Cog, Alzheimer's Disease Assessment Scale–Cognitive Subscale scores for treatment compared with placebo;

‡ADL, activities of daily living assessed with Alzheimer's Disease Cooperative Study-Activities of Daily Living (ADCS-ADL).

Source: Data from McShane et al. [32].

benefits the global clinical state compared with placebo, effect size 1.84 (95% CI 1.47–2.30), NNT 10 (95% CI 8–13). More adverse events were observed in the treatment groups compared with the placebo group, NNH 4 (95% CI 3–4). The adverse events of abdominal pain, anorexia, dizziness, nausea, vomiting, diarrhea, headache, and insomnia were most frequently found when data were pooled.

N-methyl-D-aspartate receptor antagonist – Memantine

Evidence
A Cochrane systematic review identified three studies that evaluated the efficacy and safety in patients with mild to moderate AD who were treated with memantine compared with patients treated with placebo [32]. All included trials were parallel group designs. Primary outcomes were change in global clinical state, cognition, and ADL. Secondary outcomes were adverse events.

Summary of results
Memantine improves cognitive function compared to placebo at 6 months as shown on the ADAS-Cog, effect size 0.99 (95% CI 0.21–1.78) (Table 18.2). There are benefits favoring memantine on the global clinical state compared with placebo clinician's interview-based impression of change, plus caregiver input (CIBIC-plus scale), effect size 0.13 (95% CI 0.01–0.25). There was no benefit between the two groups on ADL and behavior. Dropout rate was low, indicating the drug appears to be well tolerated in both the placebo (13%) and treatment groups (14%) [32].

Commentary
A limitation of the analysis is the small number of studies in each of the different severity subtypes, which reduces the statistical power to identify heterogeneity. It is unclear whether the small effect size in the earlier stages of AD for memantine on ADL and behavior merits its cost.

Clinical bottom line outcomes
A small treatment effect for 20 mg per day of memantine on cognitive function (1.0 ADAS-Cog point) and a small positive effect in the clinical impression of change (0.1 CIBIC +point) were found. However, the differences between treatment groups were not consistently significant. There was no significant difference in adverse events observed in the treatment groups compared with the placebo group, NNH 19 (95% CI 10–1034).

Implication for practice

Longer term studies with a focus on clinically significant end points need to be linked to economic analyses to generate information on cost utility. Further important issues are duration of treatment, severity of dementia, and effects of withdrawal at the end of the treatment period.

Treatment of moderate to severe Alzheimer's disease

A rapid decline of cognitive function and life skills characterizes the moderate to severe stage of AD. Treatment strategies aimed at prolonging both cognitive performance and daily function skills become increasingly important in preserving quality of life for both the patient and caregiver at this stage. Cholinesterase inhibitors have been the mainstay of dementia therapy for years, but were initially approved only for treatment of mild to moderate dementia [33]. Recently, donepezil in 23 mg per day strength was approved for moderate to severe AD [34]. The NMDA receptor antagonist, memantine hydrochloride, has been approved for moderate to severe dementia due to AD [35].

Clinical scenario

An 85-year-old man with a 5-year history of progressive cognitive decline was diagnosed with AD about 3 years ago and is being treated with a stable dose of a cholinesterase inhibitor. He is generally pleasant and cooperative, but requires constant supervision because of a tendency to wander. He requires prompting for bathing and toileting. His wife would like to continue caring for him at home, but finds that she is having difficulty keeping up with all the household and caregiver responsibilities. She asks if there is any other treatment available for his dementia.

Focused clinical question: *Is pharmacological treatment effective in treating moderate to severe dementia due to AD?*

N-methyl-D-aspartate receptor antagonist – Memantine

Evidence
A Cochrane systematic review was performed on three trials studying subjects with moderate to severe AD, treated with memantine in different doses (10–30 mg per day) for 6 months and compared with subjects treated with placebo [32]. The meta-analysis assessed the efficacy and safety of memantine for patients with AD. The studied subjects all had Mini-Mental Status Exam scores of 3–14. All trials used the same outcome measures to assess change in global clinical state, cognition, ADL, and behavior. Secondary outcomes were adverse events.

Summary of results
Analysis of data from the three trials showed that memantine was well tolerated with 80% of the treatment group, compared to 72% of the placebo group completing the trials. There was a significant difference in the clinical global impression of change in favor of memantine, effect size 0.28 (95% CI 0.15–0.41) (Table 18.3). Cognitive function showed improvement in the treatment group, effect size 2.97 (95% CI 1.68–4.26). There was a significant difference in ability to perform ADL in favor of memantine, effect size 1.27 (95% CI 0.44–2.09, $P = 0.003$). There was less worsening of mood

Table 18.3 Efficacy and harm of memantine for moderate to severe AD

Intervention/ dosage	Number of Trials	Outcome	Follow-up time	Treatment/ interest number/ total (%)	Placebo/ interest number/ total (%)	WMD (95% CI)	Odds ratio (%)	Relative risk (95% CI)	Absolute risk reduction (95% CI)	NNT or NNH (95% CI)	Comment
Memantine (20 mg per day)	3	Global rating†	24–28 weeks	487	477	0.28 (0.15–0.41)	–	–	–	–	Favors memantine
	3	SIB‡	24–28 weeks	–	–	2.97 (6 8–4.216)	–	–	–	–	Substantial inconsistency between studies
	3	NPI§	474	462		2.76 (0.42–0.86)§	–	–	–	–	Favors memantine to reduce behaviors
	3	ADL score**	24–28 weeks	493	485	1.27 (0.44–2.09)	–	–	–	–	Favors memantine
	3	One or more adverse events	24–28 weeks	395/506 (78)	379/499 (76)	–	1.13 (0.84–1.52)	–	–	48 (14–32)	ns
	3	Agitation	24 weeks	58/506 (12)	88/449 (18)	–	–	0.6 (0.42–0.88)	–	12 (8–28)	Favors memantine to reduce agitation

CI, confidence interval; WMD, weighted mean difference; NNT, number needed to treat; NNH, number needed to harm; ns, not statistically significant.

†Global rating an assessment of those showing improvement or no change or improvement on Clinician's Interview-Based Impression of Change, plus caregiver input (CIBIC-Plus);

‡SIB, Severe Impairment Battery scores for treatment compared with placebo;

§NPI, neuropsychiatric Inventory assess the frequency and severity of behavioral and neuropsychiatric symptoms compared to placebo;

**ADL, activities of daily living; Progressive Deterioration Scale scores for treatment compared with placebo.

Source: Data from McShane et al. [32].

and behavior, effect size 2.76 (95% CI 0.88–4.63). Reported adverse events showed memantine was well tolerated, effect size 1.13 (0.84, 1.52), NNH 48 (955 CI 14–32) [32].

Commentary

The small number of studies limits the meta-analysis. The length of the trials was short, making it difficult to assess the long-term effect on caregiver and societal burden [32]. The number of withdrawals from the placebo group compared to the memantine group could result in underestimation of effect size.

Clinical bottom line

The pooled analysis of three trials in subjects with moderate to severe AD suggests that memantine (20 mg per day) has a beneficial impact on cognition, mood, and ability to perform daily activities of living over a short 6-month period of time. Mcmantine is well tolerated.

Cholinesterase inhibitor – donepezil

A new higher dose formulation of donepezil, 23 mg per day, has recently received FDA approval for treatment of moderate to severe AD.

Evidence

A review of the literature revealed a single double-blind randomized control trial of donepezil 23 mg per day that studied the efficacy and tolerability of increasing donepezil from 10 mg per day to 23 mg per day for 24 weeks [33].

Summary of results

The single trial included 1371 patients, 981 in the 23 mg per day group and 486 in the 10 mg per day group [33]. Seventy percent of the 23 mg per day group completed the study compared with 82% of the placebo group completing the trial. At the end of the study (week 24), cognitive performance as assessed by the Severe Impairment Battery (SIB) score was significantly greater with donepezil 23 mg per day than with donepezil 10 mg per day and the least squares mean changes (LSM) in (+2.6 [0.58] vs +0.4 [0.66], respectively; difference, 2.2 (Table 18.4). The between-treatment difference in CIBIC+ score was nonsignificant (4.23 [1.07] vs 4.29 [1.07]). Adverse events were reported in 73% of patients who received donepezil 23 mg per day and in 63% of patients who received donepezil 10 mg per day. With donepezil 23 mg per day, mild, moderate, and severe adverse events were reported in 297 (30.8%), 332 (34.5%), and 81(8.4%) patients, respectively; with donepezil 10 mg per day, these proportions were 147 (31.2%), 119 (25.3%), and 34 (7.2%), respectively. The most commonly reported adverse event considered with the 23 mg per day doses was nausea (6%) compared to the 10 mg per day dose (2%). Thirteen deaths were reported during the study or within 30 days of study discontinuation (23 mg per day, 8

patients [0.8%]; 10 mg per day, 5 patients [1.1%]); all were considered unrelated to the study medication [33].

Commentary

The study appeared to show that subjects with more severe AD can achieve modest therapeutic benefits. It is unclear whether this modest impression of change in cognition would improve the caregiver burden in this population, because there was no benefit observed on functions of daily living. The study results were small with a high dropout rate and adverse event reporting. The higher rate of reported adverse events is of a concern in this more fragile population.

Clinical bottom line

Change in global assessment was not significant between the two doses. Analysis of cognitive performance favors the 23 mg per day dosing at 6 months, clinical effect size 8%. Increased side effects were reported in the 23 mg per day group compared to the 10 mg per day group, NNH 10 (95% CI 7–20) with the most common severe adverse events reported being nausea, dizziness, and vomiting. Nausea was the most frequently reported event for the 23 mg per day group NNH 10 (95% CI 7–15).

Implications for practice

The results suggest that memantine and donepezil (23 mg per day) have clinically meaningful benefit for patients with moderate to severe AD. However, all the trials were short in duration and further studies are warranted to assess long-term outcomes of such treatment in this fragile population. Cost–benefit analysis is also warranted. Additional studies are needed to further assess the benefit of higher dose donepezil in light of the large withdrawal rate and increased rate of adverse events compared to the lower dose.

Treatment of agitated behavior in Alzheimer's disease

Agitated behavior in patients with AD or other forms of dementia is a common problem that often determines the timing of a transition to a skilled care facility, as caregivers, eventually, are unable to cope with these difficult-to-manage behaviors. Behavioral problems may include delusions, restlessness, aggression (verbal and physical), and anger. Several medications have been used to manage agitated behavior in dementia. This section reviews the data available concerning the efficacy of some common therapies.

Clinical scenario

A 78-year-old man with a 2-year history of progressive decline in memory and other cognitive functions has a diagnosis of AD. In recent months, his behavior has become increasingly agitated, with episodes of verbally aggressive behavior directed at his wife. He accuses her of infidelity when she leaves the house for any length of time and

Table 18.4 Efficacy and harm of cholinesterase inhibitor (donepezil) for moderate to severe AD

Intervention/ dosage	Outcome	Follow-up time	Treatment 23 mg per day number/ total (%)	10 mg per day number/ total (%)	LSM	Odds ratio (%)	Relative risk (95% CI)	Absolute Risk reduction (95% CI)	NNT or NNH (95% CI)	Comment
Donepezil 23 mg per day	Global rating*	24 weeks	908	459	ns	–	–	–	–	ns
	SIB†	24 weeks	907	462	2.2	–	–	–	–	Favors 23 mg per day
	One or more adverse events	24 weeks	710/963 (74)	300/471 (18)	–	–	–	–	10 (7–20)	Favors lower dosing
	Vomiting	24 weeks	89/963 (9)	12/300 (2.5)	–	–	–	–	20 (13–52)	Favors lower 10 mg per day

LSM, least squares mean changes; CI, confidence interval; WMD, weighted mean difference; NNH, number needed to harm; NNT, number needed to treat; ns, not statistically significant;
*Global rating an assessment of those showing improvement or no change or improvement on Clinician's Interview-Based Impression of Change, plus caregiver input (CIBIC- Plus;
†SIB, Severe Impairment Battery scores for treatment compared with lower dose; values are number/total (percentage) unless indicated otherwise.
Source: Data from Farlow et al. [34].

he is convinced that his family is conspiring against him. Even though there have been no physical altercations, he has thrown objects during his more agitated episodes. The patient has no history of psychiatric illness and was previously considered to be pleasant and soft-spoken. Routine laboratory tests demonstrated no major abnormalities, and repeat imaging of the brain is notable only for generalized cerebral atrophy. The patient's wife and children are concerned about the sustainability of his current living situation and ask how to deal with these behavioral problems.

Focused clinical question: *Which pharmacological treatment is effective in controlling agitated behavior in patients with dementia?*

Neuroleptics – haloperidol
Neuroleptics, particularly haloperidol, have been widely used for many years to control agitated states in dementia or psychosis. Significant side effects continue to be a problem with this medication and include over-sedation, hypotension, and extrapyramidal symptoms and on rare occasions neuroleptic malignant syndrome.

Evidence
A Cochrane systematic review identified five randomized, double-blind, placebo-controlled studies of differing duration. Three studies included AD and two studies included other forms of dementia; four of the studies described the subjects as having mild to moderate dementia [36]. Primary outcomes were global improvement, control of behavioral symptoms, reduced agitation, and functional status. Secondary outcomes were adverse events and dropout rates (Table 18.5).

Summary of results
Of the behavioral symptoms assessed in three trials, only aggression exhibited a benefit associated with haloperidol, effect size 0.31 (95% CI −0.49, −0.13) [36]. Four trials assessed agitation and general behavioral symptoms, and no evidence of an effect of haloperidol compared with placebo was found, effect size 0.12 (95% CI −0.33 to 0.08). No benefit was noted in global clinical state, effect size 1.50 (95% CI 0.88–2.55). There was no evidence of a significant difference of the rate of withdrawal due to adverse events between the treated and placebo groups. Seventy-five percent of the haloperidol and placebo subjects completed the study. Only two trials reported withdrawal numbers of patients suffering from at least one adverse event, favoring placebo (NNH 13). While it was not possible to pool the adverse events, there was a significant difference in favor of placebo for the number suffering at least one extrapyramidal symptom.

Commentary
The heterogeneity in dementia severity outcome measures used, as well as the varying dosage and duration of haloperidol treatment created major limitations in conducting the meta-analysis.

Clinical bottom line
No evidence was found for any significant general improvement with haloperidol treatment for symptoms of agitation other than aggression in subjects with dementia. An increase in the adverse event rate and dropouts (NNH 13; 95% CI 6–1632) was noted in the treatment groups compared with placebo. Significant side effects continue to be a problem with this medication including extrapyramidal symptoms, hypotension, and sedation.

Atypical antipsychotics
Second-generation (atypical) antipsychotic drugs such as risperidone, olanzapine, and quetiapine fumarate are widely used to treat psychosis, aggression, and agitation in patients with AD. Even though atypical antipsychotics are generally viewed as better tolerated than typical neuroleptics such as haloperidol, their benefits are uncertain, and concerns about safety have surfaced [37,38].

Evidence
A Cochrane systematic review identified 16 randomized, double-blind, placebo-controlled parallel group studies, five for risperidone, three for olanzapine, three for quetiapine, three for aripiprazole, one for risperidone, and one for olanzapine from published data and unpublished data requested from pharmaceutical companies for review. None of the trials of amisulpride, sertindole or zotepine met inclusion criteria. Participants were all identified to have AD, mixed or vascular dementias and were from nursing homes or institutions, either community dwelling or living in care facilities. Treatment duration was a minimum of 6 weeks. Outcome measures were agitation and aggression using the Cohen-Mansfield Agitation Inventory (CMAI) and the Behavior Pathology in Alzheimer's Disease Rating Scale (BEHAVE-AD). The clinical global impression of change (CGI-C) was used to assess global change. Adverse events including extrapyramidal symptoms and other side effects were recorded [37].

Summary of results
Only 9 of the 16 studies had sufficient data to contribute to the meta-analysis. Risperidone and olanzapine showed significant benefit for the treatment of aggression and psychosis, but with a very high placebo response rate in dementia (30–40%) (Table 18.6). Serious adverse cerebrovascular events (including stroke), extrapyramidal side effects, and other adverse outcomes were reported for both risperidone (1 mg per day, NNH 25 and 2 mg per day, NNH 27) and olanzapine (5–10 mg per day, NNH 8). Dropouts were more frequent in the higher dose risperidone, 2.0 mg per day (42%) compared to placebo (30%). The withdrawal rate for olanzapine was significant compared to placebo (11% and 3%). Results were available from only one 10-week study on aripiprazole. The 2–15 mg per day dosing of aripiprazole showed benefit compared with placebo for

Table 18.5 Efficacy and harm of neuroleptics for agitation in AD

Intervention/ dosage	Number of trials	Outcome	Follow-up time	Treatment number/ total (%)	Placebo number/ total (%)	MD (95% CI)	Odds ratio (%)	Relative risk (95% CI)	Absolute risk reduction (95% CI)	NNT or NNH (95% CI)	Comment
Neuroleptic Haloperidol	2	Global improvement CGIC*	16 weeks	9/135 (66)	82/139 (58)	–	1.50 (0.88–2.55)	–	0.52 (0.42–0.61)	1	No significant difference
	4	Agitation CMAI†	16 weeks	194	175	–0.12 (–0.33 to 0.08)	–	–	–	–	Slightly favors haloperidol
	4	Behavior BEHAVE-AD‡	16 weeks	194	175	–0.19 (–0.40 to 0.01)	–	–	–	–	Favors haloperidol
	5	One or more adverse events	16 weeks	169/216 (78)	152/217 (70)	–	1.53 (1–2.35)	–	–0.62 (0.163–0.01)	13 (–6 to 1632)	Favors placebo
	1	Extrapyramidal symptoms	16 weeks	34/101	18/103	–	2.34 (1.25–4.38)	–	0.162 (0.276–0.042)	7 (4–24)	Favors placebo

CI, confidence interval; WMD, weighted mean difference; NNT, number needed to treat; NNH, number needed to harm;
*CGIC, Clinical Global Impression of Change: a scale to assess improvement in overall condition;
†CMAI, Cohen-Mansfield Agitation Inventory: indicates no change or improvement in behaviors;
‡BEHAVE-AD, Behavioral Pathology in Alzheimer's Disease: treatment compared with placebo.
Source: Data from Lonergan et al. [36].

Table 18.6 Efficacy and harm of atypical antipsychotics for agitation in AD

Intervention/ dosage	Number of trials	Outcome	Follow-up time	Treatment number/ total (%)	Placebo number/ total (%)	MD (95% CI)	Odds ratio (%)	Relative risk (95% CI)	Absolute risk reduction (95% CI)	NNT or NNH (95% CI)	Comment
Atypical antipsychotics	—	CMAI†	NA	—	—	—	—	—	—	—	—
Aripiprazole (2–15 mg per day)	1	BEHAVE-AD‡	10 weeks	106	102	—	−1.03 (−2.50 to 0.44)	—	—	—	Favors aripiprazole
	1	One or more adverse events	10 weeks	8/106	7/102	—	1.11 (0.39–3.18)	—	−0.007 (−0.082 to 0.069)	147 (−12 to 15)	Favors placebo
	—	Cerebrovascular events	10 weeks	—	—	—	—	—	—	—	—
	1	Death	10 weeks	4/106 (4)	0/102 (0)	—	9 (0.48–169.32)	—	−0.033 (−0.088 to 0.013)	31 (−11 to 75)	Favors placebo
Quetiapine (50–100 mg per day)	1	CMAI†	26	27	30	—	0.90 (−6.70 to 8.50)	—	—	—	Favors quetiapine
	—	BEHAVE-AD‡	NA	—	—	—	—	—	—	—	—
	1	SIB	26 weeks	15	19	14.61 (25.71 to −3.49)	—	—	—	—	Favors quetiapine
	—	One or more adverse events	NA	—	—	—	—	—	—	—	—
	—	Cerebrovascular events	NA	—	—	—	—	—	—	—	—
Risperidone (1 mg per day)	3	CMAI†	10–13 weeks	453	356	1.17 (2.02–0.32)	—	—	—	—	Favors risperidone
	5	BEHAVE-AD or NPI‡	10–13 weeks	602	518	0.17 (0.29–0.05)	—	—	—	—	Favors risperidone
	5	One or more adverse events	10–13 weeks	453/550 (82)	447/571 (78)	1.33 (0.98–1.80)	—	—	0.041 (0.087–0.006)	25 (11–171)	Favors placebo
Risperidone (2 mg per day)	1	CMAI†	10–13 weeks	—	—	−1.17 (−2.02 to −0.32)	—	—	—	—	Favors risperidone
	1	BEHAVE-AD‡	10–13 weeks	—	—	−1.5 (−2.05 to −0.95)	—	—	—	—	Favors risperidone
	3	One or more adverse events	8–13 weeks	146/165 (88)	138/163 (85)	1.39 (0.73–2.64)	1.11 (0.90–1.38)	—	0.36 (0.113–0.036)	27 (9–27)	Favors placebo
Risperidone all doses (0.5–2 mg)	5	Cerebrovascular events	8–13 weeks	37/1175 (3)	8/779 (1)	—	3.64 (1.72–7.69)	—	—	48 (30–123)	Favors placebo
	5	Deaths	8–13 weeks	37/1175 (3)	8/779 (1)	—	1.25 (0.73–2.16)	—	—	48 (30–123)	Favors placebo

Olanzapine (5–10 mg per day)									Favors olanzapine
2	NPI-NH	6–10 weeks	51	45	0.70 (−10.66 to 11.46)	–	–	–	Favors placebo
2	One or more adverse events	6–10 weeks	9/53 (17)	2/47 (4)	–	4.60 (0.94–22.51)	0.127 (0.254–0.001)	8 (4–1654)	–
NA	Cerebrovascular events	6–10 weeks	–	–	–	–	–	–	Favors placebo
2	Death	6–10 weeks	14/460 (3)	22/223 (9)	–	2.31 (0.66–8.13)	0.068 (0.03–0.116)	14 (9–33)	

CI, confidence interval; WMD, weighted mean difference; NNT, number needed to treat; NNH, number needed to harm;

†CMAI, Cohen-Mansfield Agitation Inventory: indicates no change or improvement in behaviors;

‡NPI, Neuropsychiatric Inventory to show improvement scores for treatment compared with placebo; BEHAVE-AD, Behavioral Pathology in Alzheimer's Disease treatment compared with placebo.

Source: Data from Ballard et al. [37].

psychosis. Out of four studies on quetiapine, only one was used for meta-analysis. The effect size on agitation was 0.90, which was not statistically significant, and showed harm compared to placebo at 26 weeks [37].

Commentary

Appraisal of the data uncovered methodological problems that could result in overestimation of the effect size. Data were noted to be incomplete, not allowing for a full pooling of data. The behavioral and neuropsychiatric symptoms of AD are complex and the trials had a low threshold for behavioral symptoms, making it difficult to determine the improvement in clinically significant agitation. Two studies combined patients with clinical diagnoses of either AD or vascular dementia, but did not present outcome data separately, making it impossible to assess outcomes specifically for AD.

Clinical bottom line

Risperidone and olanzapine are beneficial in reducing aggression in dementia, effect size −1.05 (95% CI −2.05 to −0.95). There are insufficient data to conduct a meaningful evaluation of the efficacy of any of the therapies on cognition. There is an increased mortality for people with AD who are treated with atypical neuroleptics compared to those receiving placebo. Both are associated with serious adverse cerebrovascular events and extrapyramidal symptoms. Additional meta-analysis similarly found an increase in mortality, OR 1.54 (95% CI 0.004−0.02) for this class of drug [36]. This is in line with the meta-analysis conducted by the Food and Drug Administration suggesting an increase in mortality (OR 1.7), prompting a black box warning on atypical neuroleptics. The use of atypical neuroleptics is not recommended for routine use of behavioral symptoms of AD, but rather clinicians may find case-by-case applications necessary when aggressive behaviors are the primary symptom.

Antiepileptics – valproic acid

The mechanism of action to treat agitation in dementia is unclear for the antiepileptic drug valproic acid. Yet it has been used over the last two decades to stabilize mood and manage agitation in dementia. Divalproex sodium is thought to be better tolerated.

Evidence

A Cochrane systematic review meta-analysis was conducted on an updated systematic review from 2008 on two additional randomized placebo-controlled trials on the effect of valproate on agitation in demented institutionalized patients [39]. Study interventions included either sodium valproate or divalproex sodium tablets over a duration of 3−6 weeks. Outcome measures were effects on behavioral disturbance (agitation, aggression, and mania), overall functional status, adverse events, tolerability, and safety.

Summary of results

High-dose divalproex sodium (median dose, 1000 mg per day) is not tolerated in this patient population, and low-dose divalproex sodium (480 mg per day) is ineffective for agitation. Meta-analysis of efficacy in treating agitation and aggression was not feasible, given variations in methods, valproic acid formulation, duration of treatment, and patient assessment methods. In the pooled data from three studies comparing divalproex 148/197 (75%) and placebo 119/197 (60%), the total number of patients who suffered any serious events at 6 weeks favored placebo, effect size 1.99 (95% CI 1.29−3.08), NNH 22 (95% CI 6−13) [39].

Commentary

The high dropout rates and the heterogeneity of drug dosing, duration of treatment and patient assessment, and treatment response measures created flaws that limited the ability to pool data for analysis.

Clinical bottom line

The results of two studies could not be interpreted, and the third showed no benefit relative to placebo in overall global improvement. Behavioral symptoms of agitation and aggression showed no significant improvement, effect size −2.20 (95% CI −6.38 to 1.99). In one study, 54% of treated patients versus 29% of control patients dropped out because of adverse effects, prompting discontinuation of the study. In another study, no significant difference in adverse effects was noted between treatment and placebo groups. In the third study, 68% of treated patients experienced adverse effects compared with 33% of the placebo group, although no adverse effects prompted withdrawal. Overall, high-dose divalproex sodium (median dose, 1000 mg per day) was associated with an unacceptable frequency of adverse effects.

Antidepressants – SSRIs and trazodone

Given the limited benefits associated with antipsychotics, there is an increasing interest in treating the behavioral symptoms of AD with antidepressant therapy. It is estimated that 30−40% of dementia patients receive antidepressants [40]. Selective serotonin reuptake inhibitors (SSRIs) are considered to be a safer alternative by many clinicians. Other psychoactive compounds with antidepressant properties such as trazodone are of interest for managing agitation in dementia. There are several studies on the subject that provide data for a comprehensive review.

Evidence

A Cochrane systematic review identified nine randomized-controlled comparison trials of antidepressants to either placebo or other psychotropic medications from published data and unpublished data requested from pharmaceutical companies. There were five studies comparing SSRIs to

Table 18.7 Efficacy and harm of antidepressant for agitation in AD based on reference

Intervention/ dosage	Number of trials	Outcome	Follow-up time	Treatment number/ total (%)	Placebo number/ total (%)	MD (95% CI)	Odds ratio (%)	Relative risk (95% CI)	Absolute risk reduction (95% CI	NNT or NNH (95% CI)	Comment
Antidepressants											
SSRIs (sertraline, citalopram fluvoxamine)	2	CMAI[†]	4–12 weeks	126	124	0.89 (–1.22 to 0.57)	–	–	–	–	Favors SSRI
	1	NPI[‡]	4–12 weeks	121	119	1.80 ns	–	–	–	–	No statistical difference
	1	BEHAVE-AD**	4–12 weeks	–	–	–0.70 ns	–	–	–	–	No statistical difference
	3	Withdrawals[§]	4–12 weeks	45/177 (25)	44/166 (27)	–0.70 ns	–	0.91 (0.65–1.26)	–	–	Unknown
	3	One or more adverse events	4–12 weeks	24/200 (14)	21/199 (11)	–	–	1.07 (0.55–2.11)	–	–	No difference
Trazadone (50–300 mg per day)	1	CAMI[†]	–	37	36	5.18 ns	–	–	–	–	No significant difference
	–	BEHAVE-AD[‡]	NA	–	–	–	–	–	–	–	–
	–	SIB**	NA	–	–	–	–	–	–	–	–
	1	Withdrawals[§]	NA	12/37 (32)	11/36 (30)	–	–	–	1.06 (0.54–2.09)	–	Unknown
	–	One or more adverse events	NA	–	–	–	–	–	–	–	–

CI, confidence interval; WMD, weighted mean difference; NNT, number needed to treat; NNH, number needed to harm; ns, not statistically significant;

*CGIC, Clinical Global Impression of Change: a scale to assess improvement in overall condition;

[†]CMAI, Cohen-Mansfield Agitation Inventory: indicates no change or improvement in behaviors;

[‡]NPI, Neuropsychiatric Inventory showing improvement scores for treatment compared with placebo; BEHAVE-AD, Behavioral Pathology in Alzheimer's Disease: treatment compared with placebo;

[§]Withdrawals any reason.

Source: Data from Seitz S. [41].

placebo (sertraline, citalopram): three comparing SSRIs to typical antipsychotics (haloperidol) and two studies comparing trazodone to haloperidol, with a total of 692 individuals. Primary outcome was the treatment of psychosis, agitation or neuropsychiatric symptoms in subjects with dementia. Individuals diagnosed with AD, vascular or mixed AD, dementia with Lewy bodies and dementia not otherwise specified were included in the review [41].

Summary of results

Five studies compared SSRIs to placebo and two studies were combined in a meta-analysis for the outcome of change in agitation (Table 18.7). There was a significant difference between antidepressants and placebo on measures of agitation as reported on the change in CMAI total score, although the results were heavily weighted by one large study. In meta-analysis of two studies, there were no statistically significant differences in changes in CMAI total scores. There were no differences in the rates of trial withdrawals due to adverse events for SSRIs compared to placebo for four studies reporting this outcome or in the number of trial withdrawals due to any cause in the three studies reporting this outcome. There was also no difference in trial withdrawals due to any cause or due to adverse events for SSRIs compared to typical antipsychotics. One study of trazodone compared to placebo did not find any significant difference in change in CMAI total score or trial withdrawals due to any cause. Two studies comparing trazodone to haloperidol also failed to detect any difference in change in CMAI total scores [41].

Commentary

Only a small number of studies exist with varied methodology, reducing the number of trials that could be included in a meta-analysis. Withdrawal in both the SSRI (25%) and placebo (27%) groups was higher, limiting interpretability and validity of trials. Adverse events were not uniformly reported in the trials, making it difficult to determine the true frequency of adverse events. Further studies are required to determine the effectiveness and safety of SSRIs and trazodone in managing agitation and other behavioral symptoms in AD.

Clinical bottom line

Reduced symptoms of agitation favored sertraline and citalopram compared to placebo with an effect size of 0.89 (95% CI −1.22 to −0.057). There was no evidence that trazodone provides any clinical improvement in symptoms of agitation in AD. The SSRIs appear to be well tolerated, but adverse events may have been under-reported.

Other – Memantine

In the Cochrane systematic review on memantine and dementia, data suggest that patients taking memantine were slightly less likely to develop agitation (134/1739, [7.7%] vs 175/1873, [9.3%] OR 0.78, 95% CI 0.61–0.99, $P=0.04$). This effect was slightly larger, but still small, in moderate to severe AD (58/506 [12%] vs 88/499 [18%]; OR = 0.6, 95% CI 0.42–0.86, $P=0.005$). There is no evidence either way about whether it has an effect on agitation, as previously reviewed in Question 2. Memantine is well tolerated [32].

Clinical implications

Our clinical question cannot be clearly answered by the evidence; there are no FDA-approved drugs for behavioral symptoms of AD. The trials are small, of short duration, and indicate only weak benefit with increased serious adverse events including death. The lifetime risk of developing significant psychopathology in dementia is thought to be nearly 100% and yet treatment options remain insufficiently studied and controversial [42]. The clinician is left with modest trial results, clinical experience, and caregiver preference to guide them. The need for increased research in this area is apparent.

Conclusion

Beginning, as always, with familiar clinical scenarios and vignettes, this evidence-based review of therapies for mild cognitive impairment and Alzheimer's disease has carefully outlined the central clinical question related to treatment of cognitive decline in the setting of probable AD. We have emphasized the clinical bottom-line messages by including both the statistical and clinically relevant measures in our analysis. This evidence-based appraisal is intended to better equip clinicians to combine this best evidence with their own clinical experience and the wishes of their patients to arrive at sensible answers during the clinical decision-making process.

References

1 Kokmen, E., Beard, C.M., O'Brien, P.C. *et al.* (1996) Epidemiology of dementia in Rochester, Minnesota. *Mayo Clinic Proceedings*, **71**, 275–282.

2 Hebert, L.E., Scherr, P.A., Bienias, J.L. *et al.* (2003) Alzheimer disease in the US population: prevalence estimates using the 2000 census. *Archives of Neurology*, **60**, 1119–1122.

3 Bower, J.H., Maraganore, D.M., McDonnell, S.K. *et al.* (1999) Incidence and distribution of Parkinsonism in Olmsted County, Minnesota, 1976–1990. *Neurology*, **52**, 1214–1220.

4 Sherrington, R., Rogaev, E.I., Liang, Y. *et al.* (1995) Cloning of a gene bearing missense mutations in early-onset familial Alzheimer's disease. *Nature*, **375**, 754–760.

5 Wisniewski, K.E., Wisniewski, H.M. & Wen, G.Y. (1985) Occurrence of neuropathological changes and dementia of Alzheimer's disease in Down's syndrome. *Annals of Neurology*, **17**, 278–282.

6 Levy-Lahad, E., Wasco, W., Poorkaj, P. *et al.* (1995) Candidate gene for the chromosome 1 familial Alzheimer's disease locus. *Science*, **269**, 973–977.

7 Hardy, J.A. & Higgins, G.A. (1992) Alzheimer's disease: the amyloid cascade hypothesis. *Science*, **256**, 184–185.

8 Corder, E.H., Saunders, A.M., Strittmatter, W.J. *et al.* (1993) Gene dose of apolipoprotein E type 4 allele and the risk of Alzheimer's disease in late onset families. *Science*, **261**, 921–923.

9 Corbo, R.M. & Scacchi, R. (1999) Apolipoprotein E (APOE) allele distribution in the world: is APOE4 a 'thrifty' allele? *Annals of Human Genetics*, **63**(Pt 4), 301–310.

10 U.S. Congress Office of Technology Assessment (1987) *Losing a Million Minds: Confronting the Tragedy of Alzheimer's Disease and Other Dementias, OTA-BA-323.* U.S. Government Printing Office, Washington, DC.

11 Rice, D.P., Fillit, H.M., Max, W. *et al.* (2001) Prevalence, costs, and treatment of Alzheimer's disease and related dementia: a managed care perspective. *The American Journal of Managed Care*, **7**, 809–818.

12 Shumaker, S.A., Legault, C., Rapp, S.R. *et al.* (2003) WHIMS Investigators. Estrogen plus progestin and the incidence of dementia and mild cognitive impairment in postmenopausal women: the Women's Health Initiative Memory Study: a randomized controlled trial. *JAMA*, **289**, 2651–2662.

13 Aisen, P.S., Schafer, K.A., Grundman, M. *et al.* (2003) Alzheimer's Disease Cooperative Study. Effects of rofecoxib or naproxen vs placebo on Alzheimer disease progression: a randomized controlled trial. *JAMA*, **289**, 2819–2826.

14 Petersen, R.C., Thomas, R.G., Grundman, M. *et al.* (2005) Alzheimer's Disease Cooperative Study Group. Vitamin E and donepezil for the treatment of mild cognitive impairment. *New England Journal of Medicine*, **9**(352), 2379–2388.

15 Aisen, P.S., Schneider, L.S., Sano, M., Diaz-Arrastia, R., van Dyck, C.H. *et al.* (2008) High-dose B vitamin supplementation and cognitive decline in Alzheimer disease: a randomized controlled trial. *JAMA*, **300**(15), 1774–1783.

16 Snitz, B.E., O'Meara, E.S., Carlson, M.C. *et al.* (2010) Ginkgo biloba for preventing cognitive decline in older adults: a randomized trial. *JAMA*, **302**(24), 2663–2670.

17 Rogers, S.L., Farlow, M.R., Doody, R.S. *et al.* (1998) Donepezil Study Group. A 24-week, double-blind, placebo-controlled trial of donepezil in patients with Alzheimer's disease. *Neurology*, **50**, 136–145.

18 Reisberg, B., Doody, R., Stoffler, A. *et al.* (2003) Memantine Study Group. Memantine in moderate-to-severe Alzheimer's disease. *New England Journal of Medicine*, **348**, 1333–1341.

19 Dubinsky, R.M., Stein, A.C. & Lyons, K. (2000) Practice parameter: risk of driving and Alzheimer's disease (an evidence-based review): report of the quality standards subcommittee of the American Academy of Neurology. *Neurology*, **54**, 2205–2211.

20 Petersen, R.C., Knopman, D., Boeve, B. *et al.* (2009) Mild cognitive impairment: ten years later. *Archives of Neurology*, **66**(22), 1447–1455.

21 Gauthier, S., Reisberg, B., Zaudig, M. *et al.* (2006) Mild cognitive impairment. *Lancet*, **367**, 1262–1270.

22 Birks, J. & Flicker, L. (2010) Donepezil for mild cognitive impairment. *Cochrane Database of Systematic Reviews*,(**3**), CD006104 DOI: 10.1002/14651858.CD006104.

23 Loy, C. & Schneider, L. (2006) Galantamine for Alzheimer's disease and mild cognitive impairment. *Cochrane Database of Systematic Reviews*,(**25**), DOI: 10.1002/14651858.CD001747.pub3.

24 Sobów, T. & Ktoszewskai, I. (2007) Cholinestrase inhibitors in mild cognitive impairment; a met-analysis of randomized controlled trials. *Neurologia i Neurochirurgia Polska*, **41**, 13–21.

25 Raschetti, R., Albanese, E., Vancore, N., Maggini, M. *et al.* (2007) Cholinesterase inhibitiors in mild cognitive impairment: a systematic review of randomized trials. *PLoS Medicine*, **4**(**11**), 1818–1828.

26 Diniz, B.S., Pinto, J.A., Gonzaga, M.L.C. *et al.* (2009) To treat or not to treat? A meta-analysis of the use of cholinesterase inhibitors in mild cognitive impairment for delaying progression to Alzheimer's disease. *European Archives of Psychiatry and Clinical Neuroscience*, **259**, 248–256.

27 Jadad, A.R., Moore, R.A., Carroll, D. *et al.* (1996) Assessing the quality of reports of randomized clinical trials: is blinding necessary? *Controlled Clinical Trials*, **17**(**1**), 1–12.

28 Malouf, R. & Collins, H. (2009) Tramiprosate (Alzhemed) for Alzheimer's disease (Protocol). *Cochrane Database of Systematic Reviews*,(**1**), CD007549 DOI: 10.1002/14651858.CD007549.

29 Whitehead, A., Perdomo, C., Pratt, R.D. *et al.* (2004) Donepezil for the symptomatic treatment of patients with middle to moderate Alzheimer's disease: meta-analysis of individual patient data from randomized controlled trials. *International Journal of Geriatric Psychiatry*, **19**, 624–633.

30 Hussar, D.A. (2003) New drugs. *Journal of the American Pharmacists Association*, **44**(**2**), 168–206.

31 Birks, J. (2006) Cholinesterase inhibitors for Alzheimer's disease. *Cochrane Database of Systematic Reviews*,(**1**), CD005593 DOI: 10.1002/14651858.CD005593.

32 McShane, R., Areosa Sastre, A. & Minakaran, N. (2006) Memantine for dementia. *Cochrane Database of Systematic Reviews*,(**2**), CD003154 DOI: 10.1002/14651858.CD003154.pub5.

33 Farlow, M.R. (2004) Utilizing combination therapy in the treatment of Alzheimer's disease. *Expert Review of Neurotherapeutics*, **4**(**5**), 799–808.

34 Farlow, M.R., Salloway, S., Tariot, P.N. *et al.* (2010) Effectiveness and tolerability of high-dose (23 mg/d) versus standard-dose (10 mg/d) donepezil in moderate to severe Alzheimer's disease: A 24–week, randomized, double-blind study. *Clinical Therapeutics*, **32**(**7**), 1234–1251.

35 Winblad, B., Jones, R.W., Wirth, Y. *et al.* (2007) Memantine in moderate to severe Alzheimer's disease: a meta-analysis of randomized clinical trials. *Dementia and Geriatric Cognitive Disorders*, **24**, 20–27.

36 Lonergan, E., Luxenberg, J. & Colford, J. (2002) Haloperidol for agitation in dementia. *Cochrane Database of Systematic Reviews*,(**2**), CD002852 DOI: 10.1002/14651858.CD002852.

37 Ballard, C.G., Waite, J. & Birks, J. (2008) Atypical antipsychotics for aggression and psychosis in Alzheimer's disease. *Cochrane Database of Systematic Reviews*, **4**, CD003476.

38 Schneider, L.S., Tariot, P.N., Dagerman, K.S. *et al.* (2006) Effectiveness of atypical antipsychotic drugs in patients with Alzheimer's disease. *JAMA*, **355**(15), 1525–1537.

39 Lonergan, E.T. & Luxenberg, J. (2004) Valproate preparations for agitation in dementia. *Cochrane Database of Systematic Reviews*, (**2**), CD003945 DOI: 10.1002/14651858.CD003945.pub2.

40 Pitkala, K.H., Laurila, J.V., Stradber, T.E. *et al.* (2004) Behavioral symptoms and the administration of psychotropic drugs to aged patients with dementia in nursing homes and in acute geriatric wards. *International Psychogeriatrics*, **16**(1), 61–74.

41 Seitz, D.P., Adunuri, N., Gill, S.S., Gruneir, A., Herrmann, N. & Rochon, P. (2011) Antidepressants for agitation and psychosis in dementia. *Cochrane Database of Systematic Reviews*, (**2**), CD008191 DOI: 10.1002/14651858.CD008191.pub2.

42 Burke, A.D. & Tariot, P.N. (2009) Atypical antipsychotics in the elderly: a review of therapeutic trends and clinical outcomes. *Expert Opinion on Pharmacotherapy*, **10**(15), 2408–2414.

CHAPTER 19

Evidence-based treatment of Parkinson's disease

Nicholas D. Child[1] and Bryan T. Klassen[2]
[1]*Department of Neurology, Mayo Clinic College of Medicine, Rochester, MN, USA*
[2]*College of Medicine, Mayo Clinic, Rochester, MN, USA*

Background

Parkinson's disease (PD) is one of the most common neurodegenerative disorders and is associated with neuronal loss in the dopaminergic neurons of the substantia nigra pars compacta, with resultant loss of striatal dopaminergic input. The cardinal motor features of this disease include asymmetric rest tremor, bradykinesia, rigidity, and postural instability. Particularly in advanced PD, non-motor manifestations of disease can be significant and may include cognitive decline or dementia, mood disorders such as depression and anxiety, sleep disorders, and dysautonomia.

Levodopa therapy was the first treatment able to effect substantial improvement in motor symptoms and remains the most efficacious treatment for PD. However, over time, motor complications such as clinical fluctuations and drug-induced dyskinesia may emerge. Multiple adjunctive medications, as well as surgical therapies including deep brain stimulation have been used in an attempt to normalize motor function and improve quality of life. Given the myriad approaches one could adopt to treat PD in its early and later stages a thorough understanding of the evidence supporting the various treatments is critical.

Clinical questions

1 In patients with early PD, how do the first-line pharmacological treatments change the UPDRS motor score and affect the probability of motor fluctuations and dyskinesia?

2 In patients with PD and levodopa-induced motor complications, to what extent do adjunctive pharmacologic therapies improve motor fluctuations or dyskinesia.

3 In patients with PD and levodopa-induced motor complications, to what extent does deep brain stimulation targeting the subthalamic nucleus or globus pallidus interna improve motor fluctuations, dyskinesia, and quality of life.

Search strategy

We conducted a systematic search of the literature, using the MEDLINE electronic database (1966–2013) and the reference lists from evidence-based review reports [1–3]. Papers were selected for review if they met the following criteria: (1) randomized study, (2) non-randomized controlled or non-controlled prospective or retrospective study, (3) patients with a diagnosis of PD, (4) end points including establish rating scales, (5) ≥20 patients, (6) ≥3 weeks treatment period, and (7) paper published in English. Exclusion criteria included (1) outcome measures non-validated or unconventional, (2) duplicated reports, (3) uncertain length of follow-up, (4) non-English publications, (5) report in the form of an abstract, and (6) head-to-head trials comparing different dopamine agonists.

Critical review of the evidence

Early Parkinson's disease

In patients with early PD, how do the first-line pharmacological treatments change the UPDRS motor score and affect the probability of motor fluctuations and dyskinesia?

Levodopa immediate release

The ELLDOPA trial, a randomized, double-blind, placebo-controlled trial of 361 patients with early PD were randomized to either carbidopa/levodopa at 37.5/150 mg, 75/300 mg, or 150/600 mg per day or matching placebo for 40 weeks followed by withdrawal of treatment for 2 weeks [4]. The primary outcome was the change in UPDRS score

Evidence-Based Neurology: Management of Neurological Disorders, Second Edition. Edited by Bart M. Demaerschalk and Dean M. Wingerchuk.
© 2015 John Wiley & Sons, Ltd. Published 2015 by John Wiley & Sons, Ltd.

between baseline and 42 weeks. At 42 weeks, the mean difference between the total UPDRS score was 7.8, 1.9, 1.9, and −1.4 in the placebo for 150-, 300-, and 600-mg groups, respectively. The 600-mg group had more frequent dyskinesia, nausea, infection hypertonia, and headache. A subset of the patients had [^{123}I]β-CIT studies, which showed that at 40 weeks compared to baseline the mean percent decline was significantly greater with levodopa than placebo, (percent change: −2.6, −4.7, −3.7, and −6.9 for placebo, 150 mg, 300 mg, and 600 mg per day, respectively; $P = 0.15$).

Levodopa-controlled release formulations

A total of 618 patients were studied in a blinded randomized parallel study comparing immediate-release (IR) and sustained-release (CR) carbidopa/levodopa in early PD [5]. At 5 years, 20.6% of the IR and 21.8% of the CR group had motor fluctuations or dyskinesia, and the UPDRS Part II score was slightly better in the CR group than the IR group (8.4 vs 8.8; $P = 0.031$).

A new novel extended release oral formation of carbidopa/levodopa in a 1:4 ratio has recently been developed to attain rapid levodopa concentrations and then maintain the concentration of levodopa in the therapeutic range for a prolonged duration [6,7]. Pharmacokinetic data show that IPX066 results in a similarly rapid peak concentration as immediate-release carbidopa-levodopa, and is sustained above 50% of peak concentration for 4 hours versus 1.4 hours ($P < 0.001$) [8]. IPX066 had lower dosing frequency, yet had reduced plasma levodopa concentration variability. A randomized, double-blind, placebo-controlled study of 381 levodopa-naive patients assigned to either placebo or IPX066 reported a mean improvement in UPDRS Parts II + III at 30 weeks compared to baseline of 11.7, 12.9, and 14.9 points for dosages of 145, 245, or 390 mg of levodopa, respectively versus 0.6 points for placebo ($P < 0.0001$, for all doses) [9]. IPX066 has recently been approved by the FDA and is marketed under the tradename Rytary.

Dopamine agonists

Pramipexole

A delayed-start randomized, double-blind trial of pramipexole in early PD (PROUD) to identify whether early versus delayed pramipexole initiation had clinical or neuroimaging benefits in 261 patients with PD recruited to either placebo or pramipexole and followed for 15 months, with the placebo group allowed to switch to pramipexole at 9 months or 6 months if necessary, found no significant difference in UPDRS total score between the two groups (−0.4 points, 95% CI −2.2 to 1.4, $P = 0.65$) [10]. Neuroimaging with striatal dopamine-transporter binding assessed by SPECT found a differential ^{123}I-FP-CIT binding of −0.5 percentage points, 95% CI −5.4 to 4.4, $P = 0.84$ between the groups.

The 2- and 4-year data of the CALM-PD, a multicenter, parallel-group, double-blind, randomized, controlled trial of initial treatment of pramipexole versus levodopa in 301 patients with early PD has been published [11,12]. Patients were randomized to either pramipexole 0.5 mg three times daily with placebo or carbidopa/levodopa three times daily with placebo with open-label levodopa allowed after 10 weeks to treat residual motor symptoms. At 2 years, the mean improvement in total UPDRS score from baseline was 9.2 vs 4.5 points ($P < 0.001$) for levodopa compared to pramipexole group; however, those in the pramipexole group had less wearing off, dyskinesia, or on–off motor fluctuations (28%) compared to levodopa (51%) (hazard ratio 0.45, 95% CI 0.30–0.66, $P < 0.001$) [12]. At 48 months, the mean score reduction in total UPDRS from baseline was 2±15.4 points vs −3.2±17.3 points, $P = 0.003$ in the levodopa versus pramipexole groups [11]. However, 45% of patients in the pramipexole group versus 33% in the levodopa group had dropped out by this stage (somnolence: pramipexole = 11; levodopa = 1; edema: pramipexole = 5). More patients developed motor complications in the levodopa group than the pramipexole group (74% vs 52% levodopa and pramipexole respectively; hazard ratio 0.48, 95% CI, 0.35–0.66, $P < 0.001$). A substudy of 82 patients in CALM-PD underwent dopamine transporter imaging using single-photon emission computed tomography with 2β-carboxymethoxy-3β(4-iodophenyl)tropane (β-CIT) labeled with iodine 123 to asses rates of dopamine neuron degeneration [13]. Sequential imaging demonstrated a reduction in loss of striatal [^{123}I]β-CIT uptake, a marker of dopamine neuron degeneration in those initially treated with pramipexole compared to levodopa, 16.0% vs 25.5% at 46 months ($P = 0.01$). There was a correlation of the percentage loss of striatal [^{123}I]β-CIT uptake from baseline with change in total UPDRS score from baseline in all patients.

A study of 311 patients with early PD who were randomized to either placebo or pramipexole at doses of either 0.5 or 0.75 mg twice daily or 0.5 mg three times daily [14] was conducted in 2011. Treatment was efficacious compared to placebo with mean reduction in total UPDRS score comparable among the three active treatment groups: 0.75 mg bid: 4.7 (95% confidence interval [CI] 2.5–6.9); 0.5 mg bid: 4.4 (95% CI 2.3–6.5); 0.5 mg tid: 4.4 (95% CI 2.3–6.5), $P < 0.0001$ for each comparison to placebo. Side effects were similar in all three active arms and more common than placebo and were typical of dopamine agonists.

There are three other placebo-controlled trials of pramipexole [15–17]. An initial parallel, placebo-controlled trial in 55 patients using an ascending dose of pramipexole up to a maximum of 4.5 mg per day with all subjects receiving selegiline (10 mg per day) found a statistically significant improvement in the UPDRS Part II (activities of daily living) of 5.19 vs 2.16 ($P = 0.002$), and a trend favoring pramipexole for the UPDRS Part III 11.97 vs 8.31 at 9 weeks [15]. There was a relatively strong placebo effect in this study. Two further placebo-controlled studies in early PD were published in 1997. In the first study, 264 patients were randomized to pramipexole doses of either 1.5, 3.0, 4.5, and 6.0 mg per day or matching placebo, with a 6-week dose escalation period followed by a 4-week maintenance period [16]. The mean difference between baseline and end total UPDRS scores for each group were −0.9 for placebo, −6.3, −5.9, −6.5, and −7.0 for 1.5, 3.0, 4.5, and 6.0 mg per day groups, respectively which were all statistically significant ($P < 0.005$). There was a trend toward both greater efficacy but also more clinical adverse events in the higher dose groups. A longer randomized, double-blind, placebo-controlled, parallel-group study with a 24-week period of maintenance treatment involving 335 patients with a mean dose of 3.8 mg of pramipexole found a significant improvement in UPDRS Part II and III (motor score) of 8.2 versus end maintenance 6.4 and 18.8 versus end maintenance 14.1 compared to placebo [17].

Ropinirole

A study comparing the now-discontinued sumanirole, a dopamine agonist, and ropinirole to placebo in 614 patients with early PD in a flexible-dose, double-blind, double-dummy, parallel-group of 40-week duration comparing change in UPDRS Parts II + III found a mean change of −5.20 in the ropinirole group versus a 0.38 increase in the placebo arm, $P < 0.001$ [18]. Twenty-four percent of patients in the ropinirole group and 8% in the placebo group withdrew because of side effects with the commonest in the ropinirole arm being daytime sleepiness and nausea.

There are two placebo-controlled [19,20] and three levodopa-controlled [21–23] studies of ropinirole for management of early PD. A randomized, placebo-controlled, double-blind, parallel-group study of 241 patients compared ropinirole to placebo, with the mean total daily dose of medicine at end point 15.6 mg per day, found an improvement in UPDRS Part III (motor score) from 17.9 to 13.4 points, a statistically significant improvement of 24% in the ropinirole arm compared with placebo [19]. In a second double-blind trial, patients were randomized to either ropinirole or placebo. There was a 43.4% improvement in UPDRS Part III scores in the ropinirole group compared to 21.0% in the placebo group, a statistically significant difference ($P = 0.018$, ANOVA; 95% CI −40.8%, −4.0) [20].

When compared to levodopa, ropinirole is not as efficacious but has reduced risk of dyskinesia. In the REAL-PET, a randomized, double-blind, 2-year study of [18]Fluro-dopa uptake (Ki) with positron emission tomography scans, comparing ropinirole and levodopa, found that the initial improvement in UPDRS motor scores was retained for levodopa but not ropinirole with the mean UPDRS motor score increasing by 0.70 points compared to a decrease of 5.64 for the levodopa group [23]. There was, however, significantly

fewer patients in the ropinirole arm who experienced dyskinesia (3.4% vs 26.7%; OR 0.09, 95% CI 0.02–0.29; $P < 0.001$) [23]. The PET scans showed a difference in the decline of putaminal Ki values in favor of ropinirole (13.4 vs 20.3% ($P < 0.022$).

A 5-year randomized, double-blind, parallel study of 268 patients with newly diagnosed PD of the effect of ropinirole versus levodopa found that the incidence of dyskinesia was 20% vs 45% for ropinirole and levodopa, respectively [22]. The time to dyskinesia was significantly in favor of ropinirole (hazard ratio for remaining free of dyskinesia being 2.82; 95% CI, 1.78–4.44, $P < 0.001$). There was no significance difference in the UPDRS motor score between ropinirole and levodopa groups at 5 years; however, there is a difference in favor of levodopa in the change from baseline.

Pramipexole and ropinirole prolonged release formulations

Extended release formations of pramipexole and ropinirole have also become available in recent years. Once-daily extended-release pramipexole has similar pharmacokinetics and tolerability profile to three times daily pramipexole [24]. A randomized (2:2:1; pramipexole ER, pramipexole IR TID, or placebo), double-blind, placebo and active comparator-controlled trial in subjects with early PD conducted in 259 patients found a change in adjusted mean UPDRS Part II + III scores at 18 weeks from baseline of −5.1, −8.1, and −8,4 in placebo, pramipexole ER, and pramipexole IR, respectively (including those that required levodopa rescue) [25]. In data censored post-levodopa rescue, the scores were −2.7, −7.4, and −7.5 in placebo, pramipexole ER ($P = 0.0010$), and pramipexole IR ($P = 0.006$), respectively. Adverse events were more common in pramipexole ER than placebo group, but similar to the IR formation and included somnolence, nausea, constipation, and fatigue.

Ropinirole ER has a smooth plasma concentration–time profile over 24 hours with similar dose-normalized area under the curve compared to ER versus IR formations [26]. EASE-PD, a multicenter, double blind non-inferiority crossover study of 161 patients randomized to one of four different formulation sequences compared ropinirole 24-hour prolonged release to ropinirole immediate release [27]. Following a 12-week dose titration period, patients then entered a consecutive, flexible-dose, 8-week maintenance period which at the end of the first maintenance period, half of the patients in each formulation group switched to the same or closest dose of the alternative formulation with the remaining patients switching at the end of the second maintenance period. Overall, mean total improvement in UPDRS motor scores were 13.7 (9.33) points for ropinirole 24-hour prolonged release and 12.4 (8.49) points for ropinirole immediate release. The primary end point of non-inferiority of ropinirole ER versus IR was reached (≤3 points on the upper limit of 95% CI for difference in motor UPDRS change from baseline). Adverse effects were similar in the ER and IR groups.

Rotigotine

A novel transdermal delivery system for rotigotine, a new non-ergot D3 > D2 > D1 dopamine agonist, has been developed which allows stable plasma levels over 24 hours [28,29]. There have been six randomized controlled trials of rotigotine transdermal patch, with three in patients with early Parkinson's disease, two in advanced, and one in mixed patients [30–35].

The SURE-PD study investigated the efficacy and safety in early Parkinson's disease in a randomized, double-blind, double-dummy placebo, and ropinirole-controlled study [32]. The study had a double-blind dose-titration period (up to 13 weeks for ropinirole and 4 weeks for rotigotine), followed by a minimum maintenance phase of 33 weeks for ropinirole and 24 weeks for rotigotine. The primary end point was the proportion of patients with a minimum 20% decrease in UPDRS Part II and III scores with 52% responding in the rotigotine group versus 30% in the placebo group ($P < 0.0001$). Transdermal rotigotine at doses ≤ 8 mg per day did not show non-inferiority to ropinirole at doses ≤ 24 mg per day. Application site reactions occurred in 38 of 215 patients versus 11 of 118 and 7 of 228 of the placebo and ropinirole arms, respectively. Other adverse events were comparable between rotigotine and the ropinirole arms.

A long-term open-label follow-up of rotigotine transdermal system with a mean follow-up of 5 years and 3 months with 47% still on rotigotine at the time of study closure, 74% of patients started levodopa during the study at a median time of 374 days [36]. Ninety-nine percent of patients reported at least one adverse event, the most common being somnolence (23.4% per patient-year), falls (16.5%), peripheral edema (14.2%), and application site reactions (11.7%). Seventy-five percent of patients did not develop dyskinesia during the study and of those that did 83% occurred after initiation of levodopa.

Cabergoline

There are no recent studies assessing the efficacy of cabergoline in the management of early PD patients. Bracco *et al.* conducted a randomized, double-blind, parallel-group trial comparing cabergoline with levodopa in 419 early PD [37]. At 5 years, the motor complications were significantly delayed in the cabergoline-treated group (22.3% vs 33.3%, $P = 0.0175$), with dyskinesia only occurring in 9.5% of patients compared to 21.2% of the levodopa group. Cox model proportional hazards regression showed that the relative risk of developing motor complications was >50% lower with cabergoline compared with levodopa. Dropout rates were similar for both arms, 16% and 13%, respectively for cabergoline and levodopa arms. However mean motor UPDRS scores favored levodopa at 16.3 points versus 19.2 points for cabergoline ($P < 0.01$). Even though the

overall rate of adverse events was similar for the two arms, peripheral edema was more frequent in the cabergoline arm than levodopa arm (16/1% vs 3.4%, respectively).

Bromocriptine

The Parkinson's Disease Research Group of the United Kingdom (PDRG-UK) trial has reported the 3-, 10-, and 14-year follow-up data of an open-label, randomized, multicenter study of 782 patients with three initial treatment arms (levodopa, levodopa plus selegiline, and bromocriptine) [38–40]. At 3 years, the levodopa arms were significantly more effective than bromocriptine and had fewer side effects; however, dyskinesia and motor fluctuations were significantly lower in the bromocriptine arm (2% and 5%, respectively) than in the levodopa arm (27% and 33%, respectively) [39]. At 14 years, only 21% of the initial patients were able to be contacted, and there was no statistically significant difference in the prevalence of dyskinesia or motor fluctuations [38]. UPDRS scores were not reported in this study.

The Sydney Multicenter Study of Parkinson's disease has reported 5-year, 10-year, and 15-year data on 149 patients randomized to either levodopa or bromocriptine [41–43]. At 5 years, 126 patients were reported on, with no patients able to remain on bromocriptine alone by this time; the median bromocriptine monotherapy time was 12.1 months (95% CI 8.5–17.7 months) with lack of efficacy being the main reason for the addition of other medications [43]. No patients developed dyskinesia while on bromocriptine alone. One patient developed retroperitoneal fibrosis and two patients developed pulmonary fibrosis in the bromocriptine arms. At 15 years, there were 52 survivors of the original cohort; Ninety-four percent of these patients had experienced dyskinesia with the mean duration of treatment before the onset of dyskinesia being 4.2 years (SD = 2.9) for the L-dopa group and 6.9 years (SD = 4.0) for the bromocriptine group, a significant difference (*t* test, $P = 0.009$) [41]. There was no sustained benefit from the early use of bromocriptine in preventing end of dose failure once levodopa was added.

In addition to the aforementioned trials, there are three trials where patients were randomized to bromocriptine as an adjunct treatment in addition to levodopa monotherapy, which all reported lower rates of motor fluctuations or dyskinesia with the combination of levodopa and bromocriptine [44–46].

MAO-B inhibitors
Rasagiline

MAO-B inhibitors prolong the action of levodopa by reducing metabolic breakdown. Rasagiline is a selective irreversible monoamine oxidase type-B inhibitor. The TEMPO study in 404 patients with early PD was a multicenter, parallel-group, randomized, double-blind, placebo-controlled clinical trial of rasagiline mesylate at dosages of 1 or 2 mg per day with a 1-week escalation period followed by a 25-week maintenance period [47]. At both 1 and 2 mg, rasagiline improved the total UPDRS; at 1 mg, −4.20 points compared to placebo (95% CI: −5.66 to 2.73, $P < 0.001$) and at 2 mg, −3.56 compared to placebo (95% CI: −5.04 to −2.08, $P < 0.001$). There was no statistically significant difference in the rates of adverse events between the arms. In an extension of this study, patients randomized to placebo were started on 2 mg per day of rasagiline at the end of the 26 weeks, while those on 1 and 2 mg per day were continued on this dosage, and patients were then analyzed at 1 year as a randomized delayed-start clinical trial [48]. A total of 371 initial subjects completed and were included in the intention-to-treat analysis at 52 weeks, or last observation carried forward, of this phase of the study which showed that patients treated with rasagiline 2 mg per day for 1 year had a reduction of 2.29 in mean adjusted total UPDRS score compared to subjects initially treated with placebo for 6 months. This suggests that patients initially treated with rasagiline had lesser functional decline at 12 months than those delayed treatment by 6 months.

A total of 56 patients in a 10-week (3 weeks of dose escalation followed by 7-week steady state) multicenter, parallel-group, double-blind randomized, placebo-controlled study with early PD were assigned to rasagiline mesylate 1, 2, or 4 mg per day or placebo [49]. At the end of the study, the mean (±SE) change from baseline in total UPDRS score were −1.8 (±1.3), −3.6 (±1.7), −3.6 (±1.2), and −0.5(±0.8) in the 1, 2, and 4 mg per day, and placebo groups, respectively. Reported adverse effects were similar for rasagiline and placebo.

The ADAGIO study, an 18-month double-blind, placebo-controlled, multicenter trial using a delayed-start design to assess the possibility that rasagiline has disease-modifying effects, randomized 1176 untreated PD patients to rasagiline at doses of either 1 or 2 mg per day for 72 weeks (early-start group) or 36 weeks (delayed-start group) [50]. To determine efficacy, the early-start group had to meet three hierarchical end points based on total UPDRS; superiority to placebo in rate of change in UPDRS scores between weeks 12 and 36; superiority to delayed-start treatment in the change of score between baseline and week 72; and non-inferiority to delayed-start treatment in the rate of change between weeks 48 and 72. The early-start dose of 1 mg rasagiline met all primary end points with a smaller mean increase in UPDRS between weeks 12 and 36 compared to placebo (0.009 vs 0.14 points per week, $P = 0.01$), less worsening of score between baseline and week 72 (2.82 vs 4.52 points, $P = 0.02$), and non-inferiority between the two groups (0.085 vs 0.085 points per week between weeks 48 and 72, $P < 0.001$). None of the three end points were met by the 2-mg dose.

Catechol-O-methyltransferase (COMT) inhibitors

STRIDE-PD (Stalevo Reduction In Dyskinesia Evaluation in Parkinson's Disease) conducted by Stocchi et al. was a prospective double-blind study to assess the effects of early entacapone combined with levodopa/carbidopa (LCE) versus placebo combined with levodopa/carbidopa (LC) on preventing the development of dyskinesia over 134 weeks on 747 PD patients [51]. Patients had to have had PD for less than 5 years. Patients treated with LCE had an increased risk of developing dyskinesia compared to those receiving LC (hazard ratio 1.29, $P = 0.04$). This effect was particularly pronounced in patients receiving dopamine agonists; LCE-treated patients had a greater risk of dyskinesia (hazard ratio 1.55, $P = 0.006$) and a greater frequency of dyskinesia (41.9% vs 31.3%). However, there was no difference in the time to onset (hazard ratio 0.99, 95% CI, 0.68–1.45, $P = 0.96$) or frequency (34% vs 35.5%) of dyskinesia between patients in the LCE and LC groups for those not receiving dopamine agonists. This study therefore suggests that there is no benefit in the early introduction of entacapone when delaying the onset of dyskinesia.

Hauser et al. conducted a randomized, double-blind, multicenter study of treatment of 423 early PD patients with a combination of LCE and LC [52]. The primary outcome was a combined UPDRS Part II and III scores < 90 minutes before the third levodopa dose of the day which did show a small but significant difference in favor of LCE; however, there was no difference in UPDRS Part III motor subscores.

Overall, these two studies suggest that there is no benefit in motor symptoms and dyskinesia with the early addition of entacapone to levodopa/carbidopa.

Conclusion

The evidence supports the notion that dopamine agonists are associated with a lower incidence of motor fluctuations and dyskinesia than levodopa. However, levodopa has been proved superior to agonists and other therapies in all comparative trials evaluating the degree of improvement in motor parkinsonism. In addition, dopamine agonists are associated with more frequent adverse events. MAO-B inhibitors may be effective in early PD and are not associated with significant motor complications; however, there is insufficient evidence to support a neuroprotective effect. There is no evidence to support the addition of a COMT inhibitor (entacapone) to levodopa in early PD.

PD patients with levodopa-induced motor complications

In patients with PD and levodopa-induced motor complications, to what extent do adjunctive pharmacologic therapies improve motor fluctuations or dyskinesia.

Controlled-release levodopa formulations

A number of studies have shown minor improvements in "on" time in patients with advanced PD on standard controlled-release levodopa formulations [53–57]. Lieberman et al. conducted a 16-week double-blind crossover study in 24 PD patients with a mean duration of disease of 9.3 years with all patients having "weaning-off" [53]. Even though patients on the CR4 formulation took lesser tablets pcr day of Sinemet CR4 (mean 5.0, range 3–8) than of Sinemet 25/100 (mean 6.2, range 4–11 doses per day), the mean daily dose of CR4 was higher and there was no significant differences between mean UPDRS scores and "on" and "off" duration between the two arms.

Ahlskog et al. conducted a similar study in 23 patients who were experiencing a short-duration response to standard Sinemet, and found that half the patients had a prolonged "on" response along with a favorable effect on end of dose "wearing off" [54].

Wolters et al. compared Sinemet CR to standard Sinemet in 170 patients with fluctuating PD during an 8-week open-label dose-finding phase followed by a 24-week double-blind double-dummy treatment phase [55]. The mean daily number of "off" periods was significantly decreased in the CR arm, with the "on" time being greater in the CR arm (69% of the waking day at week 24) compared to the standard arm (64% of the waking day at week 24).

A double-blind crossover study with two 8-week crossover periods preceded by two 4-week phases for drug titration of 202 PD patients with motor fluctuations found that the CR formulation significantly reduced "off" time at 4 and 6 weeks and again showed a reduced daily dosing frequency of 33% compared to standard Sinemet, although the total daily intake of levodopa was increased by 25% [56]. The side effect profile was similar for the two formulations.

Jankovic et al. conducted a study of 20 patients with "wearing-off" with a mean duration of PD symptoms of 8.3 years in a 12-week double-blind study or CR4 versus standard Sinemet [57]. There was statistically significant reduction in the "on" time without dyskinesia in the CR4 arm from 9.3 ± 4.6 to 7.5 ± 4.3 ($P < 0.05$), although the total "on" time was not significantly different. There was a reduction in the daily average number of tablets taken (5.7 ± 1.2 to 3.8 ± 0.7).

The newer controlled-release formulation IPX066 has also been studied in advanced PD. A single phase-three randomized, double-blind, double-dummy study has been conducted in 471 participants (83% randomized) who had a least 2.5 hours per day of off time and were randomized to 13 weeks of either IPX066 or immediate-release carbidopa-levodopa plus matched placebos [58]. Those on IPX066 had a reduction in mean daily off time by an average of 1.17 hours (95% CI, −1.69 to −0.66, $P < 0.0001$) compared with immediate-release carbidopa-levodopa. Those treated with the extended-release version also had a reduced number of mean doses per day (3.6 vs 5.0). A potential criticism of this paper is that the optimization phase was unbalanced with a more prolonged dose-conversion phase of 6 weeks for IPX066 compared to only 3 weeks for the immediate-release version, discrepancy potentially favoring IPX066.

Continuous duodenal levodopa infusion

Duodopa (levodopa–carbidopa 20/5 mg/ml in a carboxymethylcellulose mix) that is infused directly into the duodenum via a percutaneous endogastric gastrostomy and portable infusion pump has been assessed in patients with advanced PD with motor fluctuations and/or dyskinesia [59–61]. The duodenum infusion results in a much smoother pharmacokinetic profile than oral levodopa which should theoretically improve motor complications in patients with advanced PD [62]. DIREQT study enrolled 24 patients with advanced PD who were experiencing motor fluctuations and dyskinesia in spite of optimized treatment to a randomized crossover study comparing individualized conventional treatment versus intraduodenal infusion of levodopa/carbidopa gel for 3 + 3 weeks, there was no placebo arm [60]. The primary outcome was based on a blinded video assessment using a novel but non-validated rating scale, the Treatment Response Scale (TRS), which ranges from −3 (severe off) to +3 (on with severe dyskinesia) with 0 being *on* without any dyskinesia with the primary end point being the percentage of ratings spent within a range of −1 to +1 (which represents a functional *on* state between either mild parkinsonism or mild dyskinesia. A total of 18 patients qualified for the per protocol population. The median percentage increased from 81% to 100% with infusion treatment ($P < 0.01$), which was accompanied by a decrease in the off state. The most common adverse event was dyskinesia (seven in the conventional arm, four in the infusional arm); other reported events include constipation (6 vs 2), depression (5 vs 3), insomnia (5 vs 1), and somnolence (4 vs 3).

The interim results of a prospective open-label international study of levodopa–carbidopa intestinal gel conducted in 192 patients with advanced PD experiencing motor fluctuations reported a mean reduction in *off* time of 3.9 (±3.2) hours per day from a baseline of 6.7 hours per day and *on* time without troublesome dyskinesia increased by 4.6 (±3.5) hours per day at week 12 compared to baseline [61]. The most common adverse events were abdominal pain, device insertion complication; although, of note, four patients developed a polyneuropathy, which has been reported in other studies [63].

COMT inhibitors

There are four studies for the use of entacapone in patents with levodopa with motor fluctuations as a treatment for wearing off [64–67]. Fung et al. conducted a randomized, double-blind study comparing LCE and LC over 12 weeks on 184 patients with PD with less than 3 hours of wearing off and no dyskinesia. They found no significant difference between UPDRS-IV scores and wearing off as assessed by questionnaire [64]. A total of 270 PD patients, with a mean disease duration of 7 years, in a double-blind, randomized, placebo-controlled study received either entacapone 200 mg or placebo added on to their current levodopa regimen, which could be altered at treating clinician discretion [65]. The authors report that the UPDRS Part III score was significantly improved in the levodopa plus entacapone arm compared to placebo, although there was no statistically significant differences in "off" or "on" time between the treatment groups as recorded in patient diaries (off time decreased: -1.0 ± 1.9 and -0.9 ± 2.0 hours; on time increased: 1.1 ± 2.1 and 0.9 ± 2.0 hours; entacapone versus placebo arm, respectively). There was no significant difference in UPDRS Part IVA (dyskinesia sun score) score between the baseline and the different arms (95% CI: 0.0 [-0.3 to 0.3]), although the fluctuation sum score (UPDRS Part IVB) did decrease significantly in the entacapone arm compared to placebo arm ($P = 0.02$, 95% CI, -0.5 to 0.1). Adverse events occurred in 65% of the entacapone group and 49% of the placebo group with significantly more patients in the entacapone group experiencing nausea and discoloration of urine.

Mizuno *et al.* conducted a placebo-controlled, double-blind, parallel-group study of 341 fluctuating Japanese PD patients with >3 hours off time. The patients were randomized in a 1:1:1 fashion to either placebo, entacapone 100 mg or entacapone 200 mg per dose of levodopa plus dopa decarboxylase inhibitor (DCI) for 13 weeks [66]. The primary efficacy outcome was "on" time change as assessed by patient diaries. In the final assessment, the mean "on" time had improved in both entacapone arms by 1.4 hours compared to 0.5 hours for placebo ($P < 0.05$), a relative increase of 17% from baseline for the entacapone arms versus 6% for the placebo arm. "Off" time was decreased by 1.3, 1.1, and 0.4 hours (entacapone 100 mg, entacapone 200 mg, and placebo, respectively). Overall, there was no significant difference between the entacapone 100 mg and 200 mg groups. Adverse events occurred in 70%, 72.6%, and 86% of the placebo, entacapone 100 mg, entacapone 200 mg groups, respectively with the difference being statistically significant in the 200-mg group versus placebo. The most common adverse events were dyskinesia, somnolence, aggravation of diarrhea, and urine discoloration.

The LARGO study, an 18-week, randomized, placebo-controlled, double-blind, double-dummy, parallel-group trial, compared rasagiline, entacapone 200 mg per dose of levodopa, and placebo in 687 PD patients [67]. Patients had PD for an average of 8.9 years with an average off time of 5.57 hours. The mean total daily off time was reduced in the entacapone arm from baseline to treatment by almost three times more than the reduction with placebo, -1.2 hour entacapone versus placebo 0.4 hour, $P < 0.001$. There was an increase in daily on time without troublesome dyskinesia of 0.85 hours versus placebo 0.03 hours, $P = 0.0005$.

Amantadine

Amantadine is a low-affinity non-competitive antagonist of NMDA receptors used in the treatment of dyskinesia [68]. There are two recent studies evaluating the effect of amantadine on dyskinesia [69,70]. Wolf *et al.* conducted a randomized, placebo-controlled, parallel-group study of 32 patients who had been stable on amantadine for one year and were then switched in a double-blind fashion to either amantadine or placebo. Dyskinesia duration and intensity were assessed by UPDRS IV items 32 and 33 [70]. There was a significant increase in the score in patients treated with placebo from 3.06 (95% CI, 2.1–4.03) at baseline to 4.28 (95% CI, 3.1–5.4) at 3-week follow-up (P 5 0.02) compared with no significant change between baseline 3.2 (95% CI, 2.1–4.4) and follow-up 3.6 (95% CI, 2.3–4.8) in patients staying on amantadine. These results would be consistent with a long-term effect on dyskinesia by amantadine. A multicenter, placebo-controlled, double-blinded, randomized, crossover trial of 36 patients who had Parkinson's disease and dyskinesia to amantadine (300 mg per day) or placebo found an adjusted odds ratio for improvement by amantadine of 6.7 (95% CI, 1.4–31.5) [69]. UPDRS-IVa was improved to a significantly greater degree in amantadine-treated patients [mean (SD) of 1.83 (1.56)] compared with placebo-treated patients [0.03 (1.51)]. Side effects were noted in nine patients: six amantadine arm, one placebo arm, and two during the washout phase. The most common side effect was visual hallucinations occurring in the amantadine arm.

A randomized, double-blind study of 40 patients, who had been treated with levodopa for 7.5 years with levodopa who had dyskinesia, found that after 15 days of active arm there was a 45% reduction in total dyskinesia [71]. The effect of amantadine lasted on average 4.9 months, compared with only 1.3 months for the placebo effect ($P = 0.001$).

MAO-B inhibitors
Selegiline

Two studies have been conducted of an orally disintegrating selegiline that dissolves on contact with saliva, allowing pre-gastric absorption, which therefore minimizes first-pass metabolism which allows for high plasma concentrations and reduces amphetamine metabolites. Ondo *et al.* conducted a 12-week double-blind, placebo-controlled, parallel-design trial of orally disintegrating selegiline in 148 PD patients with mild to moderate motor fluctuations and at least 3 hours of off time daily [72]. The primary efficacy point was a reduction in the percentage of daily "off" time. There was a non-significant reduction in percentage of daily off time at weeks 10 and 12 of 11.6% for the selegiline arm versus a 9.8% reduction for placebo. On time without dyskinesia at combined weeks 10 and 12 was the same between the two arms. Overall adverse events were similar for the two arms, 73% vs 72% for selegiline and placebo, respectively; although, 7% of the selegiline arm discontinued compared to 0% in the placebo arm, particular differences occurred with dizziness in 13% vs 6%, and dyskinesia 8% vs 4% in the selegiline arms and placebo arms, respectively.

In contrast to the aforementioned study, a similarly designed study of orally disintegrating selegiline by Waters *et al.* in 140 PD patients with mild to moderate motor fluctuations with at least 3 hours of "off" time per day found significant reductions in daily "off" time of 13.2% reduction versus 3.8% for the selegiline and placebo, respectively ($P < 0.001$) at weeks 10–12 [73]. The total number of "off" hours was reduced by 2.2 hours per day versus a 0.6 reduction per day from baseline for the selegiline and placebo groups, respectively, with a corresponding improvement in dyskinesia free "on" time of 9.5% vs 3.3% for the selegiline and placebo groups, respectively ($P = 0.038$). Overall adverse events were similar for the two arms with three patients in the selegiline arms withdrawing due to an adverse event versus one in the placebo arm. The most frequent adverse events in the selegiline group were dizziness (6%), dyskinesia (4%), headache (4%), and dyspepsia (4%).

There have not been any recent studies in the role of standard selegiline, but three early studies have shown motor improvements but no consistent effect on "off" time with selegiline [74–76]. Lees *et al.* conducted a double-blind, crossover trial in 41 patients already felt to be on the maximum-tolerated dose of levodopa added either selegiline or placebo [74]. Even though the selegiline arm was effective in mild "on–off" disability, it had no effect on patients with severe "on–off" disability.

Lieberman *et al.* conducted an 8-week randomized, double-blind, placebo-controlled, parallel-group trial in 33 patients [75]. There was no significant difference in "on" time between the two groups, although patients reported less-abrupt transitions between "on" and "off" states. Adverse events were similar for the two treatment arms.

Ninety-six PD patients who were experiencing motor fluctuations and were on optimized levodopa/carbidopa were randomized by Golbe *et al.* to either selegiline or placebo [76]. There was a significant improvement in self-reported gait and symptom control scores, but objective rating of the "on" period quality did not differ between groups.

Rasagiline
The PRESTO study was a multicenter, randomized, placebo-controlled, double-blind, parallel-group study of rasagiline in 472 PD patients with at least 2.5 hours of daily "off" time despite optimized treatment [77]. The primary outcome measure was the change from baseline in mean total daily off time as measured by home diaries over 26 weeks. In patients treated with rasagiline, mean

adjusted total daily off time decreased from baseline by 1.85, 1.41, and 0.91 hours for 1.0 mg per day of rasagiline, 0.5 mg per day of rasagiline and placebo, respectively. Compared to placebo, patients treated with rasagiline had significantly reduced off time: rasagiline 0.5 mg per day had 0.49 hours (95% CI, 0.08–0.91 hours, $P = 0.02$) less off time; rasagiline 1.0 mg per day had 0.94 hours (95% CI, 0.51–1.36 hours, $P < 0.001$) less off time. However, in the 1 mg per day rasagiline group, 32% of the increase in "on" time resulted in troublesome dyskinesia. There was no significant difference between the numbers of patients in the treatment groups discontinuing due to an adverse events. Adverse events that were more common in the rasagiline arms include weight loss, vomiting, anorexia, and balance difficulty.

The LARGO study, an 18-week, randomized, placebo-controlled, double-blind, double-dummy, parallel-group trial, compared rasagiline 1 mg per day (with entacapone as a comparator, see above) to placebo in patients with at least 1 hour every day in the off state [67]. The primary outcome measure was change in total daily off time with the intention-to-treat population. Rasagiline reduced mean daily off time by 1.18 hours versus placebo $P = 0.0001$ and increased daily "on" time without troublesome dyskinesia by 0.85 hours compared to placebo, $P = 0.0005$. Adverse events occurred in 50% of all patients with rates similar for the three arms.

Dopamine agonists
Ropinirole
Barone *et al.* compared sumanirole, a highly selective D2 dopamine receptor agonist, to ropinirole and placebo in 948 PD patients who were experiencing motor fluctuations while receiving a stable dose of levodopa/carbidopa in a 40-week double-blind, double-dummy, parallel-group study [78]. The primary outcome was the change in baseline combined UPDRS Parts II and III. There was a statistically significant decrease in UPDRS Part II and III scores in the ropinirole arm compared to placebo (−13.4 vs −4.55, $P < 0.001$). Rates of adverse events were similar across different arms, with 71% and 67% of the ropinirole and placebo arms having at least one adverse event. High rates of nausea, dizziness, and somnolence were reported in the ropinirole arm.

The STRONG was a randomized, double-blind, placebo-controlled 16-week study of ropinirole as an adjunct to levodopa in 243 PD patients who had motor fluctuations or had insufficient therapeutic effect [79]. The primary outcome was change in UPDRS total motor score from baseline. The UPDRS total motor score was significantly greater for the ropinirole group than placebo (−9.5 vs −4.5, $P = 0.00001$). The mean duration of time spent "off" decreased from 4.3 hours per day at baseline to 3.1 hours per day at final evaluation in the ropinirole arm compared to no change in the placebo group. Patients stopping the study because of adverse events were similar for the two arms with the most frequent adverse events in the ropinirole arm being nausea (25%), somnolence (13%), nasopharyngitis (12%), and dyskinesia (12%).

Two further studies have investigated the role of ropinirole in patients with levodopa-induced motor fluctuations [80,81]. In Rascol *et al.* 46 PD patients with motor fluctuations received ropinirole as an adjunctive to levodopa treatment in a 3-month randomized, placebo-controlled trial [80]. The mean percentage awake time spent "off" decreased from 47% at baseline to 24% at 12 weeks and 44% to 40% in the ropinirole and placebo arms, respectively.

Lieberman *et al.* conducted a similar prospective randomized, double-blind, placebo-controlled study of ropinirole as an adjunct to levodopa in 149 PD patients with motor fluctuations for 6 months [81]. A significant proportion of patients treated with ropinirole achieved a 20% or greater reduction in levodopa dose and a 20% or greater reduction in the percentage of time spent "off" (35% vs 13%, ropinirole and placebo, respectively; $P = 0.002$).

Ropinirole ER

Watts *et al.* performed a multicenter, randomized, double-dummy, flexible-dose study of effect of additional ropinirole ER in 104 PD patients not optimally controlled with levodopa, with an initial planned study duration of 107 weeks, although the trial was terminated early because of low enrollment with a mean duration of exposure to study medication of approximately 11 months [82]. The primary end point was time to onset of dyskinesia with a significant delay in subjects treated with ropinirole ER compared to L-dopa (hazard ration [HR] 6.46; log-rank test, $P < 0.001$). During the study period, 3% of patients in the ropinirole ER group and 17% in the L-dopa group developed dyskinesia while there was no significant difference in mean change of UPDRS Part III scores from baseline between the two groups.

Pramipexole

A double-blind, placebo-controlled study of 354 PD patients with motor fluctuations compared pramipexole to placebo as add on treatment to levodopa over 24-weeks with the primary outcome measure being change from baseline to end-of-maintenance of the average UPDRS Part II score during "on" and "off" and the average UPDRS Part III score during "on" [83]. The UPDRS Part II score (average of "on" and "off") in the pramipexole group improved from 12.3 to 8.0 (baseline and end-of-maintenance, respectively) compared with placebo changes of 13.6 and 11.8, respectively ($P = 0.0001$). There was a significant change in the "off" time with pramipexole of 2.5 hours compared to 10 minutes with placebo. The most commonly reported adverse effects were dyskinesia (30% vs 8.7%; pramipexole and placebo, respectively), asymptomatic orthostatic hypotension (23.3%

vs 20.2%), nausea (16.1% vs 12.0%), visual hallucinations (11.1% vs 4.4%), and dizziness (10.6% vs 7.1%).

The CLEOPATRA-PD study, a randomized, double-blind, double-dummy, controlled trial, compared the efficacy of rotigotine with an active comparator pramipexole and placebo in 506 PD patients with wearing off type motor fluctuations of an average of at least 2.5 hours per day over 6 months [31]. Mean absolute change in off time from baseline was 2.8 hours with pramipexole compared to 0.9 hours for placebo, $P < 0.0001$. The mean change in daily off time from baseline compared to placebo at end-of-maintenance was −1.94 hours (−2.63 to −1.25, $P < 0.0001$). Rates of adverse events were similar for the three groups (66% vs 69%; placebo and pramipexole, respectively).

Mizuno *et al.* conducted a randomized, double-blind, parallel-group study of 325 PD patients comparing pramipexole, bromocriptine, and placebo over 12 weeks [84]. There was a significant reduction in UPDRS Part II and III scores in the pramipexole arm compared to placebo (−3.98 vs −2.03 UPDRS Part II; pramipexole and placebo, respectively; $P < 0.001$; −11.75 vs −5.55 UPDRS Part III; pramipexole and placebo, respectively; $P < 0.001$).

In a double-blind, placebo-controlled, randomized study, 78 PD patients with advanced disease and motor fluctuations were treated with pramipexole or placebo for 11 weeks with the primary end point being change from baseline in the total UPDRS score [85]. Mean UPDRS total score decreased by 37.3% vs 12.2% (pramipexole and placebo, respectively), with patients treated with pramipexole reporting a 12% reduction in "off" periods, which corresponds to 1.7 hours of more "on" time a day compared to an increase in "off" periods of 2% with placebo.

Rotigotine

In PREFER study, a randomized, double-blind placebo-controlled study, patients with advanced Parkinson's disease were randomized to either placebo, rotigotine 8 or 12 mg per day with primary efficacy being change in the number of "off" hours at 24 weeks [30]. Compared to placebo, there was a significant decrease in mean "off" time of 1.8 hours per day (95% CI: −2.6, −1.0; $P < 0.001$) and 1.2 hours per day (95% CI: −2.0, −0.4; $P = 0.003$) for the 8 and 12 mg per day, respectively. There were increases in "on" time without troublesome dyskinesia in both groups of rotigotine compared to placebo of 3.5 and 2.2 hours (8 and 12 mg, respectively) versus 1.1 for placebo.

The CLEOPATRA-PD study, described previously, found that with rotigotine transdermal patch, patients had a mean absolute change in mean "off" time from baseline of −2.5 hours with the absolute change compared to placebo being −1.58 hours (95% CI −2.27 to −0.90, $P < 0.0001$) [31]. There was an increase in "on" time without troublesome dyskinesia of 2.8 hours compared to 1.4 hours with placebo, $P < 0.001$.

Subcutaneous apomorphine
A 4-week randomized, double-blind, placebo-controlled trial of subcutaneously injected apomorphine in 29 PD patients with motor fluctuations found a reduction in mean UPDRS motor score of 23.9 versus 0.1 points (apomorphine and placebo, respectively) [86]. Apomorphine also significantly aborted "off" states (95% vs 23% of "off" periods, $P < 0.01$) and significantly decreased daily "off" period duration. Frequent adverse events were injection site reactions, yawning somnolence, dyskinesia, and nausea.

Conclusion

There is insufficient evidence to suggest that standard controlled-release levodopa formulations substantially improve motor complications in advanced PD. Continuous duodenal infusion of levodopa is associated with significant improvements in motor fluctuations, but also has a higher rate of therapy complications than oral agents. The dopamine agonists, ropinirole, pramipexole, and rotigotine, are more efficacious than placebo in improving motor fluctuations. However, agonists are associated with a higher rate of dyskinesia and dopaminergic side effects than placebo. Rasagiline is effective to reduce "off" time duration and increase "on" time without troublesome dyskinesia. Entacapone is also efficacious in improving motor scores in fluctuators and reducing "off" time, but is associated with a higher frequency of dyskinesia than placebo. Intermittent apomorphine infusion is effective in correcting "off" states and improving motor scores.

Deep brain stimulation

In patients with PD and levodopa-induced motor complications, to what extent does deep brain stimulation targeting the subthalamic nucleus or globus pallidus interna improve motor fluctuations, dyskinesia, and quality of life?

Deep brain stimulation (DBS) targeting either the subthalamic nucleus (STN) or globus pallidus pars interna (Gpi) has become a standard-of-care therapy for treatment of advanced PD with motor fluctuations and/or dyskinesia. Often dramatic and near-immediate improvement can be observed in individual patients after activation of the DBS system. While these types of results initially propelled the field forward, a rigorous evidence basis for the therapy has been slow in coming, and only over the last few years have well-controlled trials compared this invasive treatment against best medical therapy. Multiple challenges in trial design still exist, including the high cost of surgery and devices and difficulty in blinding patients and examiners to surgical and stimulation status.

Pre-2006
Before 2006, no large, randomized, well-controlled DBS trials had been performed. The smaller, often uncontrolled and open-label trials, which initially supported the regulatory approval and clinical use of bilateral STN DBS in PD, were reviewed in a 2006 meta-analysis [87]. Reports were considered for analysis if standard outcomes from at least 10 subjects with at least 6 months of follow-up were detailed. Of the 680 original citations identified in the literature search, 32 articles were found to meet the inclusion criteria. Overall, 37 cohorts comprising 921 patients were included. The mean age at surgery was 58.6 ± 2.4 years, and average duration of PD before surgery was 14.1 ± 1.6 years. The summary estimate of decrease in medication OFF UPDRS Part III motor scores after surgery was 27.55 points (95% CI = 24.23–30.87 points), corresponding to a 52% (95% CI = 48.1–56.5%) reduction compared to pre-surgical baseline. There existed significant between-study heterogeneity. Multivariable meta-regression analyses showed that the magnitude improvement in motor scores after DBS correlated with the magnitude of improvement to preoperative medication challenge and was also greater in those with higher baseline UPDRS Part III scores, increased disease duration, and interestingly studies published before 2002. No evidence for a significant publication bias was found on analysis using Begg's method. The average reduction in dyskinesia following surgery was 69.1% (95% CI 62.0–76.2%); however, there were multiple instruments used between the various reports. Analysis of motor diaries and/or item 39 on the UPDRS yielded an average decrease in duration of daily OFF time of 68.2% (95% CI 57.6–78.9%). Only a few studies assessed quality of life, most commonly using the Parkinson's Disease Questionnaire (PDQ-39) in which case, an average improvement of $34.5 \pm 15.3\%$ on the summary index was noted. While 778 patients reported adverse outcomes of any type, only around 11% of patients experienced an adverse event directly related to the surgery. While this meta-analysis helped to provide a more rigorous evidence base justifying DBS in advanced PD, it also highlighted the need for larger randomized controlled DBS trials.

Deuschl *et al.*
The first well-controlled trial to compare STN DBS with medical management alone was published in 2006 and involved 156 patients in Germany and Austria who had PD for at least 5 years that was insufficiently treated with medications [88]. Subjects were randomized in pairs to DBS STN versus best medical management and followed up for 6 months in an unblinded fashion. Primary end points included change from baseline to 6 months in quality of life as assessed by the Parkinson's Disease Questionnaire (PDQ-39) summary index and improvement in motor parkinsonism as measured by medication-OFF UPDRS Part III scores. Secondary end points included a dyskinesia scale, UPDRS-II, ON-medication UPDRS Part III, Schwab and England Scale for ADLs, home motor diaries, and neuropsychometric testing.

According to the intention-to-treat analysis, those with bilateral STN DBS had greater improvement in quality of life than those in the medical group (mean PDQ-39 change of −9.5 vs 0.2, $P = 0.02$). Medication OFF state parkinsonism improved by a mean of 19.5 points (from 48.0 ± 12.3 to 28.3 ± 14.7) in the stimulation group compared to essentially no change (0.4 points) in those treated with medication alone ($P < 0.001$). There was a far milder improvement in medication ON state UPDRS Part III scores (from 18.9 ± 9.3 to 14.6 ± 8.5) in the DBS group, and no improvement in the medical arm. Motor diaries showed that OFF time was reduced by 4.2 hours in the DBS group and was unchanged in the medication group ($P < 0.001$), and time spent ON with troublesome dyskinesia was reduced by 1 hour in the DBS group while remaining the same in the medication group ($P = 0.003$). Overall, these changes resulted in a gain of 4.4 hours of ON time without dyskinesia in the DBS group versus a loss of 0.5 hours in the medical group ($P < 0.001$). Levodopa-equivalent daily doses fell by 593 mg per day (representing a 50% reduction) in the DBS group and only 95 mg per day (8% reduction) in the medical group ($P < 0.001$). Emotional and cognitive measures did not differ significantly between the groups.

Serious adverse events were reported in 12.8% of the DBS group versus 3.8% of the medical group ($P = 0.04$) and including a fatal intracerebral hemorrhage and a case of suicide among the DBS cohort. Overall adverse events were, however, more common in the medical group (64.1% vs 50.0%, $P = 0.08$).

While this trial was the first to include a prospective control group, the lack of blinded assessments was a significant weakness that would be better addressed in future trials.

COMPARE

The first study to randomize target selection among PD patients was developed to compare cognitive and mood effects between the sites of stimulation [89]. The COMPARE trial analyzed 45 patients (23 Gpi, 22 STN) with co-primary end points of the Visual Analog Mood Scale and verbal fluency at 7 months post-DBS compared to pre-DBS. No significant differences in the mood or cognitive measures were present between targets at the optimal DBS setting; however, adverse mood effects occurred with ventral stimulation at either target. A similar degree of improvement in the UPDRS motor scores was seen in both groups.

PD-SURG

The PD-SURG trial out of the United Kingdom is the second published large randomized trial to compare DBS to medical therapy in patients with advanced PD [90]. Patients with PD for whom current medical therapy was inadequate were randomized to immediate surgery or continued medical therapy (183 patients each). Selection of the surgical target, and all treatment decisions other than randomization were left in the hands of the local clinicians. The primary end point was between-group difference in quality of life measured by the PDQ-39. Medication ON and OFF UPDRS Part III scores and the Dementia Rating Scale-II were secondary outcome measures.

Baseline characteristics were similar for the two groups and included a mean age of 59 years and mean duration of PD of 11 years. The intention-to-treat analysis demonstrated improvement in quality of life at 1 year of 5.0 points on the PDQ-39 summary score versus essentially no change in the medical group (between-group difference −4.7 points, 95% CI −7.6 to −1.8, $P = 0.001$). The medication OFF UPDRS Part III score decreased at 1 year by 27.4 points in the DBS group and was essentially unchanged in the medical group (difference of −26.6 points, 95% CI −32.3 to −20.9, $P < 0.0001$). At 1 year, those in the DBS group had a 34% lower levodopa equivalent daily dose (894 mg per day vs 1347 mg per day, difference = 453 mg per day, 95% CI 328–580).

The Dementia Rating Scale-II score worsened by 0.4 points in both groups ($P = 0.90$). Neuropsychological assessments were not uniformly obtained; however, analysis of available data suggested a decline in verbal fluency in the DBS group while these measures were largely unchanged in the medical group.

Veterans Affairs Cooperative DBS Study

The Veterans Affairs Cooperative Studies Program 468 study of deep brain stimulation represents one of the largest randomized trials to date evaluating this therapy in advanced PD [91–93]. The multicenter trial enrolled subjects with levodopa-responsive PD, classified at Hoehn and Yahr stage 2 or greater, and experiencing persistent disabling motor fluctuations and/or dyskinesia for at least 3 hours daily despite maximal medical therapy. As in most previous trials, patients with previous surgery for PD or with comorbid dementia were excluded. Initially 255 patients were randomized with age-stratification to surgery or best medical therapy under the care of movement disorder neurologists. The 121 patients initially randomized to surgery were further randomized to the subthalamic nucleus (STN) (60 subjects) or globus pallidus (61 subjects) targets and were blinded to the selected target [91]. An interim analysis revealed that a sample of 255 patients was sufficient for comparison between medical therapy and surgery, and hence the remaining patients were directly randomized to one of the two surgical groups [92]. In addition, 117 of the 134 patients initially assigned to medical therapy went on to receive DBS under this randomized protocol.

Primary outcome measures in the initial analysis detailing surgery (at either target) versus best medical therapy included both patient-completed motor diaries and medication OFF and ON state UPDRS Part III scores [91]. Those undergoing DBS gained a mean of 4.6 hours per day of on time without troubling dyskinesia, versus a mean change of 0 hours in those randomized to best medical therapy ($P < 0.001$). This was by way of both a reduction in OFF time and a reduction in ON time with troubling dyskinesia. In the subset of subjects aged 70 years or more, the DBS group gained a mean of 3.8 hours daily while the medical group lost 0.5 hours daily ($P < 0.001$).

The UPDRS Part III evaluations were conducted by raters blinded to surgery status. Medication OFF scores improved by a mean of 12.3 points in the surgical group, whereas the medical therapy group experienced an only 1.7-point improvement on average ($P < 0.001$). Medication decreased by 296 mg per day levodopa equivalents (23% reduction) in the DBS group, but increased by 15 mg per day (1% increase) in the medical therapy group ($P < 0.001$).

Quality of life, as assessed by the PDQ-39 summary measure and on seven of the eight subscales, was significantly improved in the DBS group compared to the medical group. The social support scale scores were not significantly different between groups.

Analysis of neurocognitive function demonstrated mild but statistically significant decline in performance of working memory ($P = 0.005$), processing speed ($P = 0.006$), phonemic fluency ($P < 0.001$), and delayed recall ($P = 0.03$) among the DBS group, while these measures improved slightly in the medical therapy group. Significant changes on the Mattis Dementia or Beck depression scales were not seen in either group.

Adverse events more common in the DBS group over the 6-month study period included falls ($P < 0.01$), gait disturbance ($P = 0.03$), depression ($P = 0.03$), and dystonia ($P < 0.01$). The most common serious adverse event was surgical site infection which occurred in 9.9% of the DBS group; 1 death secondary to cerebral hemorrhage was reported. The overall incidence risk of a serious adverse event was 3.8 times higher (95% CI, 2.3–6.3) in the DBS group than the medical group.

The VA cooperative trial's 6-month outcomes described above pooled STN and Gpi surgical groups as it was felt that any differences between the targets would not likely be apparent at this early time point and because blinded analyses between them were ongoing. A subsequent manuscript detailed the comparison of these targets among 299 patients randomized to either Gpi (152 patients) or STN (147 patients) stimulation [92]. The primary outcome for the comparison was change in the OFF-medication UPDRS Part III scores from baseline to 24 months. The motor assessments were scored by investigators blinded to stimulation target. Secondary outcomes included self-reported function (motor diaries), quality of life, neurocognitive function, and adverse events.

The OFF-medication ON-stimulation UPDRS Part III motor scores at 24 months improved by 11.8 points in the Gpi group and 10.7 points in the STN group, a non-significant difference ($P = 0.50$). Interestingly, the OFF-medication OFF-stimulation UPDRS Part III scores improved by a mean of 3.7 points in the Gpi group and worsened by 2.2 points in the STN group ($P < 0.001$) suggesting that there may be a longer washout period after deactivation of Gpi versus STN stimulation. While the main analysis used the intention-to-treat principle, subsequent mixed-model analysis, analysis limited to complete data, assignment of no-change to missing data, and worse-case scenario analyses all were consistent with the primary intention-to-treat analysis.

The equivalence of motor outcomes for stimulation at the two targets was further supported by patients' motor diaries, which showed no significant difference between targets according to time spent in any of the four states (OFF, ON with and without troublesome dyskinesia, and asleep).

The average medication use decreased to a greater extent in the STN group (408 mg per day representing a 32% reduction) than the Gpi group (243 mg per day representing an 18% reduction, $P = 0.02$). Stimulation amplitudes and pulse widths were lower among those with STN DBS compared with Gpi DBS.

At month 24, end point quality of life improved on six of eight PDQ-39 subscales in both groups, and none of the between-group differences was significant.

Analysis of neurocognitive functioning showed similar decrements in all measures of neurocognitive function, except for the processing speed index which was reduced to a greater extent after STN DBS than Gpi DBS ($P = 0.03$). The Beck Depression Inventory II improved slightly for the Gpi group, but worsened slightly for the STN group ($P = 0.02$). There were no significant differences in the type or frequency of adverse events between the two study groups at 24 months.

Thirty-six-month outcomes were reported for 159 patients who had undergone surgery per the original VA Cooperative Study design [93]. Those completing the 36-month follow-up were younger than the full sample (60.6 vs 63.2 years, $P = 0.01$), but were otherwise similar at baseline. The primary outcome was change in OFF medication UPDRS Part III scores between baseline and the 36-month follow-up. Scores improved from 41.1 to 27.1 (95% CI −16.4 to −10.8, $P < 0.001$) in the Gpi group and from 42.5 to 29.7 (95% CI −15.8 to −9.4, $P < 0.001$) in the STN group. These improvements were similar between targets and stable over the study interval. Motor diaries also revealed stable improvement in ON time without troublesome dyskinesia. PDQ-39 scores improved in both groups at 6 months, but then worsened over the remaining period; by 36 months, subscales for social support and cognition were worse than those at baseline. There were statistically significant differences between targets on the Mattis Dementia Rating Scale and the Hopkins Verbal Learning Test, which worsened in the STN group but were unchanged in the Gpi group;

however, differences in the baseline cognitive assessments between groups complicate interpretation. Overall, this extended follow-up demonstrated that both Gpi and STN DBS yield persistent motor benefits, but underscore the idea that quality of life is significantly affected by non-motor symptoms, which tend to progress despite intervention with DBS.

Another trial comparing neurostimulation to medical therapy in PD was designed in an effort to prove efficacy of a novel constant-current neurostimulation system. This prospective, randomized, multicenter controlled trial was conducted at 15 sites in the United States [94]. Inclusion criteria were: PD duration at least 5 years, favorable levodopa response as defined by 33% improvement on UPDRS Part III, 6 hours or greater OFF time, and moderate to severe dyskinesia during waking hours. In this study, all patients were implanted with a bilateral STN DBS system and then randomized in a 3:1 ratio of immediate stimulation to stimulation after a 3-month delay. Patients were aware of their group assignment. The primary outcome measure was based on motor diaries, specifically the change in the duration of ON time without bothersome dyskinesia at 3 months.

Of the 136 patients randomized, 101 were allocated to immediate stimulation (intervention) and the other 35 to delayed stimulation (controls). At 3 months, the DBS group accrued an additional 4.27 hours of good quality ON time, versus an additional 1.77 hours in the control group (between-group difference 2.51, 95% CI, 0.87–4.16, $P = 0.003$). Secondary analysis showed a reduction in medication OFF UPDRS Part III scores of 16.1 points in the stimulation group versus 2.1 points in the control group (between-group difference 14.0, 95% CI, 10.5–17.5, $P < 0.0001$). Rates of adverse events were largely in line with those reported in previous trials. This trial demonstrated the safety and efficacy of constant-current STN neurostimulation.

EARLYSTIM

The EARLYSTIM trial was designed to test the hypothesis that neurostimulation at an earlier stage of PD is associated with an improvement in quality of life {Schuepbach 2013}. Inclusion criteria covered patients between 18 and 60 years of age who had levodopa-responsive PD for at least 4 years and were below Hoen and Yahr stage 3 in the on-medication condition. In contrast to the previous studies, the presence of motor fluctuations or dyskinesia for more than 3 years was an exclusion criteria. Thus, this trial enrolled patients at an earlier stage of PD than did previous large controlled trials.

Patients were randomized to undergo either bilateral STN DBS or best medical management. Assessments continued through to 24 months. The primary end point was the between-group difference in change in quality of life over the study period as assessed by the PDQ-39 summary

index. Additional assessments included blinded evaluation of pre- and postoperative UPDRS Part III scores based on videotaped exams, activities of daily living (UPDRS-II), treatment-related complications (UPDRS-IV), motor diaries, and levodopa-equivalent daily doses. Depression scales and adverse events were collected.

A total of 251 patients were enrolled, randomized to neurostimulation (124) or medical therapy (127), and included in the intention-to-treat analysis. Baseline characteristics were similar between groups and included a mean disease duration of 7.5 years (versus 11.7 years in the VA Cooperative trial), and a mean duration of motor complications of 1.7 years. The primary outcome analysis revealed a between-group difference of 8.0 points on the PDQ-39 summary index score ($P = 0.002$), corresponding to a 26% improvement in PDQ-39 summary index score in the neurostimulation group versus a 1% decline in the medical group. All PDQ-39 subscores except communication and social support were significantly improved in the DBS versus medical group.

Medication OFF UPDRS Part III scores improved by 9.6 ± 0.8 points (38%, $P < 0.05$) in the DBS group versus no significant change in the medication group, resulting in a between-group difference of 8.6 ± 1.1 points favoring neurostimulation ($P < 0.001$). Both the UPDRS-IV scores for motor fluctuations and dyskinesia, and scores on an additional dyskinesia scale, improved to a significantly greater extent in the DBS group versus medical group. Motor diaries further confirmed beneficial effects, with a between-group difference of 1.9 hours ($P = 0.01$) more time with good mobility and no troublesome dyskinesia in the DBS group, which also experienced 1.8 hours ($P = 0.006$) less time with bad mobility versus the medical group. Levodopa-equivalent daily doses were reduced to an average of 39% in the neurostimulation group versus increased by 21% in the medical group resulting in a between-group difference of 609 mg ($P < 0.001$).

There were no significant between-group differences in the Mattis Dementia Rating Scale scores. Changes in mood as assessed by the Montgomery and Asberg Depression Rating Scale ($P = 0.004$) and Beck Depression Inventory II ($P = 0.02$) were in favor of neurostimulation. Numbers of all adverse events were not significantly different between groups, and 68 patients in the DBS group versus 56 in the medical group have at least one serious adverse event. There were three deaths, all due to suicide, two of which were in the DBS group and one of which was in the medical group. Four additional suicide attempts were split evenly between the groups.

Overall, the EARLYSTIM trial demonstrated that bilateral STN DBS at an earlier stage of motor fluctuations and/or dyskinesia improves quality of life and motor outcomes to a degree similar to that reported in earlier trials investigating DBS approximately 4–6 years further into the disease progression.

While DBS is an established symptomatic treatment for PD motor complications, it has neither been proved nor disproved to be neuroprotective. A general principle of disease-modifying strategies is that they be applied as early as possible in the course of disease; hence, future DBS trials are likely to focus on evaluating the procedure in even earlier stages of disease. A pilot study evaluating the safety of DBS in PD patients at the earliest stage of disease, before the development of either motor fluctuations or dyskinesia, has been detailed in a publication within our search window [95], though the report detailing final results was just published in 2014 [95]. Thirty subjects aged 50–70, on medication for ≥6 months but ≤4 years, and without motor fluctuations or dyskinesia were randomized to DBS + medical therapy (15) or medical therapy alone (15). A primary end point was the time to reach a 4-point worsening from baseline on the medication OFF UPDRS Part III score, a measure designed to ensure that early stimulation did not hasten disease progression. A co-primary end point was the change in levodopa-equivalent daily dose from baseline to 24 months. As the investigators hypothesized, it would be the case at this early stage of disease, there were no significant differences in the UPDRS Part III scores between groups either ON or OFF medications. Levodopa equivalents were lower in the DBS group at all time points. Two subjects in the DBS group suffered serious adverse events. On the basis of this pilot trial, the investigators have designed and gained FDA approval for a pivotal randomized trial testing DBS in this early disease stage.

Conclusion

Partly because of its perceived immediate and dramatic effects treating motor parkinsonism, DBS of the STN or Gpi rapidly because a standard-of-care therapy, even before there was a rigorous evidence base to support its use. Over the last few years, several well-designed controlled trials have demonstrated the efficacy of DBS in improving the severity of the motor symptoms, in reducing the time spent in the OFF state or with troublesome dyskinesia, and in improving quality of life. Future studies will attempt to establish evidence for or against a neuroprotective effect.

References

1 Fox, S.H., Katzenschlager, R., Lim, S.-Y. *et al.* (2011) The movement disorder society evidence-based medicine review update: Treatments for the motor symptoms of Parkinson's disease. *Movement Disorders*, **26(Suppl 3)**, S2–S41.

2 Ferreira, J.J., Katzenschlager, R., Bloem, B.R. *et al.* (2013) Summary of the recommendations of the EFNS/MDS-ES review on therapeutic management of Parkinson's disease. *European Journal of Neurology*, **20**, 5–15.

3 Goetz, C.G., Poewe, W., Rascol, O. & Sampaio, C. (2005) Evidence-based medical review update: pharmacological and surgical treatments of Parkinson's disease: 2001 to 2004. *Movement Disorders*, **20**, 523–539.

4 Fahn, S., Oakes, D., Shoulson, I. *et al.* (2004) Levodopa and the progression of Parkinson's disease. *New England Journal of Medicine*, **351**, 2498–2508.

5 Koller, W.C., Hutton, J.T., Tolosa, E. & Capilldeo, R. (1999) Immediate-release and controlled-release carbidopa/levodopa in PD: a 5-year randomized multicenter study. Carbidopa/Levodopa Study Group. *Neurology*, **53**, 1012–1019.

6 Hauser, R.A. (2012) IPX066: a novel carbidopa-levodopa extended-release formulation. *Expert Review*, **12**, 133–140.

7 Mao, Z., Hsu, A., Gupta, S. & Modi, N.B. (2013) Population pharmacodynamics of IPX066: an oral extended-release capsule formulation of carbidopa-levodopa, and immediate-release carbidopa-levodopa in patients with advanced Parkinson's disease. *Journal of Clinical Pharmacology*, **53**, 523–531.

8 Hauser, R.A., Ellenbogen, A.L., Metman, L.V. *et al.* (2011) Crossover comparison of IPX066 and a standard levodopa formulation in advanced Parkinson's disease. *Movement Disorders*, **26**, 2246–2252.

9 Pahwa, R., Lyons, K.E., Hauser, R.A. *et al.* (2014) Randomized trial of IPX066, carbidopa/levodopa extended release, in early Parkinson's disease. *Parkinsonism & Related Disorders*, **20**, 142–148.

10 Schapira, A.H.V., McDermott, M.P., Barone, P. *et al.* (2013) Pramipexole in patients with early Parkinson's disease (PROUD): a randomised delayed-start trial. *Lancet Neurology*, **12**, 747–755.

11 Holloway, R.G., Shoulson, I., Fahn, S. *et al.* (2004) Pramipexole vs levodopa as initial treatment for Parkinson disease: a 4-year randomized controlled trial. *Archives of Neurology*, **61**, 1044–1053.

12 Parkinson, S.G. (2000) Pramipexole vs levodopa as initial treatment for Parkinson disease: A randomized controlled trial. Parkinson Study Group. *JAMA*, **284**, 1931–1938.

13 Parkinson Study Group (2002) Dopamine transporter brain imaging to assess the effects of pramipexole vs levodopa on Parkinson disease progression. *JAMA*, **287**, 1653–1661.

14 Kieburtz, K. & Parkinson Study Group Prami BIDI (2011) Twice-daily, low-dose pramipexole in early Parkinson's disease: a randomized, placebo-controlled trial. *Movement Disorders*, **26**, 37–44.

15 Hubble, J.P., Koller, W.C., Cutler, N.R. *et al.* (1995) Pramipexole in patients with early Parkinson's disease. *Clinical Neuropharmacology*, **18**, 338–347.

16 Group, P.S. (1997) Safety and efficacy of pramipexole in early Parkinson disease. A randomized dose-ranging study. Parkinson Study Group. *JAMA*, **278**, 125–130.

17 Shannon, K.M., Bennett, J.P. Jr., & Friedman, J.H. (1997) Efficacy of pramipexole, a novel dopamine agonist, as monotherapy in mild to moderate Parkinson's disease. The Pramipexole Study Group. *Neurology*, **49**, 724–728.

18 Singer, C., Lamb, J., Ellis, A., Layton, G. & Sumanirole for Early Parkinson's Disease Study Group (2007) A comparison of sumanirole versus placebo or ropinirole for the treatment of

patients with early Parkinson's disease. *Movement Disorders*, **22**, 476–482.

19 Adler, C.H., Sethi, K.D., Hauser, R.A. *et al.* (1997) Ropinirole for the treatment of early Parkinson's disease. The Ropinirole Study Group. *Neurology*, **49**, 393–399.

20 Brooks, D.J., Abbott, R.J., Lees, A.J. *et al.* (1998) A placebo-controlled evaluation of ropinirole, a novel D2 agonist, as sole dopaminergic therapy in Parkinson's disease. *Clinical Neuropharmacology*, **21**, 101–107.

21 Rascol, O., Brooks, D.J., Brunt, E.R., Korczyn, A.D., Poewe, W.H. & Stocchi, F. (1998) Ropinirole in the treatment of early Parkinson's disease: a 6-month interim report of a 5-year levodopa-controlled study. 056 Study Group. *Movement Disorders*, **13**, 39–45.

22 Rascol, O., Brooks, D.J., Korczyn, A.D., De Deyn, P.P., Clarke, C.E. & Lang, A.E. (2000) A five-year study of the incidence of dyskinesia in patients with early Parkinson's disease who were treated with ropinirole or levodopa. 056 Study Group. *New England Journal of Medicine*, **342**, 1484–1491.

23 Whone, A.L., Watts, R.L., Stoessl, A.J. *et al.* (2003) Slower progression of Parkinson's disease with ropinirole versus levodopa: The REAL-PET study. *Annals of Neurology*, **54**, 93–101.

24 Jenner, P., Konen-Bergmann, M., Schepers, C. & Haertter, S. (2009) Pharmacokinetics of a once-daily extended-release formulation of pramipexole in healthy male volunteers: three studies. *Clinical Therapeutics*, **31**, 2698–2711.

25 Hauser, R.A., Schapira, A.H.V., Rascol, O. *et al.* (2010) Randomized, double-blind, multicenter evaluation of pramipexole extended release once daily in early Parkinson's disease. *Movement Disorders*, **25**, 2542–2549.

26 Tompson, D.J. & Vearer, D. (2007) Steady-state pharmacokinetic properties of a 24-hour prolonged-release formulation of ropinirole: Results of two randomized studies in patients with Parkinson's disease. *Clinical Therapeutics*, **29**, 2654–2666.

27 Stocchi, F., Hersh, B.P., Scott, B.L., Nausieda, P.A., Giorgi, L. & Ease, P.D.M.S.I. (2008) Ropinirole 24-hour prolonged release and ropinirole immediate release in early Parkinson's disease: a randomized, double-blind, non-inferiority crossover study. *Current Medical Research and Opinion*, **24**, 2883–2895.

28 Metman, L.V., Gillespie, M., Farmer, C. *et al.* (2001) Continuous transdermal dopaminergic stimulation in advanced Parkinson's disease. *Clinical Neuropharmacology*, **24**, 163–169.

29 Elshoff, J.-P., Braun, M., Andreas, J.-O., Middle, M. & Cawello, W. (2012) Steady-state plasma concentration profile of transdermal rotigotine: An integrated analysis of three, open-label, randomized, phase I multiple dose studies. *Clinical Therapeutics*, **34**, 966–978.

30 LeWitt, P.A., Lyons, K.E., Pahwa, R. & Group, S.P.S. (2007) Advanced Parkinson disease treated with rotigotine transdermal system: PREFER Study. *Neurology*, **68**, 1262–1267.

31 Poewe, W.H., Rascol, O., Quinn, N. *et al.* (2007) Efficacy of pramipexole and transdermal rotigotine in advanced Parkinson's disease: a double-blind, double-dummy, randomised controlled trial. *Lancet Neurology*, **6**, 513–520.

32 Giladi, N., Boroojerdi, B., Korczyn, A.D. *et al.* (2007) Rotigotine transdermal patch in early Parkinson's disease: a randomized, double-blind, controlled study versus placebo and ropinirole. *Movement Disorders*, **22**, 2398–2404.

33 Jankovic, J., Watts, R.L., Martin, W. & Boroojerdi, B. (2007) Transdermal rotigotine: double-blind, placebo-controlled trial in Parkinson disease. *Archives of Neurology*, **64**, 676–682.

34 Parkinson Study G (2003) A controlled trial of rotigotine monotherapy in early Parkinson's disease. *Archives of Neurology*, **60**, 1721–1728.

35 Trenkwalder, C., Kies, B., Rudzinska, M. *et al.* (2011) Rotigotine effects on early morning motor function and sleep in Parkinson's disease: a double-blind, randomized, placebo-controlled study (RECOVER). *Movement Disorders*, **26**, 90–99.

36 Elmer, L.W., Surmann, E., Boroojerdi, B. & Jankovic, J. (2012) Long-term safety and tolerability of rotigotine transdermal system in patients with early-stage idiopathic Parkinson's disease: A prospective, open-label extension study. *Parkinsonism & Related Disorders*, **18**, 488–493.

37 Bracco, F., Battaglia, A., Chouza, C. *et al.* (2004) The long-acting dopamine receptor agonist cabergoline in early Parkinson's disease: final results of a 5-year, double-blind, levodopa-controlled study. *CNS Drugs*, **18**, 733–746.[Erratum appears in CNS Drugs. 2005;19(7):633].

38 Katzenschlager, R., Head, J., Schrag, A. *et al.* (2008) Fourteen-year final report of the randomized PDRG-UK trial comparing three initial treatments in PD. *Neurology*, **71**, 474–480.

39 Parkinson's Disease Research Group in the United Kingdom (1993) Comparisons of therapeutic effects of levodopa, levodopa and selegiline, and bromocriptine in patients with early, mild Parkinson's disease: three year interim report.. *BMJ*, **307**, 469–472.

40 Lees, A.J., Katzenschlager, R., Head, J. & Ben-Shlomo, Y. (2001) Ten-year follow-up of three different initial treatments in de-novo PD: A randomized trial. *Neurology*, **57**, 1687–1694.

41 Hely, M.A., Morris, J.G.L., Reid, W.G.J. & Trafficante, R. (2005) Sydney multicenter study of Parkinson's disease: non-L-dopa-responsive problems dominate at 15 years. *Movement Disorders*, **20**, 190–199.

42 Hely, M.A., Morris, J.G., Traficante, R., Reid, W.G., O'Sullivan, D.J. & Williamson, P.M. (1999) The sydney multicentre study of Parkinson's disease: progression and mortality at 10 years. *Journal of Neurology, Neurosurgery, and Psychiatry*, **67**, 300–307.

43 Hely, M.A., Morris, J.G., Reid, W.G. *et al.* (1994) The sydney multicentre study of Parkinson's disease: a randomised, prospective five year study comparing low dose bromocriptine with low dose levodopa-carbidopa. *Journal of Neurology, Neurosurgery, and Psychiatry*, **57**, 903–910.

44 Przuntek, H., Welzel, D., Gerlach, M. *et al.* (1996) Early institution of bromocriptine in Parkinson's disease inhibits the emergence of levodopa-associated motor side effects. Long-term results of the PRADO study. *Journal of Neural Transmission*, **103**, 699–715.

45 Gimenez-Roldan, S., Tolosa, E., Burguera, J.A., Chacon, J., Liano, H. & Forcadell, F. (1997) Early combination of bromocriptine and levodopa in Parkinson's disease: a prospective randomized study of two parallel groups over a total follow-up period of 44 months including an initial 8-month double-blind stage. *Clinical Neuropharmacology*, **20**, 67–76.

46 Nakanishi, T., Mizuno, Y., Goto, I. *et al.* (1991) A nationwide collaborative study on the long-term effects of bromocriptine in patients with Parkinson's disease. The fourth interim report. *European Neurology*, **31(Suppl 1)**, 3–16.

47 Parkinson Study Group (2002) A controlled trial of rasagiline in early Parkinson disease: the TEMPO Study. *Archives of Neurology*, **59**, 1937–1943.

48 Parkinson Study Group (2004) A controlled, randomized, delayed-start study of rasagiline in early Parkinson disease. *Archives of Neurology*, **61**, 561–566.

49 Stern, M.B., Marek, K.L., Friedman, J. *et al.* (2004) Double-blind, randomized, controlled trial of rasagiline as monotherapy in early Parkinson's disease patients. *Movement Disorders*, **19**, 916–923.

50 Olanow, C.W., Rascol, O., Hauser, R. *et al.* (2009) A double-blind, delayed-start trial of rasagiline in Parkinson's disease. *New England Journal of Medicine*, **361**, 1268–1278.

51 Stocchi, F., Rascol, O., Kieburtz, K. *et al.* (2010) Initiating levodopa/carbidopa therapy with and without entacapone in early Parkinson disease: the STRIDE-PD study. *Annals of Neurology*, **68**, 18–27.

52 Hauser, R.A., Panisset, M., Abbruzzese, G. *et al.* (2009) Double-blind trial of levodopa/carbidopa/entacapone versus levodopa/carbidopa in early Parkinson's disease. *Movement Disorders*, **24**, 541–550.

53 Lieberman, A., Gopinathan, G., Miller, E., Neophytides, A., Baumann, G. & Chin, L. (1990) Randomized double-blind cross-over study of Sinemet-controlled release (CR4 50/200) versus Sinemet 25/100 in Parkinson's disease. *European Neurology*, **30**, 75–78.

54 Ahlskog, J.E., Muenter, M.D., McManis, P.G., Bell, G.N. & Bailey, P.A. (1988) Controlled-release Sinemet (CR-4): a double-blind crossover study in patients with fluctuating Parkinson's disease. *Mayo Clinic Proceedings*, **63**, 876–886.

55 Wolters, E.C. & Tesselaar, H.J. (1996) International (NL-UK) double-blind study of Sinemet CR and standard Sinemet (25/100) in 170 patients with fluctuating Parkinson's disease. *Journal of Neurology*, **243**, 235–240.

56 Hutton, J.T., Morris, J.L., Bush, D.F., Smith, M.E., Liss, C.L. & Reines, S. (1989) Multicenter controlled study of Sinemet CR vs Sinemet (25/100) in advanced Parkinson's disease. *Neurology*, **39**, 67–72.discussion 72–73.

57 Jankovic, J., Schwartz, K. & Vander Linden, C. (1989) Comparison of Sinemet CR4 and standard Sinemet: double blind and long-term open trial in parkinsonian patients with fluctuations. *Movement Disorders*, **4**, 303–309.

58 Hauser, R.A., Hsu, A., Kell, S. *et al.* (2013) Extended-release carbidopa-levodopa (IPX066) compared with immediate-release carbidopa-levodopa in patients with Parkinson's disease and motor fluctuations: A phase 3 randomised, double-blind trial. *Lancet Neurology*, **12**, 346–356.

59 Nilsson, D., Nyholm, D. & Aquilonius, S.M. (2001) Duodenal levodopa infusion in Parkinson's disease--long-term experience. *Acta Neurologica Scandinavica*, **104**, 343–348.

60 Nyholm, D., Nilsson Remahl, A.I.M., Dizdar, N. *et al.* (2005) Duodenal levodopa infusion monotherapy vs oral polypharmacy in advanced Parkinson disease. *Neurology*, **64**, 216–223.

61 Fernandez, H.H., Vanagunas, A., Odin, P. *et al.* (2013) Levodopa-carbidopa intestinal gel in advanced Parkinson's disease open-label study: Interim results. *Parkinsonism & Related Disorders*, **19**, 339–345.

62 Nyholm, D., Askmark, H., Gomes-Trolin, C. *et al.* (2003) Optimizing levodopa pharmacokinetics: Intestinal infusion versus oral sustained-release tablets. *Clinical Neuropharmacology*, **26**, 156–163.

63 Antonini, A., Isaias, I.U., Canesi, M. *et al.* (2007) Duodenal levodopa infusion for advanced Parkinson's disease: 12-month treatment outcome. *Movement Disorders*, **22**, 1145–1149.

64 Fung, V.S.C., Herawati, L., Wan, Y. & Movement Disorder Society of Australia Clinical R, Trials G, Group Q-AS (2009) Quality of life in early Parkinson's disease treated with levodopa/carbidopa/entacapone. *Movement Disorders*, **24**, 25–31.

65 Reichmann, H., Boas, J., Macmahon, D. *et al.* (2005) Efficacy of combining levodopa with entacapone on quality of life and activities of daily living in patients experiencing wearing-off type fluctuations. *Acta Neurologica Scandinavica*, **111**, 21–28.

66 Mizuno, Y., Kanazawa, I., Kuno, S., Yanagisawa, N., Yamamoto, M. & Kondo, T. (2007) Placebo-controlled, double-blind dose-finding study of entacapone in fluctuating parkinsonian patients. *Movement Disorders*, **22**, 75–80.

67 Rascol, O., Brooks, D.J., Melamed, E. *et al.* (2005) Rasagiline as an adjunct to levodopa in patients with Parkinson's disease and motor fluctuations (LARGO, Lasting effect in Adjunct therapy with Rasagiline Given Once daily, study): a randomised, double-blind, parallel-group trial. *Lancet*, **365**, 947–954.

68 Kornhuber, J., Bormann, J., Hubers, M., Rusche, K. & Riederer, P. (1991) Effects of the 1-amino-adamantanes at the MK-801-binding site of the NMDA-receptor-gated ion channel: a human postmortem brain study. *European Journal of Pharmacology*, **206**, 297–300.

69 Sawada, H., Oeda, T., Kuno, S. *et al.* (2010) Amantadine for dyskinesias in Parkinson's disease: a randomized controlled trial. *PLoS ONE*, **5**, e15298.

70 Wolf, E., Seppi, K., Katzenschlager, R. *et al.* (2010) Long-term antidyskinetic efficacy of amantadine in Parkinson's disease. *Movement Disorders*, **25**, 1357–1363.

71 Thomas, A., Iacono, D., Luciano, A.L., Armellino, K., Di Iorio, A. & Onofrj, M. (2004) Duration of amantadine benefit on dyskinesia of severe Parkinson's disease. *Journal of Neurology, Neurosurgery, and Psychiatry*, **75**, 141–143.

72 Ondo, W.G., Sethi, K.D. & Kricorian, G. (2007) Selegiline orally disintegrating tablets in patients with Parkinson disease and "wearing off" symptoms. *Clinical Neuropharmacology*, **30**, 295–300.

73 Waters, C.H., Sethi, K.D., Hauser, R.A., Molho, E., Bertoni, J.M. & Zydis Selegiline Study Group (2004) Zydis selegiline reduces off time in Parkinson's disease patients with motor fluctuations: a 3-month, randomized, placebo-controlled study. *Movement Disorders*, **19**, 426–432.

74 Lees, A.J., Shaw, K.M., Kohout, L.J. *et al.* (1977) Deprenyl in Parkinson's disease. *Lancet*, **2**, 791–795.

75 Lieberman, A.N., Gopinathan, G., Neophytides, A. & Foo, S.H. (1987) Deprenyl versus placebo in Parkinson disease: a double-blind study. *New York State Journal of Medicine*, **87**, 646–649.

76 Golbe, L.I., Lieberman, A.N., Muenter, M.D. *et al.* (1988) Deprenyl in the treatment of symptom fluctuations in advanced Parkinson's disease. *Clinical Neuropharmacology*, **11**, 45–55.

77 Parkinson Study Group (2005) A randomized placebo-controlled trial of rasagiline in levodopa-treated patients with Parkinson disease and motor fluctuations: the PRESTO study. *Archives of Neurology*, **62**, 241–248.

78 Barone, P., Lamb, J., Ellis, A. & Clarke, Z. (2007) Sumanirole versus placebo or ropinirole for the adjunctive treatment of patients with advanced Parkinson's disease. *Movement Disorders*, **22**, 483–489.

79 Mizuno, Y., Abe, T., Hasegawa, K. *et al.* (2007) Ropinirole is effective on motor function when used as an adjunct to levodopa in Parkinson's disease: STRONG study. *Movement Disorders*, **22**, 1860–1865.

80 Rascol, O., Lees, A.J., Senard, J.M., Pirtosek, Z., Montastruc, J.L. & Fuell, D. (1996) Ropinirole in the treatment of levodopa-induced motor fluctuations in patients with Parkinson's disease. *Clinical Neuropharmacology*, **19**, 234–245.

81 Lieberman, A., Olanow, C.W., Sethi, K. *et al.* (1998) A multicenter trial of ropinirole as adjunct treatment for Parkinson's disease. Ropinirole Study Group. *Neurology*, **51**, 1057–1062.

82 Watts, R.L., Lyons, K.E., Pahwa, R. *et al.* (2010) Onset of dyskinesia with adjunct ropinirole prolonged-release or additional levodopa in early Parkinson's disease. *Movement Disorders*, **25**, 858–866.

83 Moller, J.C., Oertel, W.H., Koster, J., Pezzoli, G. & Provinciali, L. (2005) Long-term efficacy and safety of pramipexole in advanced Parkinson's disease: results from a European multicenter trial. *Movement Disorders*, **20**, 602–610.

84 Mizuno, Y., Yanagisawa, N., Kuno, S. *et al.* (2003) Randomized, double-blind study of pramipexole with placebo and bromocriptine in advanced Parkinson's disease. *Movement Disorders*, **18**, 1149–1156.

85 Pinter, M.M., Pogarell, O. & Oertel, W.H. (1999) Efficacy, safety, and tolerance of the non-ergoline dopamine agonist pramipexole in the treatment of advanced Parkinson's disease: a double blind, placebo controlled, randomised, multicentre study. *Journal of Neurology, Neurosurgery, and Psychiatry*, **66**, 436–441.

86 Dewey, R.B., Hutton, J.T., LeWitt, P.A. & Factor, S.A. (2001) A randomized, double-blind, placebo-controlled trial of subcutaneously injected apomorphine for parkinsonian off-state events. *Archives of Neurology*, **58**, 1385–1392.

87 Kleiner-Fisman, G., Herzog, J., Fisman, D.N. *et al.* (2006) Subthalamic nucleus deep brain stimulation: summary and meta-analysis of outcomes. *Movement Disorders*, **21**(**Suppl 14**), S290–S304.

88 Deuschl, G., Schade-Brittinger, C., Krack, P. *et al.* (2006) A randomized trial of deep-brain stimulation for Parkinson's disease. *The New England Journal of Medicine*, **355**, 896–908.

89 Okun, M.S., Fernandez, H.H., Wu, S.S. *et al.* (2009) Cognition and mood in Parkinson's disease in subthalamic nucleus versus globus pallidus interna deep brain stimulation: the COMPARE trial. *Annals of Neurology*, **65**, 586–595.

90 Williams, A., Gill, S., Varma, T. *et al.* (2010) Deep brain stimulation plus best medical therapy versus best medical therapy alone for advanced Parkinson's disease (PD SURG trial): a randomised, open-label trial. *Lancet Neurology*, **9**, 581–591.

91 Weaver, F.M., Follett, K., Stern, M. *et al.* (2009) Bilateral deep brain stimulation vs best medical therapy for patients with advanced Parkinson disease: a randomized controlled trial. *JAMA : The Journal of the American Medical Association*, **301**, 63–73.

92 Follett, K.A., Weaver, F.M., Stern, M. *et al.* (2010) Pallidal versus subthalamic deep-brain stimulation for Parkinson's disease. *The New England Journal of Medicine*, **362**, 2077–2091.

93 Weaver, F.M., Follett, K.A., Stern, M. *et al.* (2012) Randomized trial of deep brain stimulation for Parkinson disease: thirty-six-month outcomes. *Neurology*, **79**, 55–65.

94 Okun, M.S., Gallo, B.V., Mandybur, G. *et al.* (2012) Subthalamic deep brain stimulation with a constant-current device in Parkinson's disease: an open-label randomised controlled trial. *Lancet Neurology*, **11**, 140–149.

95 Charles, P.D., Dolhun, R.M., Gill, C.E. *et al.* (2012) Deep brain stimulation in early Parkinson's disease: enrollment experience from a pilot trial. *Parkinsonism & Related Disorders*, **18**, 268–273.

CHAPTER 20
Therapies for multiple sclerosis

Greg Thaera[1] and Dean M. Wingerchuk[2]
[1]*Mayo Clinic, Scottsdale, AZ, USA*
[2]*Department of Neurology, Mayo Clinic College of Medicine, Scottsdale, AZ, USA*

Introduction

Multiple sclerosis (MS) is an idiopathic inflammatory demyelinating disease of the central nervous system. It is one of the leading causes of neurologic disability, particularly in young adults, and is presumed to be autoimmune. There are several recognized clinical patterns of MS. Most patients, about 85%, have relapsing-remitting disease (RRMS), which is defined by the fact that they experienced an acute or subacute episode of neurological dysfunction at clinical disease onset. Such an event is known as an attack (relapse, exacerbation, or flare). Attack symptoms depend on the neuroanatomic site of inflammatory demyelination, but the most common types include optic neuritis, diplopia, vertigo, and other brain stem symptoms, and spinal cord dysfunction. Attacks typically evolve over days to weeks, plateau, and usually improve or resolve completely, especially early in the disease. A patient who experience such an attack for the first time and who has brain MRI evidence of lesions suggestive of MS is said to have a "clinically isolated syndrome" with high risk for future confirmed RRMS, which would be established by subsequent new clinical attacks or MRI lesions. The disease appears to be quiescent during clinical remissions (the periods between relapses), though magnetic resonance imaging (MRI) scans often detect subclinical disease activity. The remaining 15% of MS patients present with neurological impairment that is progressive from onset (e.g., gradually worsening gait disorder from myelopathy) rather than attack-related; such patients are said to have primary progressive multiple sclerosis (PPMS). About two-thirds of RRMS patients will ultimately convert to a secondary progressive course (SPMS) over the course of years or decades. The courses of established PPMS and SPMS are fundamentally similar; relapses may occur during either, but are uncommon.

Disease-modifying therapies (DMTs) are medications that have been shown to affect the course of RRMS by reducing relapse rate and, in some cases, slowing accumulation of disability. Pivotal RCTs have established standard methodologies for assessment of relapses, neurological disability (using the 10-point Expanded Disability Status Scale (EDSS)), and confirmed disease progression (typically, a 3-month or 6-month confirmed increase in EDSS score by 0.5 point or more for those with a baseline score of 5.0 or less, or 1.0 point or more for those subjects with a baseline score of 5.5 or greater). In the United States, eight DMTs have been approved by the Food and Drug Administration (FDA) for treatment of RRMS or "relapsing forms" of MS (Table 20.1). An additional medication, intravenous mitoxantrone (Novantrone®), was approved by the FDA in 2000 for worsening RRMS or SPMS. The FDA also approved oral extended-release dalfampridine (Ampyra®) in 2009; this medication is not a DMT but a symptomatic therapy specifically approved for treatment of gait impairment due to multiple sclerosis. This chapter will discuss the evidence supporting the use of these MS therapies.

Methods

Literature searches were performed using the MEDLINE database from 1946 to 2013 and EMBASE from 1988 to 2013. Medical subject headings (MeSHs) used for each search included the term "multiple sclerosis" as well as the generic names of the drugs being evaluated. Searches were limited to randomized controlled trials (RCTs) published in English. Summary results are presented based on the main RCT outcome measure(s) that address each question. We avoided attempts to draw conclusions by comparing efficacy results (absolute or relative risk/rate reductions or numbers needed to treat) of different pivotal trials because the details of the study subjects, study methodology, outcome measures, study durations, and statistical analysis methods differ enough to provide uncertainty. However, we describe the data and conclusions for head-to-head DMT trials, where available.

Evidence-Based Neurology: Management of Neurological Disorders, Second Edition. Edited by Bart M. Demaerschalk and Dean M. Wingerchuk.
© 2015 John Wiley & Sons, Ltd. Published 2015 by John Wiley & Sons, Ltd.

Table 20.1 Disease-modifying therapies for multiple sclerosis

Subcutaneous interferon-β1b	(Betaseron®)	1993
Intramuscular interferon-β1a	(Avonex®)	1996
Subcutaneous glatiramer acetate	(Copaxone®)	1996
Subcutaneous interferon-β1a	(Rebif®)	2002
Intravenous natalizumab	(Tysabri®)	2006
Subcutaneous interferon-β1b	(Extavia®)	2009
Oral fingolimod	(Gilenya®)	2010
Oral teriflunomide	(Aubagio®)	2012
Oral dimethyl fumarate	(Tecfidera®)	2013

This table lists currently approved MS disease-modifying therapies, their US trade names, and the year each received US regulatory approval.

Clinically isolated syndrome

Clinical scenario

An otherwise healthy 26-year-old man experienced diplopia, his first-ever neurological symptom. Consistent with a clinically isolated syndrome (CIS), his brain MRI revealed multiple nonenhancing periventricular and juxtacortical lesions. He inquires whether disease-modifying therapies would help prevent a second clinical attack.

Clinical question: Interferon-beta and CIS

Compared to placebo, does treatment with interferon-beta (IFNB) reduce the likelihood of a second clinical attack in CIS and thus progression to RRMS?

Evidence

The CHAMPS trial compared weekly intramuscular IFN-β1a to placebo following diagnosis of CIS in 383 patients. The primary clinical outcome was a subsequent diagnosis of clinically definite multiple sclerosis, reached by 35% on treatment group and 50% on placebo group (relative risk 0.56, $p = 0.002$). The primary radiologic outcome was increase in T2-weighted MRI brain lesion volume; at 18 months this was 1% for the treatment group and 16% for the placebo group ($p < 0.001$) [1].

The ETOMS trial compared subcutaneous IFN-β1a 22 μg weekly to placebo in 308 CIS patients over 2 years. The primary outcome, conversion to clinically definite multiple sclerosis, was met by 34% of patients on interferon and 45% on placebo ($p = 0.047$). Secondary outcomes included annualized relapse rate of 0.33 for interferon and 0.43 for placebo ($p = 0.045$), as well as total T2-weighted lesion volume on brain MRI ($p = 0.002$) [2].

The BENEFIT trial compared subcutaneous IFN-β1b 8 million international units (8 MIU) every other day to placebo in 468 patients with CIS over 2 years. The primary outcomes were time to conversion to clinically definite multiple sclerosis (CDMS) as defined by a second clinical attack or define MS as defined by the McDonald diagnostic criteria, which incorporates both clinical and radiologic findings

[3]. CDMS was diagnosed in 28% of patients on interferon and 45% on placebo ($p < 0.0001$) while McDonald criteria were used to diagnose MS in 69% on interferon and 85% on placebo ($p < 0.00001$). Secondary radiologic outcomes included change in T2-weight lesion volume on brain MRI, which also favored the interferon group ($p < 0.05$) [4].

Clinical bottom line

Compared to placebo, conversion of CIS to clinically definite RRMS is reduced by treatment with intramuscular interferon-β1a, subcutaneous interferon-β1a, and subcutaneous interferon-β1b.

Clinical question: Glatiramer acetate and CIS

Compared to placebo, does treatment with glatiramer acetate (GA) reduce the likelihood of a second clinical attack in CIS and thus progression to RRMS?

Evidence

The PreCISe study evaluated daily subcutaneous GA versus placebo in 481 patients for 3 years. Conversion to clinically definite multiple sclerosis, the primary outcome measure, was reduced by 45% ($p = 0.0005$); the secondary outcome of a second clinical attack occurred in 24.7% of GA and 42.9% of placebo patients. GA was superior with regard to secondary MRI measures including T2 lesion volume ($p = 0.0002$) and number of new T2 lesions on last visit of 0.7 vs 1.8 for placebo ($p < 0.0001$) [5].

Clinical bottom line

Compared to placebo, GA reduces the rate of conversion from CIS to MS.

Synthesis and application of evidence

In this patient with CIS and evidence of multiple lesions on MRI, treatment either with IFNB or GA is recommended to prevent a second attack and additional lesions on MRI. He is informed about the side effects of interferon, including flu-like symptoms such as malaise and myalgias with the injections, risk of injection site reactions, and need for monitoring with blood counts and liver enzymes. The risk of development of antibodies to IFNB is also discussed because such antibodies would render the medication less effective [6]. For GA, he is informed about risk of injection site reactions including welts, chest discomfort, and hyperventilation. After discussion of adverse effects, he elects to initiate subcutaneous daily GA for CIS.

Interferon-beta and glatiramer acetate for relapsing-remitting multiple sclerosis

Clinical scenario

An otherwise healthy 29-year-old woman recently experienced her second clinical attack, confirming RRMS. She has been offered a choice between various IFNB therapies and GA. She inquired how effective the drugs are for prevention acute relapses and protecting neurological function.

Clinical question: Interferon-beta and relapses

Compared to placebo, does treatment with IFNB reduce relapse rate in RRMS?

Evidence

The IFNB MS study group compared subcutaneous IFN-β1b at doses of 1.6 and 8 million international units (MIU) every other day versus placebo in 372 subjects. Primary outcomes were annual relapse rate and proportion of patients without an exacerbation during a 2-year period. The higher dose (8 MIU) of IFN-β reduced the annual relapse rate compared to placebo over 2 years, 0.84 vs 1.27 ($p = 0.0001$). Secondary outcome measures included T2 lesion volume on MRI, which increased by 17.1% on placebo but decreased by 6.6% on 8 MIU of IFN-β [7].

The Multiple Sclerosis Collaborative Research Group (MSCRG) studied weekly intramuscular IFN-β1a at a dose of 30 μg versus placebo ($n = 301$). The primary outcome measure was time to sustained disability progression, defined as an increase of 1.0 or more points on the expanded disability status scale (EDSS) persisting at least 6 months [8]. Annual relapse rate was 0.67 for the intramuscular IFN-β1a group and 0.82 for placebo group ($p = 0.04$). T2 lesion volume on MRI decreased by 13.1% for patients on interferon versus 3.3% on placebo ($p = 0.02$) [9]

The PRISMS trial evaluated the efficacy of subcutaneous IFN-β1a given thrice weekly in RRMS. The primary outcome was the number of relapses during a 2-year period. A total of 560 subjects were divided evenly into three groups: IFN-β1a 44 μg, IFN-β1a 22 μg, and placebo. Mean relapses during the 2-year trial were 1.73, 1.82, and 2.52, respectively ($p < 0.005$ for each treatment groups compared with placebo). Secondary outcome measures include median change in T2 lesion volume on brain MRI, which was −3.8%, −1.2%, and 10.9%, respectively ($p < 0.0001$ for each treatment group compared with placebo) [10].

Clinical bottom line

Compared to placebo, annual relapse rate in RRMS is reduced by treatment with intramuscular interferon-β1a, subcutaneous interferon-β1a, and subcutaneous interferon-β1b.

Clinical question: Interferon-beta and disability progression for RRMS

Compared to placebo, does treatment with IFN-β reduce the rate of disability progression in RRMS?

Evidence

The Multiple Sclerosis Collaborative Research Group (MSCRG) studied weekly intramuscular IFN-β1a at a dose

of 30 μg versus placebo ($n = 301$). The primary outcome measure was time to sustained disability progression, defined as an increase of 1.0 or more points on the EDSS persisting at least 6 months. After 2 years, time to sustained disability progression was longer in the group versus placebo ($p = 0.02$). A total of 172 patients were on study medication for at least 2 years. Of these, 21.2% of the treatment group and 33.3% on the placebo group had sustained disability progression [3].

The PRISMS trial evaluated the efficacy of subcutaneous IFN-β1a given thrice weekly in RRMS. The primary outcome was the number of relapses during a 2-year period. A total of 560 subjects were divided equally into three groups: IFN-β1a 44 μg, IFN-β1a 22 μg, and placebo. Time to disability progression was favorably influenced by both IFN doses; at 12 months, 25% of placebo subjects experienced sustained progression (confirmed by two examinations performed 3 months apart) at 12 months compared with 18 months for the IFN-β1a 22 μg group and 21 months for the IFN-β1a 44 μg group ($p < 0.05$) [4].

Clinical bottom line

Compared to placebo, short-term disability over a 2-year period as measured by the EDSS is reduced by treatment with intramuscular or subcutaneous interferon-β1a.

Clinical question: Glatiramer acetate for relapses

Compared to placebo, does treatment GA reduce relapse rate in RRMS?

Evidence

Glatiramer acetate, administered by subcutaneous injection at a dose of 20 mg daily, was studied in an RCT versus placebo during a 2-year period ($n = 251$). The primary outcome of reduced relapse rate was met, with 1.19 relapses in the treatment group over 2 years compared to 1.68 for placebo ($p = 0.007$) [11].

A second RCT evaluated the effect of GA in 239 patients with RRMS over 9 months using monthly brain MRIs. The primary outcome, total number of enhancing lesions on MRI, averaged 25.96 for GA and 36.80 for placebo ($p = 0.003$). Change in total T2 lesion volume favored GA ($p = 0.006$). Annual relapse rate was 0.51 for GA and 0.76 for placebo ($p = 0.012$) [12].

Clinical bottom line

Compared to placebo, treatment with GA reduces annual relapse rate for a period of 2 years.

Clinical question: Glatiramer acetate for clinical disability in RRMS

Compared to placebo, does treatment GA reduce the rate of disability progression in RRMS?

Evidence

Glatiramer acetate subcutaneous injection at a dose of 20 mg daily was studied in an RCT versus placebo during a 2-year period ($n = 251$). Mean EDSS change from baseline was −0.05 for GA and 0.21 for placebo ($p = 0.023$). It was found that 20.8% of patients on GA and 28.8% on placebo experienced sustained disability progression as measured by at least a 1.0 point change on the EDSS ($p = 0.037$) [5].

Clinical bottom line

In a single RCT, treatment with GA over a 2-year period reduced short-term disability compared to placebo.

Clinical question: comparative studies of relapse rate

Among the available forms of IFN-β or GA, are any superior for reducing relapse rate?

Evidence

IFN-β and GA have been compared for efficacy in three RCTs. The REGARD study was an open-label study comparing subcutaneous IFN-β1a versus GA over 96 weeks in 764 patients with RRMS. The primary outcome, time to first relapse, was not different between groups ($p = 0.64$). Other clinical outcomes of relapse rate and disability progression were not different between groups. However, in secondary outcome measures, the IFN-β1a group had significantly fewer gadolinium (GAD) enhancing lesions per MRI scan at 0.24 vs 0.41 for GA ($p = 0.0002$). By contrast, decrease in brain volume favored GA over IFN-β (−1.073% vs −1.240%, $p = 0.018$). The total volume of T1-hypointense, T2-hyperintense, and GAD-enhancing lesions on MRI were similar between the two groups [13].

The BEYOND trial compared subcutaneous IFN-β1b at the licensed dose of 250 μg as well as a higher dose of 500 μg every other day and GA in RRMS ($n = 2244$) in a 2:2:1 ratio over 2.0–3.5 years. The primary outcome was relapse risk as defined by new neurologic symptoms starting at least 30 days from a prior episode and lasting at least 24 hours. Relapse risk and annualized relapse rate did not significantly differ among either dose of IFN-β1b or GA. In secondary imaging outcome measures, total MRI disease burden was significantly lower in both IFN-β1b groups compared to GA during the first year only ($p = 0.0001$ and 0.0008 for 250 μg). As in the REGARD study, GA showed a smaller decrease in total brain volume compared to IFN-β1b ($p = 0.02$ for 250 μg, $p = 0.007$ for 500 μg). Overall, the two doses of IFN-β1b were not significantly different from each other, while clinical outcomes between IFN-β1b and GA were similar [14].

The BECOME study compared subcutaneous IFN-β1b 250 μg thrice weekly versus subcutaneous GA 20 mg daily over 2 years in 75 patients with RRMS or CIS. The primary outcome measure was new combined active lesions, a summation of new GAD-enhancing and new nonenhancing T2/fluid-attenuated inversion recovery (FLAIR) lesions on MRI. No difference was found between the two groups ($p = 0.58$). Clinically, annualized relapse rate was 0.37 for IFN-β1b versus 0.33 for GA; this difference was not significant ($p = 0.68$) [15].

Different formulations of IFNB have also been compared in two RCTs. The EVIDENCE study evaluated subcutaneous IFN-β1a 44 μg thrice weekly versus intramuscular IFN-β1a 30 μg weekly in 677 patients with RRMS. The primary clinical outcome, proportion of relapse-free patients at 24 weeks, was met in 74.9% of subcutaneous and 63.3% of intramuscular IFN-β1a patients (OR 1.9, $p = 0.0005$). Subcutaneous interferon also showed superior results over intramuscular interferon on the primary radiologic outcome, active lesions on MRI at 24 weeks ($p < 0.001$) [16].

The INCOMIN study compared subcutaneous IFN-β1b 250 μg thrice weekly to intramuscular IFN-β1b 30 μg weekly in 188 patients with RRMS over 2 years. The primary clinical outcome measure was proportion of relapse-free patients; this comprised 51% of the subcutaneous and 36% of the intramuscular interferon groups at 2 years ($p = 0.03$). The primary radiologic outcome was the proportion of patients without new T2-hyperintense lesions on MRI. Fifty-five percent of patients on subcutaneous and 26% on intramuscular interferon groups developed no new T2 lesions ($p < 0.0003$). The secondary outcome measure of clinical progression, defined by a sustained increase in EDSS of 1.0 or greater, was seen in 13% of the subcutaneous interferon group, a significant difference compared to 30% in the intramuscular interferon group ($p = 0.005$) [17].

Clinical bottom line

1 In the available head-to-head studies, subcutaneous IFNB and GA do not significantly differ in primary clinical and imaging outcome measures.

2 More patients remained relapse-free on subcutaneous IFNB thrice weekly compared with intramuscular IFNB weekly.

Synthesis and application of evidence

Our patient is informed that treatment with any of the IFNB drugs or GA can reduce her risk of relapse by approximately one-third over 2–3 years. Intramuscular and subcutaneous interferon-β1a preparations as well as subcutaneous GA also reduce the risk of disability progression over that time. Head-to-head trials show that she is more likely to remain relapse-free on subcutaneous over intramuscular IFNB. However, these studies suggest that the differences between these first-line injectable medications are small, and in most instances, the route and frequency of administration and adverse effect profiles have more influence on patient decision-making. After discussion, she elects to initiate intramuscular IFN-β1a.

Natalizumab and fingolimod

Natalizumab (Tysabri) and fingolimod (Gilenya) are newer therapies with novel mechanisms of action. Natalizumab is an intravenous humanized monoclonal antibody against alpha-4 integrin; this medication prevents entry of lymphocytes past the blood–brain barrier into the CNS. Fingolimod is an oral sphingosine 1-phosphate (S1P) receptor modulator that effectively traps circulating lymphocytes in lymphoid tissues. Both therapies effectively reduce CNS lymphocyte trafficking; because lymphocyte entry into the CNS is a key event in the pathobiology of MS relapses, they reduce relapse risk.

Clinical scenario

A 34-year-old man with RRMS experiences multiple relapses while taking IFNB therapy. He inquires whether natalizumab or fingolimod would be effective in treating his MS.

Clinical question: Natalizumab for RRMS

When compared to placebo, IFNB, or GA, does treatment with natalizumab reduce relapse rate or prevent disability progression in RRMS?

Evidence

Natalizumab was studied in the 2-year randomized placebo-controlled AFFIRM trial in 942 RRMS patients. The primary outcomes were defined as the rate of relapse at 1 year and rate of sustained disability progression at 2 years. The annual relapse rate at 1 year was 0.26 for natalizumab and 0.81 for placebo, a relative risk reduction of 68% ($p < 0.001$). Sustained disability progression at 2 years was observed in 17% of natalizumab and 29% of placebo patients ($p < 0.001$). Radiologically, new or enlarging T2-hyperintense lesions on MRI were reduced by 83% in the treatment arm compared to placebo ($p < 0.001$) [18].

The SENTINEL study compared natalizumab to placebo in 1171 patients over 2 years. Both study groups were simultaneously treated with intramuscular IFN-β1a weekly. Primary clinical outcomes were again defined as the rate of relapse at 1 year and rate of sustained disability progression at 2 years as defined by an increase in EDSS of at least 1.0 for at least 12 weeks. Annual relapse rate at 1 year was 0.38 for combination therapy versus 0.82 for interferon alone, a relative risk reduction of 54% ($p < 0.001$). The probability of sustained disability progression at 2 years was 23% for combination therapy versus 29% for interferon monotherapy, a reduction of 24% favoring natalizumab ($p < 0.001$). Radiologically, new or enlarging T2-hyperintense lesions on MRI were reduced by 83% in the treatment arm compared to placebo ($p < 0.001$) [19].

Clinical bottom line

1 Natalizumab reduces annual relapse rate in RRMS compared to placebo.

2 Natalizumab reduces disability progression in RRMS compared to placebo.

Synthesis and application of evidence

The patient is informed that natalizumab reduces both relapse rate and disability progression compared to placebo. There have been no randomized controlled trials directly comparing the efficacy of natalizumab with either IFN-beta or GA.

The main risk of natalizumab is the potential development of progressive multifocal leukoencephalopathy (PML) from reactivation of JC virus. PML has a 20% mortality rate and high morbidity with progressive neurologic decline and multifocal T2-hyperintense lesions with scant enhancement on MRI. The patient is informed that serologic testing is available, and if negative, his risk of PML approaches zero. He subsequently tests positive, thus the risk of PML depends on exposure to prior immunosuppressant agents and duration of treatment with natalizumab. Since he has had no prior immunosuppressant therapy, his estimated risk of PML is 0.056% during the first 24 months of treatment and 0.46% thereafter. If he had prior immunosuppressant use, the risk of PML would be 0.16% during the first 24 months and 1.11% following [20].

Clinical question: Fingolimod for RRMS

When compared to placebo, IFNB, or GA, does treatment with fingolimod reduce relapse rate or prevent disability progression in RRMS?

Evidence

Fingolimod was studied in the FREEDOMS RCT over 2 years in 1272 patients. Two separate doses of 0.5 mg and 1.25 mg orally daily were evaluated. The primary end point of annual relapse rate was 0.18 for the 0.5 mg fingolimod group, 0.16 for 1.25 mg, and 0.40 for the placebo group; thus fingolimod reduced the relapse rate by 54–60% ($p < 0.0001$ for both fingolimod groups versus placebo). A secondary clinical end point was time to disease progression confirmed after 3 months. The hazard ratio of this outcome was 0.70 for the 0.5 mg dose and 0.68 for the 1.25 mg dose compared to placebo ($p < 0.02$). Radiologically, both fingolimod groups were superior to placebo when comparing new or enlarged T2-hyperintense lesions, enhancing lesions with gadolinium contrast administration, and decrease in brain volume ($p < 0.001$ for all) [21].

The TRANSFORMS study compared the two doses of oral fingolimod to weekly IFN-β1a 30 μg weekly over 1 year in 1292 RRMS patients. The annual relapse rate was 0.16 for the 0.5 mg fingolimod group, 0.20 for 1.25 mg fingolimod, and 0.33 for intramuscular IFN-β1a 30 μg weekly ($p < 0.001$ for both fingolimod groups versus interferon). There was no difference in disability progression. MRI outcomes also showed fewer new T2-hyperintense or enhancing lesions in both fin-golimod groups compared to interferon [22].

Clinical bottom line
1 Fingolimod reduces annual relapse rate in RRMS compared to placebo.
2 Fingolimod reduces annual relapse rate in RRMS compared to weekly intramuscular interferon-β1a.

Synthesis and application of evidence
Fingolimod reduced annual relapse rate compared to both placebo and weekly intramuscular interferon-β1a and would certainly be a reasonable option for efficacy in this particular patient given persistent relapses on his current therapy. There are no RCTs that directly compare fingolimod to GA or natalizumab. Potential side effects, including first-dose bradycardia, macular edema, and immunosuppression are discussed. Monitoring with complete blood counts and liver enzymes is needed, as is electrocardiogram before and after the first dose, first-dose monitoring to evaluate for bradycardia or heart block, ophthalmologic evaluation at baseline and in 3–6 months, annual dermatologic evalua-tion, baseline pulmonary function testing, and evaluation for immunity to varicella-zoster virus.

The newest oral therapies: Teriflunomide and dimethyl fumarate

Teriflunomide is an oral pyrimidine synthesis inhibitor that blocks the enzyme dihydro-orotase. Dimethyl fumarate is an oral immunomodulator that appears to work by influencing the NRF-2 pathway, which is a key cellular defense.

Clinical scenario

A 32-year-old woman with early RRMS has avoided injectable therapies and has not considered fingolimod because of need for beta-blocker therapy for a cardiac arrhythmia. She inquires whether the new oral medications teriflunomide or dimethyl fumarate would be effective in treating her MS.

Clinical question: Teriflunomide for RRMS

Compared to placebo or other disease-modifying therapies, does treatment with teriflunomide reduce relapse rate or dis-ability progression in RRMS?

Evidence
Teriflunomide was studied against placebo in one RCT by the TEMSO study group. A total of 1088 patients with RRMS, aged 18–55 years and having EDSS scores from 0.0 to 5.5, were randomly assigned in a 1:1:1 ratio to 14 mg oral teriflunomide daily, 7 mg oral teriflunomide daily, or placebo for 108 weeks. The primary outcome was annualized relapse rate. Annual relapse rates were 0.37 for either teriflunomide

group and 0.54 for placebo with relative risk reduction of 31% for both treatment arms ($p < 0.001$). The key secondary end point was confirmed disability progression, sustained for at least 12 weeks. The proportion of patients experi-encing disability progression at 108 weeks was 20.2% for 14 mg teriflunomide ($p = 0.03$ vs placebo), 21.7% for 7 mg teriflunomide ($p = 0.08$ vs placebo) compared with 27.3% for placebo [23].

Clinical bottom line
1 Teriflunomide 7 mg or 14 mg reduces annual relapse rate in RRMS compared to placebo.
2 Teriflunomide 14 mg reduces disability progression in RRMS compared to placebo.

Synthesis and application of evidence
The patient is informed that treatment with oral teriflu-no-mide is effective over placebo in reducing the relapse rate and that the higher available dose of 14 mg daily also reduces pro-gression of disability. She is also informed of currently known side effects including teratogenicity, hair loss, and risk of hep-atotoxicity, the latter requiring regular blood monitoring.

Clinical question: Dimethyl fumarate for RRMS

Compared to placebo or other disease-modifying therapies, does treatment with dimethyl fumarate reduce relapse rate or disability progression in RRMS?

Evidence
The DEFINE RCT compared oral dimethyl fumarate at doses of 240 mg twice daily, 240 mg thrice daily, and placebo in a 1:1:1 ratio in 1234 RRMS patients. The primary outcome was the proportion of patients with a clinical relapse during the 2-year trial. Twenty-six percent of the thrice daily fumarate group, 27% of the twice daily fumarate group, and 47% on placebo experienced a relapse ($p < 0.001$ for each group versus placebo). Relative risk reduction of an acute relapse was 50% for fumarate thrice daily and 49% for twice daily compared to placebo. Annual relapse rates were 0.19 for fumarate thrice daily, 0.17 for fumarate twice daily, and 0.36 for placebo ($p < 0.001$ for each treatment group versus placebo). The hazard ratio for progression of disability sustained for 12 weeks for fumarate was 0.66 thrice daily ($p = 0.01$) and 0.62 twice daily ($p = 0.005$) compared to placebo [24].

The CONFIRM RCT compared oral dimethyl fumarate at doses of 240 mg twice and thrice daily, subcutaneous injection of 20 mg GA daily, and placebo in a 1:1:1:1 ratio for 1417 RRMS patients over 2 years. The primary outcome measure, annual relapse rate, was 0.20 for fumarate thrice daily, 0.22 for fumarate twice daily, 0.29 for GA, and 0.40 for placebo ($p < 0.001$ for both fumarate groups versus placebo, $p = 0.01$ for glatiramer versus placebo). Relative reductions in sustained disability progression compared to placebo were not significant at 24% for thrice daily fumarate, 21% for twice daily fumarate, and 7% for GA ($p > 0.05$ for all the three treatment groups). Results did not significantly differ between either dosing regimen for fumarate versus GA [25].

Clinical bottom line

1 Fumarate reduces risk of relapse compared to placebo.

2 Fumarate reduces disability progression compared to placebo.

Synthesis and application of evidence

Fumarate is effective for reducing relapse rate and possibly for disability progression and is an effective option for this patient with RRMS. Side effects including flushing, nausea, and diarrhea as well as the need for monitoring with complete blood counts are discussed.

Secondary progressive MS

Clinical scenario

A 50-year-old man was diagnosed with RRMS at the age of 30 years. Over the last 3 years, he had experienced gradually progressive worsening of gait and was diagnosed with SPMS. He had no other medical conditions. He inquired whether the currently available injectable disease-modifying therapies for RRMS or mitoxantrone are beneficial for SPMS.

Clinical question: DMTs for SPMS

Compared to placebo, does treatment with IFNB, GA, or mitoxantrone reduce disability progression in SPMS?

Evidence

The European study group on Interferon-β1b in Secondary Progressive MS performed an RCT comparing subcutaneous IFN-β1b every other day to placebo in 718 patients with SPMS and EDSS 3.0–6.5 over 3 years. The primary outcome measure was time to sustained disability progression as measured by an increase in EDSS of at least 1 point, 0.5 point if previously at EDSS 6.0 or higher, lasting at least 3 months. Time to sustained disability progression was delayed in the treatment group compared to placebo, with a delay of up to 9 months ($p = 0.0008$). Compared to 49.7% of patients in the placebo group (OR = 0.63, $p = 0.0048$), 38.9% of patients in the interferon group had sustained disability progression. Mean T2 lesion volume on MRI was decreased by 5% in the treatment arm and increased by 8% for placebo ($p < 0.0001$) [26].

The North American study group on Interferon beta-1b in Secondary Progressive MS also compared subcutaneous IFN-β1b every other day in two doses of 250 µg and 160 µg/m² versus placebo in 939 SPMS patients with EDSS 3.0–6.5 over 3 years. The primary outcome measure was time to sustained disability progression as measured by an increase in EDSS of at least 1 point, 0.5 point if previously

at EDSS 6.0 or higher, confirmed at 6 months. In this primary outcome measure, there was no difference between either treatment arm compared to placebo ($p = 0.71$ pooled). Change in mean EDSS was not affected by treatment with interferon. Secondary outcome measures showed relative reductions of 36% in the annual relapse rate and 93% in change of total volume of T2-hyperintense lesions on MRI ($p < 0.0001$) with interferon therapy [27].

A combined analysis of the two previous RCTs was performed given their disparate results. Patients in the European study were found to be in earlier stages of MS disease activity compared to those in the North American study based on age, duration of disease, number of relapses over the last 2 years, and relapse rate during the study (all $p < 0.001$). A pooled analysis demonstrated reduced risk of disability progression favoring subcutaneous IFN-β1b over placebo with a relative risk reduction of 20% ($p = 0.008$) [28].

The SPECTRIMS RCT evaluated subcutaneous IFN-β1a thrice weekly at doses of 22 µg and 44 µg versus placebo over 3 years in 618 patients with SPMS. The primary outcome was time to confirmed disability progression, defined as EDSS change as above persisting for at least 6 months. There was no significant difference between either the 22 µg ($p = 0.305$) or 44 µg ($p = 0.146$) over placebo. Pre-planned subgroup analysis suggested benefit in female patients on interferon ($p = 0.038$ for 22 µg, $p = 0.006$ for 44 µg); there were no difference in baseline characteristics between male and female patients in the study [29].

The MIMS study group compared intravenous mitoxantrone every 3 months at doses of 5 and 12 mg/m² to placebo in a 2-year RCT evaluating 194 patients with SPMS or worsening RRMS. The primary outcome measure was a multivariate analysis of five factors, including time to first relapse as well as change in EDSS. The multivariate comparison favored mitoxantrone 12 mg/m² over placebo ($p < 0.0001$), with a longer time to first relapse ($p = 0.0004$) and lower annualized relapse rate ($p < 0.0001$) [30]. However, it is not clear whether disability progression was delayed in SPMS for patients on mitoxantrone independent of its effects on acute relapses.

Clinical bottom line

1 It is uncertain whether IFNB-1b slows disability progression compared to placebo in SPMS, but it may for those patients with more rapid disability progression and continued relapses superimposed on a gradually progressive course.

2 Mitoxantrone reduces measures of MS disease activity including relapse rate in patients with RRMS or worsening SPMS.

Synthesis and application of evidence

No therapy has proven efficacy in reducing accumulation of disability in SPMS without relapses. No additional medication was initiated for our patient. However, post-hoc analyses of the discrepant IFNB-1b SPMS studies suggest that some patients may gain benefit from the drug if they continue to have active inflammatory disease (essentially, a transitional stage where SPMS is accompanied by relapses). The patient was also informed of the risks associated with use of mitoxantrone, including cardiac systolic dysfunction in 12% (number needed to harm or NNH = 8), congestive heart failure in 0.4%, and therapy-related acute leukemia in 0.8% (NNH = 123) [31].

Primary progressive MS

Clinical scenario

A 55-year-old woman has had gradually progressive left leg weakness over the last 5 years without any acute episodes suggestive of relapses. She is diagnosed with primary-progressive multiple sclerosis (PPMS). She inquires whether the currently available injectable therapies or rituximab, which he read about, would slow the progression of her disease.

Clinical question: Primary progressive MS

Compared to placebo, does treatment with IFNB, GA, or rituximab reduce disability progression in PPMS?

Evidence

A single RCT compared weekly intramuscular IFN-β1a at doses of 30 and 60 μg to placebo in 50 patients with PPMS over 2 years. The primary outcome measure, time to disability progression, did not differ between interferon and placebo groups. There was no significant treatment effect on secondary clinical outcomes, timed 10-m walk and 9-hole peg test or secondary imaging outcomes, volume of T1-hypointense and T2-hyperintense lesions on MRI [32].

The PROMISE study was an RCT comparing subcutaneous daily GA to placebo in 943 PPMS patients over 3 years. The primary outcome measure, time to disability progression, was defined as an increase in EDSS by at least 1.0 for patients at baseline EDSS 3.0–5.0 or 0.5 for baseline 5.5–6.5 that was sustained after 3 months. There was no significant effect of glatiramer over placebo on time to disability progression (hazard ratio 0.87, $p = 0.1753$). A post-hoc analysis of 455 male patients suggested a significant benefit for glatiramer over placebo (HR = 0.71, $p = 0.0193$) [33].

The OLYMPUS RCT evaluated the anti-CD20+ B-cell monoclonal antibody rituximab, given as a two 1000 mg intravenous infusion 2 weeks apart for 24 weeks, versus placebo in 439 PPMS patients for 96 weeks. Time to disease progression, the primary outcome measure, did not differ between rituximab and placebo ($p = 0.1442$). With regard to secondary end points, the rituximab group had less increase in T2-weighted lesion volume on MRI ($p < 0.001$) compared to placebo, but there was no difference in the change of total brain volume ($p = 0.62$) [34].

Clinical bottom line

There is currently no treatment that prolongs time to disability progression in PPMS when compared to placebo.

Synthesis and application of evidence

No therapy has proven efficacy for slowing PPMS. Disease-modifying therapy was not recommended for the patient.

Dalfampridine

Clinical scenario

A 47-year-old woman with multiple sclerosis reports difficulty walking. She has no other past or present medical conditions. She has a spastic paraparetic gait and requires a walker for ambulation. She walks 25 feet in 10.4 seconds. She inquires whether dalfampridine would help her with her gait impairment from MS.

Clinical question: Dalfampridine for gait improvement

Compared to placebo, does oral extended-release dalfampridine improve gait in patients with multiple sclerosis?

Evidence

One RCT compared oral extended-release dalfampridine 10 mg twice daily to placebo in a 3:1 ratio over 14 weeks in 301 patients with multiple sclerosis. Inclusion criteria were ages 18–70 years and a baseline timed 25-foot walk of 8–45 seconds. The primary outcome measure was proportion of positive responders in each group, and a positive response was defined as an increase in walking speed during the timed 25-foot walk. Thirty-five percent of patients treated with dalfampridine and 8% of placebo were positive responders ($p < 0.0001$). Positive responders on dalfampridine increased walking speed by 25.2%, negative responders on dalfampridine by 7.4%, and the placebo group by 4.7% ($p < 0.0001$ for each treatment group versus placebo) [35].

Clinical bottom line

Compared to placebo, dalfampridine significantly decreases 25-foot walk time in MS patients with gait impairment.

Synthesis and application of evidence

The patient has MS-related gait impairment and requires greater than 8 seconds to complete the timed 25-foot walk. She would benefit from oral extended-release dalfampridine and was prescribed this medication.

Conclusions

Disease-modifying therapies are all effective for reducing the annual relapse rate of RRMS. Several DMTs also delay conversion from a CIS to established RRMS. Subcutaneous IFNB, GA, natalizumab, teriflunomide, and dimethyl fumarate have demonstrated efficacy for reducing disability progression in RRMS. There are relatively little head-to-head comparative data; therefore, individual treatment decisions for RRMS depend heavily on disease duration, history of recent relapses, current neurological impairment and the rate of its accumulation, as well as factors such as a patient's concomitant medical diseases and medications and his/her personal preferences (e.g., for route of administration). No therapy to date has shown efficacy against disability progression for PPMS or SPMS without relapses. Dalfampridine is an effective treatment for increasing walking speed in patients with multiple sclerosis. In summary, substantial progress has been made toward halting inflammatory disease activity in RRMS but future therapies will need to focus on SPMS and PPMS in order to meet the major unmet needs, particularly accumulation of neurological disability, of patients with multiple sclerosis.

References

1 Jacobs, L.D., Beck, R.W., Simon, J.H. *et al.* (2000) Intramuscular interferon- beta-1a therapy initiated during a first demyelinating event in multiple sclerosis. *New England Journal of Medicine*, **343**, 898–904.

2 Comi, G., Filippi, M., Barkhof, F. *et al.* (2001) Effect of early interferon treatment on conversion to multiple sclerosis: a randomized study. *Lancet*, **357**, 1576–1582.

3 McDonald, W.I., Compston, A., Edan, G. *et al.* (2001) Recommended diagnostic criteria for multiple sclerosis: Guidelines from the international panel on the diagnosis of multiple sclerosis. *Annals of Neurology*, **50**, 121–127.

4 Kappos, L., Polman, C.H., Freedman, M.S. *et al.* (2006) Treatment with interferon beta-1b delays conversion to clinically definite and McDonald MS in patients with clinically isolated syndromes. *Neurology*, **67**, 1242–1249.

5 Comi, G., Martinelli, V., Rodegher, M. *et al.* (2009) Effect of glatiramer acetate on conversion to clinically definite multiple sclerosis in patients with clinically isolated syndrome (PreCISe study): a randomised, double-blind, placebo-controlled trial. *Lancet*, **374**, 1503–1511.

6 Kappos, L., Clanet, M. & Sandberg-Wollheim, M. (2005) Neutralizing antibodies and efficacy of interferon β-1a. *Neurology*, **65**, 40–47.

7 The IFNB Multiple Sclerosis Study Group (1993) Interferon beta-1b is effective in relapsing-remitting multiple sclerosis. I. Clinical results of a multicenter, randomized, double-blind, placebo-controlled trial. *Neurology*, **43**, 655–661.

8 Kurtzke, J.F. (1983) Rating neurologic impairment in multiple sclerosis: an expanded disability status scale (EDSS). *Neurology*, **33**, 1444–1452.

9 Jacobs, L.D., Cookfair, D.L., Rudick, R.A. *et al.* (1996) Intramuscular interferon beta-1a for disease progression in relapsing multiple sclerosis. *Annals of Neurology*, **39**, 285–294.

10 PRISMS Study Group (1998) Randomised double-blind placebo-controlled study of interferon β-1a in relapsing/remitting multiple sclerosis. *Lancet*, **352**, 1498–1504.

11 Johnson, K.P., Brooks, B.R., Cohen, J.A. *et al.* (1995) Copolymer 1 reduces relapse rate and improves disability in relapsing-remitting multiple sclerosis. *Neurology*, **45**, 1268–1276.

12 Comi, G., Filippi, M., Wolinsky, J.S. *et al.* (2001) European/Canadian multicenter, double-blind, placebo-controlled study of the effects of glatiramer acetate on magnetic resonance imaging-measured disease activity and burden in relapsing multiple sclerosis. *Annals of Neurology*, **49**, 290–297.

13 Mikol, D.D., Barkhof, F., Chang, P. *et al.* (2008) Comparison of subcutaneous interferon beta-1a with glatiramer acetate in relapsing-remitting multiple sclerosis (the REbif vs Glatiramer Acetate in Relapsing MS Disease [REGARD] study): a multicentre, randomized, parallel, open-label trial. *Lancet Neurology*, **7**, 903–914.

14 O'Connor, P., Fillippi, M., Amason, B. *et al.* (2009) 250μg or 500μg interferon beta-1b versus 20mg glatiramer acetate in relapsing-remitting multiple sclerosis: a prospective, randomized, multicentre study. *Lancet Neurology*, **8**, 889–897.

15 Cadavid, D., Wolansky, L.J., Skurnick, J. *et al.* (2009) Efficacy of treatment of MS with IFN-β1b or glatiramer acetate by monthly brain MRI in the BECOME study. *Neurology*, **72**, 1976–1983.

16 Panitch, H., Goodin, D.S., Francis, G. *et al.* (2002) Randomized, comparative study of interferon beta-1a treatment regiments in MS: the EVIDENCE trial. *Neurology*, **59**, 1496–1506.

17 Durelli, L., Verdun, E., Barbero, P. *et al.* (2002) Every-other-day interferon beta-1b versus once-weekly interferon beta-1a for multiple sclerosis: results of a 2-year prospective randomized multicenter study (INCOMIN). *Lancet*, **359**, 1453–1460.

18 Polman, C.H., O'Connor, P.W., Havrdova, E. *et al.* (2006) A randomized, placebo-controlled trial of natalizumab for relapsing multiple sclerosis. *New England Journal of Medicine*, **354**, 899–910.

19 Rudick, R.A., Stuart, W.H., Calabresi, P.A. *et al.* (2006) Natalizumab plus interferon beta-1a for relapsing multiple sclerosis. *New England Journal of Medicine*, **354**, 911–923.

20 Bloomgren, G., Richman, S., Hotermans, C. *et al.* (2012) Risk of natalizumab-associated progressive multifocal leukoencephalopathy. *New England Journal of Medicine*, **366**, 1870–1880.

21 Kappos, L., Radue, E.-W., O'Connor, P. *et al.* (2010) A placebo-controlled trial of oral fingolimod in relapsing multiple sclerosis. *New England Journal of Medicine*, **362**, 387–401.

22 Cohen, J.A., Barkhof, F., Comi, G. *et al.* (2010) Oral fingolimod or intramuscular interferon for relapsing multiple sclerosis. *New England Journal of Medicine*, **362**, 402–415.

23 O'Connor, P., Wolinsky, J., Confavreux, C. *et al.* (2011) Randomized trial of teriflunomide for relapsing multiple sclerosis. *New England Journal of Medicine*, **365**, 1293–1303.

24 Gold, R., Kappos, L., Arnold, D. *et al.* (2012) Placebo-controlled phase 3 study of oral BG-12 for relapsing multiple sclerosis. *New England Journal of Medicine*, **367**, 1098–1107.

25 Fox, R., Miller, D., Phillips, J. *et al.* (2012) Placebo-controlled phase 3 study of oral BG-12 or glatiramer in multiple sclerosis. *New England Journal of Medicine*, **367**, 1087–1097.

26 European Study Group on Interferon β-1b in Secondary Progressive MS (1998) Placebo-controlled multicentre trial of interferon β-1b in treatment of secondary progressive multiple sclerosis. *Lancet*, **352**, 1491–1497.

27 The North American Study Group on Interferon beta-1b in Secondary Progressive MS (2004) Interferon beta-1b in secondary progressive MS: Results from a 3-year controlled study. *Neurology*, **63**, 1788–1795.

28 Kappos, L., Weinshenker, B., Pozzilli, C. *et al.* (2004) Interferon beta-1b in secondary progressive MS – a combined analysis of the two trials. *Neurology*, **63**, 1779–1787.

29 Secondary Progressive Efficacy Clinical Trial of Recombinant Interferon-beta-1a in MS (SPECTRIMS) Study Group (2001) Randomized controlled trial of interferon beta-1a in secondary progressive MS. *Neurology*, **56**, 1496–1504.

30 Hartung, H.-P., Gonsette, R., König, N. *et al.* (2002) Mitoxantrone in progressive multiple sclerosis: a placebo-controlled, double-blind, randomised, multicenter trial. *Lancet*, **360**, 2018–2025.

31 Marriott, J.J., Miyasaki, J.M., Gronseth, G. & O'Connor, P. (2010) Evidence report: The efficacy and safety of mitoxantrone in multiple sclerosis. *Neurology*, **74**, 1463–1470.

32 Leary, S.M., Miller, D.H., Stevenson, V.L. *et al.* (2003) Interferon β-1a in primary progressive MS: an exploratory, randomized, controlled trial. *Neurology*, **60**, 44–51.

33 Wolinsky, J.S., Narayana, P.A., O'Connor, P. *et al.* (2007) Glatiramer acetate in primary progressive multiple sclerosis: results of a multinational, multicenter, double-blind, placebo-controlled trial. *Annals of Neurology*, **61**, 14–24.

34 Hawker, K., O'Connor, P., Freedman, M.S. *et al.* (2009) Rituximab in patients with primary progressive multiple sclerosis: results of a randomized double-blind placebo-controlled multicenter controlled trial. *Annals of Neurology*, **66**, 460–471.

35 Goodman, A., Brown, T., Krupp, L. *et al.* (2009) Sustained-release oral fampridine in multiple sclerosis: a randomized, double blind, controlled trial. *Lancet*, **373**, 732–738.

21 CHAPTER 21
Amyotrophic lateral sclerosis

Cumara B. O'Carroll[1], Amelia K. Adcock[2], and Bart M. Demaerschalk[1]

[1] *Department of Neurology, Mayo Clinic, Phoenix, AZ, USA*
[2] *West Virginia University, Morgantown, West Virginia, USA*

Background

Motor neuron disorders encompass a group of neurode-generative conditions in which the premature loss of motor neurons (upper and lower) is the essential pathological feature. Amyotrophic lateral sclerosis (ALS), also known as motor neuron disease (MND) in the United Kingdom, is the most common of these conditions. The classic pathological features of ALS include the loss of anterior horn cells and motor cells in the lower cranial motor nuclei, and degeneration of the corticospinal tracts [1]. As a result, patients present with progressive limb paralysis, later developing dysphagia, dysarthria, and respiratory insufficiency. It is an inexorably progressive disease with a fatal outcome. Median survival time is approximately 36 months [2], and death usually results from respiratory failure. Adverse prognostic indicators include older age at onset, low forced vital capacity, short time from first symptom onset to presentation, and bulbar onset [3,4]. In addition, survival is significantly shorter in patients who have bulbar involvement at first assessment regardless of the site of onset [5].

The incidence of ALS is fairly uniform worldwide, and is between 1.5 and 2.0 per 100,000 population per year, with a prevalence of approximately 6 per 100,000. There is a slight male predominance with a 1.6:1 sex ratio [3]. It is generally a disease of the late middle-aged and elderly, but can certainly occur in younger age groups. While ALS is arguably one of the most devastating diseases known to medical science, the pathophysiology remains unknown. There is growing evidence to suggest a multifactorial and likely multigenetic disease. Even though the majority of cases are sporadic, 5–10% of patients have a positive family history, and these familial forms may provide additional insights into potential basic etiological mechanisms. Most show an autosomal-dominant pattern of inheritance, though there are autosomal-recessive forms described in highly consanguineous populations in northern Africa. Of those patients with a dominant autosomal pattern, 10–20% have mutations in the copper/zinc superoxide dismutase (SOD1) gene on chromosome 21 [3].

Hosts of putative disease-modifying therapies have been reported, but only one (riluzole) has so far been licensed. The thrust of the treatment of ALS/MND is thus mainly symptomatic and palliative. Other putative disease-modifying therapies have included nerve growth factors such as recombinant human insulin-like growth factor 1 (IGF-1), ciliary neurotrophic growth factor (CNTF), and bovine-derived nerve growth factor (BDNF) as well as xaliproden, a drug given orally and thought to enhance nerve growth factor gene expression. Further potential disease-modifying treatments including stem cell therapy are still in their infancy, and evidence from randomized clinical trials (RCTs) is not yet available.

Criteria for the diagnosis of ALS/MND were initially aimed at providing a tool which could be used to facilitate multicenter international clinical trials and further investigations of familial ALS/MND. These were based on the outcome of a Workshop held under the auspices of the World Federation of Neurology in 1990 and are known as the Escorial Criteria. They were updated following further Workshops at Airlie House in 1994 and 1998 (the "Revised Criteria for the Diagnosis of Amyotrophic Lateral Sclerosis," www.wfnals.org/guidelines/1998elescorial/elescorial1998). A schema for the use of these criteria is given in Table 21.1 and Figure 21.1.

Framing answerable clinical questions

Major current therapeutic issues in ALS/MND can most conveniently be summarized as follows for the purposes of

Table 21.1 Summary of modified Escorial criteria (Airlie House Revision) of diagnosis of ALS/MND

	Category of diagnosis					
	Suspected	Possible	Definite familial, laboratory supported	Probable, laboratory supported	Probable	Definite
Clinical requirements	Lower motor neurone signs only in one or more regions or upper motor neurone signs in one or more regions	Lower + upper motor neurone signs in only one region	Lower + upper motor neurone signs in only one region	Lower + upper motor neurone signs in only one region or upper motor neurone signs in one or more regions	Lower + upper motor neurone signs in two region	Lower + upper motor neurone signs in three region
Laboratory requirement			Gene identified	Electromyography (EMG) shows acute denervation in two or more limbs		

To make a diagnosis of ALS/MND under any of the above criteria there *must* also be:

1 Evidence of progression over time;

2 No objective sensory signs which cannot be explained on the basis of a co-morbidity.

Source: Adapted from www.wfnals.org/guidelines/1998elescorial/elescorial1998schema.htm. Reproduced with permission of WFN-ALS.

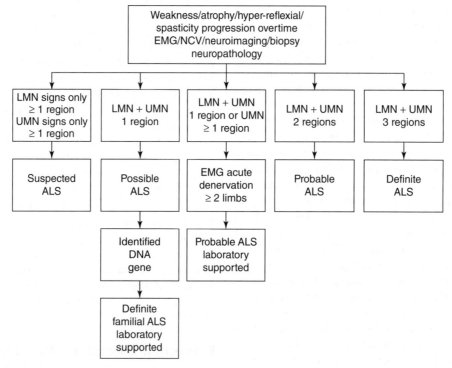

Figure 21.1 Criteria for the diagnosis of ALS/MND. EMG: electromyography; NCV: nerve conduction velocity; LMN: lower motor neurone; MN: upper motor neurone. Source: Reproduced with permission from WFN-ALS.

framing the core questions to be addressed in the remainder of this chapter:

1 Do any pharmacological treatments prolong survival in patients with possible or definite ALS/MND?

2 How does noninvasive ventilatory support affect probability of survival and quality of life (QoL) in patients with ALS/MND? If noninvasive ventilatory support is to be used, when is it best to start?

3 How does long-term mechanical ventilation (LTMV) affect survival and QoL in patients with ALS/MND with respiratory insufficiency?

4 Does mechanical insufflation–exsufflation (MI-E) alleviate respiratory symptoms in patients with ALS/MND who have excessive secretions?

5 How does feeding gastrostomy improve nutritional state and probability of survival in patients with ALS/MND with bulbar involvement?

6 What symptomatic treatments are available for patients with ALS/MND?

7 Is multidisciplinary care (MDC) an effective means of symptomatic and supportive management in patients with ALS/MND?

General approach to the search for evidence

High-quality evidence was first sought in the Cochrane Database of Systematic Reviews (CDSR) searching for reviews relating to ALS, MND, and motoneurone disease. The Cochrane Central Database of Controlled Trials was also searched for clinical trials relevant to ALS/MND. This was followed by searches on MEDLINE using search strings "MND" and "ALS" to identify papers relevant to ALS/MND and "riluzole," "IGF-1," "CNTF," "BDNF," "amino acid," "lamotrigine," "gabapentin," "minocycline," "lithium," "xaliproden," "creatine," "vent*," "resp*," "sniff," "nippv," "insuffl*," "exsuffl*," "cough," "dysphagia," "bulbar," "peg," and "gastrost*" to identify papers relevant to the questions asked in this chapter.

Critical review of the evidence for each question

Pharmacological treatment

Do any pharmacological treatments prolong survival in patients with possible or definite ALS/MND?

A whole host of drugs have been postulated as potential disease-modifying therapies in ALS/MND. The effectiveness of virtually all these drugs in prolonging survival has not been supported by evidence from RCTs. The glutamate-release inhibitor riluzole has, however, been licensed as a disease-modifying treatment in many countries. The clinical effectiveness of both riluzole and IGF-1 has been examined in Cochrane systematic reviews. Cochrane systematic reviews have also been undertaken for branched-chain amino acids, antioxidants, CNTF, and creatine.

Riluzole

Many causal and pathogenic theories for ALS/MND exist, one which suggests that chronic glutamate excitotoxicity may accumulate to toxic levels and thus lead to neuronal cell death. Since riluzole acts as a glutamate-release inhibitor, this was the basis for undertaking clinical trials testing the efficacy of this drug. The first RCT of riluzole demonstrated a modest increase in survival in patients treated with riluzole compared to those given placebo [6]. Many questions were however raised by this study, particularly the apparent disproportionate benefit observed in bulbar as opposed to limb-onset patients [7]. A larger dose ranging study also suggested a small prolongation of survival in patients receiving riluzole 100 and 200 mg daily [8]. A third trial in France and Belgium involved patients with advanced ALS/MND not included in these studies [9]. This study did not show a significant survival advantage from riluzole. A fourth trial in Japan with multiple outcome measures was also negative [10]. The Cochrane systematic review [11] concludes that riluzole 100 mg daily prolongs life by about 2–3 months in patients with probable and definite ALS/MND with symptoms of less than 5 years duration, forced vital capacity (FVC) greater than 60% and age less than 75 years. In addition, in 2009, an evidence-based practice parameter issued by the American Academy of Neurology recommended riluzole to slow disease progression for patients with ALS/MND [12]. The most frequent side effects are nausea and asthenia. Alterations of liver function tests sometimes occur and should be monitored monthly for the first 3 months, then at 3-month intervals. Riluzole should be avoided in patients with significant hepatic impairment.

Recombinant human insulin-like growth factor 1 (IGF-1)

There are four RCTs of IGF-1 in ALS/MND. Earlier trials yielded conflicting results, with the most recent and largest study showing no benefit of IGF-1 therapy in patients with ALS/MND. One trial [13] suggested slowing of progression of functional impairment and QoL, but this was not confirmed in a second, smaller trial [14]. The larger study compared IGF-1 0.05 and 0.1 mg/kg per day with placebo and the smaller IGF-1 0.1 mg/kg per day with placebo. The methodology of both trials was considered unsatisfactory due to the high risk of bias. A substantial number of patients receiving IGF-1 experienced drug-related adverse effects including injection site inflammation which could also have adversely affected blinding. IGF-1 seems otherwise a well-tolerated and safe drug. RCTs to date have been seriously compromised by details of trial design [15]. A third RCT looked at the use of intrathecal recombinant human insulin-like growth factor 1 (rhIGF-1) in human ALS, but given small study size and other design flaws, it was difficult to determine efficacy and optimum dose [15,16]. Maximizing potential efficacy of IGF-1 and other neurotrophins in ALS/MND may also depend on effective delivery of the trophin to the site of the pathology. Finally, the most recent RCT by Sorenson *et al.* [17] randomized 330 patients to receive 0.05 mg/kg body weight of rhIGF-1 administered subcutaneously twice daily or placebo for 2 years. The primary outcome measure was change in manual muscle testing score and the secondary outcome measures included rate of change in the revised ALS functional rating scale and tracheostomy-free survival. The authors concluded that IGF-1 does not provide any benefit for patients with ALS, as there was no difference between treatment groups in any outcome measure after 2 years [17]. Therefore, to date the efficacy of IGF-1 in ALS/MND remains unproven.

Ciliary neurotrophic growth factor (CNTF)

A Cochrane review has also examined the efficacy of CNTF in ALS/MND. Two randomized trials were identified including 1300 ALS/MND patients treated with subcutaneous CNTF at different concentrations. No significant differences were observed between the CNTF and placebo groups for survival, the primary outcome measure. A significant increase in adverse events occurred in patients given higher doses of CNTF. As with IGF-1, alternative delivery methods might however be usefully evaluated in the future [18].

Amino acids

Amino acid preparations have also been suggested as possible disease-modifying treatments for ALS/MND. A Cochrane review addressed the potential efficacy of amino acids in prolonging survival and/or slowing the progression in ALS/MND. No benefit could be demonstrated for either branched-chain amino acids or L-threonine in improving survival in ALS/MND. There was no evidence of an effect of any of these treatments on muscle strength or disability as measured by functional rating scales [19].

Free radicals

Free radicals and reactive oxygen species have been strongly implicated as potential etiological vectors in ALS/MND. A range of antioxidant medications have been investigated as possible disease-modifying treatments. A Cochrane review examined the effects of antioxidant medication in ALS/MND. Of 25 studies identified only 10 met the inclusion criteria. These studies included 1015 participants. There was insufficient evidence of efficacy of individual antioxidants, or antioxidants in general to justify the use of antioxidant treatment in people with ALS/MND. Many of the studies were poorly designed, underpowered, of short duration, and had low numbers of participants. Given the relatively low cost of vitamins C and E, the high tolerance and safety, and the fact that there is no clear contraindication, use continues in patients with ALS/MND [20].

Bovine-derived nerve growth factor (BDNF)

On the basis that BDNF is a potent survival factor for motor neurons 1135 ALS/MND patients were randomized to placebo, 25 or 100 μg/kg BDNF for 9 months. There

was no benefit of BDNF treatment for any of the primary end points. Among the 60% of patients with baseline FVC of ≤91% predicted, survival was significantly greater for 100 μg/kg BDNF versus placebo. In the 20% treated with BDNF, 100 μg/kg who reported altered bowel function, 9-month survival was significantly better than placebo. Further clinical trials of BDNF using either intrathecal delivery or high-dose subcutaneous administration were suggested [21]. The safety and tolerability of intrathecal BDNF has since been investigated. Twenty-five patients with probable or definite ALS/MND received either BDNF (25, 60, 150, 400, or 1000 μg per day) or placebo in a 12-week randomized, double-blinded, sequential, dose-escalation study. In each dose cohort, four patients received BDNF and one received placebo. The majority of patients receiving BDNF reported mild sensory symptoms, including paresthesia. Sleep disturbance, dry mouth, agitation, and other behavioral effects were encountered at higher doses (>150 μg per day). Cerebrospinal fluid (CSF) BDNF levels were directly related to dose. Intrathecal treatment with BDNF in doses of up to 150 μg per day was well tolerated and feasible. The number of patients and study design did not allow conclusions on efficacy to be made [22].

Lamotrigine

The suggestion that glutamate excitotoxicity might be implicated in the pathogenesis of ALS/MND led to a double-blind, placebo-controlled trial of lamotrigine 100 mg per day in which 67 patients were entered. This dose of lamotrigine did not seem to alter the course of ALS/MND [23]. A second study examined the effect of lamotrigine 300 mg per day. Thirty patients completed this double-blind, placebo-controlled, crossover study. No effect of lamotrigine on the progression of ALS/MND was found [24].

Gabapentin

A randomized, double-blind, placebo-controlled phase II trial was undertaken to evaluate the efficacy of gabapentin 2.4 g per day in slowing the rate of decline of muscle strength in 152 patients with ALS/MND. The primary outcome measure was the slope of the arm megascore and the secondary measure FVC. A nonstatistically significant trend ($P = 0.057-0.08$) was observed toward slower decline of arm strength in patients taking gabapentin compared with placebo. No effect on FVC was observed [25]. A phase III trial compared gabapentin 3.6 g and placebo daily for 9 months. The mean rate of decline in arm muscle strength was not significantly different between the groups. There was no beneficial effect upon the rate of decline of secondary measures and no symptomatic benefit [26].

Minocycline

In 2004, a double-blind, randomized, placebo-controlled feasibility trial of minocycline in ALS/MND included 19 patients who received 200 mg per day or placebo for 6 months. There were no significant differences in adverse events. In a second 8-month crossover trial, 23 ALS/MND patients received up to 400 mg per day. The mean tolerated dose was 387 mg per day. There was a trend toward more gastrointestinal symptoms ($P = 0.057$), and the urea and liver enzymes became elevated ($P < 0.05$) in the minocycline-treated patients, though not deemed to be clinically significant [27,28]. Pontieri *et al.* completed a 6-month randomized, open-label study in 2005 investigating the safety of combined minocycline and riluzole treatment in patients with ALS/MND. This study enrolled 20 patients and was not powered to determine efficacy of minocycline. Statistical analysis was performed only on 13 of the original patients, and minocycline was not associated with significant side effects or laboratory abnormalities [28,29]. These safety trials laid the foundation for a multicenter, randomized, placebo-controlled phase III trial. In 2007, Gordon *et al.* randomized 412 patients with ALS/MND to receive placebo or minocycline in escalating doses of up to 400 mg per day for 9 months. The primary outcome measure was the difference in rate of change in the revised ALS functional rating scale (ALSFRS-R). Secondary outcome measures were forced vital capacity (FVC), manual muscle testing (MMT), quality of life, survival, and safety. Patients in the minocycline group had a statistically significant faster deterioration of their ALSFRS-R scores ($P = 0.005$). They also demonstrated a trend toward faster decline in FVC ($P = 0.11$) and MMT score ($P = 0.11$), in addition to greater mortality during the 9-month treatment phase when compared to the placebo group ($P = 0.23$). There was no difference in quality-of-life scores between the two groups. These results prompted a closer look at the use of minocycline not only for the treatment of ALS, but also for other neurological disorders [30].

Xaliproden

The safety and functional efficacy of xaliproden were tested in a double-blind, placebo-controlled study, which included 54 ALS/MND patients treated for up to 32 weeks. The 6-month intent-to-treat analysis showed no statistically significant effect, but a trend toward favor of 2 mg xaliproden compared to placebo for reduction in the rate of deterioration of FVC, limb functional score and manual muscle testing. These results were thought to suggest a possible disease-modifying effect [31]. On the basis of these results, two further randomized, double-blind, placebo-controlled, multicenter, multinational studies were undertaken to assess efficacy and safety. Patients were randomly assigned to placebo, 1 or 2 mg xaliproden orally in the first study ($n = 867$ patients); or the same with riluzole 50 mg twice a day background therapy in both groups in the second study ($n = 1210$ patients). The two primary end points were time to death, tracheostomy or permanent assisted ventilation,

and time to vital capacity (VC) <50%. Significant results were not obtained in either of these studies [32].

Creatine

Creatine is found primarily in skeletal muscle and is a naturally occurring nitrogenous organic acid that helps in adenosine triphosphate production. In mouse models of ALS, it has been shown to increase survival [33], and this prompted clinical trials in humans. A Cochrane review examined the efficacy of creatine in prolonging ALS/MND survival and slowing disease progression. Three randomized trials were included, with a total of 386 ALS/MND patients, receiving either creatine monohydrate 5–10 g per day or placebo. The primary outcome measure was tracheostomy-free survival time and secondary outcomes were change in ALS functional rating revised scores (ALSFRS-R) over time and change in percent predicted FVC over time. No significant differences were observed between the creatine and placebo groups for either primary or secondary outcome measures across all three studies. The creatine was well tolerated in all three studies, without serious adverse events, but there was no beneficial effect on prolonging survival time or slowing disease progression in ALS/MND patients [34].

Lithium

In a small pilot study in Italy, lithium carbonate and riluzole reportedly delayed neurological decline in patients with ALS/MND as measured by the ALS functional rating scale revised (ALSFRS-R), FVC, and survival time. Lithium was tested on the basis that it induces autophagy in animal models at a serum concentration range of 0.4–0.8 mEq/L. This pilot study had its limitations given that only 16 subjects received lithium, that the subjects were not masked to treatment allocation, and the fact that the cohort of patients enrolled in the study appeared to have a less aggressive disease course when compared to the general ALS/MND population. Despite these limitations, the results of this study laid the foundation for future studies investigating lithium as a potential treatment for ALS/MND [35].

In 2010, Aggarwal *et al.* published the results of a double-blind, placebo-controlled trial with a time-to-event design, evaluating the safety and efficacy of lithium in combination with riluzole in patients with ALS/MND. Eighty-four patients on stable doses of riluzole for at least 30 days were randomized to receive either lithium or placebo. The primary end point was defined as a decrease of at least 6 points on the ALSFRS-R or death. Interim analyses were planned for when 84 patients had been allocated treatment, 6 months later or after 55 events, and after 100 events. The stopping boundary for futility at the first interim analysis was a P value of at least 0.68. The study was actually stopped at the first interim analysis because criterion for futility was met ($P = 0.78$). The difference in the mean decline in the ALSFRS-R between lithium and placebo groups was 0.15 (95% CI −0.43 to 0.73, $P = 0.61$), and it was concluded that there was no evidence to suggest that lithium in combination with riluzole slows progression in ALS/MND more than riluzole alone [36].

Another randomized, double-blind, placebo-controlled trial by Verstraete *et al.* looked at the safety and efficacy of lithium carbonate, at target blood levels of 0.4–0.8 mEq/L, in 133 ALS/MND patients. Patients were randomized to receive either lithium carbonate or placebo as adjunctive therapy to riluzole. The primary end point was survival, defined as death, tracheostomal ventilation, or noninvasive ventilation for more than 16 hours a day, while secondary outcome measures consisted of ALSFRS-R and FVC. This trial did not demonstrate any beneficial effect of lithium carbonate over placebo, on either survival or functional decline in patients with ALS/MND, at 12 months or 16 months [37].

Assessment of respiratory function

How does noninvasive ventilatory support affect probability of survival and QoL in patients with ALS/MND? If noninvasive ventilatory support is to be used, when is it best to start?

The assessment of respiratory function in ALS/MND has tended to focus on VC, FVC, and forced expiratory volume (FEV1), the usual procedure being to compare readings from individual patients with those predicted for persons of the same age, sex, height, and weight. These physiological parameters are thus expressed as percentages of the predicted value (i.e., "% predicted"). More recently, novel methods such as sniff pressures have been evaluated.

An early indication that respiratory function monitoring might be valuable in following the course of ALS/MND came from a study of 218 patients. Most patients were found to have characteristic abnormalities in pulmonary function, including reduced FVC. FVCs as low as 50% predicted were commonly missed by clinical evaluation [38]. Subsequent experience has confirmed the importance of monitoring respiratory function in the routine care of people with ALS/MND and established the vital role of pulmonary function testing in trials of putative disease-modifying treatments.

Jackson *et al.* noted that there was no consensus on the physiological marker of choice to trigger the initiation of noninvasive positive pressure ventilation (NIPPV) in ALS/MND. Advice at that time recommended that the decision should be based on FVC. Twenty ALS/MND patients with FVC 70–100% predicted were reviewed. Baseline measurements included the ALS functional rating scale-respiratory version (ALSFRS-R), SF-36, FVC%, maximal inspiratory pressure (MIP), maximal expiratory pressure (MEP), and nocturnal oximetry. The patients were randomized to receive NIPPV based on either nocturnal oximetry studies suggesting oxygen desaturation <90% for one cumulative minute ("early intervention") or FVC <50% ("standard of care"). At enrollment, there was no significant correlation between FVC% and the ALSFRS-R, MEP, MIP, or duration of nocturnal desaturation <90%. An increase in the vitality subscale of the SF-36 was demonstrated in five out of six patients randomized to "early intervention" with NIPPV. The data indicated that FVC% did not correlate well with respiratory symptoms and suggested that MIP and nocturnal oximetry may be more sensitive measures of early respiratory insufficiency. It was suggested that earlier institution of NIPPV might result in improved QoL [39,40].

Lyall *et al.* related physiological measurements to biochemical markers of respiratory failure. Respiratory muscle strength (RMS) was measured in 81 ALS/MND patients to evaluate the relationship between RMS and the presence of ventilatory failure, defined as a carbon dioxide tension of 6 kPa or less. Parameters studied included VC, static inspiratory and expiratory mouth pressures (MIP, MEP), maximal esophageal, transdiaphragmatic, and nasal sniff (SNP) pressures. No test had significant predictive power for hypercapnia in patients with significant bulbar weakness. It was concluded that in ALS/MND patients without significant bulbar involvement, novel tests of RMS have greater predictive power for hypercapnia than conventional tests. In particular, the noninvasive SNP is more sensitive than VC and MIP, suggesting that SNP could usefully be included in tests of RMS in ALS/MND [41].

The potential utility of SNP in testing RMS in ALS/MND was also tested in 16 patients who were examined monthly over 8–28 months. SNP was recorded in parallel with maximal inspiratory pressure (PI(max)) and maximal expiratory pressure (PE(max)). It was concluded that SNP was the single respiratory test best combining linear decline, sensitivity in mild disease, and feasibility of use in advanced disease [42]. In Morgan *et al.*, 98 patients with ALS/MND were followed trimonthly for 3 years and the observation was made that a sniff nasal-inspiratory force less than 40 cmH$_2$O was significantly related with nocturnal hypoxemia. In addition, they found that when the sniff nasal-inspiratory force was less than 40 cmH$_2$O, the hazard ratio for death was 9.1 ($P = 0.001$) and the median survival was 6 ± 0.3 months. While the sensitivity of FVC <50% for predicting 6-month mortality was 58% with a specificity of 96%, the sensitivity of the sniff nasal-inspiratory force <40 cmH$_2$O was 97% with a specificity of 79% for death within 6 months. Thus, not only is the sniff nasal-inspiratory force test a good measure of respiratory muscle strength in ALS/MND, but it may also provide prognostic information [43].

Attention has also been drawn to the possible use of respiratory function testing as a predictor of QoL in ALS/MND. Most ALS/MND patients have evidence of respiratory muscle weakness at diagnosis. Sleep disruption, due to apnea, hypopnea, orthopnea, or REM-related desaturation, is common. The relative impact of these factors on QoL was studied in 23 people with ALS/MND. QoL was assessed using generic and specific instruments and RMS by measurement of VC, maximum static pressures, and SNP. Overall limb and axial muscle strength was estimated using a summated muscle score based on the MRC scale. There were moderate to strong correlations between QoL and all measurements of respiratory muscle function. Multivariate analysis suggested that maximum static inspiratory pressure was the strongest independent predictor of QoL [44].

NIPPV

How do we decide when to institute NIPPV?

ALS/MND patients with alveolar hypoventilation were reviewed in order to demonstrate variability in symptoms, physiological status, and outcome, following the institution of NIPPV. There were 27 consecutive patients who tolerated NIPPV for more than 4 hours per 24-hour period for more than 2 weeks. All met the El Escorial Criteria for the diagnosis of ALS/MND. Spirometry was measured in the sitting and when possible, the supine positions. Resting arterial blood gases were available in 22. Orthopnea was the most common symptom at the commencement of NIPPV. No correlation existed between age at institution of NIPPV, duration of effective use of NIPPV, or VC and duration of effective use of NIPPV. The lack of correlation between VC at the institution of NIPPV and duration of its effectiveness suggest that more sensitive indicators for the onset of alveolar hypoventilation should be defined, particularly since the principal benefit from its use is relief of symptomatic alveolar hypoventilation. No clear guidance was thus given on the optimum timing for the institution of NIPPV [45]. In the absence of clearer indications, attention should be given to the occurrence of orthopnea in following up patients with ALS/MND, and the possible need for respiratory support considered when this symptom is reported.

Cognitive dysfunction is present in a proportion of non-demented patients with ALS/MND, and respiratory muscle weakness can lead to nocturnal hypoventilation, resulting in sleep disturbance and excessive daytime somnolence. Nocturnal sleep deprivation might contribute to impaired cognitive function. Cognitive function was evaluated in 9 MND patients with sleep disturbance caused by nocturnal hypoventilation (NIPPV group) and 10 similar patients without ventilation problems (control group). The NIPPV group then started nocturnal NIPPV. After about 6 weeks, cognitive function was reassessed. Statistically significant improvement in two of the seven cognitive tests was demonstrated in the NIPPV group, with a trend toward significant improvement in two others. Scores in the control group did not improve significantly. Nocturnal hypoventilation and sleep disturbance may be associated with cognitive dysfunction and this might be helped by NIPPV. These

observations have important implications for the investigation of cognitive dysfunction in non-demented patients with ALS/MND, and the effect of ventilation on QoL [46].

A further study examined the potential effect of NIPPV on QoL in ALS/MND more specifically. QoL was prospectively studied using the SF-36 in 16 ventilated ALS/MND patients. NIPPV improved scores in the "vitality" domain by as much as 25% for up to 15 months. NIPPV was not associated with reduced QoL [47]. Even though it is suggested that NIPPV probably improves survival in ALS/MND, the magnitude and duration of any improvement in QoL and the optimal criteria for initiating treatment are unclear. QoL was serially evaluated using the SF-36 scale, chronic respiratory disease questionnaire, sleep apnea, QoL index, respiratory function, and polysomnography in 22 ALS/MND patients. A trial of NIPPV was offered when subjects had orthopnea, daytime sleepiness, unrefreshing sleep, daytime hypercapnia, nocturnal desaturation, or an apnea–hypopnea index >10. Of 17 subjects offered NIPPV, 15 accepted and 10 continued treatment subsequently. Outcome was assessed by changes in QoL and NIV (noninvasive ventilation) compliance. Subjects were followed to death or for at least 26 months. QoL domains assessing sleep-related problems and mental health improved. Median survival following successful initiation of NIPPV was 512 days. Survival and duration of improved QoL were strongly related to NIPPV compliance. VC declined more slowly following initiation of NIPPV. Orthopnea was the best predictor of benefit from, and compliance with, NIPPV. Moderate or severe bulbar weakness was associated with lower compliance and less improvement in QoL. NIPPV may thus be associated with improved QoL and survival. Subjects with orthopnea and preserved bulbar function showed the largest benefit [40,48].

A more recent study by the same group monitored a cohort of 92 patients for orthopnea, maximum inspiratory pressure <60% predicted or symptomatic hypercapnia. When one of these criteria had been met, patients were randomly allocated to NIV or "standard care" not including NIV. Median survival of the NIV-treated patients was 219 days as opposed to 171 days for those given "standard" care. Primary end points were time to 75% of baseline level for the mental component summary of the SF36 (168 days for NIV-treated, 99 days for "standard" care) and sleep apnea, QoL; index symptoms domain (192 days for NIV-treated, 46 days for "standard" care). The authors commented that NIV increased patient survival and QoL, and that the survival advantage was much greater than that from currently available neuroprotective therapy [49].

A Cochrane review examining the efficacy of mechanical ventilation (noninvasive ventilation and tracheotomy) in improving survival and quality of life in ALS/MND identified two randomized controlled trials, Jackson *et al.* and Bourke *et al.* [39,49]. Though both trials were originally included, Jackson *et al.* was eventually excluded given incomplete data. No other RCTs were identified. The authors concluded that survival and some measures of QoL were improved in ALS/MND patients using noninvasive ventilation, as long as they had intact bulbar function [50].

Invasive assisted ventilation

How does Long-Term Mechanical Ventilation (LTMV) affect probability of survival and QoL in patients with ALS/MND with respiratory insufficiency?

This is a controversial issue and considerable differences exist in approach and practice in different countries. Acute respiratory insufficiency (ARI) with alveolar hypoventilation or incapacitating dyspnea without peripheral muscle involvement can both be early features in ALS/MND. It has been suggested that such patients might benefit from more invasive assisted ventilation (LTMV).

Moss *et al.* examined advance care planning and outcomes of patients with ALS/MND receiving LTMV in a population-based study in homes and chronic care facilities. Seventy-five ALS/MND patients were identified; 50 of the 58 (86%) who were able to communicate consented to structured interviews, 36 at home, and 14 in an institution. Thirty-eight had completed advance directives, and 96% wanted them. Thirty-eight also wished to stop LTMV in certain circumstances. Those who had completed advance directives were more likely to have communicated their preference to stop LTMV to their family and physician than those who had not (76% vs 29%; $P = 0.05$). Patients living at home rated their QoL as being better than those in an institution (7.2 vs 5.6; $P = 0.0052$). Their annual expenses were also less ($136,560 vs $366,852; $P = 0.0018$). Most patients receiving LTMV would want to stop it under certain circumstances, and advance care planning enhances communication of patient preferences to family and physicians. Home-based LTMV is less costly and associated with greater patient satisfaction [51].

A further study made a retrospective analysis of the results of LTMV in 10 ALS/MND patients. LTMV outside the intensive care unit (ICU) was found to be possible in these patients and seven of them returned home. Return to the home environment was however found to be very difficult for ventilator-dependent patients lacking family support [52].

Moss *et al.* conducted a further study to better inform ALS/MND patients about home ventilation. They gathered data on the prevalence of ALS/MND patients on home ventilation in northern Illinois and the percentage who chose it, and asked patients, families, and physicians about attitudes toward home ventilation. Fewer than 10% of ALS/MND patients had chosen home ventilation, and less than 5% remained on it for any length of time. Seventeen (90%) were however glad to have chosen home ventilation and would choose it again. Family caregivers reported major burdens. Only half said they would choose it for themselves.

The mean yearly cost of home ventilation was estimated at $153,252. Home ventilation thus seems effective for a small number of ALS/MND patients but imposes significant burdens on families [53].

A more recent retrospective study evaluated a protocol for early respiratory assessment of ALS/MND patients who might be helped by LTMV in their homes and investigated the effects of the protocol and bulbar involvement on the survival of patients receiving NIPPV. LTMV was indicated in 86 ALS/MND patients, 22 of whom presented with bulbar involvement. Treatment with LTMV had been initiated in one group of patients before and in a second group after protocol initiation. The majority of patients in the first group began treatment with LTMV during an acute episode requiring ICU admission ($P = 0.001$) and tracheal ventilation ($P = 0.025$), with a lower percentage of patients beginning LTMV treatment without ARI ($P = 0.013$). No significant differences in survival were found between the groups, but greater survival was observed in the second group ($P = 0.03$) when patients with bulbar involvement were excluded. Multivariate analysis showed bulbar involvement to be an independent prognostic factor for survival (relative risk 1.6, 95% confidence interval, 1.01–2.54, $P = 0.04$). It was concluded that early and systematic respiratory evaluation is necessary to improve the results of LTMV in patients with ALS/MND [54].

The implementation of LTMV varies widely in different countries. LTMV appears sometimes to be helpful in small number of ALS/MND patients but imposes considerable additional burdens on families and caregivers. LTMV may also be less useful in patients with substantial bulbar involvement.

Cough assist devices (insufflation/exsufflation)

Does mechanical insufflation–exsufflation (MI-E) alleviate respiratory symptoms in patients with ALS/MND who have excessive secretions?

There has been interest in cough assist devices (insufflation/exsufflation) in the alleviation of respiratory symptoms in ALS/MND. Elimination of airway secretion is a major issue in the care of patients with ALS/MND. Bulbar muscle weakness is often a reason for failure of NIPPV and may lead to tracheotomy. Expiratory aids may help to overcome these problems, at least for a while. Lahrmann *et al.* reported a patient with advanced ALS/MND, receiving nocturnal NIPPV, who was reported to benefit from regular use of an MI-E device [55]. Other studies have included other disorders associated with excessive secretions and have not focused exclusively on ALS/MND. One examined the physiological effects and tolerance of MI-E prospectively in patients with chronic ventilatory failure from various causes in 13 ALS/MND patients, 9 with severe COPD and 7 with other neuromuscular disorders. The results suggested good tolerance and physiological improvement in patients with restrictive and obstructive disease, suggesting that MI-E may be a useful complement to NIPPV for patients with a wide variety of neuromuscular diseases [56]. A further investigation focused on 26 consecutive patients with ALS/MND, 15 of whom had severe bulbar dysfunction. Even though both groups had a similar time from ALS/MND symptom onset to diagnosis, differences ($P < 0.05$) were found between non-bulbar and bulbar patients in lung function and cough capacity parameters: MI-E is able to generate clinically effective peak cough flows in stable ALS/MND patients except for those with bulbar dysfunction who also have a maximum insufflation capacity >11 and peak cough flow maximum insufflation capacity <2.7 L/s who probably have severe dynamic collapse of the upper airways during the exsufflation cycle. Clinically stable patients with mild respiratory dysfunction might not benefit from MI-E except during an acute respiratory illness [57].

Feeding gastrostomy

How does feeding gastrostomy improve nutritional state and probability of survival in patients with ALS/MND with bulbar involvement?

In the natural progression of ALS/MND, a state of malnutrition often develops, associated with reduced oral intake, caused by difficulties with swallowing and/or anorexia. The issue of when and how a feeding tube should be inserted remains controversial.

It is well established that bulbar involvement in ALS/MND is an adverse prognostic indicator on account of a higher risk of aspiration and consequences of dysphagia. One study assessed the effects of percutaneous endoscopic gastrostomy (PEG) in 31 ALS/MND patients with bulbar involvement at 3-month intervals over 2 years following PEG insertion. The data were compared with a control group of 35 ALS/MND patients who refused PEG. Mortality did not differ significantly between the two groups during the first 6 months, but after this time, mortality was lower in the PEG group. In the patients who had PEG, the body mass index showed a mild but statistically significant improvement, while in the controls it decreased significantly. It was suggested that PEG could improve survival in elderly and young ALS/MND patients with bulbar involvement, enhance QoL, and help integration in social and family surroundings [58].

In a further study, safety and factors related to survival after PEG were reviewed in a series of 50 consecutive ALS/MND patients. No major acute or long-term complications were observed. Stabilization or increase in weight was observed after PEG. Median survival after PEG was 185 days, with a worse outcome in patients with weight loss ≥10% healthy body weight and FVC <65%. It was noted that PEG may be a useful option in the symptomatic treatment of dysphagia in ALS/MND [59].

PEG insertion has been considered a reliable route for nutrition and hydration in ALS/MND patients with dysphagia. A retrospective analysis of the CNTF and BDNF databases was made to determine the clinical status of ALS/MND patients during the 30 days preceding PEG insertion. By comparing the rate of decline pre- and post-PEG, nutritional supplementation via PEG seemed to stabilize the weight loss otherwise experienced. Death within 30 days of PEG was associated with a marked reduction in FVC and identified a group of patients in whom PEG should be inserted with caution. These data were thought to emphasize the importance of sequential measurement of FVC in managing ALS/MND patients to guide the timing of PEG insertion [60].

Thirty-three ALS/MND patients with erect or supine FVC <50% predicted underwent attempted PEG placement using NIPPV, oxygen support, and conscious sedation anesthesia. Gastrostomy tubes were successfully placed in all patients. Mean survival was 211 days with 67% surviving >180 days. FVC at the time of PEG placement did not predict survival [61].

A retrospective evaluation of gastrostomy placement in 36 ALS/MND patients over a 3.5-year period attempted to determine the optimal insertion method. Twenty patients were referred for PEG and 16 for percutaneous radiologic gastrostomy (PRG)/radiologically inserted gastrostomy (RIG). Gastrostomy method, success rate of each technique, and reason for procedure failure were reviewed in each patient. Preoperative FVC was recorded. The log-rank test was used to compare survival rates after PRG and PEG, and the Wilcoxon-rank sum test to evaluate the influence of declining FVC on PEG success. The Kaplan–Meier product limit method was used to estimate survival probabilities. Of 20 patients referred for PEG, 11 were successful. The nine failures resulted from failure to transilluminate the abdominal wall. All 16 patients initially referred for PRG were successful. The nine patients in whom PEG failed subsequently had a successful PRG. In patients with diaphragmatic palsy and a high subcostal stomach, an angled subcostal approach or intercostal approach was recommended for PRG insertion. One aspiration-related death occurred in the PEG group and a second patient from the PEG group required laparotomy for postoperative peritonitis. One death occurred in the PRG group because of inadvertent placement of the tube in the peritoneal cavity. There was no significant difference between PEG and PRG in terms of patient survival, and FVC did not have a statistically significant influence on PEG failure. It was however suggested that PRG was the method of choice on the basis of these observations [62]. A more recent retrospective study compared PRG and PEG in terms of tolerance, efficacy, and survival in 40 patients with ALS/MND. General success rates were 85.7% for PEG and 100% for PRG, with successful and well-tolerated placement seen in 81.8% of PRGs and 57.1% of PEGs ($P = 0.1$).

Advanced age ($P = 0.02$) and PRG ($P = 0.07$) were predictive of successful and well-tolerated placement. The ability to perform spirometry ($P = 0.002$) and interval from diagnosis to gastrostomy placement ($P = 0.001$) were predictors of survival. Oximetry measurements ($P = 0.007$) and interval from diagnosis to placement ($P = 0.02$) were predictive of mortality at 6 months. Thus, Blondet et al. concluded that PRG is both better tolerated and more efficacious than PEG, because it avoids respiratory decompensation that may occur with PEG, and survival is linked to disease evolution, not to the choice of PRG or PEG placement [63].

Data from patients with and without PEG with ALS functional rating scale-bulbar subscale (ALSFRSb) scores ≤5 were evaluated to compare characteristics of ALS/MND patients with and without PEG. PEG use was markedly increased as ALSFRSb scores declined. PEG patients used significantly more assistive devices, multidisciplinary care, home care nurses, and aides, had more frequent physician visits, emergency department visits, and hospital admissions ($P < 0.0001$), as well as lower health status based on the mini-SIP scale ($P = 0.0047$). PEG use varied greatly between centers. PEG was thought to have a positive impact in 79% of patients as a whole but only in 37.5% of patients who received PEG later. Even though only a small number of patients were studied, PEG use showed no survival benefit. It was thought that patients generally did not receive PEG until bulbar function was severely reduced. Aggressive proactive nutritional management was considered essential in patients with ALS/MND to try and secure better outcomes [64].

As PEG may not be practicable in patients with severe respiratory impairment, the alternative method of PRG was evaluated for safety, effect on survival, and respiratory function in 25 ALS/MND patients with respiratory failure. These 25 consecutive ALS/MND patients with severe dysphagia and FVC <50% were compared with 25 consecutive patients with FVC <50% who underwent PEG. Respiratory function was evaluated before and after each procedure. The two groups were broadly similar. PRG placement was successful in all cases, PEG in 23/25. One patient in each group died after the procedure. The mean survival time after gastrostomy placement was 204 days in the PRG group and 85 days in the PEG group ($P < 0.004$). Respiratory function decreased more in the PEG group than in the PRG group ($P < 0.02$). PRG appeared to be safer than PEG in MND patients with moderate to severe respiratory impairment, and seemed to be associated with longer survival [65].

Data seeking further insights into the frequency, timing, and outcomes following PEG insertion from gastrostomy in ALS/MND were obtained from the Scottish MND Register. Descriptive statistics of patients undergoing PEG were extracted. Survival analysis used Kaplan–Meier and Cox proportional hazards methods. For patients diagnosed between 1989 and 1998, 142 PEGs were placed in 1226 patients of whom 130 were done before the censoring date.

Approximately 5% of patients underwent gastrostomy every year, but this rate appeared to double between 1989 and 1998. Mean age at insertion was 66.8 years, following mean disease duration of 24 months. Median survival from PEG insertion was 146 days. The 1-month mortality after PEG was 25%. PEG did not confer a survival advantage compared with no PEG. The authors concluded that PEGs were being inserted more frequently in people with ALS/MND. An unexpectedly high early mortality was detected, which probably reflected a lack of selection bias compared with previously published data. It was suggested that changes in practice surrounding PEG placement since 1998 might have resulted in better outcomes for patients with ALS/MND [66].

Complications after PEG and RIG along with their effects on survival were evaluated in 50 patients having definite or probable ALS/MND. RIG was considered first-line therapy when the slow vital capacity (SVC) was less than 50% predicted or when PEG was refused by the patient. Thirty patients had a PEG and 20 an RIG. The two populations were comparable in age, gender ratio, and disease duration before gastrostomy. SVC was lower in those patients having RIG than PEG. The frequency of complications at gastrostomy insertion and during the first month was not significantly different between the two groups. Kaplan–Meier survival curves from the date of gastrostomy were not different in univariate or multivariate analysis. The authors suggested that the main benefit of RIG is its utility in patients who have a relatively higher level of ventilatory compromise [67].

The American Academy of Neurology (AAN) practice parameter guidelines recommend that PEG should be considered for prolonging survival in patients with ALS. Furthermore, it is stated that there are insufficient data to support or refute specific timing of PEG insertion or PEG for improving quality of life [12]. A Cochrane review examined the efficacy of percutaneous endoscopic gastrostomy placement or other tube feeding placement on survival, nutritional status, and quality of life, as well as the minor and major complications of PEG. No randomized controlled trials were found evaluating whether enteral tube feeding is beneficial compared to continuation of oral feeding for any of the outcome measures. The authors analyzed several retrospective and prospective studies, and 15 were included in the final discussion. Many of these studies are discussed earlier [58–62,64–66]. They conclude that the best evidence to date suggests a survival advantage for some patients with ALS/MND who pursue enteral tube feeding, though are careful to point out that these conclusions are tentative. Likewise, evidence for improved nutrition is also incomplete, but tentatively favorable. Emphasis is placed on the need for further studies looking at quality of life. Finally, based on a number of recent non-randomized studies comparing surgical and radiographic approaches to feeding tube insertion, they conclude that the two procedures appear to be equivalent [68].

Symptom control

What symptomatic treatments are available for patients with ALS/MND?

Cramps

Cramps often affect ALS/MND patients during the course of their illness. Treatment thus far has largely been empirical without any evidence from RCTs. A recent Cochrane review assessed the effect of different interventions on muscle cramps as a primary or secondary end point, or adverse events in people with ALS/MND. Twenty randomized and quasi-randomized trials of oral, subcutaneous, and intravenous medications in 4789 patients with ALS/MND were identified. Only a trial of tetrahydrocannabinol (THC) assessed cramps as a primary end point, while 13 studies including vitamin E, baclofen, riluzole, indinavir, xaliproden, L-threonine, and memantine assessed cramps as a secondary end point. The studies assessing cramps as an adverse event totaled six and evaluated creatine, gabapentin, lithium, dextromethorphan, and quinidine. The authors concluded that none of the trials provided evidence to support any of the above-mentioned interventions for muscle cramps in ALS/MND, though they emphasized that many studies were underpowered [69].

The 2012 European Federation of Neurological Societies (EFNS) guidelines make recommendations for a trial of levetiracetam for the treatment of cramps in patients with ALS/MND, based on a small open-label pilot study [70,71]. The dose range was 500–1500 mg twice daily, and it was well tolerated. Patients experienced a significant reduction in cramp severity and frequency, which lasted the duration of this year-long study. Another option is quinine sulfate taken at a dose of 200 mg twice daily, though it has been banned by the FDA because of safety concerns. However, a recent Cochrane review of cramps in non-ALS patients found quinine sulfate to be effective, with no difference in adverse events between placebo and those taking quinine sulfate [72]. In addition, EFNS guidelines suggest physical exercise, physiotherapy, and/or hydrotherapy may be helpful. Where there was lack of evidence but consensus was clear, they stated their recommendations as "good clinical practice points."

Spasticity

Spasticity is commonly found in patients with ALS/MND and may lead to worsening muscle function and greater difficulty performing activities of daily living. A Cochrane review systematically assessed treatments for spasticity in the ALS/MND population, with the primary outcome measure being a reduction in spasticity at 3 months or greater as measured by the Ashworth scale. Secondary outcome measures were analyzed at 1 month or greater and included validated measures based on history, physical examination, function, spasticity, and quality of life, in addition to adverse events and measures of cost. Only one RCT was indentified, and this trial included 25 patients with ALS/NMD and looked at the effect of moderate intensity, endurance-type exercise versus "usual activities." Unfortunately, given the small size of the study, they were unable to determine whether individualized moderate intensity endurance exercises for the trunks and limbs are beneficial or harmful in patients with ALS/MND [73].

Even though not formally tested in ALS/MND, EFNS guidelines make recommendations based on good clinical practice to use gabapentin (900–2400 mg daily), tizanidine (6–24 mg daily), memantine (10–60 mg daily), dantrolene (25–100 mg daily), tetrazepam (100–200 mg daily), and diazepam (10–30 mg daily). Additional recommendations are made for regular physical therapy, hydrotherapy with exercises in warm pools (32–34 °C), and cryotherapy. If spasticity is so severe that it does not respond to oral medications, then intrathecal baclofen may be considered [70].

Pain

Unfortunately, pain is a common symptom in ALS/MND and occurs in up to 73% of patients, especially in advanced stages [3]. This is a result of lack of mobility of the joints, skin pressure, muscle atrophy, and contractures. A Cochrane review aimed to analyze the evidence for the efficacy of drug therapy in relieving pain in ALS in addition to evaluating possible side effects associated with different drugs and the effect on survival and quality of life. No randomized controlled trials were found regarding the management of pain in ALS/MND. The authors found that acetaminophen or NSAIDs were usually used as first-line treatment, with some success in the earlier stages of the disease process. However in later stages, opioids were more effective for pain management, as well as having beneficial effects on dyspnea and insomnia. Data regarding the characteristics of pain in ALS/MND and the effectiveness of different analgesics are scarce, highlighting the need for further research into this important aspect of palliative care [74].

Pseudobulbar emotional lability

Pathological laughing and crying occurs in up to 50% of ALS/MND patients, irrespective of bulbar motor involvement [3,70,75]. This emotional lability is not a mood disorder and does not correlate with cognitive impairment, but can often be quite socially disabling. Two randomized controlled trials involving 466 patients with ALS/MND and pseudobulbar affect, evaluated a fixed dose combination of dextromethorphan and quinidine. Both trials showed efficacy in improving emotional lability and quality of life in this patient population [76,77]. In October 2010, dextromethorphan/quinidine received approval from the US FDA as first-in-class pseudobulbar affect pharmacotherapy [78]. Antidepressants such as amitriptyline, fluvoxamine, and citalopram are also recommended as good clinical practice by the EFNS [70].

Multidisciplinary care

Is multidisciplinary care (MDC) an effective means of symptomatic and supportive management in patients with ALS/MND?

Given that there is no curative treatment for ALS/MND, the focus of management is on symptomatic, rehabilitative, and palliative therapy. This care is usually delivered by a team of specialists from different disciplines (e.g., physicians, nurses, and therapists) working together in an organized and collaborative manner to form a multidisciplinary team [1]. A Cochrane review assessed the effectiveness of MDC in patients with ALS/MND and looked at the types of approaches that were most effective and the outcomes affected. This review did not find any randomized controlled trials or controlled clinical trials, but did result in the analysis of five observational studies, that were considered "low quality" and "very low quality" studies. The evidence from these studies suggests that MDC may improve some aspects of quality of life (i.e., mental health), reduce the frequency of hospitalizations and length of stay, and improve disability. There is conflicting evidence on survival. The authors emphasize the need for further research into outcome measurement, caregiver needs, and the evaluation of optimal settings, type, intensity, frequency, and cost-effectiveness of MDC in the ALS/MND population [79].

EFNS guidelines suggest that multidisciplinary care should be available to patients with ALS/MND and that attendance at MDC clinics may extend survival, decrease medical complications (level B), and improve quality of life (level C). On the basis of good clinical practice consensus, they recommend that the following specialists should make up the MDC team: neurologist, rehabilitation medicine specialist, pulmonologist, gastroenterologist, occupational therapist, respiratory therapist, physical therapist, social worker, speech therapist, dietitian, specialized nurse, psychologist, dentist, and palliative care physician. They suggest that ALS/MND patients should be reviewed by the MDC team at least every 2–3 months, and emphasize the importance of good communication between MDC team members and the patient's primary care physician [70].

Conclusions

Riluzole remains the only licensed disease-modifying treatment for ALS/MND. RCT evidence suggests only modest effectiveness. The National Institute for Health and Clinical Excellence (NICE) suggested that further studies were desirable following the dose ranging trial [8], but these have never been done and seem unlikely to happen in the future. In the meantime any further insights are likely to come from observational studies rather than prospective randomized investigations.

Similar sentiments apply to IGF-1. RCTs so far completed have not had the ability to definitively demonstrate the potential efficacy of IGF-1 as a disease-modifying treatment for ALS/MND. There is hope that novel delivery methods, such as viral vectors, may lead to new insights into the possible effectiveness of IGF-1 as well as other neurotrophins in ALS/MND.

While stem cell therapy has been identified as having huge potential as a disease-modifying treatment for ALS/MND and other neurodegenerative diseases, it is too early to make further comment. Interest in respiratory interventions as symptomatic treatments for ALS/MND has developed considerably in recent years. NIPPV may favorably influence QoL and survival and cough exsufflator/insufflator devices may also be useful. Optimum methods of monitoring respiratory function during the course of ALS/MND remain uncertain. SNP has been suggested as a possible alternative to traditional methods such as FVC.

Whatever the role of respiratory function monitoring in determining the use of respiratory interventions, it seems increasingly clear that such monitoring is important in judging the timing of feeding gastrostomy in ALS/MND. The morbidity and mortality of PEG insertion probably increases as FVC% predicted declines. If an endoscopic technique is to be used, FVC should probably be at least 50%, certainly 40% predicted. PRG/RIG may however be preferable to PEG when feeding gastrostomies need to be established in patients with more severe levels of respiratory impairment.

References

1 Demaerschalk, B.M. & Strong, M.J. (2000) Amyotrophic lateral sclerosis. *Current Treatment Options in Neurology*, **2**(1), 13–22.

2 Rowland, L.P. & Shneider, N.A. (2001) Amyotrophic lateral sclerosis. *New England Journal of Medicine*, **344**, 1688–1700.

3 Mitchell, J.D. & Borasio, G.D. (2007) Amyotrophic lateral sclerosis. *Lancet*, **369**, 2031–2041.

4 Chio, A., Logroscino, G., Hardiman, O. *et al.* (2009) Prognostic factors in ALS: a critical review. *Amyotrophic Lateral Sclerosis*, **10**, 310–323.

5 Weikamp JG, Schelhaas HJ, Hendriks JC, de Swart BJ, Geurts AC. Prognostic value of decreased tongue strength on survival time in patients with amyotrophic lateral sclerosis. *Journal of Neurology* 2012 doi: 10.1007/s00415-012-6503-9. Epub 2012 Apr 24.

6 Bensimon, G., Lacomblez, L., Meininger, V. *et al.* (1994) A controlled trial of riluzole in amyotrophic lateral sclerosis. *New England Journal of Medicine*, **330**, 585–591.

7 Rowland, L.P. (1994) Riluzole for the treatment of amyotrophic lateral sclerosis – too soon to tell? *New England Journal of Medicine*, **330**, 636–637.

8 Lacomblez, L., Bensimon, G., Leigh, P.N. *et al.* (1996) Dose ranging study of riluzole in amyotrophic lateral sclerosis. *Lancet*, **37**, 1425–1431.

9 Bensimon, G., Lacomblez, L., Delumeau, J.C. *et al.* (2002) A study of riluzole in the treatment of advanced stage or elderly patients with amyotrophic lateral sclerosis. *Journal of Neurology*, **249**, 609–615.

10 Yanagisawa, N., Tashiro, K., Tohgi, H. *et al.* (1997) Efficacy and safety of riluzole in patients with amyotrophic lateral sclerosis: double blind placebo-controlled study in Japan. *Igakuno Ayumi*, **182**, 851–866.

11 Miller, R.G., Mitchell, J.D. & Moore, D.H. (2012) Riluzole for amyotrophic lateral sclerosis (ALS)/motor neuron disease (MND) (Cochrane Review). *Cochrane Database of Systematic Reviews*, **3**.

12 Miller, R.G., Jackson, C.E., Kasarkis, E.J. *et al.* (2009) Practice parameter update: the care of the patient with amyotrophic lateral sclerosis: drug, nutritional, and respiratory therapies (an evidence-based review): report of the Quality Standards Subcommittee of the American Academy of Neurology. *Neurology*, **73(15)**, 1218–1226.

13 Lai, E.C., Felice, K.J., Festoff, B.W. *et al.* (1997) Effect of recombinant human insulin-like growth factor-1 on progression of ALS. A placebo-controlled study. *Neurology*, **49**, 1621–1630.

14 Borasio, G.D., Robberecht, W., Leigh, P.N. *et al.* (1998) A placebo controlled trial of insulin-like nerve growth factor-1 in amyotrophic lateral sclerosis. *Neurology*, **51**, 583–586.

15 Mitchell, J.D., Wokke, J.H.J. & Borasio, G. (2011) Recombinant human insulin-like growth factor I (rhIGF-I) for amyotrophic lateral sclerosis/motor neuron disease (Cochrane Review). *Cochrane Database of Systematic Reviews*,(**10**).

16 Nagano, I., Shiote, M., Murakami, T. *et al.* (2005) Beneficial effects of intrathecal IGF-I administration in patients with amyotrophic lateral sclerosis. *Neurological Research*, **27(7)**, 768–772.

17 Sorenson, E.J., Windbank, A.J., Mandrekar, J.N. *et al.* (2008) Subcutaneous IGF-1 is not beneficial in 2-year ALS trial. *Neurology*, **71**, 1770–1775.

18 Bongioanni, P., Reali, C. & Sogos, V. (2011) Ciliary neurotrophic factor (CNTF) for amyotrophic lateral sclerosis/motor neuron disease. *Cochrane Database of Systematic Reviews*, **8**.

19 Parton, M., Mitsumoto, H. & Leigh, P.N. (2009) Amino acids for amyotrophic lateral sclerosis/motor neuron disease. *Cochrane Database of Systematic Reviews*, **1**.

20 Orrell, R.W., Lane, R.J.M. & Ross, M. (2011) Antioxidant treatment for amyotrophic lateral sclerosis/motor neuron disease. *Cochrane Database of Systematic Reviews*, **6**.

21 BDNF Study Group (1999) (Phase III) A controlled trial of recombinant methionyl human BDNF in ALS. *Neurology*, **52**, 1427–1433.

22 Ochs, G., Penn, R.D., York, M. *et al.* (2000) A phase I/II trial of recombinant methionyl human brain derived neurotrophic factor administered by intrathecal infusion to patients with amyotrophic lateral sclerosis. *Amyotrophic Lateral Sclerosis and Other Motor Neuron Disorders*, **1**, 201–206.

23 Eisen, A., Stewart, H., Schulzer, M. & Cameron, D. (1993) Anti-glutamate therapy in amyotrophic lateral sclerosis: a trial using lamotrigine. *Canadian Journal of Neurological Sciences*, **20**, 297–301.

24 Ryberg, H., Askmark, H. & Persson, L.I. (2003) A double-blind randomized clinical trial in amyotrophic lateral sclerosis using lamotrigine: effects on CSF glutamate, aspartate, branched-chain amino acid levels and clinical parameters. *Acta Neurologica Scandinavica*, **108**, 1–8.

25 Miller, R.G., Moore, D., Young, L.A. *et al.* (1996) Placebo-controlled trial of gabapentin in patients with amyotrophic lateral sclerosis. *Neurology*, **47**, 1383–1388.242 Part 3: Neurological diseases c22.qxd 3/16/09 12:29 PM Page 242.

26 Miller, R.G., Moore, D.H. II,, Gelinas, D.F. *et al.* (2001) Phase III randomized trial of gabapentin in patients with amyotrophic lateral sclerosis. *Neurology*, **56**, 843–848.

27 Gordon, P.H., Moore, D.H., Gelinas, D.F. *et al.* (2004) Placebo-controlled phase I/II studies of minocycline in amyotrophic lateral sclerosis. *Neurology*, **62**, 1845–1847.

28 Sathasivam, S., Addison-Jones, R., Miller, R.G., Moore, D.H. & Young, C.A. (2009) Minocycline for amyotrophic lateral sclerosis or motor neuron disease (Protocol). *Cochrane Database of Systematic Reviews*, **1**.

29 Pontieri, F.E., Ricci, A., Pellicano, C., Benincasa, D. & Buttarelli, F.R. (2005) Minocycline in amyotrophic lateral sclerosis: a pilot study. *Neurological Science*, **26(4)**, 285–287.

30 Gordon, P.H., Moore, D.H., Miller, R.G. *et al.* (2007) Efficacy of minocycline in patients with amyotrophic lateral sclerosis: a phase III randomized trial. *Lancet Neurology*, **6(12)**, 1045–1053.

31 Lacomblez, L., Bensimon, G., Douillet, P., Doppler, V., Salachas, F. & Meininger, V. (2004) Xaliproden in amyotrophic lateral sclerosis: early clinical trials. *Amyotrophic Lateral Sclerosis and Other Motor Neuron Disorders*, **5**, 99–106.

32 Meininger, V., Bensimon, G., Bradley, W.R. *et al.* (2004) Efficacy and safety of xaliproden in amyotrophic lateral sclerosis: results of two phase III trials. *Amyotrophic Lateral Sclerosis and Other Motor Neuron Disorders*, **5**, 107–117.

33 Klivenyi, P., Ferrante, R.J., Matthews, R.T. *et al.* (1999) Neuroprotective effects of creatine in a transgenic animal model of amyotrophic lateral sclerosis. *Nature Medicine*, **5(3)**, 347–350.

34 Pastula, D.M., Moore, D.H. & Bedlack, R.S. (2010) Creatine for amyotrophic lateral sclerosis/motor neuron disease. *Cochrane Database of Systematic Reviews*, **8**.

35 Fornai, F., Longone, P., Cafaro, L. *et al.* (2008) Lithium delays progression of amyotrophic lateral sclerosis. *Proceedings of the National Academy of Sciences of the United States of America*, **105**, 2052–2057.

36 Aggarwal, S.P., Zinman, L., Simpson, E. *et al.* (2010) Safety and efficacy of lithium in combination with riluzole for treatment of amyotrophic lateral sclerosis: a randomised, double-blind, placebo-controlled trial. *Lancet Neurology*, **9**, 481–488.

37 Verstraete, E., Veldink, J.H., Huisman, M.H. *et al.* (2012) Lithium lacks effect on survival in amyotrophic lateral sclerosis; a phase IIb randomized sequential trial. *Journal of Neurology, Neurosurgery and Psychiatry*, **83**, 557–564.

38 Fallat, R.J., Jewitt, B., Bass, M., Kamm, B. & Norris, F.H. Jr., (1979) Spirometry in amyotrophic lateral sclerosis. *Archives of Neurology*, **36**, 74–80.

39 Jackson, C.E., Rosenfeld, J., Moore, D.H. *et al.* (2001) A preliminary evaluation of a prospective study of pulmonary function studies and symptoms of hypoventilation in ALS/MND patients. *Journal of Neurological Sciences*, **191**, 75–78.

40 Miller, R.G., Jackson, C.E., Kasarskis, E.J. *et al.* (2009) Quality Standards Subcommittee of the American Academy of Neurology. Practice parameter update: the care of the patient with amyotrophic lateral sclerosis: drug, nutritional, and respiratory therapies (an evidence-based review): report of the Quality Standards Subcommittee of the American Academy of Neurology. *Neurology*, **73**, 1218–1226.

41 Lyall, R.A., Donaldson, N., Polkey, M.I., Leigh, P.N. & Moxham, J. (2001) Respiratory muscle strength and ventilatory failure in amyotrophic lateral sclerosis. *Brain*, **124**, 2000–2013.

42 Fitting, J.W., Paillex, R., Hirt, L., Aebischer, P. & Schluep, M. (1999) Sniff nasal pressure: a sensitive respiratory test to assess progression of amyotrophic lateral sclerosis. *Annals of Neurology*, **46**, 887–893.

43 Morgan, R.K., McNally, S., Alexander, M., Conroy, R., Hardiman, O. & Costello, R.W. (2005) Use of Sniff nasal-inspiratory force to predict survival in amyotrophic lateral sclerosis. *American Journal of Respiratory and Critical Care Medicine*, **171**, 269–274.

44 Bourke, S.C., Shaw, P.J. & Gibson, G.J. (2001) Respiratory function vs. sleepdisordered breathing as predictors of QOL in ALS. *Neurology*, **57**, 2040–2044.

45 Sivak, E.D., Shefner, J.M., Mitsumoto, H. & Taft, J.M. (2001) The use of noninvasive positive pressure ventilation (NIPPV) in ALS patients. A need for improved determination of intervention timing. *Amyotrophic Lateral Sclerosis and Other Motor Neuron Disorders*, **2**, 139–145.

46 Newsom-Davis, I.C., Lyall, R.A., Leigh, P.N., Moxham, J. & Goldstein, L.H. (2001) The effect of non-invasive positive pressure ventilation (NIPPV) on cognitive function in amyotrophic lateral sclerosis (ALS): a prospective study. *Journal of Neurology, Neurosurgery and Psychiatry*, **71**, 482–487.

47 Lyall, R.A., Donaldson, N., Fleming, T. *et al.* (2001) A prospective study of quality of life in ALS patients treated with non-invasive ventilation. *Neurology*, **57**, 153–156.

48 Bourke, S.C., Bullock, R.E., Williams, T.L., Shaw, P.J. & Gibson, G.J. (2003) Noninvasive ventilation in ALS: indications and effect on quality of life. *Neurology*, **61**, 171–177.

49 Bourke, S.C., Tomlinson, M., Williams, T.L., Bullock, R.E., Shaw, P.J. & Gibson, G.J. (2006) Effects of non-invasive ventilation on survival and quality of life in patients with amyotrophic lateral sclerosis: a randomised controlled trial. *Lancet Neurology*, **5**, 140–147.

50 Radunovic, A., Annane, D., Jewitt, K. & Mustfa, N. (2009) Mechanical ventilation for amyotrophic lateral sclerosis/motor neuron disease. *Cochrane Database of Systematic Reviews*, **4**.

51 Moss, A.H., Oppenheimer, E.A., Casey, P. *et al.* (1996) Patients with amyotrophic lateral sclerosis receiving long-term mechanical ventilation. Advance care planning and outcomes. *Chest*, **110**, 249–255.

52 Escarrabill, J., Estopa, R., Farrero, E., Monasterio, C. & Manresa, F. (1998) Long-term mechanical ventilation in amyotrophic lateral sclerosis. *Respiratory Medicine*, **92**, 438–441.

53 Moss, A.H., Casey, P., Stocking, C.B., Roos, R.P., Brooks, B.R. & Siegler, M. (1993) Home ventilation for amyotrophic lateral sclerosis patients: outcomes, costs, and patient, family, and physician attitudes. *Neurology*, **43**, 438–443.

54 Farrero, E., Prats, E., Povedano, M., Martinez-Matos, J.A., Manresa, F. & Escarrabill, J. (2005) Survival in amyotrophic lateral sclerosis with home mechanical ventilation: the impact of systematic respiratory assessment and bulbar involvement. *Chest*, **127**, 2132–2138.

55 Lahrmann, H., Wild, M., Zdrahal, F. & Grisold, W. (2003) Expiratory muscle weakness and assisted cough in ALS. *Amyotrophic Lateral Sclerosis and Other Motor Neuron Disorders*, **4**, 49–51.

56 Winck, J.C., Goncalves, M.R., Lourenco, C., Viana, P., Almeida, J. & Bach, J.R. (2004) Effects of mechanical insufflation–exsufflation on respiratory parameters for patients with chronic airway secretion encumbrance. *Chest*, **126**, 774–780.

57 Sancho, J., Servera, E., Diaz, J. & Marin, J. (2004) Efficacy of mechanical insufflation–exsufflation in medically stable patients with amyotrophic lateral sclerosis. *Chest*, **125**, 1400–1405.

58 Mazzini, L., Corra, T., Zaccala, M., Mora, G., Del Piano, M. & Galante, M. (1995) Percutaneous endoscopic gastrostomy and enteral nutrition in amyotrophic lateral sclerosis. *Journal of Neurology*, **242**, 695–698.

59 Chio, A., Finocchiaro, E., Meineri, P., Bottacchi, E. & Schiffer, D. (1999) Safety and factors related to survival after percutaneous endoscopic gastrostomy in ALS. *Neurology*, **53**, 1123–1125.

60 Kasarskis, E.J., Scarlata, D., Hill, R., Fuller, C., Stambler, N. & Cedarbaum, J.M. (1999) A retrospective study of percutaneous endoscopic gastrostomy in ALS patients during the BDNF and CNTF trials. *Journal of Neurological Sciences*, **169**(**1–2**), 118–125.

61 Gregory, S., Siderowf, A., Golaszewski, A.L. & McCluskey, L. (2002) Gastrostomy insertion in ALS patients with low vital capacity: respiratory support and survival. *Neurology*, **58**, 485–487.

62 Thornton, F.J., Fotheringham, T., Alexander, M., Hardiman, O., McGrath, F.P. & Lee, M.J. (2002) Amyotrophic lateral sclerosis: enteral nutrition provision – endoscopic or radiologic gastrostomy? *Radiology*, **224**, 713–717.

63 Blondet, A., Lebigot, J., Nicolas, G. & Boursier, J. (2010) Radiologic versus endoscopic placement of percutaneous gastrostomy in amyotrophic lateral sclerosis: multivariate analysis of tolerance, efficacy, and survival. *Journal of Vascular and Interventional Radiology*, **21**, 527–533.

64 Mitsumoto, H., Davidson, M., Moore, D. *et al.* (2003) Percutaneous endoscopic gastrostomy (PEG) in patients with ALS and bulbar dysfunction. *Amyotrophic Lateral Sclerosis and Other Motor Neuron Disorders*, **4**, 177–185.

65 Chio, A., Galletti, R., Finocchiaro, C. *et al.* (2004) Percutaneous radiological gastrostomy: a safe and effective method of nutritional tube placement in advanced ALS. *Journal of Neurology, Neurosurgery and Psychiatry*, **75**, 645–647.

66 Forbes, R.B., Colville, S. & Swingler, R.J. (2004) Scottish Motor Neurone Disease Research Group. Frequency, timing and outcome of gastrostomy tubes for amyotrophic lateral sclerosis/motor neurone disease – a record linkage study from the Scottish Motor Neurone Disease Register. *Journal of Neurology*, **251**, 813–817.

67 Desport, J.C., Mabrouk, T., Bouillet, P., Perna, A., Preux, P.M. & Couratier, P. (2005) Complications and survival following radiologically and endoscopically-guided gastrostomy in patients with amyotrophic lateral sclerosis. *Amyotrophic Lateral Sclerosis and Other Motor Neuron Disorders*, **6**, 88–93.

68 Katzberg, H.D. & Benatar, M. (2011) Enteral tube feeding for amyotrophic lateral sclerosis/motor neuron disease. *Cochrane Database of Systematic Reviews*, **1**.

69 Baldinger, R., Katzberg, H.D. & Weber, M. (2012) Treatment for cramps in amyotrophic lateral sclerosis/motor neuron disease. *Cochrane Database of Systematic Reviews*, **4**.

70 Andersen, P.M., Abrahams, S., Borasio, G.D. *et al.* (2012) EFNS guidelines on the clinical management of amyotrophic lateral sclerosis (MALS)- revised report of an EFNS task force. *European Journal of Neurology*, **19**(**3**), 360–375.

71 Bedlack, R.S., Pastula, D.M., Hawes, J. & Heydt, D. (2009) Open-label pilot trial of levetiracetam for cramps and spasticity in patients with motor neuron disease. *Amyotrophic Lateral Sclerosis*, **10**(**4**), 210–215.

72 El-Tawil, S., Al Musa, T., Valli, H. *et al.* (2010) Quinine for muscle cramps. *Cochrane Database of Systematic Reviews*, **12**.

73 Ashworth, N.L., Satkunam, L.E. & Deforge, D. (2012) Treatment for spasticity in amyotrophic lateral sclerosis/motor neuron disease. *Cochrane Database of Systematic Reviews*, **2**.

74 Brettschneider, J., Kurent, J., Albert, L. & Mitchell, J.D. (2010) Drug therapy for pain in amyotrophic lateral sclerosis or motor neuron disease. *Cochrane Database of Systematic Reviews*, **11**.

75 Corcia, P. & Meininger, V. (2008) Management of amyotrophic lateral sclerosis. *Drugs*, **68**(**8**), 1037–1048.

76 Brooks, B.R., Thisted, R.A., Appel, S.H. *et al.* (2004) Treatment of pseudobulbar affect in ALS with dextromethorphan/quinidine: a randomized trial. The AVP-923 ALS Study Group. *Neurology*, **63**, 1364–1370.

77 Pioro, E.P., Brooks, B.R., Cummings, J. *et al.* (2010) Dextromethorphan plus ultra low-dose quinidine reduces pseudobulbar affect. *Annals of Neurology*, **68**, 693–702.

78 Pioro, E.P. (2011) Current concepts in the pharmacotherapy of pseudobulbar affect. *Drugs*, **71**(**9**), 1193–1207.

79 Ng, L. & Khan, F. (2011) Multidisciplinary care for adults with amyotrophic lateral sclerosis or motor neuron disease. *Cochrane Database of Systematic Reviews*, **12**.

CHAPTER 22

Peripheral nerve disorders

Jennifer A. Tracy and P. James B. Dyck

Department of Neurology, Mayo Clinic, Rochester, MN, USA

Introduction

Peripheral nervous system disorders are common, and there is a vast range of potential causes, including metabolic, nutritional, inflammatory, and inherited. For this chapter, we will focus on the evidence for treatment of chronic inflammatory demyelinating polyradiculoneuropathy (CIDP), Guillain–Barré syndrome (acute inflammatory demyelinating polyradiculoneuropathy (AIDP)), multifocal motor neuropathy, and diabetic polyneuropathy.

Critical review of the evidence for each disorder will be presented.

Treatment for CIDP

In patients with CIDP, what is the evidence for benefit of immunotherapy options?

CIDP is an immune-mediated primarily demyelinating disorder, though secondary axonal loss is also common. It can present in either a progressive or relapsing-remitting form, and unlike Guillain–Barré syndrome, it is a chronic condition, which in most patients requires long-term immunotherapy for management. While CIDP is generally thought of as a motor-predominant symmetric process with both proximal and distal weakness, as well as of sensory loss, it has been recognized that subtypes exist which are very focal in terms of body regions involved (e.g., Lewis–Sumner syndrome) or in types of nerve fibers involved (e.g., chronic immune sensory polyradiculopathy (CISP)). Most data available are for the treatment of the more classical CIDP phenotype, and it is unclear to what extent they can be extrapolated to the less common subtypes.

The data for selecting a specific type of immunotherapy are limited, but the treatments generally employed are corticosteroids (either oral or intravenous), intravenous immunoglobulin, plasma exchange, and a variety of steroid-sparing oral immunosuppressive agents.

While corticosteroids are often a first-line treatment, the evidence-based data for their efficacy is not extensive. A study of 28 patients with CIDP treated with oral prednisone showed some improvement in strength and disability parameters [1]. In a prospective study of 10 patients with CIDP treated with oral methylprednisolone, 6 of 9 of the patients who completed the study went into remission [2]. A retrospective study of CIDP patients treated with oral prednisone, intravenous methylprednisolone, oral cyclosporine, or IVIG showed no significant differences in treatment outcomes between the groups, suggesting that intravenous corticosteroids may be as effective as oral prednisone [3]. However, Attarian *et al.* [4] caution that in their retrospective study of patients with Lewis–Sumner syndrome, two of the four who received steroid medications (initial daily dose of 1 mg/kg for at least 6 weeks) experienced a dramatic neurological decline while on steroids. This may indicate that the less classical, more focal forms of CIDP may respond differently to treatment.

The first controlled study to show efficacy of IVIG was when Dyck *et al.* [5] compared IVIG to plasmapheresis in a crossover designed study with a washout period and found that both treatments were effective for CIDP. A large placebo-controlled, double-blinded prospective study of IVIG in CIDP, which included 117 patients, showed an improved INCAT disability score in 54% of the IVIG-treated patients (statistically significant compared to placebo) [6]. Other studies include a placebo-controlled trial of IVIG (0.4 g/kg IV for 5 days) versus placebo in 30 patients and noted improvement in the treatment group in disability score and grip strength [7]. Another study treated 53 CIDP patients with 1 g/kg IVIG on days 1, 2, and 21 versus placebo, and there were significant improvement in the average muscle score in the IVIG group on day 42 [8]. There is increased interest in subcutaneous immunoglobulin administration, for the purposes of ease of administration in the home setting. A small prospective study of five CIDP patients who were IVIG responsive, switched them to subcutaneous immunoglobulin administration, and found no difference in muscle strength, grip strength, or on a disability scale [9].

Dyck *et al.* [10] prospectively treated 29 CIDP patients with either plasmapheresis or sham exchange, and found improved nerve conduction parameters in the treated patients. Hahn *et al.* [11] treated 18 CIDP patients with plasmapheresis and found that 80% of the 15 patients who finished the trial had significant improvement. Dyck *et al.* [5], as previously noted, treated 20 patients with either IVIG or plasma exchange, with a crossover component to the study, and found improvement in disease status in both, but no significant difference between the two groups.

Several steroid sparing oral immunomodulatory agents have been studied for the treatment of CIDP. A recent large trial of 60 CIDP patients with methotrexate versus placebo as an add-on to either baseline IVIG or corticosteroid failed to show a significant difference between methotrexate or placebo in the end point of reducing the mean weekly dose of steroids or IVIG by 20% [12]. A randomized controlled study of 27 patients treated with prednisone or prednisone and azathioprine did not show any significant difference between the two groups 9 months later [13]. One treatment study of 13 patients treated with mycophenolate mofetil did not show significant improvement in either strength, sensory, or disability scores, but 3 of the patients were felt to have clinical improvement [14]. A retrospective study of 19 patients with treatment-refractory CIDP showed that the group with progressive CIDP treated with cyclosporine A had decreased disability scores [15]. A retrospective review of 15 cases treated with intravenous cyclophosphamide showed that 11 had a complete remission [16].

A retrospective study of 13 patients with CIDP unresponsive or only partially responsive to other therapies, who were ultimately treated with rituximab, showed some response in 9, and 6 of them had some clinical improvement [17]. Chin *et al.* [18] reviewed 10 patients with CIDP who were either treatment-refractory or intolerant to other medical treatments, who were treated with etanercept, and found that 3 had significant improvement and 3 had possible improvement. Marsh *et al.* [19] reported on seven treatment-refractory CIDP patients who were treated with alemtuzumab; they noted that two patients had prolonged remission and two had a partial response, the mean monthly IVIG use was 202 g before treatment, and decreased to 149 g after treatment. While the initial data for alemtuzumab seem promising, there is an increased risk of development of autoimmune disease, with one study of alemtuzumab in multiple sclerosis patients showing that 23% developed autoimmune thyroid disease [20].

At present, three treatments are considered first-line treatments in CIDP – IVIG, plasma exchange, and corticosteroids. The practice of most neuromuscular physicians is to use corticosteroids and/or IVIG initially for the treatment of CIDP. Plasma exchange is a good treatment but is more invasive and usually has to be given in a hospital setting. While corticosteroids are inexpensive, the side effect profile for long-term use is high. In most cases, IVIG and plasma exchange are better tolerated, but are expensive therapies. Data of efficacy for most steroid sparing agents are limited, sometimes to case reports and small case series alone. Rituximab, etanercept, and alemtuzumab are promising, but the side effect profiles can be severe, and hence their use must be limited.

Treatment for Guillain–Barré syndrome

What is appropriate initial treatment for Guillain–Barré syndrome, and is there a role for repeated treatments?

Guillain–Barré syndrome, also known as acute inflammatory demyelinating polyradiculoneuropathy (AIDP), is a primarily demyelinating disorder which is usually of rapid onset, with maximal severity of disease within 4 weeks from initial symptoms. This is usually a monophasic syndrome, characterized by progressive severe weakness, which can involve respiratory and bulbar muscles, and there can be marked associated autonomic dysfunction. Supportive care (e.g., respiratory and hemodynamic support) is crucial for survival in many patients.

As GBS typically presents in a monophasic fashion, study of treatments has primarily focused on quick-acting immunomodulatory agents rather than longer-term oral immunosuppressive therapies. As such, most of the data available regarding treatments are for corticosteroids, plasma exchange, and IVIG.

Swick *et al.* [21] performed a small study of GBS patients receiving either placebo or ACTH treatment and reported that the mean duration to recovery was 4.4 months in the treated patients and 9.0 months in the untreated patients ($p = 0.05$); they studied a larger group of 38 patients which included the subjects in the double-blind trial as well as other historical patients at their institution, and in this larger group, the mean duration to recovery was 4.1 months in steroid-treated patients, and 7.7 months in nontreated patients, which was a statistically significant difference. Hughes *et al.* [22] treated 21 GBS patients with prednisolone (60 mg daily for 1 week, then 40 mg daily for 4 days, then 30 mg daily for 3 days) and compared these to 19 untreated patients, with assessments at 1, 3, and 12 months. Interestingly, at all time points there were greater improvements in the control than in the corticosteroid group, these differences however were nonsignificant except for the 3-month assessment of patients enrolled within a week of their illness. These findings were interpreted as showing a lack of efficacy of corticosteroids, but also raised the issue of potential harm with their use. The role of corticosteroids as add-on agents in the treatment of GBS with either IVIG or plasma exchange will be discussed below.

Kennard *et al.* [23] treated 12 consecutive GBS patients with plasma exchange (mean 7 treatments) and examined them 2 weeks after their treatment; 9 patients experienced some improvement, though the authors felt that in only 4 was there clearly improvement beyond that expected from the natural history of the disease. Greenwood *et al.* [24] performed a small randomized controlled trial comparing patients treated with plasma exchange and no exchange, with standard supportive care in both groups, and did not find a significant benefit from plasma exchange. Mendell *et al.* [25] also performed a randomized controlled trial of patients receiving plasma exchange (nine treatments) and prednisone (starting at 100 mg daily, with a taper) versus supportive therapy alone, and failed to find a difference in the mean of the average muscle scores for each week of the 24-week study. They hypothesize that either the small size of their study (25 patients) may have resulted in the failure to find a significant difference, or that the addition of prednisone may have had a deleterious effect. Osterman *et al.* [26] however studied 38 patients in a controlled trial (18 receiving plasma exchange), and found significantly better outcome in the treated patients in time to the onset of improvement (mean 8.5 days versus 17.1 days in the untreated group) and in the course of muscular weakness. Farkkila *et al.* [27] found significantly better hand grip force (using a strain-gauge dynamometer) in patients treated with plasma exchange than in patients in the control group. A much larger study (245 patients) randomized patients to either plasmapheresis (200–250 cc plasma per kilogram body weight over 7–14 days) or conventional treatment and found significant improvement in the treated group in percentage of patients who improved by at least 1 clinical grade at a 4-week assessment (54% of the treated group versus 39% of the controls), the time to improve 1 clinical grade, the time until able to walk unassisted, and the outcome at 6 months after randomization [28].

Kleyweg *et al.* [29] performed an open study treating patients with intravenous gammaglobulin (0.4 g/kg per day for 5 days); four out of six treated patients were considered to be responders. Most trials of intravenous immunoglobulin are in comparison to plasma exchange, which was considered the standard of care at the time these trials took place. Van der Meche *et al.* [30] randomized patients to either IVIG (0.4 g/kg per day for 5 treatments) or plasma exchange (200–250 mL/kg for 5 treatments); data analysis after accrual of 150 subjects showed that strength improved by 1 or more grade at 4 weeks in 53% of IVIG and 34% of plasma exchange patients – this difference was statistically significant. The median time to improvement by 1 grade was 27 days in the IVIG group and 41 days in the plasma exchange group ($p = 0.05$). Bril *et al.* [31] randomized 50 GBS patients to either IVIG (0.5 g/kg daily for 4 days) or plasma exchange (200–250 mL/kg for 5 treatments over 7–10 days) and found similar improvement, with 61% of the plasma exchange and 69% of the IVIG patients improving

by 1 disability grade at 1 month; this difference was not significant, and there was no significant difference in the rate of complications between the groups. Van Koningsveld *et al.* [32] studied 233 patients with GBS who received IVIG 0.4 g/kg per day for 5 days, and randomized them to receive either methylprednisolone 500 mg or placebo daily for 5 days (started within 48 hours of the first IVIG dose), and found no significant differences in change from baseline disability score of one or more at the 4-week time point.

A single study (P.E. Trial Group) [33] randomized 379 GBS patients into treatments with (1) plasma exchange (5 50 mg/kg exchanges over 8–13 days), (2) IVIG 0.4 g/kg per day for 5 days, and (3) the plasma exchange followed by the IVIG treatment. There was no significant difference between the groups on disability score 4 weeks later, and there were no significant differences between groups to time of recovery of unassisted walking or to no longer needing a ventilator. On the basis of this, most clinicians do not treat with plasma exchange followed by IVIG.

However, an important issue is whether there are groups of patients who may benefit from either repeated doses of treatment or more aggressive initial treatment, and there is not yet a consensus on this issue. Farcas *et al.* [34] described 12 patients with GBS treated with IVIG in a 2-year period at their institution – 8 had stabilization and then improvement, but 4 were stable without improvement at 14–21 days after IVIG. These four patients were treated with a second course of IVIG and all had a good response, with improvements on a disability scale. Kuitwaard *et al.* [35] measured serum IgG levels in 174 GBS patients before and after a standard course of IVIG and found that patients with a lesser change in IgG levels recovered more slowly and were less likely to be ambulating without assistance at 6-month follow-up. The authors suggest that in patients with a lower change in serum IgG, changes in dosing and perhaps repeat dosing could be considered. These are very intriguing ideas and further research needs to be done to assess whether individualized IVIG treatment plans should be considered on this basis.

At present, based on the data, standard recommendations are for plasma exchange for nonambulant patients within 4 weeks of symptoms or ambulant patients within 2 weeks of symptom onset, or IVIG for nonambulant patients within 2 and possibly within 4 weeks. The use of corticosteroids is not recommended [36].

Treatment for multifocal motor neuropathy

What is the best treatment strategy for multifocal motor neuropathy?

Multifocal motor neuropathy is a rare disorder causing progressive asymmetric weakness without associated sensory loss. The characteristic pattern on nerve conductions/electromyography is isolated involvement of motor fibers, with conduction block along motor nerves, without sensory involvement. The natural history is that of a progressively worsening disorder over time, without spontaneous improvement [37].

Multiple reports have shown a lack of response to corticosteroids in MMN patients. Pestronk et al. [38] described two patients with MMN who failed to respond to prednisone (100 mg daily for 4–6 months). Feldman et al. [39] reported a lack of response to steroids in 13 patients with MMN. In addition, there is the suggestion that in some patients worsening can occur as a result of corticosteroid use. Donaghy et al. [40] reviewed the course of four patients with MMN treated with oral prednisolone (60 mg per day with planned slow taper starting 2–4 weeks after treatment) and noted that all four had marked motor deterioration within 4 weeks above what would have been expected by the baseline rate of disease progression. Van den Berg et al. [41] treated two MMN patients with pulsed high-dose dexamethasone (40 mg per day for 4 days every 28 days), and they continued to deteriorate, and they report the weakness was most severe 1 week after the medication was taken; both patients declined further dexamethasone after six cycles, and then both had improvements with subsequent IVIG.

Azulay et al. [42] performed a double-blind, placebo-controlled crossover study for the use of IVIG in 12 patients with lower motor neuron associated with anti-GM1 antibodies – 5 of these had multifocal motor neuropathy. All the five MMN patients had improvements after 5 days of IVIG (0.4 g/kg daily), two had improvements by day 5, and three by day 28, though the improvements were statistically significant at day 28. Interestingly, the authors noted there was no change in GM1 antibody levels with the IVIG treatment. The patients with lower motor neuron syndromes (not MMN) did not show a statistically significant change in strength with IVIG. Federico et al. [43] studied 16 patients with MMN in a randomized, double-blind, crossover trial with IVIG (0.4 g/kg/day for 5 days) and placebo. Nine patients reported subjective functional improvement as dramatic or very good with IVIG, and with IVIG treatment, there were significant improvements in neurological disability score, grip strength, and in conduction block. Leger et al. [44] treated 19 patients with MMN with IVIG (500 mg/kg per day daily for 5 days, once a month for 3 months) or placebo, with a crossover for nonresponders at month 4 (for 3 further months). Seven of the nine patients who received IVIG (and only two of the nine with placebo) were responders at month 4. Responders were defined as having 1 or more MRC point in two affected muscles and 1 point less in two activities of daily living (out of a 0–5 self evaluation scale, 0 being normal) compared to baseline. There was no significant difference in overall MRC score, or in motor electrophysiological studies or anti-GM1 titers between the patients with IVIG and placebo. Of previously IVIG-naïve patients, six of nine were responders by the end of the trial, and of patients who had been treated successfully previously with IVIG before entering the trial, eight of nine had responded to IVIG by the end of the trial.

Van den Berg et al. [45] evaluated long-term outcome of the use of IVIG in MMN; they studied seven patients with MMN, all of whom had good response to IVIG, and extended this to one treatment with IVIG per week for 6 and to intermittent as-needed treatments in 1 (who had a longer response period after the initial treatment with IVIG), for 2–4 years. They found that IVIG continued to have benefit in most muscle groups, but in three, there continued to be some degree of decline in a minority of muscle groups. Electrophysiologically, there was improvement in conduction block, but in the course of treatment there were new sites of conduction block identified as well as ongoing axonal degeneration, indicating that while IVIG was beneficial in these patients, the underlying process was not halted. Azulay et al. [46] reported on 18 MMN patients with variable interval treatments of IVIG with a mean follow-up time of 25.3 months, and found the clinical improvement (final strength increase of at least 30%) in 12 of the patients.

Pestronk et al. [38] reported on two patients with MMN who had dramatic improvement in strength after treatment with cyclophosphamide. Feldman et al. [39] reported on nine patients with MMN treated with cyclophosphamide, eight of whom had clinical improvement, as well as decreases in anti-GM1 antibody titers. Brannagan et al. [47] reported on a treatment-refractory MMN patient who responded to high-dose cyclophosphamide (50 mg/kg daily for 4 days), with improvement in strength on a 6-month follow-up, despite being taken off IVIG after her cyclophosphamide treatment. Axelson et al. [48] treated an MMN patient responsive to IVIG but needing frequent infusions, with high-dose cyclophosphamide and autologous blood stem cell transplant, and his clinical status declined markedly after this treatment, though again improved after subsequent IVIG treatment.

Meucci et al. [49] followed up six patients who were responsive to an initial course of IVIG, who were treated with oral cyclophosphamide (1–3 mg/kg per day) with periodic IVIG (0.4 g/kg per day for 2 days) with worsening, and found that at mean follow-up of 47 months, there were significant improvements in Rankin score, and upper and lower limb disability scores. They noted that all patients continued to periodically need IVIG infusions, but that they were able to extend their treatment interval while on cyclophosphamide.

Feldman et al. [39] described four patients with MMN, treated with plasma exchange, with no clinical response. Kaji et al. [50] also described an MMN patient, ultimately responsive to IVIG, who had previously failed to respond to steroids, plasma exchange, or cyclophosphamide. Nemni et al. [51] reported on two MMN patients with improvements in strength with cyclosporine A. Bouche et al. [52] commented on a single MMN patient, unresponsive to IVIG, who stabilized on azathioprine. Krarup *et al.* [53] described a patient with MMN who did not respond to azathioprine (200 mg per day for 8 months). Toscano *et al.* [54] described a patient with MMN on IVIG, who had a reduced frequency of disease exacerbations after azathioprine was started, but it ultimately needed to be discontinued secondary to elevated liver transaminases. Benedetti *et al.* [55] reported on four patients with MMN (classified as two definite, one probable, and one possible) who were on high-dose IVIG and had mycophenolate mofetil 1 g twice a day added to their regimen for an average of 9 months. In two patients, IVIG could be discontinued after 4 months, and in one, the IVIG dose could be reduced to half after 4 months; none of these three patients had a deterioration in the MRC sum score or INCAT disability score. In the last patient, the IVIG could transiently be reduced, but ultimately the patient needed to return to the prior IVIG schedule (though the patient also had azathioprine discontinued after 3 months). Piepers *et al.* [56] subsequently performed a randomized, controlled trial assessing MMN patients already receiving IVIG to see if the addition of mycophenolate mofetil would decrease the IVIG maintenance dose. Twenty-eight patients were in this trial, and only one of the patients in the mycophenolate mofetil group was able to reduce the IVIG dose by 50% at 12 months, which was the primary end point; there were no significant differences between the two groups as a whole in terms of mean IVIG doses or dose reduction.

Pestronk *et al.* [57] treated 14 MMN patients (all with elevations of IgM ganglioside antibodies, 11 with conduction block) with rituximab, and there was a mean improvement in strength of 22% at 2 years. Stieglbauer *et al.* [58] reported on three MMN patients with decreasing responsiveness to IVIG, who were placed on rituximab monotherapy, and had sustained benefit. A more recent open-label trial (Chaudhry *et al.*) [59] of rituximab in six MMN patients, with a primary outcome of difference in IVIG requirement in the 12 months following therapy compared to the 12 months before therapy, did not show a significant change in IVIG requirement, and in addition, showed no significant differences in MRC sum scores, grip strength, and overall disability sum score.

At this point, IVIG is considered the best treatment option for MMN, with cyclophosphamide for patients who are either poor responders, or for whom ongoing very high dose of IVIG is needed to maintain clinical function.

Treatment for diabetic polyneuropathy

What are the data to assess role of tight glucose control in the prevention of diabetic neuropathy? What are the data for the use of alpha-lipoic acid in diabetic polyneuropathy?

Diabetic polyneuropathy usually presents as a length-dependent sensory greater than motor-deficit, often with significant pain. This is the most common type of neuropathy in diabetic patients, though many of these patients are in fact asymptomatic, but with findings detectable on clinical and/or electrophysiological examination (Dyck *et al.*) [60]. Because of the known association of diabetic polyneuropathy with prolonged and severe hyperglycemic exposure (Dyck *et al.*) [61], there has been much attention given to the role tight glycemic control could play in the prevention and/or progression of diabetic polyneuropathy. There has also been much interest in the possible beneficial effects of alpha-lipoic acid in diabetic polyneuropathy.

There are several studies on other agents attempting to modify the development or progression of peripheral neuropathy, including aldose reductase inhibitors and recombinant human nerve growth factor, but these studies have primarily shown conflicting or negative results, and these agents are not being used in the clinical realm for treatment of diabetic polyneuropathy. While these studies deserve attention in their own right, we will not address them further here.

A large trial of 1441 patients with diabetes mellitus was performed, which randomized them to either intensive therapy (three or more insulin injections per day or insulin pump, with four or more blood sugar checks daily) or conventional therapy (one to two daily insulin injections) and followed them long term (mean duration of follow-up time of 6.5 years) for diabetic complications. In intensively treated patients, there was a 64% risk reduction for development of confirmed clinical neuropathy (defined as abnormal history, physical examination, or both, and unequivocal nerve conduction or autonomic nervous system abnormalities) [62]. This is encouraging that the neuropathic abnormalities that occur over time may be modifiable – either preventable or delayed. Albers *et al.* [63] reassessed 1186 of these patients 13–14 years after closeout of the former trial, and repeated clinical evaluation and nerve conduction studies, and found that in the prior intensively treated group, the prevalence of confirmed clinical neuropathy increased from 9 to 25%, and in the prior conventionally treated group, the prevalence of confirmed clinical neuropathy increased from 17 to 35%. The final difference in prevalence remained statistically significant.

Alpha-lipoic acid, an antioxidant, has been extensively studied, with the thought that it may improve underlying nerve function. Ziegler *et al.* [64] performed a randomized, double-blind, placebo-controlled study of type 2 diabetics with symptomatic diabetic polyneuropathy, treating them with either IV alpha-lipoic acid (600 mg IV daily for 3 weeks) followed by oral alpha-lipoic acid (600 mg thrice a day for 6 months), IV alpha-lipoic acid followed by oral placebo, or IV placebo followed by oral placebo, and at 7-month follow-up, there was no significant difference in change in Total Symptom Score or Neuropathy Impairment Score between the groups. Ametov *et al.* [65] performed a double-blind trial of 120 patients with diabetic sensorimotor peripheral neuropathy, and treated them with either alpha-lipoic acid 600 mg IV daily (5 days per week, for a total of 14 treatments) or a placebo. After 14 treatments, there was a significant improvement from baseline in the Total Symptom Score – a combined measure of positive neuropathic sensory symptoms. Ziegler et al. [66] performed a randomized, double-blind trial of 181 diabetics with diabetic polyneuropathy, with four treatment groups, alpha-lipoic acid 600 mg by mouth daily, 1200 mg by mouth daily, 1800 mg by mouth daily, or placebo, for 5 weeks. All the alpha-lipoic acid-treated groups had significant improvement in Total Symptom Score versus placebo, and the highest rate of a ≥50% drop in the Total Symptom Score was in the 600 mg per day group.

At this point in time, the best data would indicate that tight glucose control is most helpful for prevention of the development of diabetic polyneuropathy. There may be benefit in positive neuropathic symptoms from alpha-lipoic acid.

References

1 Dyck, P.J., O'Brien, P.C., Oviatt, K.F. et al. (1982) Prednisone improves chronic inflammatory demyelinating polyradiculoneuropathy more than no treatment. *Annals of Neurology*, **11**, 136–141.

2 Muley, S.A., Kelkar, P. & Parry, G.J. (2008) Treatment of chronic inflammatory demyelinating polyneuropathy with pulsed oral steroids. *Archives of Neurology*, **65**, 1460–1464.

3 Lopate, G., Pestronk, A. & Al-Lozi, M. (2005) Treatment of chronic inflammatory demyelinating polyneuropathy with high-dose intermittent intravenous methylprednisolone. *Archives of Neurology*, **62**(2), 249–254.

4 Attarian, S., Verschueren, A., Franques, J. et al. (2011) Response to treatment in patients with Lewis-Sumner syndrome. *Muscle & Nerve*, **44**(2), 179–184.

5 Dyck, P.J., Litchy, W.J., Kratz, K.M. et al. (1994) A plasma exchange versus immune globulin infusion trial in chronic inflammatory demyelinating polyradiculoneuropathy. *Annals of Neurology*, **36**(6), 838–845.

6 Hughes, R.A.C., Donofrio, P., Bril, V. et al. (2008) Intravenous immune globulin (10% caprylate-chromatography purified) for the treatment of chronic inflammatory demyelinating polyradiculoneuropathy (ICE study): a randomized, placebo-controlled trial. *Lancet Neurology*, **7**, 136–144.

7 Hahn, A.F., Bolton, C.F., Zochodne, D. et al. (1996) Intravenous immunoglobulin treatment in chronic inflammatory demyelinating polyradiculoneuropathy. A double-blind, placebo-controlled, cross-over study. *Brain*, **119**, 1067–1077.

8 Mendell, J.R., Barohn, R.J., Freimer, M.L. et al. (2001) Randomized controlled trial of IVIg in untreated chronic inflammatory demyelinating polyneuropathy. *Neurology*, **56**, 445–449.

9 Cocito, D., Serra, G., Falcone, Y. et al. (2011) The efficacy of subcutaneous immunoglobulin administration in chronic inflammatory demyelinating polyneuropathy responders to intravenous immunoglobulin. *Journal of the Peripheral Nervous System*, **16**(2), 150–152.

10 Dyck, P.J., Daube, J., O'Brien, P. et al. (1986) Plasma exchange in chronic inflammatory demyelinating polyradiculoneuropathy. *New England Journal of Medicine*, **314**, 461–465.

11 Hahn, A.F., Bolton, C.F., Pillay, N. et al. (1996) Plasma-exchange therapy in chronic inflammatory demyelinating polyneuropathy. A double-blind, sham-controlled, cross-over study. *Brain*, **119**, 1055–1066.

12 RMC Trial Group (2009) Randomised controlled trial of methotrexate for chronic inflammatory demyelinating polyradiculoneuropathy (RMC trial): a pilot, multi-centre study. *Lancet Neurology*, **8**, 158–164.

13 Dyck, P.J., O'Brien, P., Swanson, C. et al. (1985) Combined azathioprine and prednisone in chronic inflammatory demyelinating polyneuropathy. *Neurology*, **35**, 1173–1176.

14 Gorson, K.C., Amato, A.A. & Ropper, A.H. (2004) Efficacy of mycophenolate mofetil in patients with chronic immune demyelinating polyneuropathy. *Neurology*, **63**, 715–717.

15 Barnett, M.H., Pollard, J.D., Davies, L. et al. (1998) Cyclosporin A in resistant chronic inflammatory demyelinating polyradiculoneuropathy. *Muscle & Nerve*, **21**, 454–460.

16 Good, J.L., Chehrenama, M., Mayer, R.F. et al. (1998) Pulse cyclophosphamide therapy in chronic inflammatory demyelinating polyneuropathy. *Neurology*, **51**, 1735–1738.

17 Benedetti, L., Briani, C., Franciotta, D. et al. (2011) Rituximab in patients with chronic inflammatory demyelinating polyradiculoneuropathy: a report of 13 cases and review of the literature. *Journal of Neurology, Neurosurgery, and Psychiatry*, **82**(3), 306–308.

18 Chin, R.L., Sherman, W.H., Sander, H.W., Hays, A.P. & Latov, N. (2003) Etanercept (Enbrel) therapy for chronic inflammatory demyelinating polyneuropathy. *Journal of the Neurological Sciences*, **210**(1–2), 19–21.

19 Marsh, E.A., Hirst, C.L., Llewelyn, J.G. et al. (2010) Alemtuzumab in the treatment of IVIG-dependent chronic inflammatory demyelinating polyneuropathy. *Journal of Neurology*, **257**(6), 913–919.

20 The CAMMS223 Trial Investigators. (2008) Alemtuzumab vs. interferon beta-1a in early multiple sclerosis. *New England Journal of Medicine*, **359**, 1786–1801.

21 Swick, H.M. & McQuillen, M.P. (1976) The use of steroids in the treatment of idiopathic polyneuritis. *Neurology*, **26**, 205–212.

22 Hughes, R.A.C., Newsom-Davis, J.M. et al. (1978) Controlled trial of prednisolone in acute polyneuropathy. *Lancet*, **2**, 750–753.

23 Kennard, C., Newland, A.C. & Ridley, A. (1982) Treatment of the Guillain-Barre syndrome by plasma exchange. *Journal of Neurology, Neurosurgery, and Psychiatry*, **45**, 847–850.

24 Greenwood, R.J., Newsom-Davis, J., Hughes, R.A. et al. (1984) Controlled trial of plasma exchange in acute inflammatory polyradiculoneuropathy. *Lancet*, **1**(8382), 877–879.

25 Mendell, J.R., Kissel, J.T., Kennedy, M.S. et al. (1985) Plasma exchange and prednisone in Guillain-Barré syndrome: a controlled randomized trial. *Neurology*, **35**(11), 1551–1555.

26 Osterman, P.O., Fagius, J., Lundemo, G. *et al.* (1984) Beneficial effects of plasma exchange in acute inflammatory polyradiculoneuropathy. *Lancet*, **2**(**8415**), 1296–1299.

27 Farkkila, M., Kinnunen, E., Haapanen, E. *et al.* (1987) Guillain Barré syndrome: quantitative measurement of plasma exchange therapy. *Neurology*, **37**(**5**), 837–840.

28 The Guillain-Barré Syndrome Study Group. (1985) Plasmapheresis and acute Guillain-Barré syndrome. *Neurology*, **35**, 1096–1104.

29 Kleyweg, R.P., van der Meche, F.G.A. & Meultree, J. (1988) Treatment of Guillain-Barré syndrome with high-dose gammaglobulin. *Neurology*, **38**, 1639–1641.

30 van der Meche, F.G. & Schmitz, P.I. (1992) A randomized trial comparing intravenous immune globulin and plasma exchange in Guillain-Barré syndrome. Dutch Guillain-Barré Study. Group. *New England Journal of Medicine*, **326**(**17**), 1123–1129.

31 Bril, V., Ilse, W.K., Pearce, R. *et al.* (1996) Pilot trial of immunoglobulin versus plasma exchange in patients with Guillain-Barré syndrome. *Neurology*, **46**, 100–103.

32 van Koningsveld, R., Schmitz, P.I.M., Meche, F.G. *et al.* (2004) Effect of methylprednisolone when added to standard treatment with intravenous immunoglobulin for Guillain-Barré syndrome: randomized trial. *Lancet*, **363**(**9404**), 192–196.

33 Plasma Exchange/Sandoglobulin Guillain-Barré Syndrome Trial Group. (1997) Randomised trial of plasma exchange, intravenous immunoglobulin, and combined treatments in Guillain-Barré syndrome. *Lancet*, **349**, 225–230.

34 Farcas, P., Avnun, L., Frisher, S. *et al.* (1997) Efficacy of repeated intravenous immunoglobulin in severe unresponsive Guillain-Barré syndrome. *Lancet*, **350**(**9093**), 1747.

35 Kuitwaard, K., de Gelder, J., Tio-Gillen, A.P. *et al.* (2009) Pharmacokinetics of intravenous immunoglobulin and outcome in Guillain-Barré syndrome. *Annals of Neurology*, **66**(**5**), 597–603.

36 Hughes, R.A., Wijdicks, E.F., Barohn, R. *et al.* (2003) Practice parameter: immunotherapy for Guillain Barré syndrome: report of the Quality Standards Subcommittee of the American Academy of Neurology. *Neurology*, **61**(**6**), 736–740.

37 Taylor, B.V., Wright, R.A., Harper, C.M. *et al.* (2000) Natural history of 46 patients with multifocal motor neuropathy with conduction block. *Muscle & Nerve*, **23**(**6**), 900–908.

38 Pestronk, A., Cornblath, D.R., Ilyas, A.A. *et al.* (1988) A treatable multifocal motor neuropathy with antibodies to GM1 ganglioside. *Annals of Neurology*, **24**(**1**), 73–78.

39 Feldman, E.L., Bromberg, M.B., Albers, J.W. *et al.* (1991) Immunosuppressive treatment in multifocal motor neuropathy. *Annals of Neurology*, **30**(**3**), 397–401.

40 Donaghy, M., Mills, K.R., Boniface, S.J. *et al.* (1994) Pure motor demyelinating neuropathy: deterioration after steroid treatment and improvement with intravenous immunoglobulin. *Journal of Neurology, Neurosurgery, and Psychiatry*, **57**(**7**), 778–783.

41 Van den Berg, L.H., Lokhorst, H. & Wokke, J.H. (1998) Pulsed high-dose dexamethasone is not effective in patients with multifocal motor neuropathy. *Neurology*, **50**(**1**), 314–315.

42 Azulay, J.P., Blin, O., Pouget, J. *et al.* (1994) Intravenous immunoglobulin treatment in patients with motor neuron syndromes associated with anti-GM1 antibodies: a double-blind, placebo-controlled study. *Neurology*, **44**(**3 Pt 1**), 429–432.

43 Federico, P., Zochodne, D.W., Hahn, A.F. *et al.* (2000) Multifocal motor neuropathy improved by IVIg: randomized, double-blind, placebo-controlled study. *Neurology*, **55**(**9**), 1256–1262.

44 Leger, J.M., Chassande, B., Musset, L. *et al.* (2001) Intravenous immunoglobulin therapy in multifocal motor neuropathy: a double-blind, placebo-controlled study. *Brain*, **124**(**Pt 1**), 145–153.

45 Van den Berg, L.H., Franssen, H. & Wokke, J.H. (1998) The long-term effect of intravenous immunoglobulin treatment in multifocal motor neuropathy. *Brain*, **121**(**Pt 3**), 421–428.

46 Azulay, J.P., Rihet, P., Pouget, J. *et al.* (1997) Long term follow up of multifocal motor neuropathy with conduction block under treatment. *Journal of Neurology, Neurosurgery, and Psychiatry*, **62**(**4**), 391–394.

47 Brannagan, T.H. 3rd, Alaedini, A. & Gladstone, D.E. (2006) High-dose cyclophosphamide without stem cell rescue for refractory multifocal motor neuropathy. *Muscle & Nerve*, **34**(**2**), 246–250.

48 Axelson, H.W., Oberg, G. & Askmark, H. (2008) No benefit of treatment with cyclophosphamide and autologous blood stem cell transplantation in multifocal motor neuropathy. *Acta Neurologica Scandinavica*, **117**(**6**), 432–434.

49 Meucci, N., Cappellari, A., Barbieri, S. *et al.* (1997) Long term effect of intravenous immunoglobulins and oral cyclophosphamide in multifocal motor neuropathy. *Journal of Neurology, Neurosurgery, and Psychiatry*, **63**(**6**), 765–769.

50 Kaji, R., Shibasaki, H. & Kimura, J. (1992) Multifocal demyelinating motor neuropathy: cranial nerve involvement and immunoglobulin therapy. *Neurology*, **42**(**3 Pt 1**), 506–509.

51 Nemni, R., Santuccio, G., Calabrese, E. *et al.* (2003) Efficacy of cyclosporine treatment in multifocal motor neuropathy. *Journal of Neurology*, **250**(**9**), 1118–1120.

52 Bouche, P. & Moulonguet, A. (1995) Ben Younes Chennoufi A. Multifocal motor neuropathy with conduction block: a study of 24 patients. *Journal of Neurology, Neurosurgery, and Psychiatry*, **59**, 38–44.

53 Krarup, C., Stewart, J.D., Sumner, A.J. *et al.* (1990) A syndrome of asymmetric limb weakness with motor conduction block. *Neurology*, **40**(**10**), 118–127.

54 Toscano, A., Rodolico, C., Benvenga, S. *et al.* (2002) Multifocal motor neuropathy and asymptomatic Hashimoto's thyroiditis: first report of an association. *Neuromuscular Disorders*, **12**(**6**), 566–568.

55 Benedetti, L., Grandis, M., Nobbio, L. *et al.* (2004) Mycophenolate mofetil in dysimmune neuropathies: a preliminary study. *Muscle & Nerve*, **29**, 748–749.

56 Piepers, S., Van den Berg-Vos, R., Van der Pol, W.-L. *et al.* (2007) Mycophenolate mofetil as adjunctive therapy for MMN patients: a randomized, controlled trial. *Brain*, **130**, 2004–2010.

57 Pestronk, A., Florence, J., Miller, T. *et al.* (2003) Treatment of IgM antibody associated polyneuropathies using rituximab. *Journal of Neurology, Neurosurgery, and Psychiatry*, **74**(4), 485–489.

58 Stieglbauer, K., Topakian, R., Hinterberger, G. & Aichner, F.T. (2009) Beneficial effect of rituximab monotherapy in multifocal motor neuropathy. *Neuromuscular Disorders*, **19**(7), 473–475.

59 Chaudhry, V. & Cornblath, D.R. (2010) An open-label trial of rituximab (Rituxan[REGISTERED] in multifocal motor neuropathy. *Journal of the Peripheral Nervous System*, **15**(3), 196–201.

60 Dyck, P.J., Kratz, K.M., Karnes, J.L. *et al.* (1993) The prevalence by staged severity of various types of diabetic neuropathy, retinopathy, and nephropathy in a population-based cohort: the Rochester Diabetic Neuropathy Study. *Neurology*, **43**(4), 817–824.

61 Dyck, P.J., Davies, J.L., Wilson, D.M. *et al.* (1999) Risk factors for severity of diabetic polyneuropathy: intensive longitudinal assessment of the Rochester Diabetic Neuropathy Study cohort. *Diabetes Care*, **22**(9), 1479–1486.

62 Anonymous. (1995) The effect of intensive diabetes therapy on the development and progression of neuropathy. The Diabetes Control and Complications Trial Research Group. *Annals of Internal Medicine*, **122**(8), 561–568.

63 Albers, J.W., Herman, W.H., Pop-Busui, R. *et al.* (2010) Effect of prior intensive insulin treatment during the Diabetes Control and Complications Trial (DCCT) on peripheral neuropathy in type 1 diabetes during the Epidemiology of Diabetes Interventions and Complications (EDIC) Study Group. *Diabetes Care*, **33**(5), 1090–1096.

64 Ziegler, D., Hanefeld, M., Ruhnau, K.-J. *et al.* (1999) Treatment of symptomatic diabetic polyneuropathy with the antioxidant alpha-lipoic acid: a 7-month multicenter randomized controlled trial (ALADIN III study). *Diabetes Care*, **22**(8), 1296–1301.

65 Ametov, A.S., Barinov, A., Dyck, P.J. *et al.* (2003) The sensory symptoms of diabetic polyneuropathy are improved with alpha-lipoic acid: the SYDNEY trial. *Diabetes Care*, **26**(3), 770–776.

66 Ziegler, D., Ametov, A., Barinov, A. *et al.* (2006) Oral treatment with alpha-lipoic acid improves symptomatic diabetic polyneuropathy: the SYDNEY 2 trial. *Diabetes Care*, **29**(11), 2365–2370.

23

CHAPTER 23

Critical illness neuromyopathy

Brent P. Goodman[1] and Andrea J. Boon[2]

[1]*Department of Neurology, Mayo Clinic, 13400 East Shea Boulevard, Scottsdale, AZ, 85259, USA*
[2]*Department of Physical Medicine, Mayo Clinic, 200 1st Street SW, Rochester MN, 55905, USA*

Background

Improvements in the survival of critically ill patients over the past few decades have resulted in an increasing number of patients with neuromuscular complications of critical illness. Muscle weakness and atrophy in a patient with sepsis was described by Osler toward the end of the nineteenth century [1], and a disseminated neuropathy following coma was later ascribed to metabolic and ischemic peripheral nervous system lesions [2]. However, it was not until the seminal work of Bolton and colleagues in 1984, that the clinical, electrodiagnostic, and pathological features of neuromuscular weakness associated with critical illness were described, and the term critical illness polyneuropathy (CIP) was introduced [3]. Pathological and electrodiagnostic studies in patients with CIP suggested a degenerative, axonal process without features of inflammation or primary demyelination [4–6].

Since these initial studies describing CIP, it has become increasingly apparent that muscle involvement, termed critical illness myopathy (CIM), is a frequent complication of critical illness. There is evidence to suggest that CIM is a more frequent cause of weakness in critically ill patients than CIP. In one prospective study, 23 of 24 quadriplegic, critically ill patients showed myopathic features on muscle biopsy, with abnormalities on sural nerve biopsy in only 8 of them [7]. In another prospective study of 22 patients with nerve conduction studies (NCS) suggesting CIP, all patients who underwent muscle biopsy had myopathic abnormalities indicating CIM [8]. Given that neuropathy and myopathy may often occur together in the same patient, the term critical illness neuromyopathy (CINM) may be the most appropriate clinical designation of acquired neuromuscular weakness in the critically ill patient [9].

Incidence and prevalence rates of CINM are not precisely known. A number of factors influence the estimated frequency of CINM including the nature of the condition responsible for critical illness, number and type of risk factors to which critically ill patients are exposed, and the type and timing of the diagnostic evaluation performed [10]. Recent estimates suggest that 70–80% of critically ill patients develop CIP and/or CIM [11–13], and may reach 100% in patients with multiorgan failure and sepsis [13].

A number of factors have been recognized as independent risk factors for the development of CIP or CIM, including illness severity [14,15], duration of multiorgan dysfunction [16,17], duration of vasopressor and catecholamine support [18], duration of ICU stay [18,19], hyperglycemia [15,18,20], female sex [8], renal failure [21], hypersomolality [21], parenteral nutrition [21], low serum albumin [19], and neurological failure [22]. Neuromuscular blocking agents and corticosteroids have been identified in some studies as increasing risk, but not in others [23]. Prolonged immobility may also have significant deleterious effects on skeletal muscle, resulting in muscle weakness [24]. Length of mechanical ventilation may be used as a surrogate marker for immobilization, and is associated with limb weakness severity [8], or electrodiagnostic evidence of CIP [18,19].

Clinical features and diagnosis

Critical illness polyneuropathy is characterized as an axonal sensorimotor peripheral neuropathy with the potential to affect limb and respiratory muscles. Muscle weakness is characteristically symmetrical, lower limb-predominant, and often affects distal more than proximal muscles [24]. Typically, the neuromuscular complications of critical illness are preceded by an encephalopathy [25], which may complicate the clinical recognition of neuromuscular impairment. If possible to assess, sensory loss may be evident in the distal extremities. Failure to wean from mechanical ventilation is common and may be the predominant feature that leads to the clinical recognition of CINM.

CIM presents similarly to CIP, and particularly when the sensory examination is unreliable due to altered mental status, these conditions cannot be distinguished clinically.

Evidence-Based Neurology: Management of Neurological Disorders, Second Edition. Edited by Bart M. Demaerschalk and Dean M. Wingerchuk.
© 2015 John Wiley & Sons, Ltd. Published 2015 by John Wiley & Sons, Ltd.

As previously discussed, electrodiagnostic and pathological studies may confirm the presence of both polyneuropathy and myopathy in most critically ill patients with neuromuscular weakness. Patients with CIM characteristically develop a symmetrical quadriparesis, often with reduced deep tendon reflexes, normal sensation, and failure to wean from mechanical ventilation.

Electrodiagnostic testing in CIP shows a reduction in motor compound muscle action amplitudes (CMAPs), with preservation of distal latencies and conduction velocities, and fibrillation potentials on needle electromyography (EMG), consistent with axonal degeneration. Nerve conduction studies in CIM show low-amplitude, prolonged CMAP durations, and fibrillation potentials with small motor unit potentials on needle EMG [26]. Nerve or muscle biopsy is not necessary in most cases of suspected CIP or CIM. However, early histopathological studies demonstrated axonal degeneration with a decreased density of myelinated fibers in patients with CIP [4]. Muscle biopsy findings are variable in critical illness myopathy, with atrophy of type 1 or type 2 fibers, or both, and loss of myosin thick filaments reported [9]. Rat models of denervation with concomitant steroid administration have demonstrated electrical inexcitability, potentially resulting from NaV1·4 sodium channel impairment [27,28]. It is thought that this inexcitability is responsible for the electrodiagnostic findings in CINM, and is the primary cause of weakness in these patients [26].

Framing of clinical question and search strategy

The following evidence-based discussion focuses on the reduction of CINM incidence and severity, including the following three topics: (1) Reduction of CINM incidence utilizing intensive insulin therapy; (2) Treatment of CINM using early physical and occupational therapy and sedation interruption; and (3) Reduction of CINM incidence using electrical muscle stimulation. The topics are presented similarly, preceded by a clinical patient scenario that provides the foundation for a clinical question, and for each topic a subsequent critical appraisal of the literature. The general search strategy involved the use of PubMed, MEDLINE, the Cochrane Library, and the Cochrane Database of Reviews of Effectiveness utilizing the search terms "critical illness neuropathy," "critical illness polyneuropathy," "critical illness myopathy," "critical illness neuromyopathy," and "critical illness polyneuromyopathy."

Clinical scenario

A 62-year-old man with a history of hypertension and hyperlipidemia is admitted for worsening cough, dyspnea, and fever, and despite prompt administration of antibiotics, develops respiratory failure and hypotension, necessitating intubation and vasopressor support. His medical condition deteriorates further as he develops progressive renal and hepatic failure, as well as a worsening encephalopathy. As his medical condition stabilizes, the patient is noted to have little spontaneous movement of his extremities, and on formal manual muscle strength testing both proximal and distal weakness are evident. Attempts to wean the patient from mechanical ventilation have not been successful despite improving pulmonary status. The primary medical team caring for the patient is concerned about the development of neuromuscular weakness in this patient, and asks whether anything can be done to reduce the patient's risk for developing a critical illness neuromyopathy.

Critical review of the evidence for each question

Intensive insulin therapy in CINM

Does intensive insulin therapy reduce the incidence or severity of CINM in critically ill patients?

As has previously been discussed, hyperglycemia is an independent risk factor for the development of CINM [15,18,20]. It has been suggested that hyperglycemia may cause peripheral nervous system damage via increased generation of reactive oxygen species or a deficient scavenging system [29]. Avoidance of hyperglycemia may diminish nitric oxide release, thereby limiting endothelial dysfunction and reducing the extent of end-organ damage [30]. Insulin may confer other endothelial protective benefits independent of its glycemic effects, by reducing inflammation and improving dyslipidemia [29,30].

Clinical bottom line

- There is no definitive evidence that intensive insulin therapy reduces the overall incidence of CINM.
- There is evidence that intensive insulin therapy reduces the electrodiagnostic severity of CINM, but it is not clear that this results in clinically meaningful improvement in CINM incidence or severity.

Evidence

In the studies reviewed, intensive insulin therapy was compared with conventional insulin therapy, comparing the incidence of CINM between groups.

Study design

One study was a prospective, randomized, controlled one whose primary outcome measure was death, but included CIP as a secondary outcome measure [31]. A second study involved a prospective, subgroup analysis of CIP incidence and duration of mechanical ventilation dependency in a large group of critically ill patients [18]. A third study from the same group involved a subgroup analysis of a prospectively planned, randomized control trial, examining the effect of intensive insulin therapy on CINM incidence at 7 days, in a large group of critically ill patients [20]. The final study, a retrospective analysis of a large group of critically ill patients, examined the incidence of CINM as established by electrodiagnostic testing [32].

Summary of results

In a large, randomized trial of 1548 patients, there was a 34% reduction in overall mortality in those treated with intensive insulin therapy compared with conventional insulin therapy, and a 44% reduction in CIP [31]. The diagnosis of CIP was established in this trial by abnormal findings on needle EMG. The other two prospective studies from the same authors reported a significant reduction in CINM incidence from near 50% in both the conventional insulin groups to 25% [18] and 38.9% [20]. A retrospective study from the same authors reported a statistically significant reduction in CINM from 74.4% to 48.7% [32]. However, in this retrospective study, the number of electrodiagnostic studies ordered was similar between the two groups, suggesting that despite the significant differences in electrodiagnostic findings between them, the clinical manifestations (that would prompt electrodiagnostic studies) were no different between groups (Table 23.1).

Furthermore, as indicated, these four studies utilized electrodiagnostic criteria (primarily the presence of abnormal spontaneous activity on needle EMG) to establish a diagnosis of CINM. Electrodiagnostic testing alone, particularly using presence or absence of abnormal spontaneous activity on needle EMG, is not adequate to establish a diagnosis of CINM. Despite the proposal of diagnostic criteria for CIP and CIM [24], these criteria have not been widely accepted or implemented in clinical trials, and certainly were not utilized in the intensive insulin therapy trials reviewed above.

Physical and occupational therapy in critical illness neuromyopathy

Does early physical and occupational therapy reduce the incidence or severity of CINM in critically ill patients?

Mechanical ventilation and the use of sedating medications in critically ill patients often result in prolonged episodes of immobility and altered levels of awareness. Immobility, even in the absence of systemic inflammation, may contribute significantly to muscle wasting and weakness [33]. Muscle atrophy may begin within hours of bed rest, and after 10 days of bed rest, even healthy individuals may experience a large loss of muscle mass and strength [34]. Protocols to minimize sedation, utilizing daily interruptions in sedation, and early mobilization of mechanically ventilated patients have been shown to improve outcomes [35–37].

Clinical bottom line

• Early physical and occupational therapy in conjunction with interruption of sedation may improve functional outcome in critically ill patients.

• It is not clear whether this improvement results from a decrease in the incidence or severity of CINM as the presence or severity of CINM was not established in this or other studies evaluating this intervention.

Evidence

In a large, randomized control trial of 104 critically ill, mechanically ventilated patients, the primary outcome measure was independent status at hospital discharge, including ability to perform activities of daily living and to walk independently [38]. Patients were randomized to either physical and occupational therapy performed during sedation interruption or usual care. Secondary end points included delirium duration and number of ventilator-free days during the first 28 days of their hospital stay.

Summary of results

A return to a functional, independent status at hospital discharge was significantly more likely (59%) in the group receiving early physical and occupational therapy when compared to the control group (35%). Patients in the intervention group also had a significantly shorter duration of delirium (2 days versus 4 days) and experienced more ventilator-free days (23.5 days compared to 21.1 days) relative to the control group. However, there was no reported clinical or electrodiagnostic assessment of the presence or severity of CINM in these patients. Furthermore, 103 patients with a "rapidly developing neurological/neuromuscular disease" were excluded from

Table 23.1 Overview of intensive insulin therapy studies on CINM

Study	Study Type	Dx CINM	Effect of strict glucose control (SGC)		
			SGC group	Control group	p-value
Hermans *et al.* [32]	RCS	PSA	48.7% CINM	74.4% CINM	<0.00
Van den Berghe *et al.* [18]	RCT	PSA	25% CINM	49% CINM	<0.00
Hermans *et al.* [20]	RCT	PSA	38.9% CINM	50.5% CINM	<0.02
Van den Berghe *et al.* [31]	RCT	EMG	20.5% CINM	26.3% CINM	<0.007

CINM, critical illness neuromyopathy; PSA, pathological spontaneous activity; RCT, randomized control trial; RCS, retrospective cohort study.

the study. It is not clear whether this included patients with CINM. In addition, no differences in length of ICU or hospital stay were noted between groups.

Electrical muscle stimulation in CINM

Does electrical muscle stimulation reduce the incidence or severity of critical illness neuromyopathy in critically ill patients?

Electrical muscle stimulation (EMS) has been utilized in patients with congestive heart failure and chronic obstructive pulmonary disease as an alternative to exercise, and has been shown in a systematic review to improve muscle strength and exercise capacity [39]. It has been hypothesized that EMS may result in a beneficial systemic effect on peripheral microcirculation [40]. This technique involves the application of electrodes over selected muscles, with delivery of sufficient electrical impulses to result in a visible muscle contraction. A major advantage of using EMS in this patient cohort is that it does not require patient cooperation, and can therefore be performed in an encephalopathic patient.

Clinical bottom line

• There is evidence to suggest that daily EMS sessions reduce the incidence of CINM.

Evidence

There has been one randomized trial evaluating EMS in critically ill patients [41]. Patients were randomly assigned to receive daily EMS to the lower limbs or standard care while in the ICU, with the primary outcome measure involving Medical Research Council (MRC) score between groups. Secondary end points included duration of weaning from mechanical ventilation and length of ICU stay.

Summary of results

A total of 52 critically ill patients were randomized to standard care or EMS. The MRC score was significantly higher in the EMS group compared to the control group, and the weaning period was significantly shorter in the EMS group than the control group. ICU stay was shorter in the EMS group than the control group, but this difference was not statistically significant. Electrodiagnostic testing was not performed in these patients. Patients in this study were considered to have CINM if they had an MRC score of less than 48, a score used in other studies to identify "ICU-acquired paresis" [20,42]. Significantly fewer patients were diagnosed with CINM in the EMS group compared to the control group.

Conclusions

CINM is a frequent and serious complication of critically ill patients that prolongs mechanical ventilation time, lengthens ICU and hospital duration times, and may result in long-term, residual weakness that impacts quality of life. Despite the identification of multiple risk factors, the pathogenesis of this disorder remains incompletely understood. Attempts to definitively identify critical risk factors and to study the impact of various therapeutic interventions have been hampered by a lack of consistently applied diagnostic criteria. Future clinical trials, whether they involve risk factor modification, pharmacologic intervention, or rehabilitative approaches, should ideally include clinical and electrodiagnostic assessment.

References

1 Osler, W. (1892) *The Principles and Practice of Medicine*, 1st edn. D. Appleton, New York.

2 Mertens, H.G. (1961) Disseminated neuropathy following coma. On the differentiation of so-called toxic neuropathy. *Nervenarzt*, **32**, 71–79.

3 Bolton, C.F., Gilber, J.J., Hahn, A.F. & Sibbald, W. (1984) Polyneuropathy in critically ill patients. *Journal of Neurology, Neurosurgery, and Psychiatry*, **47**, 1223–1231.

4 Bolton, C.F. *et al.* (1986) Critically ill polyneuropathy: electrophysiological studies and differentiation from Guillain-Barre syndrome. *Journal of Neurology, Neurosurgery, and Psychiatry*, **49**, 563–573.

5 Bolton, C.F. (1996) Sepsis and the systemic inflammatory response syndrome: neuromuscular manifestations. *Critical Care Medicine*, **24**, 1408–1416.

6 Bolton, C.F. (2005) Neuromuscular manifestations of critical illness. *Muscle and Nerve*, **32**, 140–163.

7 Latronico, N., Fenzi, F., Recupero, D. *et al.* (1996) Critical illness myopathy and neuropathy. *Lancet*, **347**(**9015**), 1579–1582.

8 De Jonghe, B., Sharshar, T., Lefaucheur, J.P. *et al.* (2002) Paresis acquired in the intensive care unit:a prospective multicenter study. *JAMA*, **288**(**22**), 2859–2867.

9 Goodman, B.P. & Boon, A.J. (2008) Critical illness neuromyopathy. *Physical Medicine and Rehabilitation Clinics of North America*, **19**(**1**), 98–110.

10 Zinc, W., Kollmar, R. & Schwab, S. (2009) Critical illness polyneuropathy and myopathy in the intensive care unit. *Nature Reviews Neurology*, **5**, 372–379.

11 Witt, N. *et al.* (1991) Peripheral nerve function in sepsis and multiple organ failure. *Chest*, **99**, 176–184.

12 Hund, E. (2001) Neurological complications of sepsis:critical illness polyneuropathy and myopathy. *Journal of Neurology*, **248**, 929–934.

13 Tennila, A. *et al.* (2000) Early signs of critical illness polyneuropathy in ICU patients with systemic inflammatory response syndrome or sepsis. *Intensive Care Medicine*, **26**(**9**), 1360–1363.

14 de Letter, M.A., Schmitz, P.I., Visser, L.H. *et al.* (2001) Risk factors for the development of polyneuropathy and myopathy in critically ill patients. *Critical Care Medicine*, **29**, 2281–2286.

15 Nanas, S., Kritikos, K., Angelopoulos, E. *et al.* (2008) Predisposing factors for critical illness polyneuromyopathy

in a multidisciplinary intensive care unit. *Acta Neurologica Scandinavica*, **118**, 175–181.

16 Bednarik, J., Vondracek, P., Dusek, L. *et al.* (2005) Risk factors for critical illness polyneuromyopathy. *Journal of Neurology*, **252**, 343–351.

17 De Jonghe, B., Sharshar, T., Lefaucheur, J.P. *et al.* & for the Groupe de Reflexion et d'Etude des Neuromyopathies en Reanimation (2002) Respiratory weakness is associated with limb weakness and delayed weaning in critical illness. *JAMA*, **288**, 2859–2867.

18 Van den Berghe, G., Schoonheydt, K., Becx, P. *et al.* (2005) Insulin therapy protects the central and peripheral nervous system of intensive care patients. *Neurology*, **64**, 1348–1353.

19 Witt, N.J., Zochodne, D.W., Bolton, C.F. *et al.* (1991) Peripheral nerve function in sepsis and multiple organ failure. *Chest*, **99**, 176–184.

20 Hermans, G., Wilmer, A., Meersseman, W. *et al.* (2007) Impact of intensive insulin therapy on neuromuscular complications and ventilator dependency in the medical intensive care unit. *American Journal of Respiratory and Critical Care Medicine*, **175**, 480–489.

21 Garnacho-Montero, J., Madrazo-Osuna, J., Garcia-Garmendia, J.L. *et al.* (2001) Critical illness polyneuropathy: risk factors and clinical consequences. A cohort study in septic patients. *Intensive Care Medicine*, **27**, 1288–1296.

22 Latronico, N., Shehu, I. & Seghelini, E. (2005) Neuromuscular sequelae of critical illness. *Current Opinion in Critical Care*, **11**, 126–132.

23 Hermans, G., De Jonghe, B., Bruyninckx, F. & Ven den Berhe, G. (2009) Interventions for preventing critical illness polyneuropathy critical illness myopathy. *Cochrane Database of Systematic Reviews*, **1**, CD006832.

24 Latronico, N. & Bolton, C.F. (2011) Critical illness polyneuropathy and myopathy: a major cause of muscle weakness and paralysis. *Lancet Neurology*, **10**, 931–941.

25 Bolton, C.F., Young, B.G. & Zochodne, D.W. (1993) The neurological complications of sepsis. *Annals of Neurology*, **33**, 94–100.

26 Goodman, B.P., Harper, C.M. & Boon, A.J. (2009) Prolonged compound muscle action potential duration in critical illness myopathy. *Muscle and Nerve*, **40**, 1040–1042.

27 Rich, M.M. & Pinter, M.J. (2003) Crucial role of sodium channel fast inactivation in muscle fiber inexcitability in a rat model of critical illness myopathy. *Journal of Physiology*, **547**, 555–566.

28 Rich, M.M., Pinter, M.J., Kraner, S.D. & Barchi, R.L. (1998) Loss of electrical excitability in an animal model of acute quadriplegic myopathy. *Annals of Neurology*, **43**, 171–179.

29 Van den Berghe, G. (2004) How does blood glucose control with insulin save lives in intensive care? *Journal of Clinical Investigation*, **114**, 1187–1195.

30 Langouche, L., Vanhorebeck, I., Vlasselaers, D. *et al.* (2005) Intensive insulin therapy protects the endothelium of critically ill patients. *Journal of Clinical Investigation*, **115**, 2277–2286.

31 Van den Berghe, G., Wouter, P., Weekers, F. *et al.* (2001) Intensive insulin therapy in critically ill patients. *NEJM*, **345(19)**, 1359–1367.

32 Hermans, G., Schrooten, M., Van Damme, P. *et al.* (2009) Benefits of intensive insulin therapy on neuromuscular complications in routine daily clinical practice: a retrospective study. *Critical Care*, **13(1)**, 1–12.

33 Ochala, J., Ahlbeck, K., Radell, P.J. *et al.* (2011) Factors underlying the early limb muscle weakness in acute quadriplegic myopathy using an experimental ICU porcine model. *PLoS One*, **6**, e20876.

34 Kortebein, P., Ferrando, A., Lombeida, J. *et al.* (2007) Effect of 10 days of bed rest on skeletal muscle in healthy older adults. *JAMA*, **297**, 1772–1774.

35 Schweickert, W.D. & Kress, J.P. (2008) Strategies to optimize analgesia and sedation. *Critical Care*, **12**, S6.

36 Bailey, P., Thomsen, G.E., Spuhler, V.J. *et al.* (2008) Early activity is feasible and safe in respiratory failure patients. *Critical Care Medicine*, **35**, 139–145.

37 Thomsen, G.E., Snow, G.L., Rodriguez, L. *et al.* (2008) Patiens with respiratory failure increase ambulation after transfer to an intensive care unit where early activity is a priority. *Critical Care Medicine*, **36**, 1119–1124.

38 Schweickert, W.D., Pohlman, M.C., Pohlman, A.S. *et al.* (2009) Early physical and occupational therapy in mechanically ventilated, critically ill patients: a randomised controlled trial. *Lancet*, **373**, 1874–1882.

39 Sillen, M.J., Janssen, P.P., Akkermans, M.A. *et al.* (2009) Effects of neuromuscular electrical stimulation of muscles of ambulation in patients with chronic heart failure or COPD. A systematic review of the English-language literature. *Chest*, **136**, 44–61.

40 Gerovasili, V., Tripokaki, E., Karatzanos, E. *et al.* (2009) Short term systemic effect of electrical muscle stimulation in critically ill patients. *Chest*, **136**, 249–1256.

41 Routsi, C., Gerovasili, V., Vasileiadis, I. *et al.* (2010) Electrical muscle stimulation prevents critical illness polyneuromyopathy: a randomized parallel intervention trial. *Critical Care*, **14**, R74.

42 De Jonghe, B., Sharshar, T., Lefaucheur, J.P. *et al.* (2004) Does ICU-acquired paresis lengthen weaning from mechanical ventilation? *Intensive Care Medicine*, **30**, 1117–1121.

24

CHAPTER 24

Muscle disorders

Amelia K. Adcock[1], Cumara B. O'Carroll[2], and Bart M. Demaerschalk[3]

[1] *West Virginia University, Morgantown, West Virginia, USA*
[2] *Mayo Clinic College of Medicine, Phoenix, AZ, USA*
[3] *Department of Neurology, Mayo Clinic, Phoenix, AZ, USA*

Introduction

This chapter discusses updated management for the following muscular disorders: Duchenne muscular dystrophy (DMD), Limb-girdle muscular dystrophies (LGMDs), Myasthenia gravis, Polymyositis, and facioscapulohumeral muscular dystrophy (FSHD).

Critical review of the evidence for each disorder

Duchenne muscular dystrophy

The parents of a 6-year-old boy with DMD inquire if there is anything to halt his deterioration or improve muscle strength. Do they have any harmful effects? At what age should treatment be started?

Background

DMD is the most common inherited muscle disorder with a prevalence of 2 per 10,000 males [1]. Affected boys develop neck and hip flexor weakness in early childhood ultimately becoming nonambulatory between ages 7 and 12 [2]. Death typically occurs in the 20s, with some patients now surviving until age 25 mainly due to the increased use of ventilatory support [3,4]. The only proven, yet poorly understood, effective pharmacological therapy in DMD patients is steroids. Variability of response, loss of ambulation, and severity of side effects are well-known entities. Only recently has the administration of corticosteroids been subjected to full review.

Clinical scenario

Wheelchair dependence increases the likelihood of complications such as scoliosis and ventilatory impairment. Therefore, both pharmacological and non-pharmacological therapies seek to prolong ambulation and delay these expected complications. Physiotherapy techniques aim to prevent the development of fixed deformities such as limb contractures. For example, prevention or improvement of Achilles tendon contractures is an important factor in allowing walking stability to be maintained. If tendon contractures become excessively tight, then surgical release may be recommended [5].

Evidence

Since the early 1970s, corticosteroid treatment has been the main drug modality employed in efforts to alter the relentless progression of disability and death in DMD. The precise mechanism of how steroids accomplish this is unclear, although it appears unlikely to be on account of their anti-inflammatory action [6]. Notwithstanding the number of studies performed, evidence from just six randomized controlled studies was judged eligible for inclusion in the 2009 Cochrane Systematic Review [7]. Prolongation of ambulation was the primary outcome measure; however, this was an outcome measure in only one study, which furthermore did not show significant benefit of steroid use [8]. Secondary outcome measures of muscle strength and functional tests were available and therefore assessed. Five randomized controlled trials demonstrated improvement in muscle strength and function, but for a relatively short period of 6 months [9–13] with the sixth study showing improvement for up to 2 years (*8 Angelini*).

The studies reported data on a total of 249 patients treated with corticosteroids and compared with a total of 88 placebo patients. Most patients received prednisone ($n = 151$) with much smaller numbers treated with prednisolone ($n = 10$) and deflazacort ($n = 17$). The five 6-month studies used prednisone or prednisolone given daily; deflazacort was used in an alternate-day regimen at 2 mg/kg for a longer interval of 2 years [*8 Angelini*].

Prolongation of ambulation was reported by Angelini *et al.*, but Manzur *et al.* conclude that this result was not supported by the statistical methods used. Secondary

Evidence-Based Neurology: Management of Neurological Disorders, Second Edition. Edited by Bart M. Demaerschalk and Dean M. Wingerchuk.
© 2015 John Wiley & Sons, Ltd. Published 2015 by John Wiley & Sons, Ltd.

outcome measures of muscle strength assessments and tests of functional ability such as Gowers' sign, timed walking tests, and forced vital capacity were individually assessed from pooled data and all found to be better in the treated groups compared with placebo (*13 Manzur*).

The Practice parameter produced by the American Academy of Neurology [14] also reviews relevant evidence for the treatment of DMD with corticosteroids. Seven class 1 trials were included [*Griggs, Mendell, Rahman, Backman, Fenichel, Siegel*], all showing improvement in various parameters such as muscle strength, functional tests, and lung function, with minimum treatment durations of 6 months. Prednisone at three different daily doses (0.3, 0.75, or 1.5 mg/kg per day) was used and each was effective. Prednisone at a dose of 0.75 mg/kg per day produced an 11% net increase in average strength score, as well as improvement in timed functional tests. Alternate-day prednisone did not have the same effect when given at lower doses of 1.25 or 2.5 mg/kg, but appears to be of possible benefit at doses of 5 mg/kg per day [15]. Deflazacort was used in two class 1 trials [*Angelini*, [16]]. Mesa *et al.* used deflazacort at 1 mg/kg per day for 9 months, whereas Angelini *et al.* used 2mg/kg on alternate days for 2 years. Both groups showed sustained improvement in measured parameters. Short-term adverse events from steroid treatment, such as excessive weight gain and behavioral changes, were found to be more common than placebo, but not deemed severe. Deflazacort, however, was not associated with the statistically significant weight gain seen with prednisone over 6 months. Long-term evaluation was not possible. It was postulated that some of the weight gain may have been from increased muscle mass as judged from 24-hour urinary creatinine excretion [*Griggs*]. Other potential side effects such as osteoporosis and dysglycemia were not evaluated. Unfortunately, insufficient data precluded any conclusions regarding outcome and age of initiation.

Summary

The dose of prednisone recommended in the conclusion of both reviews was 0.75 mg/kg per day. Side effects of treatment may necessitate dose reduction, but even at a lower dose of 0.3 mg/kg per day, improvement is seen. Deflazacort, if available, is recommended at a dose of 0.9 mg/kg per day [*Moxley III*]. There are no class 1 studies that examine the important question of the optimal age to begin treatment. The ideal duration of treatment is also unclear, although class IV studies suggest continuation of improvement at 3 years [17].

Limb-girdle muscular dystrophies

Are there any effective interventions for these conditions and what is the evidence underlying their use?

Background

The LGMDs are all individually rare, although for some conditions clear prevalence differences between different geographical populations are emerging. Even though all the LGMDs are currently classified under one umbrella term, they are a heterogeneous group both in terms of their clinical features and molecular causation; they are classified together due to their general (but not exclusive) predilection for involvement of the proximal musculature. Establishing a precise molecular diagnosis may be a challenge and due to both this and the uncommon nature of most of the LGMDs, randomized controlled trials of specific drug interventions are a distant prospect at present. The age of onset in the LGMDs ranges from childhood to late adult life. Thus, at present there is no clear unified molecular target for drug therapy, and therefore clinical practice has emphasized the role of surveillance and timely intervention when cardiac and respiratory complications occur. These complications can be treated with standard therapies.

Evidence

There is no randomized controlled trial (RCT)-based evidence to guide in the management of these collectively rare muscular dystrophies. However, an expert panel has published useful guidelines [18]. Knowledge of the LGMD subtype may allow anticipation and timely intervention if respiratory and/or cardiac complications develop. Expert opinion currently recommends serial monitoring of respiratory function tests, to be followed up by overnight oximetry if required. Provision of noninvasive ventilatory support has been shown to prolong life in conditions such as DMD, and similar principles apply here. The frequency of monitoring may be modulated according to the expected prognosis associated with the particular LGMD subtype, as some commonly involve the respiratory muscles whereas others rarely do. For potential cardiac complications, knowledge of the underlying diagnosis also guides onward referral for cardiac monitoring. With the development of cardiomyopathy and/or cardiac dysrhythmia, intervention may be needed.

Myasthenia gravis

1 *A 60-year-old man with acetylcholine receptor positive generalized myasthenia is referred to you. What should he be treated with?*
2 *In a 20-year-old woman presenting with generalized and severe myasthenia gravis, what is the evidence for and against thymectomy? At what stage of the disease should it be employed?*

Background

By far the most common neuromuscular junction disorder is acquired myasthenia gravis and this will be encountered in everyday clinical practice by the general neurologist. A "one-size-fits-all" treatment approach however, is unlikely to be successful considering its clinical and biological heterogeneity. For example, consideration of age, onset, severity of disease, comorbidities, or a patient's childbearing potential may limit available drug and other treatment options. In addition, treatment response often differs depending on which underlying acetylcholine receptor antibodies are positive. For example, patients with positive Musk antibodies may be less responsive to acetylcholinesterase inhibitors. We focus here on maintenance therapy for generalized anti-Ach MG.

Corticosteroids

Oral corticosteroids are widely accepted as first-line immunosuppressive treatment for autoimmune myasthenia gravis, although there is surprisingly little definitive evidence for their efficacy compared with other treatments. Studies comparing corticosteroids with placebo are not possible due to ethical reasons. Evidence from RCTs was the subject of a Cochrane review [19]. A variety of primary and secondary outcome measures were assessed in order to evaluate treatment efficacy in terms of clinical improvement, remission, and adverse events. The authors found that treatment with prednisone did produce improvement in the short term compared with placebo, but remarked on serious methodological flaws contained in all the studies. Two controlled studies comparing corticosteroids with placebo [20,21] are discussed. Both studies were of small numbers of patients ($n = 13$) for 2 years and ($n = 20$) for 14 weeks, respectively. The 1998 study, which used intravenous methylprednisolone, produced the greater degree of strength enhancement with a relative rate of improvement 7.2 times as compared with the placebo group. Zhang and Wu [22] examined different doses of corticosteroid in juvenile myasthenia and found that both were efficacious, but that those receiving intravenous methylprednisolone improved more quickly and for longer.

Corticosteroids with azathioprine

Gajdos et al. compared corticosteroids with azathioprine [23] and found that similar percentages (72% and 74%, respectively) were in remission. Bromberg et al. also compared prednisone with azathioprine [24] over a year-long-study period; numbers were very small with only one of five patients on azathioprine securing "satisfactory improvement." No studies comparing azathioprine with steroids were identified by the Cochrane review, rather two studies comparing azathioprine *plus* prednisolone and prednisolone alone ($n = 75$) did not show any clinical benefit [25]. A lower dose of prednisolone, however, was required for those on combination treatment with azathioprine.

Immunosuppressive treatments

As is the case with steroids, no quality-randomized controlled data exist for any other immunosuppressant therapy. Limited evidence extrapolated from small RCTs examining cyclosporine plus steroids, cyclophosphamide plus steroids, or cyclosporine alone suggests that both agents can improve MG. Cyclophosphamide-induced remission compared with placebo in two further studies [26,27]. The latest agent to undergo close scrutiny is mycophenolate mofetil. The two studies conducted by Meriggioli et al. [28,29] were suggestive of improvement when compared with placebo,

but numbers were small. Tacrolimus at low dose has been studied in 19 patients with just under half showing improvement [30]. Overall, data from these studies are difficult to compare due to confounding factors such as whether or not the patient had undergone thymectomy and concomitant steroid use. The bottom line according to the most recent Cochrane review is that no clear benefit exists at 6 or 12 months for the drugs we routinely use for MG treatment including azathioprine (+/− steroids), mycophenolate mofetil (+/− prednisolone, cyclosporine, or both), or tacrolimus (+/− corticosteroids, plasma exchange, or both). The evidence for the use of immunosuppressive agents in myasthenia gravis is therefore mixed. Consensus guidelines [31] published by Skeie et al. recommends azathioprine together with corticosteroids, the aim of treatment being to progressively lower the steroid dose as the azathioprine becomes effective. This was a level A recommendation.

Thymectomy

Resection is indicated in thymomatous myasthenia due to the potential to spread locally, and should be followed by radiotherapy for those uncommon thymomas which are malignant.

Controversy remains in the nonthymomatous myasthenic patient. Transsternal or transcervical thymectomy is a major procedure; perioperative risk may be increased by the typical concomitant use of corticosteroids or intravenous immunoglobulin in efforts to enhance the patient's functional status preoperatively. Thymectomy ideally hopes to incite a prolonged medication-free remission or at least nominal symptoms with a minimal maintenance dose. A review of thymectomy studies in nonthymomatous myasthenia gravis published as a Practice parameter for the American Academy of Neurology [32] appeared to support the benefit of the procedure, although none of the trials reviewed were randomized controlled. Class II and III studies were evaluated and numerical adjustments were made in an attempt to reduce the impact of potential confounders. Twenty-eight articles ascertained from 1953 to 1998 were assessed; including some overlap in the individual patient cohorts. All were designated class II studies as none of the patients were assigned to thymectomy using a randomization procedure. Evaluation of the studies showed variation in patient type between cohorts (e.g., ocular myasthenia, presence or absence of thymic hyperplasia, or unknown) and study method (e.g., surgical technique, definition of remission criteria, and duration of follow-up). Outcome assessments were not blinded. The outcome in most cohorts was consistent with thymectomy patients trending toward remission as judged by medication freedom. The few exceptions to this were nonideal studies in various respects, as the authors discuss. The issue of optimal timing of thymectomy was difficult to infer due to possible confounding factors such as prior treatments, gender differences, and disease severity. Overall, adjusted median relative outcome rates showed a positive association between thymectomy and remission and improvement in myasthenia gravis. Consensus guidelines published recently concur with the above and recommend thymectomy for nonthymomatous patients below 60 years of age is a level B recommendation (*Skeie*). On account of the nonideal data and continued uncertainties regarding the role of thymectomy, a multicenter RCT comparing prednisone plus transsternal thymectomy and prednisone alone aims to ascertain whether the risks of surgery are outweighed by its benefits. The study designed by Newsom–Davis *et al.* intends to enroll 150 patients over 3 years with a follow-up time of 5 years [33]. For those patients with antibodies to muscle-specific kinase (MuSK), the impact of thymectomy (as well as medical treatment) is unknown at present. The largest published cohort to date included 39 patients who underwent thymectomy [34]. Even though pathologic changes were only confirmed in one patient, 50% were deemed to have good clinical outcomes including five in complete stable remission.

Polymyositis

Are there specific diagnostic criteria that I can apply to the diagnosis of myositis? What is the best treatment for myositis?

Background

The precise incidence of myositis is hard to determine due to the lack of agreed diagnostic criteria and thus the lack of consistency in making the diagnosis. A number of schemata have been proposed over the years and although the understanding of inflammatory myopathies has evolved, disease classification has not. This is in part due to an increasing number of conditions that must now be considered within the differential diagnosis. Myositis is generally regarded as an acquired autoimmune inflammatory muscle disease resulting in proximal muscle weakness, elevated concentrations of creatinine kinase, abnormal electromyography, and inflammation seen on muscle biopsy. Even though the mechanism is unclear, it is generally considered to be responsive to anti-inflammatory or immunosuppressive treatment. Myositis may occur in isolation or in association with autoimmune lung disease, often with Jo-1 or other antisynthetase antibodies, or with other connective tissue diseases (e.g., overlap syndrome). It can also be associated with overt or covert malignancy.

Clinical scenario

A 65-year-old woman is referred to your clinic by her general practitioner (GP). She was diagnosed as having myositis 3 months previously and has been treated with steroids, which she continues to take as prednisolone 30 mg daily. However, there has been no improvement in her symptoms, and she has put on weight. The GP asks what should be done next.

Diagnosis

In the setting of persistent symptoms despite treatment, it would be prudent to first confirm the diagnosis. However, the problem of diagnosis quickly becomes a dilemma problem of classification. Bohan and Peters devised the following most frequently referenced myositis criteria in 1975 [35]: (1) insidious onset of symmetrical weakness in the limb-girdle muscles and anterior neck flexors; (2) pathologic evidence of muscle inflammation; (3) elevated sera skeletal muscle enzymes; (4) EMG abnormalities consistent with myopathic process and exclusion of alternative neuromuscular conditions. Polymyositis (PM) and dermatomyositis (DM) were further differentiated solely on the presence of a rash. This oversimplification does not take into the account the fundamental pathologic differences between the two conditions. PM is a T cell-mediated disorder associated with circulating antibodies. DM is a complement-mediated microangiopathy [36] affecting the perimysial blood vessels. Rather than circulating antibodies, B cell -directed immune complexes collect in the vessel walls. Notwithstanding the sensible exclusion of other muscle diseases, Bohan and Peters could not have accounted for as yet unknown conditions of inclusion body myositis (IBM) or some late onset muscular dystrophies, which can also exhibit inflammation on biopsy.

IBM is currently regarded as the most common inflammatory myopathy [37]. By contrast, diagnostic criteria for IBM were agreed upon by an expert panel [38] and subsequently endorsed by others [39].

In addition to diagnostic uncertainty, the lack of a universally adopted classification system has hampered RCT's successful design and real -world implication for management in myositis patients. A multidisciplinary consensus group comprised European rheumatologists and neurologists recently urged adoption of an adapted classification scheme in efforts to standardize diagnosis and interpretation of clinical trials [40].

The most common reason for refractory PM in older people is in fact a misdiagnosis of IBM [41]. Returning to our clinical scenario, consideration of a revised diagnosis reflecting this would be particularly relevant.

Treatment

After confirming the diagnosis of PM, one might wish to review how to treat it. Is the patient's steroid dose appropriate? If so, what additional immunomodulatory agents are recommended? A search of the Cochrane Database of Systematic Reviews reveals one relevant review of treatment of PM by Choy *et al.* [42]. An updated version was released in 2009, but due to minor inconsistencies it was withdrawn and has not yet been corrected [43]. Similar to other muscle conditions, it is conspicuous for the absence of placebo-controlled data scrutinizing steroids, the typical first-line therapy. Instead, most of the studies have focused on second-line agents designed to reduce and ideally replace steroids for long-term immunotherapy. Such treatments are used in recognition of the fact that steroids, while being good short-term immunosuppressive agents, have side effects that preclude their long-term use. Even though there are no current nor likely forthcoming evidence-based guidelines summarizing the dose or duration of steroid treatment, most would agree that 30 mg of prednisone per day in our clinical scenario is too modest. A dose of 1–1.5 mg/kg per day for at least 4 weeks would be more conventional [44]. A relatively recent RCT published in 2010 by van de Vlekkert et al. compared monthly pulse dexamethasone therapy to daily prednisolone with follow-up time of 18 months. No significant difference was found between groups in either primary outcome: (1) time to relapse or remission and (2) functional status. However, pulsed dexamethasone caused substantially less side effects, justifying its use as a viable first-line alternative especially in high-risk steroid adverse patients [45].

If our patient fails a trial of adequately dosed steroids, a second-line agent will need to be pursued. Choy et al.'s review identified five qualifying trials. All used the Bohan and Peters diagnostic criteria [46–50]. Three were judged to be of high quality while two were open label with inadequate allocation concealment. The second-line treatments assessed were plasma exchange, leukapheresis or sham apheresis with 12 treatments given over a 1-month period [46], 2 mg/kg per day azathioprine or placebo for 3 months in addition to 60 mg of prednisolone daily [49], prednisolone plus either low-dose methotrexate (15 mg weekly) or azathioprine (2.5 mg/kg daily) for 1 year [47], methotrexate 7.5–15 mg (mostly 10 mg) orally weekly or cyclosporin A 3.0–3.5 mg/kg per day for at least 6 months [48], oral methotrexate up to 25 mg weekly with azathioprine 150 mg daily for 6 months, or intravenous methotrexate 500 mg/m^2 every 2 weeks for 12 treatments each with leucovorin rescue (50 mg/m^2 every 6 hours for 4 doses) [50]. Thus only two of the relevant trials assessed immunosuppressive treatment against placebo. None of the trials gave statistically significant results in favor of any of the immunosuppressive treatments. This is not to say that none of these treatments work, but rather that the trials have been inadequately powered to show benefit. Since this systematic review fails to help answer our question, we might try and seek guidance from less rigorous lines of evidence such as nonrandomized trials. Van de Vledkkert et al. conducted a MEDLINE and EMBASE search from 1966 to 2001 yielding 74 case reports and 18 case series. They assessed these reports using 10 standards that were thought important to allow any reader to recognize his/her own patient, copy the treatment, and have some idea of the treatment effect. They concluded that the majority were of dubious quality and would not allow a useful systematic review [51]. More recently, Mann et al. reviewed treatment of "idiopathic inflammatory myopathies" (IIM) which, by default, included other inflammatory myopathies in addition to DM and PM. Their efforts concluded: (1) limited data exist for efficacy of novel immunosuppressants

mycophenolate mofetil, leflunomide, and tacrolimus; (2) even though rituximab's mechanism of action lends itself to humorally mediated conditions, preliminary results of a large RCT failed to meet its end point [52]; (3) intravenous immunoglobulin in patients with esophageal involvement showed significant resolution in retrospective analysis; and (4) TNF neutralization has showed variable results and does not mirror the benefit seen in other rheumatologic conditions [53]. Thus, the decision as to what second-line immunosuppressive treatment to use is still based upon expert opinion and personal preference.

Facioscapulohumeral muscular dystrophy

Are there specific disease-modifying treatments or symptomatic treatments that can be used?

Background

Facioscapulohumeral muscular dystrophy (FSHD) is a dominantly inherited dystrophy with a characteristic pattern of muscle weakness, almost always beginning in the face. It is the third most common dystrophy following Duchenne's and myotonic dystrophy, and is defined by the loss of the D4Z4 repeat in the subtelomere of chromosome 4q. It is unclear how this alteration in chromatin structure leads to the phenotypic disease [54], although it is postulated to provoke a deleterious gain of function as 4q monosomy does not produce FSHD [55,56]. Muscle biopsy is reserved for cases with nonconfirmatory genetic or electrodiagnostic testing. Extramuscular manifestations include mild high-frequency hearing loss and retinal telangiectasias [57].

Clinical scenario

A 25-year-old man is referred to your clinic with a genetically proven diagnosis of FSHD. He wants to know if there is any treatment that can help him.

Evidence

Part of the difficulty of finding a suitable pharmacological treatment for FSHD is that its precise pathogenesis is unknown and therefore, as of yet, we do not have disease-specific therapeutic strategies. The current approach has focused on generic muscle disease or symptomatic therapies. FSHD muscle can mimic inflammatory myopathies on biopsy suggesting a potential therapeutic target. Steroid response is variable and failed to yield any improvement in the only open-label study [58]. The most recent Systematic Cochrane Review published in 2004 identified two high-quality RCTs looking at medication therapy in FHSD [59]. One RCT compared creatinine supplementation with placebo finding a nonsignificant difference in favor of creatinine [60]. The other RCT was a small pilot comparing high- and low-dose albuterol (salbutamol) with placebo. There was no significant difference in muscle strength at 1 year, but some improvement in secondary measures such as lean body mass and handgrip [61]. An updated RCT published in 2009 by Payan *et al.* again failed to show benefit of salbutamol given 3 weeks out of every 4 for the duration of 6 months [62]. Van der Kooi *et al.* performed an RCT combining albuterol with exercise, which showed limited positive effects on muscle strength and volume, but not of a sufficient degree as to justify its routine use. No discernable effect on pain, fatigue, or psychological distress was illustrated [63]. New novel therapies have been attempted including autologous stem cell transplantation with mesoangioblasts [64].

Several nonpharmacological interventions can offer functional improvement such as adequate assistance devices and serial exams monitoring for extramuscular manifestations. Currently, Voet *et al.* has proposed a protocol for a prospective double-blind RCT to investigate the potential benefits of aerobic exercise and cognitive behavioral therapy on FSHD fatigue [65]. Surgical intervention with scapular fixation can address the prominent and disabling scapular winging seen in FSHD. Periscapular weakness prevents even a relatively spared deltoid muscle from elevating the arm. It follows then that fixation would lead to worthwhile functional gains. Several retrospective reviews have suggested significant benefits [66–68], however no prospective controlled study confirms this [69]. Thus, neither the indications nor optimal techniques of scapular fixation are clearly established. Furthermore, complications include postoperative pain, loss of Function, and injury to the brachial plexus [70,71]. Most experts recommend consideration of the procedure only in patients most likely to benefit that is, those with preserved upper arm strength, slow progression, and after a successful trial of manual fixation [72].

References

1 Prevalence of Duchenne/Becker muscular dystrophy among males aged 5-24 years—four states, 2007. (2009) *MMWR. Morbidity and Mortality Weekly Report*, **58**(40), 1119–1122.

2 Moxley, R.T. III (2006) Clinical overview of Duchenne Muscular Dystrophy. In: Chamberlain, J. & Rando, T. (eds), *Duchenne Muscular Dystrophy: Advances in Therapeutics*. NY. Taylor & Francis Group, New York, pp. 1–20.

3 Eagle, M., Baudouin, S.V., Chandler, C., Giddings, D.R., Bullock, R. & Bushby, K. (2002) Survival in Duchenne muscular dystrophy: improvements in life expectancy since 1967 and the impact of home nocturnal ventilation. *Neuromuscular Disorders*, **12**(10), 926–929.

4 Bushby, K., Finkel, R., Birnkrant, D.J. *et al.* (2010) Diagnosis and management of Duchenne muscular dystrophy, part 2: implementation of multidisciplinary care. *Lancet Neurology*, **9**(2), 177–189.

5 Sussman, M. (2002) Duchenne muscular dystrophy. *Journal of the American Academy of Orthopaedic Surgeons*, **10**(2), 138–151.

6 Lit, L., Sharp, F.R., Apperson, M. *et al.* (2009) Corticosteroid effects on blood gene expression in Duchenne muscular dystrophy. *The Pharmacogenomics Journal*, **9**, 411–418.

7 Manzur, A.Y., Kuntzer, T., Pike, M. & Swan, A.V. (2008) Glucocorticoid corticosteroids for Duchenne muscular dystrophy. *Cochrane Database of Systemic Reviews*, (**1**). Art No: CD003725.

8 Angelini, C., Pegoraro, E., Turella, E. *et al.* (1994) Deflazacort in Duchenne dystrophy: study of long-term effect. *Muscle & Nerve*, **17**(4), 386–391.

9 Griggs, R.C., Moxley, R.T. III,, Mendell, J.R. *et al.* (1991) Prednisone in Duchenne dystrophy. A randomized, controlled trial defining the time course and dose response. Clinical Investigation of Duchenne Dystrophy Group. *Archives of Neurology*, **48**(4), 383–388.

10 Mendell, J.R., Moxley, R.T., Griggs, R.C. *et al.* (1989) Randomised double blind six month trial of prednisone in Duchenne's muscular dystrophy. *New England Journal of Medicine*, **320**, 1592–1597.

11 Rahman, M.M., Hannan, M.A., Mondol, B.A., Bhoumick, N.B. & Haque, A. (2001) Prednisolone in Duchenne muscular dystrophy. *Bangladesh Medical Research Council Bulletin*, **27**(1), 38–42.

12 Beenakker, E.A.C., Maurits, N.M., Fock, J.M., Brouwer, O.F. & van der Hoeven, J.H. (2005) Functional ability and muscle force in healthy children and ambulant Duchenne muscular dystrophy patients. *European Journal of Paediatric Neurology*, **9**(6), 387–393.

13 Manzur, A.Y., Kuntzer, T., Pike, S. *et al.* (2004) Glucocorticoid corticosteroids for Duchenne dystrophy. *Cochrane Database of Systematic Reviews*, **2**.: CD003725.

14 Moxley, R.T. III,, Ashwal, S., Pandya, S. *et al.* (2005) Practice parameter: corticosteroid treatment of Duchenne dystrophy: report of the Quality Standards Subcommittee of the American Academy of Neurology and the Practice Committee of the Child Neurology Society. *Neurology*, **64**(1), 13–20.

15 Siegel, I.M., Miller, J.E. & Ray, R.D. (1974) Failure of corticosteroid in the treatment of Duchenne (pseudo-hypertrophic) muscular dystrophy. Report of a clinically matched three year double-blind study. *IMJ. Illinois Medical Journal*, **145**(1), 32–33.

16 Mesa, L.E., Dubrovsky, A.L., Corderi, J., Marco, P. & Flores, D. (1991) Steroids in Duchenne muscular dystrophy–deflazacort trial. *Neuromuscular Disorders*, **1**(4), 261–266.

17 Fenichel, G.M., Florence, J.M., Pestronk, A. *et al.* (1991) Long-term benefit from prednisone therapy in Duchenne muscular dystrophy. *Neurology*, **41**(12), 1874–1877.

18 Norwood, F., de Visser, M., Eymard, B., Lochmuller, H. & Bushby, K. (2006) Limb girdle muscular dystrophies. In: Hughes, R.A.C., Brainin, M. & Gilhus, N.E. (eds), *European Handbook of Neurological Management*. Blackwell Publishing, Oxford.

19 Schneider-Gold, C., Gajdos, P., Toyka, K.V. & Hohlfeld, R.R. (2005) Corticosteroids for myasthenia gravis. *Cochrane Database of Systematic Reviews*, **2**. Article no.: CD002828.

20 Howard, F.M. Jr., Duane, D.D., Lambert, E.H. & Daube, J.R. (1976) Alternate-day prednisone: preliminary report of a double-blind controlled study. *Annals of the New York Academy of Sciences*, **274**, 596–607.

21 Lindberg, C., Andersen, O. & Lefvert, A.K. (1998) Treatment of myasthenia gravis with methylprednisolone pulse: a double blind study. *Acta Neurologica Scandinavica*, **97**(6), 370–373.

22 Zhang, J. & Wu, H. (1998) Effectiveness of steroid treatment in juvenile myasthenia. *Chinese Journal of Pediatrics*, **36**, 612–614.

23 Myasthenia Gravis Study Group (1993) A randomised clinical trial comparing prednisone and azathioprine in myasthenia gravis. Results of the second interim analysis. Myasthenia Gravis Clinical Study Group. *Journal of Neurology, Neurosurgery & Psychiatry*, **56**, 1157–1163.

24 Bromberg, M.B., Wald, J.J., Forshew, D.A., Feldman, E.L. & Albers, J.W. (1997) Randomized trial of azathioprine or prednisone for initial immunosuppressive treatment of myasthenia gravis. *Journal of Neurological Sciences*, **150**(1), 59–62.

25 Palace, J., Newsom-Davis, J. & Lecky, B. (1998) A randomized double-blind trial of prednisolone alone or with azathioprine in myasthenia gravis. Myasthenia Gravis Study Group. *Neurology*, **50**(6), 1778–1783.

26 De Feo, L.G., Schottlender, J., Martelli, N.A. & Molfino, N.A. (2002) Use of intravenous pulsed cyclophosphamide in severe, generalized myasthenia gravis. *Muscle and Nerve*, **26**(1), 31–36.

27 Perez, M.C., Buot, W.L., Mercado-Danguilan, C., Bagabaldo, Z.G. & Renales, L.D. (1981) Stable remissions in myasthenia gravis. *Neurology*, **31**(1), 32–37.

28 Meriggioli, M.N., Rowin, J., Richman, J.G. & Leurgans, S. (2003) Mycophenolate mofetil for myasthenia gravis: a double-blind, placebo-controlled pilot study. *Annals of the New York Academy of Sciences*, **998**, 494–499.

29 Meriggioli, M.N., Ciafaloni, E., Al Hayk, K.A. *et al.* (2003) Mycophenolate mofetil for myasthenia gravis: an analysis of efficacy, safety, and tolerability. *Neurology*, **61**(10), 1438–1440.

30 Konishi, T., Yoshiyama, Y., Takamori, M., Yagi, K., Mukai, E. & Saida, T. (2003) Clinical study of FK506 in patients with myasthenia gravis. *Muscle and Nerve*, **28**(5), 570–574.

31 Skeie, G.O., Apostolski, S., Evoli, A. *et al.* (2006) Guidelines for the treatment of autoimmune neuromuscular transmission disorders. *European Journal of Neurology*, **13**(7), 691–699.

32 Gronseth, G.S. & Barohn, R.J. (2000) Practice parameter: Thymectomy for autoimmune myasthenia gravis (an evidence-based review): Report of the Quality Standards Subcommittee of the American Academy of Neurology. *Neurology*, **55**, 7–15.

33 Yoshikawa, H., Iwasa, K. & Takamori, M. (2011) Current status and future prospects of therapy for myasthenia gravis: considering thymectomy. *Brain and Nerve*, **63**(7), 729–736.

34 Guptill, J., Sanders, D. & Evoli, A. (2011) Anti-MuSK antibody myasthenia gravis: clinical findings and response to treatment in two large cohorts. *Muscle and Nerve*, **44**, 36–40.

35 Bohan, A. & Peter, J.B. (1975) Polymyositis and dermatomyositis (first of two parts). *New England Journal of Medicine*, **292**, 344–347.

36 Dalakas, M.C. & Hohlfeld, R. (2003) Polymyositis and dermatomyositis. *Lancet*, **362**, 971–982.

37 Munshi, S.K., Thanvi, B., Jonnalagadda, S.J., Da Forno, P., Patel, A. & Sharma, S. (2006) Inclusion body myositis: an underdiagnosed myopathy of older people. *Age and Ageing*, **35**(1), 91–94.

38 Griggs, R.C., Askanas, V., DiMauro, S. *et al.* (1995) Inclusion body myositis and myopathies. *Annals of Neurology*, **38**, 705–713.

39 Muller-Felber W, Pongratz D, Reimers C. 64th ENMC International Workshop: therapeutic approaches to dermatomyositis, polymyositis, and inclusion body myositis 29–31.

40 Hoogendijk, J.E., Amato, A.A., Lecky, B.R. *et al.* (2004 May) 119th ENMC international workshop: trial design in adult idiopathic inflammatory myopathies, with the exception of inclusion body myositis, 10–12 October 2003, Naarden, The Netherlands. *Neuromuscular Disorders*, **14**(5), 337–345.

41 Askanas, V. & Engel, W.K. (1998) Sporadic inclusion-body myositis and hereditary inclusion-body myopathies: diseases of oxidative stress and aging? *Archives of Neurology*, **55**, 915–920.

42 Choy, E.H., Hoogendijk, J., Lecky, B.R. & Winer, J. (2012) Immunosuppressant and immunomodulatory treatment for dermatomyositis and polymyositis. *Cochrane Database of Systematic Reviews*, **8**. doi:10.1002/14651858CD003643.pub4.

43 Choy EHS, Hoogendijk JE, Lecky B, Winer JB, Gordon P. Immunosuppressant and immunomodulatory treatment for dermatomyositis and polymyositis. Cochrane Database of Systematic Reviews, 2009, **4**. Art. No.: CD003643. DOI: 10.1002/14651858.CD003643.pub3.

44 Dalakas, M.C. (2006) Therapeutic targets in patients with inflammatory myopathie: present approaches and a look to the future. *Neuromuscular Disorders*, **16**(4), 223–236.

45 van de Vlekkert, J., Hoogendijk, J.E., de Haan, R.J. *et al.* (2010) Oral dexamethasone pulse therapy versus daily prednisolone in sub-acute onset myositis, a randomised clinical trial. *Neuromuscular Disorders*, **20**(6), 382–389.. Epub 2010 Apr 25.

46 Miller, F.W., Leitman, S.F., Cronin, M.E. *et al.* (1992) Controlled trial of plasma exchange and leukapheresis in polymyositis and dermatomyositis. *New England Journal of Medicine*, **326**, 1380–1384.

47 Miller, J., Walsh, Y., Saminaden, S., Lecky, B.R.F. & Winer, J.B. (2002) Randomised double blind controlled trial of methotrexate and steroids compared with azathioprine and steroids in the treatment of idiopathic inflammatory myopathy. *Journal of Neurological Sciences*, **199**(**Suppl**), S53.

48 Vencovsky, J., Jarosova, K., Machacek, S. *et al.* (2000) Cyclosporine A versus methotrexate in the treatment of polymyositis and dermatomyositis. *Scandinavian Journal of Rheumatology*, **29**(2), 95–102.

49 Bunch, T.W., Worthington, J.W., Combs, J.J., Ilstrup, D.M. & Engel, A.G. (1980) Azathioprine with prednisone for polymyositis. A controlled, clinical trial. *Annals of Internal Medicine*, **92**(3), 365–369.

50 Villalba, L., Hicks, J.E., Adams, E.M. *et al.* (1998) Treatment of refractory myositis: a randomized crossover study of two new cytotoxic regimens. *Arthritis and Rheumatism*, **41**(3), 392–399.

51 van de Vlekkert, J., Tjin-A-Ton, M.L. & Hoogendijk, J.E. (2004) Quality of myositis case reports open to improvement. *Arthritis and Rheumatism*, **51**(1), 148–150.

52 Aggarwal, R. & Oddis, C.V. (2011) Therapeutic approaches in myositis. *Current Rheumatology Reports*, **13**(3), 182–191.

53 Mann, H. & Vencovsky, J. (2011) Clinical trials roundup in idiopathic inflammatory myopathies. *Current Opinion in Rheumatology*, **23**, 605–611.

54 Lemmers, R.J., de Kievit, P., Sandkuijl, L. *et al.* (2002) Facioscapulohumeral muscular dystrophy is uniquely associated with one of the two variants of the 4q subtelomere. *Nature Genetics*, **32**(2), 235–236.

55 Tupler, R., Berardinelli, A., Barbierato, L. *et al.* (1996) Monosomy of distal 4q does not cause facioscapulohumeral muscular dystrophy. *Journal of Medical Genetics*, **33**, 366–370.

56 Tawil, R. (2006) van der Maarel sm. Facioscapulohumeral muscular dystropy. *Muscle and Nerve*, **34**, 1–15.

57 Osborne, R.J., Welle, S., Venance, S.L. *et al.* (2007) Expression profile of FSHD supports a link between retinal vasculopathy and muscular dystrophy. *Neurology*, **68**(8), 569–577.

58 Tawil, R., McDermott, M.P., Pandya, S., King, W., Kissel, J. & Mendell, J.R. (1997) A pilot trial of prednisone in facioscapulohumeral muscular dystrophy. FSH-DY Group. *Neurology*, **48**, 46–49.

59 Rose MR, Tawil R, (2004) Drug treatment for facioscapulohumeral muscular dystrophy. *Cochrane Database of Systematic Reviews* (**2**), Article no.:CD002276.

60 Walter, M.C., Lochmuller, H., Reilich, P. *et al.* (2000) Creatine monohydrate in muscular dystrophies: A double-blind, placebo-controlled clinical study. *Neurology*, **54**(9), 1848–1850.

61 Kissel, J.T., McDermott, M.P., Natarajan, R. *et al.* (1998) Pilot trial of albuterol in facioscapulohumeral muscular dystrophy. FSH-DY Group. *Neurology*, **50**(5), 1402–1406.

62 Payan, C.A., Hogrel, J.Y., Hammouda, E.H. *et al.* (2009) Periodic salbutamol in facioscapulohumeral muscular dystrophy: A randomized controlled trial. *Archives of Physical Medicine and Rehabilitation*, **90**(7), 1094–1101.

63 van der Kooi, E.L., Kalkman, J.S., Lindeman, E. *et al.* (2007) Effects of training and albuterol on pain and fatigue in facioscapulohumeral muscular dystrophy. *Journal of Neurology*, **254**(7), 931–940. Epub 2007 Mar 14.

64 Morosetti, R., Mirabella, M., Gliubizzi, C. *et al.* (2007) Isolation and characterization of mesoangioblasts from facioscapulohumeral muscular dystrophy muscle biopsies. *Stem Cells*, **25**, 3173–3182.

65 Voet, N., Bleijenberg, G., Padberg, G. *et al.* (2010) Effect of aerobic exercise training and cognitive behavioural therapy on reduction of chronic fatigue in patients with facioscapulohumeral dystrophy: protocol of the FACTS-2-FSHD trial. *BMC Neurology*, **10**, 5656.

66 Bunch, W.H. & Siegel, I.M. (1993) Scapulothoracic arthrodesis in facioscapulohumeral muscular dystrophy. Review of seventeen procedures with three to twenty-one-year follow up. *The Journal of bone and joint surgery. American*, **75**(3), 372–376.

67 Giannini, S., Faldini, C., Pagkrati, S. *et al.* (2007) Fixation of winged scapula in facioscapulohumeral muscular dystrophy. *Clinical Medicine & Research*, **5**, 155–162.

68 Rhee, Y.G. & Ha, J.H. (2006) Long-term results of scapulothoracic arthrodesis of facioscapulohumeral muscular dystrophy. *Journal of Shoulder and Elbow Surgery*, **15**, 445–450.

69 Mummery, C.J., Copeland, S.A. & Rose, M.R. (2003) Scapular fixation in muscular dystrophy. *Cochrane Database of Systematic Reviews*, **3**. Article no. :CD003278.

70 Wolfe, G.I., Young, P.K., Nations, S.P., Burkhead, W.Z., McVey, A.L. & Barohn, R.J. (2005) Brachial plexopathy following thoracoscapular fusion in facioscapulohumeral muscular dystrophy. *Neurology*, **64**, 572–573.

71 Mackenzie, W.G., Riddle, E.C., Earley, J.L. & Sawatzky, B.J. (2003) A neurovascular complication after scapulothoracic arthrodesis. *Clinical orthopaedics and related research*, **408**, 157–161.

72 Tawil, R. (2008) Facioscapulohumeral muscular dystrophy. *Neurotherapeutics*, **5**(4), 601–606.

CHAPTER 25

Sleep disorders

Joyce K. Lee-Iannotti

Mayo Clinic Arizona, Scottsdale, AZ, USA

Background

Recent years have been marked by a renewed interest of neurologists in sleep disorders, not only primary sleep disorders such as narcolepsy with or without cataplexy, idiopathic hypersomnia with or without long sleep time, restless legs syndrome, but also sleep disorders associated with neurological conditions such as rapid eye movement (REM) sleep behavior disorder predominantly in synucleinopathies, obstructive sleep apnea syndrome in stroke patients, or in neurodegenerative conditions.

Framing clinical questions

In this chapter, we will focus on five areas of interest: obstructive sleep apnea syndrome in stroke patients, due to the high incidence of the phenomenon and the unsettled therapeutic attitude; narcolepsy, given the discovery of the role of the loss or dysfunction of hypocretin/orexin neurons, both in animal models and in humans, and the emergence of a renewed treatment, sodium oxybate; idiopathic hypersomnia and the distinction between idiopathic hypersomnia with and without long sleep time; REM sleep behavior disorder (RBD) as it relates to Parkinson's disease and other synucleinopathies; and insomnia in Parkinson's disease, because of its numerous etiological factors and complexity of treatment.

Critical review of evidence

Sleep-disordered breathing and stroke

1 *What are the consequences of sleep-disordered breathing on the severity and outcome of stroke?*

2 *What is the required treatment in a stroke patient diagnosed with obstructive sleep apnea (OSA)?*

3 *What is the outcome of stroke patients with obstructive sleep apnea syndrome treated with continuous positive airway pressure (CPAP)?*

Stroke is the leading cause of disability among adults and the prevalence of sleep-disordered breathing in patients with acute ischemic stroke is fairly high (30–70%). Growing evidence shows that sleep-disordered breathing is strongly associated with increased risk of stroke, and is independent of other known risk factors.

Scenario

A 66-year-old male shopkeeper was brought into the emergency room after being found on the floor unable to move his left side. Physical examination revealed a complete left hemiplegia equally involving face, arm, and leg, and marked inattention to the left side of the body.

Speech was normal and the patient was fully oriented. There appeared to be sensory deficit on the left to pinprick and light touch, although examination was difficult because of neglect of that side. Reflexes were decreased on the left, and left plantar response was extensive. General examination was remarkable for slight obesity with a body mass index of 28.1. Blood pressure and pulse were regular at 160/100 mmHg and 80, respectively. The patient had increased neck girth and his spouse disclosed loud snoring, nocturia, marked fatigue on awakening, and excessive daytime sleepiness for several years. Early computed tomography (CT) scan revealed a decrease in the size of the right lateral ventricle compatible with early swelling of the right hemisphere. Polysomnography demonstrated a high apnea–hypopnea index of 44 respiratory events per hour of sleep, mainly obstructive sleep apneas, with a mean oxyhemoglobin saturation of 91% and a nadir of 81%.

Evidence

1 Sleep-disordered breathing accompanied by arterial oxyhemoglobin desaturation appears to be associated with higher mortality at 1 year and lower Barthel index scores at discharge and at 3 and 12 months after stroke [1].

Evidence-Based Neurology: Management of Neurological Disorders, Second Edition. Edited by Bart M. Demaerschalk and Dean M. Wingerchuk.
© 2015 John Wiley & Sons, Ltd. Published 2015 by John Wiley & Sons, Ltd.

2 Only a few studies are available on the effects of CPAP in patients with sleep-disordered breathing and stroke. In one trial (nonrandomized), the effectiveness of nasal CPAP was studied in 105 stroke patients (75 males, 30 females) with a polysomnogram-confirmed diagnosis of moderate or severe obstructive sleep apnea syndrome (respiratory disturbance index > 15) [2]. Thirty-one patients (29.5%) rejected CPAP during the titration or shortly after, while 74 (70.5%) tolerated it and continued treatment at home. Subjective well-being was measured with a visual analogue scale in 41 unselected patients, and 24-hours blood pressure in 16 patients before and after 10 days of treatment. Differences were compared between patients who did and did not accept treatment. Among the 41 unselected patients, the compliant users showed a clear improvement in well-being in 28 patients who accepted the treatment ($P = 0.021$) in comparison with the 13 patients without acceptance; among the 16 patients, 11 showed a high compliance while 5 did not use CPAP. Only the compliant patients had a reduction in mean nocturnal blood pressure. In a second trial, 63 patients consecutively admitted to a stroke rehabilitation unit 2–4 weeks after a stroke, with an apnea–hyponea index ≥15, were randomized to either CPAP treatment ($n = 33$) or a control group ($n = 30$) [3]. Both groups were assessed at baseline and after 7 and 28 nights using the Montgomery-Asberg-Depression-Rating Scale (MADRS), Mini-Mental State Examination (MMSE) scale, and Barthel-ADL index. Compared to controls, depressive symptoms (MADRS) improved in patients randomized to CPAP treatment ($P = 0.004$). On the other hand, no significant treatment effect was found with regard to delirium, MMSE, and Barthel-ADL index. A more recent study conducted by Ryan *et al.* evaluated the influence of CPAP on outcomes of rehabilitation in stroke patients with OSA and showed that CPAP-compliant patients ($n = 22$) improved in functional and motor, but not neurocognitive outcomes at 1 month [4]. In terms of secondary stroke prevention, Martinez-Garcia *et al.* prospectively analyzed the role of long-term CPAP treatment in protecting stroke patients from new vascular events [4]. A total of 51 patients with an apnea–hyponea index (AHI) ≥ 20 were included. Two groups were defined: patients who could tolerate CPAP ($n = 15$) and patients who could not tolerate CPAP after 1 month of initial adaptation ($n = 36$). The incidence of new vascular events, evaluated through a follow-up time of 18 months, was 6.7% in the patients who tolerated CPAP and 36% in those who did not tolerate CPAP, indicating that CPAP treatment afforded significant protection against new vascular events after ischemic stroke. Furthermore, the same authors conducted a similar prospective, observational study to analyze the independent impact of long-term CPAP treatment on mortality in patients with ischemic stroke [5]. The study involved 166 patients with a follow-up time of 5 years and suggested that long-term CPAP treatment in moderate to severe OSA is associated with a reduction in excess risk of mortality in stroke victims.

3 CPAP, the main medical therapy for patients with sleep-related breathing disorders, is, in theory, the most relevant therapy for sleep apnea in stroke patients. However, compliance with CPAP treatment is a problem in stroke patients, especially when delirium and severe cognitive impairment occur. In addition, a low functional status, as measured by the Barthel index, and the presence of aphasia are of concern. In general, CPAP treatment in stroke patients requires much support from nurses or family. In conclusion, CPAP treatment offers improved prognosis in stroke patients affected with sleep-disordered breathing. This improvement concerns well-being, mood, motor and functional skills post stroke, protection against new vascular events, and reduction in mortality. On the other hand, delirium, mental state, and neurocognitive rehabilitation have not shown to be improved by CPAP therapy.

Narcolepsy with and without cataplexy

1 *In a subject suspected of narcolepsy with cataplexy, which tests should be performed before treatment?*

2 *Which treatment should be implemented? Among patients with narcolepsy with or without cataplexy, how do pharmacological treatments affect the probability of reducing daytime sleepiness and/or cataplexy?*

3 *What are the problems that can occur with time in relation with the treatment?*

Narcolepsy with cataplexy is primarily characterized by excessive daytime sleepiness and cataplexy. The former is usually the most disabling symptom and the first one to occur. It is characterized by episodes of naps or lapses into sleep across the daytime, also termed "sleep attacks." Cataplexy, a unique feature of the condition, is characterized by sudden loss of muscle tone provoked by strong emotions that are usually positive (e.g., fit of laughter, receiving a compliment, and excitement) and less often negative (e.g., anger or stress). Sleep paralysis, hypnagogic hallucinations, and sleep fragmentation commonly occur in patients with narcolepsy with cataplexy. These three symptoms, however, can occasionally, occur in normal people. Narcolepsy without cataplexy is a minor phenotype of the same condition. Narcolepsy with cataplexy affects 20–40/100,000 of the European and North American population, depending on the methodology of the surveys. Studies using both questionnaires and polysomnography find lower prevalence of the condition than those relying on questionnaire only. Both sexes are affected, with some preponderance of males. Narcolepsy without cataplexy is less frequent, but no prevalence study is available. The natural history of narcolepsy varies considerably with subjects. In most cases, excessive daytime sleepiness and irresistible sleep episodes persist throughout the lifetime, and they tend to improve with advancing age. Cataplexy may resolve with increasing age and even spontaneously disappear in some patients. Nocturnal sleep remains unchanged over the course of the lifetime, however.

Clinical scenario

A 32-year-old secretary complained of excessive daytime sleepiness and irresistible episodes of sleep occurring daily or almost daily for the last 1 year. The interview quickly showed that she had cataplexy at a rate of approximately one attack per week and hypnagogic hallucinations. The diagnosis of narcolepsy with cataplexy was confirmed by an all-night polysomnography followed by a multiple sleep latency test (MSLT) showing a mean sleep latency of 6.5 minutes and three sleep onset REM periods (SOREMPs). This woman is on the verge of being fired due to falling asleep at work.

Evidence

1 Narcolepsy can be diagnosed on purely clinical grounds. However, additional tests are useful to confirm the diagnosis. Most commonly, nocturnal polysomnography (with a minimum of 6 hours of sleep) followed by an MSLT is recommended. In a few selected cases, measurement of cerebrospinal fluid (CSF) levels of hypocretin-1 may be indicated. SOREMPs are observed in 25–50% of cases of narcolepsy with cataplexy, and is a highly specific finding. In addition, a disruption of the normal sleep pattern with repeated awakenings, termed "sleep fragmentation" is a frequent feature. The MSLT demonstrates a mean sleep latency of less than 8 minutes and two or more SOREMPs. However, a few typical cases of narcolepsy may have only one SOREMP or even none, not uncommon in elderly subjects. Measuring CSF levels of hypocretin-1 is highly specific and sensitive for the diagnosis of narcolepsy with cataplexy. Values less than 110 pg/mL are found in approximately 90% of cases of narcolepsy with cataplexy. However, because of the limited number of laboratories providing this service, the test should be used in few selected indications only: need to objectively document a diagnosis when the MSLT cannot be used (e.g., inability to withdraw antidepressants and stimulants); already treated patients if the diagnosis is in doubt; in young children and in cases with associated psychiatric or neurological disorders. This test is of much less value in narcolepsy without cataplexy as only 10% of patients show low values [6,7].

2 The two more recently introduced treatments of excessive daytime sleepiness, modafinil and sodium oxybate, are the most commonly used agents in newly diagnosed narcoleptic patients (Table 25.1, [8–13]). Modafinil is given at a daily dose of 400 mg (range 100–400 mg), with one dose in the morning and one dose early in the afternoon. One of the major advantages of modafinil is its relative lack of adverse effects. It can be administered concurrently with anticataplectic medications without concern for significant drug-to-drug interactions. Of note, a newer medication, armodafinil (NuVigil), a single isomer of modafinil, was approved for the treatment of narcolepsy-associated excessive sleepiness. In a clinical trial comparing it with placebo, armodafinil improved wakefulness, memory, attention, and fatigue in narcoleptics [14]. Sodium oxybate (not yet registered for excessive daytime sleepiness in Europe) is taken orally upon getting into bed and again 2.5–4 hours later. The current recommended starting dose is 4.5 g per day divided into two equal doses of 2.25 g. The dose may be increased to a maximum of 9 g per day by increments of 1.5 g. Two weeks are recommended between dosage increments. In addition to either modafinil or sodium oxybate, behavioral measures are always advisable. Naps during the day to counteract the effects of sleepiness is strongly recommended. This may require that letters be written to the employer to allow adjustments in the work schedule. Previous treatments included methylphenidate, 10–60 mg per day, and in case of nonresponse, dextroamphetamine, or methamphetamine under close monitoring. Treatment of cataplexy relies on sodium oxybate with the same mode of administration already recommended for excessive daytime sleepiness (Table 25.2, [12,13,16,15]). Second-line treatments include tricyclic antidepressants (e.g., clomipramine), selective serotonin reuptake inhibitors (e.g., fluoxetine or fluvoxamine), a norepinephrine uptake inhibitor (e.g., viloxazine), or a norepinephrine and serotonin uptake inhibitor (e.g., venlafaxine). However, the use of these drugs is based on no or few randomized, placebo-controlled clinical trials, and none are registered for cataplexy with the exception of clomipramine, which is registered in a few European countries. Benzodiazepines or nonbenzodiazepine hypnotics may be effective in consolidating sleep. Unfortunately, objective evidence is lacking over intermediate or long-term follow-up. According to US-based Xyrem studies [11,12], a significant decrease of nighttime awakenings is obtained with sodium oxybate 3–9 g, given in two doses, one at bedtime and another one during the night.

3 As already mentioned, adverse effects are limited with modafinil. Headache is the most common complaint followed by nausea, rhinitis, and nervousness. As for sodium oxybate, the most commonly reported adverse effects include vomiting, incontinence, sleepwalking, and confusion, but in a limited number of cases. There is a subset of patients who either do not respond to stimulants or to anticataplectic drugs, who show an insufficient response despite escalating doses of medication, or who have decreased responsiveness with long-term medications. This has sparked interest in novel therapies, such as either hypocretin- based therapies (peptide agonists, nonpeptide agonists, and cell transplantation or gene therapy) or immune-based therapies (steroid therapies, intravenous immunoglobulins, or plasmapheresis) [15].

Table 25.1 Treatment of excessive daytime sleepiness

References	Methods	Interventions	Participants	Outcome measures	Outcome
Billiard et al. [8]	12-week, placebo-controlled trial. Crossover design	Modafinil, 300 mg (2 divided doses) 100 mg in a.m. and 200 mg at noon or vice versa	50 narcolepsy with cataplexy subjects	Maintenance of Wakefulness Test (MWT) Global Symptoms Index (GSI)	Modafinil improves daytime sleepiness
Broughton et al. [9]	6-week, randomized placebo-controlled trial. Crossover design	Modafinil 200 or 400 mg in divided doses (morning and noon), versus placebo	75 narcoleptic subjects	MWT Epworth Sleepiness Scale (ESS)	Modafinil effective in keeping narcolepsy patients awake
US Modafinil in Narcolepsy Study Group [10]	9-week, randomized placebo-controlled trial	Modafinil 200 or 400 mg, versus placebo, followed by an open-label treatment period	283 narcoleptic subjects	ESS MSLT MWT GSI	Modafinil 200 mg and 400 mg significantly reduced all measures of sleepiness
US Modafinil in Narcolepsy Study Group [11]	9-week, randomized placebo-controlled trial	Modafinil 200 or 400 mg versus placebo	271 narcoleptic subjects	MSLT MWT ESS	Effective for treatment of daytime sleepiness in narcolepsy for 9 weeks
US Xyrem Multicenter Study Group [12]	4-week, randomized placebo-controlled trial	Sodium oxybate, 3, 6, or 9 g, versus placebo	136 narcolepsy with cataplexy subjects	Daily diaries (no of inadvertent naps/sleep attacks) ESS Clinical Global Impression of Change (CGI-c)	Frequency of inadvertent naps/sleep attacks and nightime awakenings, reduced at all doses, becoming significant at the 9 g dose ESS reduced at all doses, becoming significant at the 9 g dose CGI-c demonstrated a dose-related improvement, significant at the 9 g dose
US Xyrem Multicenter Study Group [13]	12-month, open-label trial	Sodium oxybate 6 g nightly, taken in equally divided doses at bedtime and 2.5–4 h later. The study protocol permitted the dose to be increased or decreased in 1.5 g increments at 2 week intervals, based on efficacy response or adverse experiences, but staying within the range of 3–9 g nightly	118 narcolepsy with cataplexy subjects previously enrolled in a 4-week double-blind sodium oxybate trial	Daily diaries (no of inadvertent naps/sleep attacks) ESS CCI-c	Overall improvement in excessive daytime sleepiness, which were significant at 4 weeks and maximal after 8 weeks

Source: Data from [8–13].

Table 25.2 Treatment of cataplexy

References	Methods	Participants	Interventions	Outcome measures	Outcome
The US Xyrem Multicenter Study Group [12]	4-week, randomized placebo-controlled trial	136 narcolepsy with cataplexy subjects	Sodium oxybate, 3, 6, or 9 g, versus placebo	Daily diaries (no of cataplectic attacks) CGI-c	Weekly cataplectic attacks were decreased by sodium oxybate at the 6 g dose and significantly at the 9 g dose. CGI-c demonstrated a dose-related improvement, significant at the 9 g dose
US Xyrem Multicenter Study Group [13]	Method: 12-month, open-label trial	118 narcolepsy subjects previously enrolled in a 4-week double-blind sodium oxybate trial	Sodium oxybate 6 g nightly, taken in equally divided doses at bedtime and 2.5–4 h later. The study protocol permitted the dose to be increased or decreased in 1.5 g increments at 2-week intervals based on efficacy response or adverse experiences, but staying within the range of 3–9 g nightly	Daily diaries (no of cataplectic attacks) CGI-c	Significant decrease in frequency of cataplexy attacks
US Xyrem Multicenter Study Group [15]	Double-blind treatment withdrawal paradigm in patients who had received continuous treatment with sodium oxybate for 7–44 months (mean 21 months)	55 narcolepsy with cataplexy subjects	Subjects enrolled in a 2-week single-blind sodium oxybate treatment phase to establish a baseline for the weekly occurrence of cataplexy, followed by a 2-week double-blind phase in which patients were randomized to receive unchanged drug therapy versus placebo	Daily diaries (no of cataplexy attacks)	The abrupt cessation of sodium oxybate therapy in the placebo patients resulted in a significant increase in the number of cataplexy attacks compared to patients who remained on sodium oxybate
Xyrem International Study Group [16]	8-week, double-blind, placebo-controlled	22 narcolepsy with cataplexy subjects	Subjects randomized to receive 4.5, 6 or 9 g sodium oxybate nightly for 8 weeks versus placebo	Daily diaries (no of cataplexy attacks)	Compared to placebo, nightly doses of 4.5, 6 and 9 g sodium oxybate resulted in statistically significant median decreases in weekly cataplexy attacks of 57.0%, 65.0% and 84.7%, respectively. The decrease in cataplexy at the 4.5 g dose represented a novel finding

Source: Data from [12,13,15,16].

Idiopathic hypersomnia with and without long sleep time

1 *In a subject complaining of excessive daytime sleepiness, prolonged night sleep, and difficulty in awakening, which diagnosis should be evoked and which tests should be performed?*
2 *Which treatment should be established?*
3 *What is the outcome of the treatment of idiopathic hypersomnia with long sleep time?*

There are two types of idiopathic hypersomnia: idiopathic hypersomnia with long sleep time and idiopathic hypersomnia without long sleep time. Both disorders usually occur before 25 years of age. Idiopathic hypersomnia with long sleep time includes a prolonged sleep episode of at least 10 hours and is remarkable for three symptoms: a complaint of constant or recurrent daily excessive sleepiness and unwanted nap(s), longer and less irresistible than in narcolepsy and nonrefreshing regardless of their duration; night sleep is sound, uninterrupted, and prolonged; morning awakening is laborious and sometimes referred to as sleep drunkenness. In addition, it is associated with symptoms suggesting autonomic nervous system dysfunction, including headaches, which may be migrainous in quality, orthostatic hypotension with syncope, and peripheral vascular complaints (Raynaud's-type phenomena with cold digits). Idiopathic hypersomnia without long sleep time stands as isolated excessive daytime sleepiness with nocturnal sleep of normal habitual duration (>6 but <10 hours). Daytime sleep episodes may be more irresistible and more refreshing than in idiopathic hypersomnia with long sleep time, establishing a bridge with narcolepsy without cataplexy. Abnormally, long sleep or severe sleep drunkenness are not classic features of this condition. Because of long-standing nosological uncertainty and the relative rarity of the condition, prevalence studies have not been conducted so far. However, a ratio of 1 to 2 patients with idiopathic hypersomnia, either with or without long sleep time, for every 10 with narcolepsy, is suggested from clinical series.

Clinical scenario

A 24-year-old department manager working on morning shift (6:00–14:00) was referred for great difficulty waking up in the morning. He first got remarks from his superiors and is now on the verge of being fired. This is all the more upsetting to him as he had good marks in his job when he was working on the afternoon shift, and had no problem being in time at his work. He developed excessive daytime sleepiness and difficulty waking up in the morning during late adolescence. He reports having to be awakened by his parents with major difficulty. At present, he lives alone. He does not wake up to the ringing of the alarm clock or to the wake-up call. He has to use a repeating alarm clock and when he eventually wakes up, he is almost confused, very slow, and unable to react adequately to any event. During daytime, he complains of being more or less drowsy, and when he takes an afternoon nap, he may sleep for up to 3–4 hours experiencing the same difficulty to wake up.

Evidence

1 The scenario refers to a typical case of idiopathic hypersomnia with long sleep time. However, laboratory tests are essential to confirm the diagnosis and rule out other hypersomnia conditions. Polysomnographic monitoring of nocturnal sleep demonstrates normal sleep except for its prolonged duration. Sleep efficiency is usually more than 85%. Non-REM (NREM) sleep and REM sleep are in normal proportions. The MSLT demonstrates a mean sleep latency less than 8 minutes, with some exceptions however, and less than two SOREMPs. However, the MSLT seems questionable. Indeed, awakening the patient in the morning in view of the first session of the test precludes documenting the abnormally prolonged night sleep, and the MSLT sessions preclude recording of prolonged unrefreshing daytime sleep episode(s) of major diagnostic value. Thus, other procedures are of potential interest: a 1-week actigraphy or a 24-hours continuous polysomnography on an ad-lib sleep/wake protocol. Hypocretin-1 concentrations in the cerebrospinal fluid are typically normal, differentiating this disease entity from narcolepsy with cataplexy. Differential diagnosis includes upper airway resistance syndrome, hence the need for monitoring esophageal pressure during sleep in the case of multiple arousals documented on polysomnography; narcolepsy without cataplexy characterized by the presence of two or more SOREMPs on the MSLT; hypersomnia associated with psychiatric disorder, in which the complaint of excessive daytime sleepiness is rather similar to that of idiopathic hypersomnia with long sleep time, with the exception of frequent poor sleep at night and typically prolonged sleep latency on the MSLT; posttraumatic hypersomnia in which past history is remarkable for recent severe head trauma; hypersomnia, following a viral infection such as pneumonia, infectious mononucleosis, or Guillain–Barré syndrome, where hypersomnia develops within months after the infection; chronic fatigue syndrome characterized by persistent or relapsing fatigue not resolving with sleep or rest and polysomnography with frequent evidence of alpha intrusion into sleep electroencephalogram (EEG).
2 Historically, the only medications that have often brought partial or intermittent relief have been the stimulants, particularly methylphenidate and amphetamine. Randomized, placebo-controlled trials are lacking in idiopathic hypersomnia with long sleep time and idiopathic hypersomnia without long sleep time. The only available study is an open-label study of modafinil in 18 patients with idiopathic hypersomnia taken globally, dating back to 1988 [17]. In this study, the clinical diagnosis was confirmed by a 24-hours polysomnography. Drowsiness and sleep episodes

were evaluated through sleep diary data. During the second month of treatment, drowsiness and sleep episodes were significantly reduced. However, duration of night sleep and difficulty in awakening were not considered. Apart from this study, there are some clinical reports of morning sleep drunkenness being reduced by administering a small dose of stimulant in the evening or immediately after morning awakening. In addition, a recent study reported decreased sleep drunkenness, shortened nocturnal sleep duration, and relieved daytime sleepiness in five of ten subjects with idiopathic hypersomnia with long sleep time treated with melatonin (2 mg of slow-release melatonin administered at bedtime) [18]. Behavioral treatment possibilities are limited. Naps are of no help as they are both lengthy and nonrefreshing. "Saturating" the subjects with sleep on weekends has been recommended, but does not seem to have a sustained effect.

3 The prognosis for spontaneous improvement of idiopathic hypersomnia is poor. The condition almost always has a stationary course and persists into old age. Clinical experience indicates that modafinil has a sustained effect in some subjects while it vanishes with time in others.

REM-Behavior Disorder in Parkinson's disease

1 *What are predisposing and precipitating factors in RBD?*
2 *What are the available treatments of RBD?*
3 *What is the outcome of RBD with the various treatments available?*

REM-Behavior disorder (RBD) is characterized by abnormal behaviors emerging during REM sleep that cause injury or sleep disruption. RBD is associated with electromyographic (EMG) abnormalities during REM sleep. The EMG demonstrates an excess of muscle tone or phasic EMG twitching activity during REM sleep. There are two forms of RBD: an idiopathic form and a form associated with neurological disorders, mainly synucleinopathies, narcolepsy, and other neurological conditions (e.g., stroke, multiple sclerosis, and brainstem neoplasms). The most remarkable aspect of the association between synucleinopathies and RBD is that the latter can precede the development of the former by years. Two-thirds of men over the age of 50 years initially diagnosed with idiopathic RBD eventually develop a parkinsonian disorder at a mean interval of 13 years from the onset of RBD. Idiopathic RBD is becoming progressively scarce (and may cease to exist) as more patients with RBD are being thoroughly evaluated and meticulously followed for prolonged periods. RBD is a male predominant disorder that usually emerges after the age of 50 years. The prevalence is not known. In a study aimed at evaluating the frequency of RBD in a large group of unselected patients with Parkinson's disease, one-third met the diagnostic criteria of RBD based on polysomnographic recordings. Only one-half of these cases could have been detected by history.

Clinical scenario

A 66-year-old architect was referred for a 7-year history of progressively severe and injurious dream-enacting behavior. He would frequently kick the wall, punch his pillow, and sometimes bite his wife in bed or grab her by the hair while dreaming that he was confronted or attacked by unfamiliar people or animals. One night, while dreaming that his daughter was attacked by a man, he violently punched his wife. This patient was diagnosed recently with Parkinson's disease. Overnight, polysomnography demonstrated classic RBD findings with intermittent loss of REM atonia and increased phasic twitching during REM sleep of the submental, anterior tibialis, and extensor digitorum muscles.

Evidence

1 RBD is associated with underlying neurological disorders, particularly synucleinopathies (e.g., Parkinson's disease, multiple system atrophy, and dementia with Lewy bodies), narcolepsy, and certain medications (e.g., venlafaxine, SSRI, mirtazapine, and other antidepressant agents).

2 The most frequently prescribed treatment of RBD is clonazepam. Treatment is usually immediately active at a dose of 0.5–1.0 mg at bedtime [19]. Despite the dramatic control of clinical symptoms, clonazepam has little effect on the characteristic polysomnographic REM sleep abnormalities. Clonazepam is generally effective and safe. All instances of drug discontinuation result in prompt relapse. An alternative treatment is desirable for those with RBD refractory to clonazepam, for those who experience disturbing adverse effects, mainly excessive daytime sleepiness or ataxia, for those who develop tolerance and for those in whom clonazepam aggravates obstructive sleep apnea syndrome. In these subjects, melatonin is of definite value. According to Boeve *et al.*, RBD was either controlled or significantly improved in 10 of 14 patients, at doses of 3–12 mg [20]. The mean duration of follow-up was 14 months (range 9–25 months), with eight patients experiencing continued benefit with melatonin beyond 12 months of therapy. However, five patients reported adverse effects, morning headaches in two, morning sleepiness in two, and delirium/hallucinations in one. These symptoms resolved with decreased dosage. Another possibility is pramipexole, a dopaminergic D2–D3 receptor agonist, which was shown to be active in five of eight patients with apparent idiopathic RBD [21].

3 Long-term outcome of RBD with available medications is unclear. The main risk of clonazepam is the development of tolerance, although little evidence of it was reported in the clinical outcome of 70 consecutive cases with RBD [19]. As for melatonin, the actual risk of protracted consumption remains unknown. Preliminary observations suggest that long-term melatonin administration is associated with decreased semen quality, but the antigonadal effects of exogenous melatonin on the reproductive hormones are not conclusively established.

Insomnia in Parkinson's disease

1 *In patients with Parkinson's disease, what should be done first for those complaining of insomnia?*
2 *In this particular patient, which therapeutic program can be proposed?*
3 *What is the outcome of insomnia?*

Parkinson's disease is primarily a disease of the elderly. The prevalence increases with age from 0.9% among persons with age 65–69 years to 5% among persons with age 80–84 years. Sleep problems are common. In one series of insomniac patients with Parkinson's disease, 67% had difficulty initiating sleep and 88% had difficulty maintaining sleep. Insomnia in patients with Parkinson's disease may depend on several factors, including Parkinson's disease-related motor symptoms occurring at night, use of sleep-altering medications, psychiatric symptoms, especially depression and dementia, and other sleep disorders.

Scenario

A 65-year-old retired bus driver, affected with Parkinson's disease for 7 years, was referred for insomnia. The subject complained of frequent awakenings throughout the night, particularly in the second half of it, of decreased total sleep time, and of daytime fatigue. Moreover, interview of the subject revealed awakenings associated with paresthesias of the legs forcing him to get up and walk around. On examination, he was found to be very slow in his movements and often sat motionless with an expressionless face. His right hand shook. There was cogwheel rigidity of his right wrist and a shuffling gait. Wearing off had developed within the last 6 months. There was no obvious cognitive impairment, but some degree of depression. The treatment was four carbidopa/levodopa (Sinemet) 250 mg, four ropinirole 3 mg, and one zolpidem tablets at night.

Evidence

1 Given the plurality of possible contributing factors, it is of utmost importance to assess the respective part of each of the factors involved in the insomnia of a patient with Parkinson's disease. Parkinson's disease-related nocturnal motor symptoms most often reflect the presence of motor fluctuations ("on off" phenomena, "wearing off") during the day, and are often due to nocturnal under-dosage of dopamine drugs. In addition, nocturia and urinary incontinence may participate in the disturbance of sleep. Accordingly, a careful description from both the patient and his/her primary caretaker is essential to determine the behavior of the patient during the night. Drug regimen and the time of day when drugs are taken must be considered, given their ability to alter sleep patterns in patients with Parkinson's disease. Another issue is underlying depression and/or cognitive impairment which are associated with sleep

fragmentation and sleep–wake cycle disruption. Finally, patients with Parkinson's disease may suffer from other sleep disorders such as restless legs syndrome, obstructive sleep apnea syndrome, or RBD. Polysomnography may be indicated in some cases.

2 The severity of nocturnal disturbances in patients with Parkinson's disease contrasts with the paucity of clinical trials specifically designed for the treatment of these Parkinson's disease-related sleep disturbances. In the aforementioned scenario, Parkinson's disease-related motor symptoms were obviously important, particularly in the second half of the night. Consequently, adding a small dose of dopaminergic medication at bedtime, such as 100 mg of L-dopa combined with 25 mg of carbidopa (Sinemet 25/100), with a second similar dose at 2 or 3 a.m., if the patient awakens is a possible option. Alternatively, a bedtime dose of a controlled-release formulation containing 200 mg of L-dopa and 50 mg of carbidopa can be proposed [22–24]. Moreover, adding a catechol-O-methyltransferase (COMT) inhibitor may be useful to provide a long-acting antiparkinsonism benefit. Because of the variability of response to dopaminergic medications, trials of several different agents in varying doses are usually warranted if sleep is not improved. Of note is that dopaminergic medications may induce sleep problems such as vivid dreams or nightmares. In addition, this patient was probably affected with restless legs syndrome responsible for awakenings with paresthesias of the legs. However, the patient was already under dopamine agonists, which have been proved to be effective in treating restless legs syndrome, and the dose required to treat restless legs syndrome tends to be lower than that used to treat motor symptoms of Parkinson's disease [25]. Finally, treatment of the associated depression may lead to an improvement of nocturnal disturbances. One possibility is tricyclic antidepressants. SSRIs can also be an option, but they have an activating effect and tend to increase disruption of normal sleep architecture [26].

3 The global evaluation of nocturnal disturbances and the chosen therapeutic intervention should improve the nocturnal disturbances experienced by this patient. However, it is important to realize that management of nocturnal disturbances may sometimes be at the expense of some other symptoms of Parkinson's disease, to the point that it may be advisable in some cases not to treat nocturnal disturbances.

Conclusion

Much effort has been invested in further identifying sleep disorders and sleep disorders associated with neurological conditions, and in designing relevant laboratory tests. On the other hand, most of the available therapeutic interventions refer to common sense-based practice, and there is still an urgent need for randomized-controlled trials in many areas of sleep disorders, to assess the validity of the current interventions.

References

1 Good, D.C., Henkle, J.Q., Gelber, D. *et al.* (1996) Sleep-disordered breathing and poor functional outcome after stroke. *Stroke*, **27**, 252–259.

2 Wessendorf, T.E., Wang, Y.M., Thilmann, A.F. *et al.* (2001) Treatment of obstructive sleep apnoea with nasal continuous positive airway pressure in stroke. *European Respiratory Journal*, **18**, 623–629.

3 Sandberg, O., Franklin, K.A., Bucht, G. *et al.* (2001) Nasal continuous positive airway pressure in stroke patients with sleep apnoea: a randomized treatment study. *European Respiratory Journal*, **18**, 630–634.

4 Ryan, C.M., Bayley, M., Green, R. *et al.* (2011) Influence of continuous positive airway pressure on outcomes of rehabilitation in stroke patients with obstructive sleep apnea. *Stroke*, **42**(4), 1062–1067.

5 Martinez-Garcia, M.A., Galiano-Blancart, R., Roman-Sanchez, P. *et al.* (2005) Continuous positive airway pressure treatment in sleep apnea prevents new vascular events after ischemic stroke. *Chest*, **128**, 2123–2129.

6 Martinez-Garcia, M.A. & Soler-Cataluna, J.J. (2009) Continuous Positive Airway Pressure Treatment reduces Mortality in patients with ischemic stroke and obstructive sleep apnea: A 5 year follow – up study. *American Journal of Respiratory and Critical Care Medicine*, **180**, 36–41.

7 Mignot, E., Lammers, G.J., Ripley, B. *et al.* (2002) The role of cerebrospinal fluid hypocretin measurement in the diagnosis of narcolepsy and other hypersomnias. *Archives of Neurology*, **59**, 1553–1562.

8 Billiard, M., Besset, A., Montplaisir, J. *et al.* (1994) Modafinil: a double blind multicenter study. *Sleep*, **17**(**Suppl**), S107–S112.

9 Broughton, R., Fleming, J.A.E., Georges, C.F.P. *et al.* (1997) Randomized, double blind, placebo-controlled crossover trial of modafinil in the treatment of excessive daytime sleepiness in narcolepsy. *Neurology*, **49**, 444–451.

10 US Modafinil in Narcolepsy Multicenter Study Group (1998) Randomized trial of modafinil for the treatment of pathological somnolence in narcolepsy. *Annals of Neurology*, **434**, 88–97.

11 US Modafinil in Narcolepsy Multicenter Study Group (2000) Randomized trial of modafinil as a treatment for the excessive daytime somnolence of narcolepsy. *Neurology*, **54**, 1166–1175.

12 US Xyrem Multicenter Study Group (2002) A randomized, doubleblind, placebo-controlled multicenter trial comparing the effects of three doses of orally administered sodium oxybate with placebo for the treatment of narcolepsy. *Sleep*, **25**, 42–49.

13 US Xyrem Multicenter Study Group (2003) A 12-month, open-label multi-center extension trial of orally administered sodium oxybate for the treatment of narcolepsy. *Sleep*, **26**, 31–35.

14 Harsh, J.R., Hayduk, R., Rosenberg, R. *et al.* (2006 Apr) The efficacy and safety of armodafinil as treatment for adults with excessive sleepiness associated with narcolepsy. *Current Medical Research and Opinion*, **22**(4), 761–774.

15 Xyrem International Study Group (2005) Further evidence supporting the use of sodium oxybate for the treatment of cataplexy: a double-blind placebo-controlled study in 228 patients. *Sleep Medicine*, **6**, 415–421.

16 US Xyrem Multicenter Study Group (2004) Sodium oxybate demonstrates long-term efficacy for the treatment of cataplexy in patients with narcolepsy. *Sleep Medicine*, **5**, 119–123.

17 Mignot E. & Nishino S. (2005) Emerging therapies in narcolepsy-cataplexy. *Sleep*, **28**(6), 754–763.

18 Bastuji, H. & Jouvet, M. (1988) Successful treatment of idiopathic hypersomnia and narcolepsy with modafinil. *Progress in Neuro-Psychopharmacology & Biological Psychiatry*, **12**, 695–700.

19 Montplaisir, J. & Fantini, L. (2001) Idiopathic hypersomnia. A diagnostic dilemma. *Sleep Medicine Reviews*, **5**, 361–362.. c09.qxd 3/16/09 12:21 PM Page 77.

20 Schenck, C.H. & Mahowald, M.W. (1990) Polysomnographic, neurologic, psychiatric, and clinical outcome report on 70 consecutive cases with REM sleep behavior disorder (RBD): sustained clonazepam efficacy in 89.5% of 57 treated patients. *Cleveland Clinic Journal of Medicine*, **57**(**Suppl**), S9–S23.

21 Boeve, B.F., Silber, M.H. & Ferman, T.J. (2003) Melatonin for treatment of REM sleep behaviour disorder in neurologic disorders: results in 14 patients. *Sleep Medicine*, **4**, 281–284.

22 Fantini, M.L., Gagnon, J.F., Filipini, M.D. *et al.* (2003) The effects of pramipexole in REM sleep behavior disorder. *Neurology*, **61**, 1418–1420.

23 Jansen, E.N. & Meerwaldt, J.D. (1990) Madopar HBS in nocturnal symptoms of Parkinson's disease. *Advances in Neurology*, **53**, 527–531.

24 Pahwa, R., Busenbark, K., Huber, S.J. *et al.* (1993) Clinical experience with controlled-release carbidopa/levodopa in Parkinson's disease. *Neurology*, **43**, 677–681.

25 Garcia-Borreguero, D., Odin, P. & Serrano, C. (2003) Restless legs syndrome and PD: a review of the evidence for a possible association. *Neurology*, **61**(**Suppl. 3**), S49–S55.

26 Force, M.D.T. (2002) Management of Parkinson's disease: an evidence based review. *Movement Disorders*, **17**(**Suppl. 4**), S1–S165.

CHAPTER 26

Acute migraine attacks

E. Anne MacGregor[1], Rashmi B. Halker[2], and Bert B. Vargas[2]

[1]*Centre for Neuroscience & Trauma, BICMS, Barts and the London School of Medicine and Dentistry, London, UK*
[2]*Department of Neurology, Mayo Clinic, Phoenix, AZ*

Background

Headache is the most common neurological condition in the world, with more than 90% of the population reporting headaches at some time in their lives [1]. All currently recognized primary and secondary headache disorders are classified within the International Classification of Headache Disorders, 3rd ed., beta (ICHD-3β), which is divided into primary headaches, secondary headaches, and neuralgias and other headaches [2] (Table 26.1). Among primary headache disorders, tension-type headache is the most prevalent worldwide, but in patients seeking medical help, migraine is by far the most frequently presenting headache subtype [3].

Migraine is more prevalent than diabetes, epilepsy, and asthma combined, affecting more than 14% (7.6% of men and 18.3% of women) of the UK population – over 6 million people [4]. Migraine has been ranked by the World Health Organization (WHO) as 19th among all diseases worldwide causing disability (12th in women) [5]. WHO has also recognized the burdens, both individual and societal, that exist as well as the enormous financial costs to society through lost productivity [6]. Research shows that in the United Kingdom alone, an estimated 5.7 working days are lost per year for every working or student migraineur and each working day up to 90,000 people are absent from work or school as a result of migraine [4]. Prevalence of migraine varies with age, rising through early adult life, and peaking during the most productive working years.

Despite all these facts, the impact of migraine is frequently minimized and is often not recognized as a public health problem; it is widely underdiagnosed and undertreated, in children and adults [7,8]. It has been estimated that in the United Kingdom and the United States around two-thirds of patients with migraine never consult their doctor, are misdiagnosed, and are treated (or treat themselves) with only nonspecific over-the-counter medication [7]. Many patients would benefit from correct diagnosis and medical management (especially when their treatment course is complicated by medication-overuse headache) or from treatment with more specific drugs (notably the triptans for migraine sufferers). Accurate diagnosis and appropriate treatment are cost-effective by minimizing time lost from work and burden placed on the families of sufferers as well as reducing personal and financial costs of headache [9].

Case scenario

A 43-year-old woman presents with headaches since her early teens. She recalls that when they first started, she had two or three severe headache attacks per year lasting at least 24 hours if untreated. She would feel nauseous and noticed that the headaches occasionally improved once she vomited. While in college, they increased in frequency and severity to the point where, in her final year, she began to have headache on most days and attempted to control them with over-the-counter analgesics. She sought medical advice and was told that she had chronic sinusitis. After graduating from college, the pattern initially reverted back to infrequent attacks but after she had children she began to experience monthly attacks with her periods. They would only last a day and would respond to the over-the-counter analgesics. For the last couple of years the headaches have again become more frequent and severe. She now has two to three severe headache attacks per month with nausea, each lasting 2–3 days even after using her usual painkillers, and she is missing many days of work. Her doctor has suggested that she is "stressed" and advised antidepressants. She was angered by this suggestion, as between attacks she feels completely well. She has asked to see you for a second opinion. She wants to know why no one has suggested a brain scan and why she cannot just have some stronger painkillers.

Framing answerable clinical questions

Even though the most likely headache disorder to present in the outpatient setting is migraine, you are concerned that the

---

Evidence-Based Neurology: Management of Neurological Disorders, Second Edition. Edited by Bart M. Demaerschalk and Dean M. Wingerchuk.
© 2015 John Wiley & Sons, Ltd. Published 2015 by John Wiley & Sons, Ltd.

Table 26.1 *The International Classification of Headache Disorders*, 3rd Edition

Primary headaches

1. Migraine, *including*:
   1.1 Migraine without aura
   1.2 Migraine with aura
2. Tension-type headache, *including*:
   2.1 Infrequent episodic tension-type headache
   2.2 Frequent episodic tension-type headache
   2.3 Chronic tension-type headache
3. Cluster headache and other trigeminal autonomic cephalalgias, *including*:
   3.1 Cluster headache
4. Other primary headaches

Secondary headaches

5. Headache attributed to head and/or neck trauma, *including*:
   5.2 Chronic post-traumatic headache
6 Headache attributed to cranial or cervical vascular disorder, *including*:
   6.2.2 Headache attributed to subarachnoid haemorrhage
   6.4.1 Headache attributed to giant cell arteritis
7. Headache attributed to non-vascular intracranial disorder, *including*:
   7.1.1 Headache attributed to idiopathic intracranial hypertension
   7.4 Headache attributed to intracranial neoplasm
8. Headache attributed to a substance or its withdrawal, *including*:
   8.1.3 Carbon monoxide-induced headache
   8.1.4 Alcohol-induced headache
   8.2 Medication-overuse headache
   8.2.1 Ergotamine-overuse headache
   8.2.2 Triptan-overuse headache
   8.2.3 Analgesic-overuse headache
9. Headache attributed to infection, *including*:
   9.1 Headache attributed to intracranial infection
10. Headache attributed to disorder of homoeostasis
11. Headache or facial pain attributed to disorder of cranium, neck, eyes, ears, nose, sinuses, teeth, mouth or other facial or cranial structures, *including*:
    11.2.1 Cervicogenic headache
    11.3.1 Headache attributed to acute glaucoma
12. Headache attributed to psychiatric disorder

Neuralgias and other headaches

13. Cranial neuralgias, central and primary facial pain and other headaches, *including*:
    13.1 Trigeminal neuralgia
14. Other headache, cranial neuralgia, central or primary facial pain

Source: Data from IHS 2013 [2].

increased frequency of her headaches might suggest underlying pathology. She has been diagnosed in the past with chronic sinusitis and, most recently, depression. Are these valid diagnoses?

You frame six specific questions to address.

1 In middle-aged people, what is the likelihood that recurrent headaches are migraine? [baseline risk]

2 In middle-aged people, what is the utility of investigations and brain scans in the diagnosis of headache? [baseline risk]
3 For people with migraine, which nonspecific acute treatments are effective in increasing the probability of response or pain-free at 2 hours? [therapy]
4 For people with migraine, which specific acute treatments are effective in increasing the probability of response or pain-free at 2 hours? How great are the adverse events? [therapy]
5 For people with migraine, which treatments for prophylaxis are effective in reducing the frequency of migraine by 50%? What are the likely adverse events? [therapy]
6 For people with migraine, what is the likelihood of attacks persisting lifelong? [prognosis]

Critical review of the evidence

1. Diagnosis

In middle-aged people, what is the likelihood that the headaches are migraine?

Migraine is the most common form of disabling headache presenting to doctors. Some studies suggest that the lifetime prevalence of migraine in women is as great as 25%, compared with only 8% in men [10]. Adults with migraine describe episodic attacks of moderate to severe headache lasting between 4 hours and 3 days, with associated nausea or vomiting and photophobia and phonophobia [2]. During attacks, activity is limited as it commonly exacerbates the pain. Less commonly, attacks are preceded by a neurological aura, typically visual, lasting 5–60 minutes typically resolving before the onset of headache. Even though migraine is equally common in both sexes before puberty, there is increased female prevalence following menarche [11]. This difference between the sexes becomes greater with increasing age, peaking during the early 40s and declining thereafter [12,13]. This sex difference during the reproductive years is generally considered to result from the additional trigger of the monthly fluctuation of estrogen with the menstrual cycle, which can be particularly exacerbated during perimenopause [14].

Daily and near-daily headaches are frequently complicated by medication overuse, as using acute analgesics for more than 2–3 days per week can often contribute to an increase in headache frequency over time [2]. Medication overuse must always be managed because it can mask the diagnosis, cause other illnesses, and make the effective treatment of primary headache disorders difficult. Furthermore, many migraine sufferers are misdiagnosed as having either sinusitis or tension-type headache.

2. CT scan

In middle-aged people, what is the utility of investigations and brain scans in the diagnosis of headache?

In clinical practice, a primary concern is differentiation of primary headaches from secondary sinister headaches.

Taking a careful history is a crucial step in diagnosis of primary headaches, together with ensuring a normal neurological examination. When first evaluating a patient for headache, it is extremely important to screen for any worrisome features. The mnemonic SNOOP4 is helpful in identifying red flags in a patient's history (Box 26.1) [15]. If red flags are present, additional investigations, including neuroimaging, are warranted. A separate history is required for each type of headache reported, particularly noting the course and duration of each. Much of the time, what patients perceive to be distinct separate headache types are simply different manifestations of migraine. Consequently, it is imperative that practitioners be familiar with the diagnostic criteria for migraine [see Box 26.1]. Many specialists advocate the use of a diary, which patients can use to establish a temporal pattern for their headache and to document important associated features which may aid in diagnosis. A review of four studies of screening questions for migraine in patients with headache identified five predictors: pulsating, duration 4–72 hours, unilateral, nausea, and disabling [15]. If three predictors are present, the likelihood ratio for migraine is 3.5 (95% CI, 1.3–9.2), increasing to 24 (95% CI, 1.5–388) if four predictors are present.

BOX 26.1: SNOOP4 Red Flags:

Systemic symptoms and signs
Neurologic symptoms or signs
Onset: peak severity at onset or within 1 minute
Older age of onset (>40 years)
Progressive: change in pattern from previous headache
Postural/positional aggravation
Precipitated by Valsalva
Papilledema
Data from Dodick D [15].

Investigations, including neuroimaging, generally do not contribute to the diagnosis [16]. Imaging is necessary only if secondary headache is suspected because of undefined headache, or the presence of red flags including atypical symptoms, persistent neurological or psychopathological abnormalities, or abnormal findings on neurologic examination [16].

3. Nonspecific acute treatments

For people with migraine, which nonspecific acute treatments are effective in increasing the probability of response or pain-free at 2 hours?

Analgesics and nonsteroidal anti-inflammatory drugs

Analgesics are the first-line acute treatment for migraine. Many analgesics have been shown in multiple trials to be more effective than placebo, including aspirin (500–1000 mg), diclofenac (50–100 mg), flurbiprofen (100–300 mg), ibuprofen (400–2400 mg), naproxen (750–1250 mg), acetaminophen (1000 mg), piroxicam (40 mg), and tolfenamic acid (200–400 mg) [17–21]. Several trials have examined the efficacy of a proprietary combination of acetaminophen, aspirin, and caffeine; each trial found that the combination analgesic was significantly more effective than placebo [21] (Table 26.2).

Antiemetics

Nausea and vomiting are commonly associated with migraine. For some individuals, these symptoms can be far more distressing and difficult to control than the headache itself and can make it difficult to treat with oral medications. Several antiemetics are commonly used although clinical trial data are limited. The recognition that gastric stasis accompanies migraine led to trials with gastroprokinetic agents metoclopramide (10 mg po, im or iv), and domperidone (20–30 mg po or pr), which may have the additional advantage of enhancing the bioavailability of concomitant drugs given orally to treat migraine [23]. Chlorpromazine (25–50 mg im), metoclopramide (10 mg iv or im), and prochlorperazine (10 mg iv or im) have also been used as single-agent therapies for migraine with success [24].

4. Specific acute treatments

For people with migraine, which specific acute treatments are effective in increasing the probability of response or pain-free at 2 hours? How great are the adverse events?

Triptans

Sumatriptan, the first triptan to become available, was initially available only in its subcutaneous form. At least 28 placebo-controlled trials have been demonstrated that 6 mg of subcutaneous sumatriptan is better than placebo in providing headache relief at 1 hour [25]. Twenty-four trials have also established that oral sumatriptan is better than placebo for the acute treatment of migraine. It is well tolerated, though minor adverse events are not uncommon [26]. Overall, the proportion of patients reporting relief with oral sumatriptan is lower than that with subcutaneous sumatriptan [27]. There is also evidence to support that a combination of sumatriptan and naproxen is more effective than either drug alone [28].

In addition to sumatriptan, six other triptans are commercially available: almotriptan, eletriptan, frovatriptan, naratriptan, rizatriptan, and zolmitriptan. A systematic review and meta-analysis that took data from 53 trials involving over 24,000 patients compared all oral triptans against sumatriptan (at a dose of 100 mg) as the comparator [22]. All the triptans were found to be more effective than placebo at relieving headache and other symptoms of migraine. The typical end point was the headache response

Table 26.2 Nonspecific acute treatments for migraine

Types of study (reference)	Intervention	Outcome	Number of patients (number of trials)	Control group risk	Absolute risk reduction	NNT (95% CI)
SR [20]	Tolfenamic acid 200 mg versus placebo	2 hours response	84 (1)	29%	48%	2.1 (1.5–3.5)
SR [20]	Aspirin 900 mg plus metoclopramide 10 mg versus placebo	2 hours response 2 hours pain-free	749 (N/A) 753 (3)	25% 7%	32% 11%	3.2 (2.6–4.0) 8.6 (6.2–14)
SR [20]	Paracetamol 500 mg plus aspirin 500 mg plus caffeine 130 mg versus placebo	2 hours response	1220 (3)	No data	No data	3.9 (3.2–4.9)
SR [20]	Paracetamol 1000 mg versus placebo	2 hours response	289 (1)	39%	19%	5.2 (3.3–13)
RCT [19]	Aspirin 1000 mg versus placebo	2 hours response 2 hours pain-free	401 (1)	34% 6%	18% 14%	5.6 7.1
RCT [17]	Ibuprofen 200 mg versus 400 mg versus 600 mg versus placebo	2 hours response 2 hours pain-free	729 (1)	50% 13%	14–22% 12–16%	4.5–7.1 6.3–8.3
RCT [18]	Diclofenac 50 mg (tablet or sachet) versus placebo	2 hours response 2 hours pain-free	328 (1)	24% 12%	17.5–22% 7–13%	4.5–5.7 7 sachet (5.5–13.4) 15.8 tablet (8.6–96.2)

SR: systematic review; RCT: randomised controlled trial; NNT: number needed to treat; CI: confidence interval.
Source: Ferrari *et al.* [22]. Reproduced with permission of International Headache Society.

at 2 hours (a positive response being defined as reduction of pain from moderate or severe at baseline to absent or mild by 2 hours) (Figures 26.1 and 26.2).

More stringent parameters are pain-free at 2 hours (reduction of pain from moderate or severe at baseline to absent by 2 hours), sustained pain-free at 24 hours (reduction of pain from moderate or severe at baseline to absent by 2 hours, headache does not return, and no other headache medication taken), and adverse event data are shown in Table 26.3.

A number of conclusions can be drawn about the efficacies of the various oral triptans:
• Fastest onset to effect is with subcutaneous sumatriptan.
• Eletriptan and rizatriptan are the most rapidly acting oral triptans, with a T_{max} of approximately 30 minutes.
• Oral almotriptan, sumatriptan, and zolmitriptan have a T_{max} of approximately 45–60 minutes.
• Frovatriptan and naratriptan are the slowest, taking up to 4 hours before effect is seen.
• Intranasal zolmitriptan is faster acting than oral zolmitriptan.
• Pain-free rates at 2 hours and sustained pain-free rates over 24 hours are higher for almotriptan, eletriptan, and rizatriptan than for sumatriptan.
• The highest likelihood of consistent success is with almotriptan, eletriptan, and rizatriptan.
• The lowest rate of adverse events is with almotriptan, eletriptan, and naratriptan.

Current guidelines suggest the following approach to symptomatic treatment of migraine, based on the available evidence and expert consensus [21,29]:
• Initial treatment with NSAID with or without a prokinetic antiemetic is a reasonable choice for mild to moderate migraine.
• Initial treatment with a triptan is a reasonable choice when the headache is moderate to severe or when the migraine, whatever its severity, has failed to respond to nonspecific medication in the past.
• It is advisable to choose a specific triptan and route of administration based on time to peak severity of headache and ability to tolerate oral medications (which can be a significant problem in migraineurs who experience significant nausea or vomiting).
• Specifically, intranasal zolmitriptan or subcutaneous sumatriptan may be useful in patients with nausea and vomiting or when a rapid response is important.

A rational hierarchy of the use of triptans has been proposed (Table 26.4).

Triptans are more effective when taken while the headache is mild.

Relapse of headache, typically the day following initial treatment, is a significant problem in clinical practice, the rate being 15–40%. The highest relapse rate is associated with subcutaneous sumatriptan and the lowest with naratriptan and frovatriptan. If migraine relapses after successful

(a)

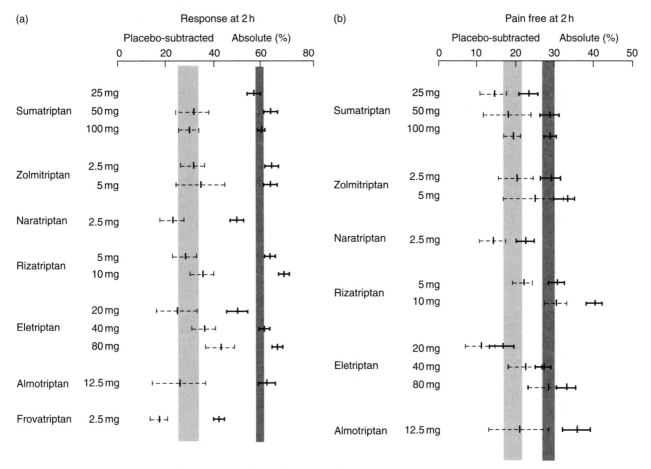

Figure 26.1 Data (mean and 95% CI) for headache response at 2 hour (a) and pain-free at 2 hour (b) are shown for each triptan. Absolute and placebo-subtracted outcomes are presented with the hatched region being the 95% CI envelope for sumatriptan 100 mg. (Source: Ferrari *et al.* [22]. Reproduced with permission of International Headache Society.)

treatment, a second dose of triptan can be given. There is also some evidence that the combination of a triptan and an NSAID reduces the likelihood of relapse [30].

Contraindications to triptans include coronary artery disease, stroke, uncontrolled hypertension, basilar-type migraine, and hemiplegic migraine.

Ergot derivatives

The evidence for the efficacy of ergot derivatives in the symptomatic treatment of migraine is inconsistent, and their use is largely based on long-standing and wide clinical experience. A review of 18 trials found that oral ergotamine was more effective than placebo for some parameters in seven trials, but no better than placebo in three trials [31].

There are few studies on non-oral routes of ergotamine (rectal, sublingual, nasal, and inhaled). Since oral bioavailability is poor, these other routes should, theoretically, be advantageous. An evidence-based expert consensus statement has brought in recommendations for the use of ergotamine (Table 26.5).

Dihydroergotamine can be administered intramuscularly, intravenously, subcutaneously, and intranasally but few trials have assessed its efficacy.

Ergot derivatives have been used less commonly since the triptans became available, but they still have a place in the management of migraine.

Contraindications to ergot derivatives are essentially the same as for the triptans. Similar to triptans, there is risk of medication overuse headache if taken too often, and hence the frequency of intake should be restricted to a maximum of 9 days per month.

5. Prophylaxis

For people with migraine, which prophylactic treatments are effective in reducing the frequency of migraine by at least 50%? What are possible adverse events?

Prophylactic drugs aim to reduce the frequency of migraine attacks, their duration, and their severity. Agents used include antihypertensives (including beta-blockers and calcium-channel blockers), antidepressants, anticonvulsants,

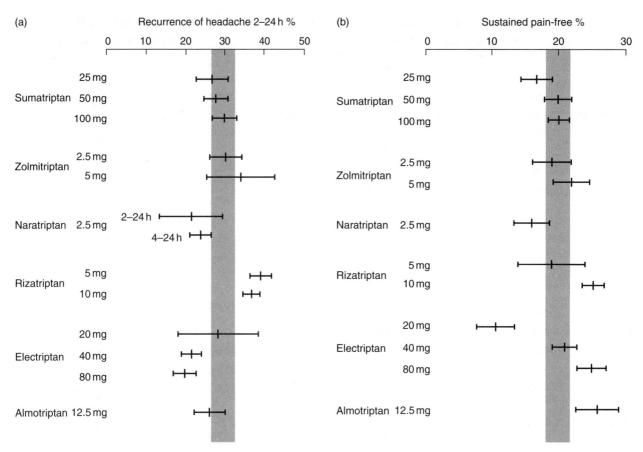

Figure 26.2 Data (mean and 95% CI) for headache recurrence from 2–24 hours (a) and sustained pain-free (b) are presented with the hatched region being the 95% CI envelope for sumatriptan 100 mg. For naratriptan, the recurrence rate is given for the interval 4–24 hours post dose (as presented in the original publications) and for 2–24 hours post dose (after recalculating the data). (Source: Ferrari *et al.* [22]. Reproduced with permission of International Headache Society.)

and NSAIDs. Overall, about one-third of patients who are treated with prophylactic agents can be expected to have a 50% reduction in the frequency of their headaches (Table 26.6).

A second or third prophylactic agent taken concomitantly may be needed in some cases.

Guidelines published by the American Academy of Neurology suggest the following indications for prophylactic treatment of migraine, based on the available evidence and expert consensus [35]:
• Recurrent migraine that, in the patient's opinion, significantly interferes with his/her daily routine in spite of acute treatment.
• Frequent headaches.
  ○ Acute therapies cannot be used because of contraindications, failure, overuse, or adverse effects.
• Cost considerations.
• Patient preference.
• The presence of uncommon migraine conditions that may predispose to permanent neurological sequelae, such as hemiplegic migraine, basilar-type migraine, migraine with prolonged aura, or migrainous infarction.

The guidelines go on to give further consensus-based recommendations for selecting the most appropriate prophylactic medication:
• Start with medications that have the highest level of evidence-based efficacy.
• With any medication, start with the lowest dose that has been shown to be effective, and increase it slowly until clinical benefits are achieved for the patient in the absence of, or until limited by, adverse effects.
• Give each medication an adequate trial, which in many cases may mean 2–3 months.
• Consider reducing the dose or even discontinuing the medication if headaches are well controlled after 3–6 months.
• Long-acting formulations may improve compliance.
• Establish that any agent chosen is not contraindicated in any coexisting illness.
• Choose an agent that may be beneficial in any coexisting illness, remembering that some conditions are more common in people with migraine (e.g., anxiety disorders, affective disorders, stroke, myocardial infarction, epilepsy, and Raynaud's phenomenon).

Table 26.3 Meta-analysis of triptans: NNTs of 2-hours pain-free and 24-hours sustained pain-free and NNH

Intervention	Number of participants (number of trials)	Outcome	Absolute risk reduction/increase (95% CI)	NNT or NNH (95% CI)	Ratio of NNH/NNT
Sumatriptan 100 mg versus placebo	2071 (9)	2 hour pain-free	19.5 (17.3; 21.8)	5.1 (4.6–5.8)	1.5
		24 hours sustained pain-free	20.0 (18.2; 21.3)	5.0 (4.7–5.5)	1.5
		Adverse events	13.2 (8.6; 17.8)	7.6 (5.6–11.6)	
Sumatriptan 50 mg versus placebo	583 (3)	2 hour pain-free	18.0 (11.7; 24.3)	5.6 (4.1–8.5)	2.3
		24 hours sustained pain-free	19.8 (17.8; 21.8)	5.1 (4.6–5.6)	2.5
		Adverse events	7.8 (2.6; 13.1)	12.8 (7.6–38)	
Zolmitriptan 2.5 mg versus placebo	1320 (3)	2 hour pain-free	20.4 (15.6; 25.1)	4.9 (4.0–6.4)	1.3
		24 hours sustained pain-free	19.0 (16.1; 21.8)	5.3 (4.6–6.2)	1.2
		Adverse events	15.9 (9.6; 22.1)	6.3 (4.5–10.4)	
Zolmitriptan 5 mg versus placebo	1596 (5)	2 hour pain-free	25.2 (16.9; 33.5)	4.0 (3.0–5.9)	1
		24 hours sustained pain-free	21.9 (19.3; 24.6)	4.6 (4.1–5.2)	0.9
		Adverse events	24.5 (15.5; 33.5)	4.1 (3.0–6.5)	
Rizatriptan 10 mg versus placebo	4437 (11)	2 hour pain-free	30.4 (27.5; 33.2)	3.3 (3.0–3.6)	2.2
		24 hours sustained pain-free	25.3 (23.7; 26.9)	3.9 (3.7–4.2)	1.9
		Adverse events	13.5 (10.6; 16.3)	7.4 (6.1–9.4)	
Eletriptan 40 mg versus placebo	2894 (7)	2 hour pain-free	27.2 (25.2; 29.2)	3.7 (3.4–4.0)	3.7
		24 hours sustained pain-free	20.9 (19.1; 22.7)	4.8 (4.4–5.2)	2.9
		Adverse events	7.3 (2.7; 11.8)	13.7 (8.5–37)	
Almotriptan 12.5 mg versus placebo	1074 (3)	2 hour pain-free	21.0 (13.3; 28.7)	4.8 (3.5–7.5)	11.7
		24 hours sustained pain-free	25.9 (22.7; 29.1)	3.9 (3.4–4.4)	14.3
		Adverse events	1.8 (−2.7; 6.2)	56 (16.1–no harm)	
Naratriptan 5 mg versus placebo	2023 (5)	2 hour pain-free	14.1 (10.7; 17.5)	7.0 (5.7–9.3)	6.0
		24 hours sustained pain-free	15.9 (13.4; 18.5)	6.3 (5.4–7.5)	6.7
		Adverse events	2.4 (−2.2; 7.0)	42 (14.2–no harm)	
Frovatriptan 2.5 mg versus placebo	2892 (5)	2 hour pain-free			Approximately 10

Source: Adapted from Ferrari *et al.* [22] with permission.

Table 26.4 Proposed rational hierarchy for the use of triptans

Use	Dose regimen
Appropriate for first use of a triptan	Almotriptan 12.5 mg, eletriptan 40 mg, sumatriptan 50 mg or zolmitriptan 2.5 mg orally
When greater efficacy is needed	Eletriptan 80 mg or rizatriptan 10 mg, sumatriptan 100 mg or zolmitriptan 5 mg orally or sumatriptan 20 mg nasal spray
When a rapid response is important above all	Sumatriptan 6 mg subcutaneously or zolmitriptan 5 mg intranasal
When nausea or vomiting precludes oral therapy	Sumatriptan 6 mg subcutaneously or zolmitriptan 5 mg intranasal
When side effects are troublesome with other triptans	Naratriptan 2.5 mg or almotriptan 12.5 mg orally or frovatriptan 2.5mg
When headache relapse is a problem	Ergotamine tartrate 1–2 mg may be helpful

Source: Data from MacGregor *et al.* [29].

Beta-blockers

There is extensive clinical experience of using beta-blockers in the prophylaxis of migraine, and multiple clinical trials have been shown to be 60–80% effective in bringing about a reduction of more than 50% in the frequency of attacks. Propranolol has been the most extensively studied, and there is consistent evidence for its effectiveness at daily doses of 120–240 mg [32]. Propranolol, metoprolol, and timolol have a level A recommendation, indicating there have been at least two class 1 trials demonstrating their effectiveness [36]. Atenolol and nadolol have a level B recommendation based on the strength of the available studies. Pindolol, a

Table 26.5 Recommendations for the use of ergotamine

Parameter	Recommendations	Comments
Which patients?	Patients requiring migraine-specific therapy	When a migraine-specific therapy is indicated, a triptan is a better choice than ergotamine for most patients.
	Patients established on ergotamine	Patients who are responding satisfactorily, have no contraindications and no signs of dose escalation, should not usually be switched to a triptan.
Special cases	Patients with very long attacks	Attacks lasting >48 hours may be usefully treated with ergotamine
	Patients with frequent headache relapse	Headache relapse is probably less likely with ergotamine
Frequency of dosing	Once a week or six times a month	Ergotamine-induced headache and rebound headache are associated with frequent use. This can be limited by restricting ergotamine consumption and encouraging use of a preventative medication as headache becomes more frequent.
		May be modified to four consecutive doses for menstrual migraine
Dose per attack	Single dose (0.5–2 mg)	Should be given as a single dose as early as practicable in the attack at a dose that produces a response with as few side effects as possible. It is useful to test this dose for tolerability for nausea between attacks.
Preferred route	Rectal	Generally better used rectally, provided it is acceptable to the patient, because of improved absorption.

Source: Tfelt-Hansen *et al.* [31]. Reproduced with permission of Oxford University Press.

Table 26.6 Prophylactic drugs with data on ≥50% reduction in migraine attacks

Intervention	Outcome	Number of participants (number of trials)	Control group risk (range)	Relative risk (95% CI)	Absolute risk increase (95% CI)	Comment
Propranolol (SR) Ref. [32]	≥50% reduction of migraine or headache index	688 (9)	30% (11–50)	1.9 (1.6–2.3)	28% (21; 35)	Parallel group and pooled crossover data (PROP CR) Main AEs: fatigue (<10%).
	Adverse effects	619 (6)	24% (4–65)	1.4 (1.2–1.8)	10% (3; 16)	
Topiramate (SR) Ref. [20]	≥50% reduction of migraine	822 (5)	22%	2.1 (1.7–2.6)	24%	21% on topiramate withdrew because of AE. Main AEs: paresthesia (50%), fatigue (15%), nausea (13%).
Sodium valproate (SR) Ref. [20]	≥50% reduction of migraine	349 (3)	18% (14–20)	2.6 (1.7–4.0)	28% (24; 34)	15% on sodium valproate withdrew because of AEs
	Adverse effects	369 (3)	35%	1.5	17%	Main AEs: weight gain (>10%), somnolence (<10%), alopecia (<10%).
Gabapentin (SR) Ref. [33]	≥50% reduction of migraine	87 (1)	16%	2.9 (1.23–6.74)	30% (12; 49)	Just one small trial. Main AEs: Dizziness (28%), somnolence (21%).
Flunarizine 5 mg versus 10 mg (RCT) Ref. [34]	≥50% reduction of migraine compared to run-in	783 (1)	No placebo control		46–53%	Propranolol 160 mg used as an active comparator with 48% responders. Main AEs: somnolence (20%), weight gain (11%).

SR: systematic review; RCT: randomised controlled trial; CI: confidence interval.

beta-blocker with intrinsic sympathomimetic activity, and the beta-1 selective beta-blocker nebivolol is level C, that is, possibly effective.

Antidepressants

The antidepressant most commonly used in the prophylaxis of migraine is amitriptyline, a tricyclic antidepressant, which also has the strongest evidence base for its use [36]. Amitriptyline can also be beneficial in the prophylaxis of chronic tension-type headache. Amitriptyline and venlafaxine, a selective serotonin-norepinephrine reuptake inhibitor, are rated as level B based on the available three class II studies supporting amitriptyline and the one class I and one class II trials in favor of venlafaxine [36].

Antiepileptic drugs/neuromodulators

Divalproex sodium and valproate have been shown in at least five studies to be effective in the prophylaxis of migraine [33]. Daily doses of 500, 1000, and 1500 mg can all be effective; titration is required. The multiple daily dosing that is needed may be able to be avoided by using extended-release preparations, and one double-blind, randomized, controlled class I trial with extended-release (ER) divalproex sodium is found to be an effective migraine prophylactic agent at a dose of 500–1000 mg per day. Despite that divalproex sodium and valproate carry a level A recommendation in migraine prevention, their use is often limited, particularly in women of childbearing potential, because of significant risks of fetal abnormalities, as well as side effects of excessive weight gain, hair loss, hirsutism, and liver function abnormalities. Topiramate has also been shown to be effective at doses of 50–200 mg per day per four class I and seven class II studies and also carries a first-line level A recommendation for migraine prophylaxis [37,36].

Calcium-channel blockers

Verapamil and nimodipine are rated level U, that is, inconclusive evidence for efficacy in migraine prophylaxis [36].

Herbs and vitamins

Often seen as "nondrug" options, herbs and vitamins are popular therapeutic options for many people with migraine and are increasingly scrutinized in randomized placebo-controlled trials.

Petasites, an extract from the butterbur plant, has been shown in two class I studies to be effective in reducing migraine frequency at a dose of 50–75 mg twice a day and consequently is the only herbal supplement to carry a level A recommendation for migraine prevention [34].

A class I trial demonstrated that feverfew (*Tanacetum parthenium*) can help reduce migraine frequency; a dose-finding study suggests that 6.25 mg thrice a day is an effective dose. No major side effects were associated with feverfew, and it carries a level B recommendation for migraine prophylaxis [34].

Riboflavin (vitamin B2), in doses of 400 mg daily (more than 20 times the recommended daily intake) has been assessed against placebo in 55 patients with migraine in a randomized trial of 3 months. Using an intention-to-treat analysis, riboflavin was significantly superior to placebo in reducing attack frequency [38]. The proportion of patients who reported at least 50% fewer headache days was at 15% for placebo and 59% for riboflavin, a significant difference. There were no serious side effects. On the basis of this single class I trial, riboflavin has also been given a level B recommendation for migraine prevention [34].

Like riboflavin, Coenzyme Q10 (CoQ10) also improves energy metabolism and 100 mg per day has been compared with placebo in 42 migraine patients in a double-blind, randomized trial [39]. The 50%-responder-rate for attack frequency was 14.4% for placebo and 47.6% for CoQ10, a significant difference. CoQ10 was well tolerated. On the basis of this single class II study, it carries a level C recommendation for migraine prevention [34].

Magnesium has been given a level B recommendation for migraine prevention based on two positive class II studies and one negative class III study, and is considered generally well tolerated [34].

A randomized, double-blind, placebo-controlled trial of a compound providing a daily dose of riboflavin 400 mg, magnesium 300 mg, and feverfew 100 mg was compared against 25 mg riboflavin ("placebo") [40]. Of 49 patients who completed the 3-month trial, there was no difference between active and "placebo" groups reporting a 50% or greater reduction in migraines (42% and 44%, respectively) neither was there a difference in 50% or greater reduction in migraine days (33% and 40%). Compared to baseline, however, both groups showed a significant reduction in the number of migraines, migraine days, and migraine index.

However, further large and rigorously conducted trials of herbs and vitamin treatments are needed before they can be recommended as an alternative to standard therapies.

Physical treatments

A number of physical treatments for migraine have been studied, including transcutaneous electrical nerve stimulation (TENS), occlusal adjustment, cervical manipulation, and acupuncture. With the exception of acupuncture, there are few studies reported on these treatments. A review of 22 acupuncture patients for migraine prophylaxis included four trials in which acupuncture was compared to a proven prophylactic drug treatment, patients receiving acupuncture tended to report more improvement and fewer side effects [38].

Behavioral therapy

Behavioral therapies that have been studied include relaxation training, biofeedback, and cognitive behavioral therapy. A review of 70 prospective controlled trials of behavioral treatments for migraine showed that, compared with controls, all of these therapies are somewhat effective in preventing migraine [39].

6. Prognosis

For people with migraine, what is the likelihood of attacks persisting lifelong?

In general, the prognosis of migraine is favorable. Studies consistently show that migraine peaks during the 40s but usually remits in later life [41]. The reason for this decline in prevalence is unknown, although it has been postulated that it could relate to a reduced vascular response with advancing years.

Conclusion

Migraine is a highly prevalent disorder and the most common headache subtype in patients presenting to outpatient primary care clinics; however, the diagnosis of all primary headache disorders should be based on criteria contained within the 3rd Edition of the International Classification of Headache Disorders (ICHD-IIIβ). The presence of red flags on history or examination of the headache patient should prompt a workup for possible underlying secondary causes of headache. The absence of red flags in combination with a headache phenotype that lacks atypical features is reassuring and the need to undertake an extensive diagnostic workup declines significantly.

Since the severity of your patient's attacks varies, there is good quality evidence to support the recommendation of an NSAID together with a prokinetic antiemetic. You also prescribe a triptan for attacks that do not respond to this and recommend that if a triptan is always required, it can be taken together with the NSAID to increase efficacy and reduce the likelihood of relapse. Given the frequency of the attacks you discuss prophylactic options and settle on a beta-blocker as being the most suitable first-line agent, as she does not wish to take an antidepressant or an anticonvulsant. You assure her that the present increased frequency of attacks is in keeping with the expected pattern of migraine for her age and sex and that the natural history of migraine is such that it is likely to improve post menopause.

Future research needs

The science of migraine continues to advance and future studies may one day discover biomarkers which can be used to diagnose headache disorders and perhaps identify treatments which may be efficacious for specific individuals.

Studies on the genetics and pathophysiology may one day yield new treatment options and the development of pharmaceuticals and devices designed specifically for migraine and other primary headache disorders.

Future research may also better define the links between migraine and other comorbid conditions such as depression, anxiety disorders, obesity, obstructive sleep apnea, and medication overuse.

References

1 Rasmussen, B.K. (1995) Epidemiology of headache. *Cephalalgia*, **15**(1), 45–68.

2 Headache Classification Subcommittee of the International Headache Society (IHS) (2013) The International Classification of Headache Disorders, 3rd edn. *Cephalalgia*, **33**(9), 629–808.

3 Lipton, R.B., Dodick, D., Sadovsky, R. *et al*. ID Migraine validation study (2003) A self-administered screener for migraine in primary care: The ID Migraine validation study. *Neurology*, **61**(3), 375–382.

4 Steiner, T.J., Scher, A.I., Stewart, W.F., Kolodner, K., Liberman, J. & Lipton, R.B. (2003) The prevalence and disability burden of adult migraine in England and their relationships to age, gender and ethnicity. *Cephalalgia*, **23**(7), 519–527.

5 World Health Organization (2001) *Mental Health: New Understanding*. WHO, Geneva. Available at: http://www.who.int/whr/2001/en/whr01_en.pdf [accessed 24 July 2014].

6 World Health Organization and Lifting the Burden (2011) *Atlas of headache disorders and resources in the world 2011*. WHO, GenevaAvailable at: http://www.who.int/mental_health/management/who_atlas_headache_disorders.pdf [accessed 24 July 2014].

7 Lipton, R.B., Scher, A.I., Steiner, T.J. *et al*. (2003) Patterns of health care utilization for migraine in England and in the United States. *Neurology*, **60**(3), 441–448.

8 Bigal, M.E., Kolodner, K.B., Lafata, J.E., Leotta, C. & Lipton, R.B. (2006) Patterns of medical diagnosis and treatment of migraine and probable migraine in a health plan. *Cephalalgia*, **26**(1), 43–49.

9 Steiner, T.J. (2004) Lifting the burden: the global campaign against headache. *Lancet Neurology*, **3**(4), 204–205.

10 Rasmussen, B.K., Jensen, R., Schroll, M. & Olesen, J. (1991) Epidemiology of headache in a general population – a prevalence study. *Journal of Clinical Epidemiology*, **44**(11), 1147–1157.

11 Bille, B. (1962) Migraine in school children. *Acta Paediatrica Scandinavica*, **51**(**Suppl. 136**), 1–151.

12 Scher, A., Stewart, W. & Lipton, R. (1999) Migraine and headache: a meta-analytic approach. In: Crombie, I. (ed), *Epidemiology of Pain*. IASP Press, Seattle.

13 Stewart, W.F., Lipton, R.B., Celentano, D.D. & Reed, M.L. (1992) Prevalence of migraine headache in the United States. Relation to age, income, race, and other sociodemographic factors. *JAMA*, **267**(1), 64–69.

14 MacGregor, E.A., Frith, A., Ellis, J., Aspinall, L. & Hackshaw, A. (2006) Incidence of migraine relative to menstrual cycle phases of rising and falling estrogen. *Neurology*, **67**(12), 2154–2158.

15 Dodick, D.W. (2010) Pearls: headache. *Seminars in Neurology*, **30**(1), 74–81.OR New England Journal of Medicine. 2006; 354, 158–165

16 Detsky, M.E., McDonald, D.R., Baerlocker, M.O., Tomlinson, G.A., McCory, D.C. & Booth, C.M. (2006) Does this patient with headache have a migraine or need neuroimaging? *JAMA*, **296**, 1274–1283.

17 Rabbie, R., Derry, S. & Moore, R.A. (2013) Ibuprofen with or without an antiemetic for acute migraine headaches in adults. *Cochrane Database of Systematic Reviews*, Issue **4**. Art. No.: CD008039. doi:10.1002/14651858.CD008039.pub3.

18 Derry, S., Rabbie, R. & Moore, R.A. (2013) Diclofenac with or without an antiemetic for acute migraine headaches in adults. *Cochrane Database of Systematic Reviews*, Issue **4**. Art. No.: CD008783. doi:10.1002/14651858.CD008783.pub3.

19 Kirthi, V., Derry, S. & Moore, R.A. (2013) Aspirin with or without an antiemetic for acute migraine headaches in adults. *Cochrane Database of Systematic Reviews*, Issue **4**. Art. No.: CD008041. doi:10.1002/14651858.CD008041.pub3.

20 Derry, S. & Moore, R.A. (2013) Paracetamol (acetaminophen) with or without an antiemetic for acute migraine headaches in adults. *Cochrane Database of Systematic Reviews*, Issue **4**. Art. No.: CD008040. doi:10.1002/14651858.CD008040.pub3.

21 US Headache Consortium. *Evidence-based guidelines for migraine headache in the primary care setting: pharmacological management of acute attacks.* Available at http://www.americanheadachesociety.org/assets/1/7/03_HAConsortium_AcuteGuideline2000.PDF: [accessed 24 July 2014].

22 Ferrari, M.D., Goadsby, P.J., Roon, K.I. & Lipton, R.B. (2002) Triptans (serotonin, 5-HT1B/1D agonists) in migraine: detailed results and methods of a meta-analysis of 53 trials. *Cephalalgia*, **22**(8), 633–658.

23 Ross-Lee, L.M., Eadie, M.J., Heazlewood, V., Bochner, F. & Tyrer, J.H. (1983) Aspirin pharmacokinetics in migraine. The effect of metoclopramide. *European Journal of Clinical Pharmacology*, **24**, 777–785.

24 Gelfand, A.A. & Goadsby, P.J. (2012) A neurologist's guide to acute migraine therapy in the emergency room. *The Neurohospitalist*, **2**(2), 51–59.

25 Derry, C.J., Derry, S. & Moore, R.A. (2012) Sumatriptan (subcutaneous route of administration) for acute migraine attacks in adults. *Cochrane Database of Systematic Reviews*, Issue **2**. Art. No.: CD009665. doi:10.1002/14651858.CD009665.

26 Derry, C.J., Derry, S. & Moore, R.A. (2012) Sumatriptan (oral route of administration) for acute migraine attacks in adults. *Cochrane Database of Systematic Reviews*, Issue **2**. Art. No.: CD008615. doi:10.1002/14651858.CD008615.pub2.

27 Derry, C.J., Derry, S. & Moore, R.A. (2014) Sumatriptan (all routes of administration) for acute migraine attacks in adults - overview of Cochrane reviews. *Cochrane Database of Systematic Reviews*, Issue **5**. Art. No.: CD009108. doi:10.1002/14651858.CD009108.pub2.

28 Law, S., Derry, S. & Moore, R.A. (2013) Sumatriptan plus naproxen for acute migraine attacks in adults. *Cochrane Database of Systematic Reviews*, Issue **10**. Art. No.: CD008541. doi:10.1002/14651858.CD008541.pub2.

29 MacGregor EA, Steiner TJ, Davies PTG. Guidelines for all health-care professionals in the diagnosis and management of migraine, tension-type, cluster and medication-overuse headache. 2010 Available at www.bash.org.uk [accessed 17th July 2014].

30 Smith, T.R., Sunshine, A., Stark, S.R., Littlefield, D.E., Spruill, S.E. & Alexander, W.J. (2005) Sumatriptan and naproxen sodium for the acute treatment of migraine. *Headache*, **45**(8), 983–991.

31 Tfelt-Hansen, P., Saxena, P.R., Dahlof, C. *et al.* (2000) Ergotamine in the acute treatment of migraine: a review and European consensus. *Brain*, **123**(**Pt 1**), 9–18.

32 Linde, K. & Rossnagel, K. (2004) Propranolol for migraine. *Cochrane Database of Systematic Reviews*, Issue **2**. Art. No.: CD003225. doi:10.1002/14651858. CD003225.pub2.

33 Linde M, Mulleners WM, Chronicle EP, McCrory DC. (2013), Valproate (valproic acid or sodium valproate or a combination of the two) for the prophylaxis of episodic migraine in adults. *Cochrane Database of Systematic Reviews*, Issue **6**. Art. No.: CD010611. DOI: 10.1002/14651858.CD010611.

34 Holland, S., Silberstein, S.D., Freitag, F., Dodick, D.W., Argoff, C. & Ashman, E. (2012) Evidence-based guideline update: NSAIDs and other complementary treatments for episodic migraine prevention in adults. *Neurology*, **78**, 1346–1353.

35 US Headache Consortium. Evidence-based guidelines for migraine headache in the primary care setting: pharmacological management for prevention of migraine. Available at http://www.americanheadachesociety.org/assets/1/7/05_HAConsortium_PreventionGuideline2000.PDF [accessed 24 July 2014].

36 Silberstein, S.D., Holland, S., Freitag, F., Dodick, D.W., Argoff, C. & Ashman, E. (2012) Evidence-based guideline update: pharmacologic treatment for episodic migraine prevention in adults. *Neurology*, **78**, 1337–1345.

37 Linde M, Mulleners WM, Chronicle EP, McCrory DC. (2013) Topiramate for the prophylaxis of episodic migraine in adults. *Cochrane Database of Systematic Reviews*, Issue **6**. Art. No.: CD010610. DOI: 10.1002/14651858.CD010610.

38 Linde, K., Allais, G., Brinkhaus, B., Manheimer, E., Vickers, A. & White, A.R. (2009) Acupuncture for migraine prophylaxis. *Cochrane Database of Systematic Reviews*, Issue **1**. Art. No.: CD001218. doi:10.1002/14651858.CD001218.pub2.

39 US Headache Consortium. Evidence-based guidelines for migraine headache: behavioral and physical treatments. Available at http://www.americanheadachesociety.org/assets/1/7/04_HAConsortium_BehavioralGuideline2000.PDF: [accessed 24 July 2014].

40 Maizels, M., Blumenfeld, A. & Burchette, R. (2004) A combination of riboflavin, magnesium, and feverfew for migraine prophylaxis: a randomized trial. *Headache*, **44**(9), 885–890.

41 Lipton, R.B., Stewart, W.F., Diamond, S., Diamond, M.L. & Reed, M. (2001) Prevalence and burden of migraine in the United States: data from the American Migraine Study II. *Headache*, **41**(7), 646–657.

27 CHAPTER 27
Therapy of vestibular disorders, nystagmus and cerebellar ataxia

Michael Strupp and Thomas Brandt

Department of Neurology, German Center for Vertigo and Balance Disorders and Institute for Clinical Neurosciences, University Hospital Munich, Campus Grosshadern, Munich, Germany

Introduction

The terms vertigo and dizziness cover a number of multisensory and sensorimotor syndromes of various etiologies and pathogeneses, which can be elucidated best by an interdisciplinary approach. After headache, it is one of the most frequent presenting symptoms, not only in neurology. The lifetime prevalence is almost 30% [1]. Vertigo and dizziness are often associated with nystagmus, other ocular motor or cerebellar disorders. Here, first, the treatment of common peripheral and central vestibular disorders, including related cerebellar disorders is described. The second part deals with the clinically most relevant forms of nystagmus, in particular downbeat and upbeat nystagmus, along with their pathophysiology and current therapy (for reference see also [2–5]). The third and final part gives an overview of current studies in the field, including those in cerebellar ataxia, and perspectives.

Principles of the pharmacotherapy of vertigo, dizziness, ocular motor disorders, and nystagmus

The prerequisites of a successful treatment of vertigo, dizziness, ocular motor disorders, and nystagmus are the *"4 Ds"*: correct diagnosis, correct drug, appropriate dosage, and sufficient duration. First, a correct *Diagnosis* which can be simply made in most patients on the basis of the patient history and the clinical examination even without any laboratory examinations (for the relative frequency of the different vestibular disorders, see Table 27.1); Second, the correct *Drug* – only a few have been proven to be effective. Third, an appropriate *Dosage* – often the dosage given is too low. Fourth, a sufficient *Duration* – often drugs are given too long, such as antivertigenous agents which delay central compensation and may cause drug addiction or not long enough as in chronic

disorders such as Menière's disease, vestibular migraine or episodic ataxias, which require a long-term treatment

Depending on the etiology, the various forms of vestibular disorders can be treated with pharmacological therapy, physical therapy, psychotherapeutic measures, or rarely surgery. Before beginning any treatment, the patient should be told that the prognosis is generally good for two reasons: (1) vertigo often takes a favorable natural course (e.g., the peripheral vestibular function improves or central vestibular compensation of the vestibular tone imbalance takes place) and (2) most forms can be successfully treated (mainly with drugs or physiotherapy). Several agents are now available for the specific treatment of certain forms of vestibular and ocular motor disorders.

Peripheral vestibular disorders

Three typical forms of peripheral vestibular disorders can be differentiated by their characteristic signs and symptoms: (1) bilateral peripheral loss of vestibular function (bilateral vestibulopathy), characterized by oscillopsia during head movements and instability of gait and posture; (2) acute/subacute unilateral failure of vestibular function, characterized by rotatory vertigo, oscillopsia, and a tendency to fall toward the affected ear (most often caused by acute unilateral vestibulopathy); and (3) paroxysmal, inadequate stimulation or inhibition of the peripheral vestibular system, characterized by attacks of vertigo and oscillopsia. This occurs in benign paroxysmal positioning vertigo, Menière's disease, vestibular paroxysmia, or vestibular migraine.

Acute unilateral vestibulopathy

Acute unilateral vestibulopathy is the second most common cause of peripheral vestibular vertigo (the first being benign paroxysmal positioning vertigo). It accounts for 7% of the

---

Evidence-Based Neurology: Management of Neurological Disorders, Second Edition. Edited by Bart M. Demaerschalk and Dean M. Wingerchuk.

Table 27.1 Relative frequency of different vertigo syndromes diagnosed in an interdisciplinary special outpatient clinic for dizziness (n = 17,718 patients)

Diagnosis	Frequency	
	n	%
1. BPPV	3036	17.1
2. Phobic postural dizziness	2661	15.0
3. Central vestibular vertigo	2178	12.3
4. Basilar vestibular migraine	2017	11.4
5. Menière's disease	1795	10.1
6. Vestibular neuritis	1462	8.3
7. Bilateral vestibulopathy	1263	7.1
8. Vestibular paroxysmia	655	3.7
9. Psychogenic vertigo	515	2.9
10. Perilymph fistula	93	0.5
Unknown vertigo syndromes	480	2.7
Other disorders	1563	8.8

Source: Brandt et al. [4]. Reproduced with permission of Springer.

patients who present at outpatient clinics specializing in the treatment of dizziness [4] and has an incidence of 3.5 per 100,000 population [6]. The key signs and symptoms are the acute onset of sustained rotatory vertigo, horizontal spontaneous nystagmus toward the unaffected ear with a rotational component, postural imbalance with Romberg's sign, that is, falls with the eyes closed toward the affected ear and nausea. Caloric testing invariably shows ipsilateral hyporesponsiveness or nonresponsiveness and the head-impulse test is pathological. In the past, either inflammation of the vestibular nerve or labyrinthine ischemia was proposed to cause vestibular neuritis. Currently, a viral cause is favored. The evidence, however, remains circumstantial. Herpes simplex virus type 1 (HSV-1) DNA has been detected on autopsy with the use of polymerase chain reaction in about two of three human vestibular ganglia [7–11]. This, as well as the expression of CD8-positive T-lymphocytes, cytokines, and chemokines, indicates that the vestibular ganglia are latently infected with HSV-1 [12].

Symptomatic therapy for nausea and vomiting. Antivertiginous drugs can be administered. They should only be given during the first days and only in cases of severe nausea and vomiting, as they act as sedatives and may delay central compensation of the peripheral vestibular deficit [13].

Causal therapy

A prospective, randomized, placebo-controlled study in 141 patients showed that monotherapy with methylprednisolone significantly improved the peripheral vestibular function of patients with vestibular neuritis [14]. With this therapy the proportion of patients who experience a functional improvement of the affected labyrinth is significantly increased from 39% to 62%. Valacyclovir had no influence on the course of the disease, neither as monotherapy nor in combination with methylprednisolone. These findings are supported by both a meta-analysis [15] and another study [16]. However, a Cochrane analysis still makes no treatment recommendation for corticosteroids, and the effects on life quality have still not been investigated sufficiently [17]. Thus, further studies on the effects on vestibular function, subjective improvement, and quality of life are required [18]. In clinical practice, currently a 3-week treatment with corticosteroids (methylprednisolone, initially 100 mg per day; dose is tapered off by 20 mg every fourth day) is recommended [14].

Improvement of central vestibular compensation

Pharmacological and metabolic studies in animals suggest that alcohol, phenobarbital, chlorpromazine, diazepam, and ACTH antagonists retard central compensation, whereas caffeine, amphetamines, and glucocorticoids accelerate it (overview in Ref. [13]). It has not yet been sufficiently investigated whether these drugs influence the central compensation in humans and if so, how much. There is an ongoing trial on the effects of betahistine-dihydrochloride on central compensation in acute vestibular neuritis, the ideal model of an acute unilateral peripheral vestibular deficit (betahistine-dihydrochloride 48 mg thrice a day versus placebo; the BETAVEST trial).

Menière's disease

Menière's disease is clinically characterized by recurrent spontaneous attacks of vertigo, fluctuating hearing loss, tinnitus, and aural fullness. Its lifetime prevalence is about 0.51% [1]. Endolymphatic hydrops is assumed to be the pathological basis of Menière's disease, either due to a too high production or a too low absorption of the endolymph. Nowadays, endolymphatic hydrops can be visualized by high-resolution MRI of the inner ear after transtympanic injections of gadolinium [19]. The increased endolymphatic pressure causes periodic rupturing or leakage (by the opening of nonselective, stretch-activated ion channels [20] of the membrane separating the endolymph from the perilymph space. Therefore, pathophysiologically it makes sense to reduce the production and increase the absorption of endolymph. The clinical aims of treatment of Menière's disease are to stop vertigo, reduce or abolish tinnitus, and preserve and even reverse hearing loss. Most studies focus on the severest symptom of Menière's disease: recurrent attacks of vertigo.

The primary goal of therapy for Menière's disease is to prevent attacks in order to prevent the progression of vestibulocochlear deficits. To date, more than 2500 articles have been published on the treatment of the disease. Accordingly, the spectrum of therapy recommendations ranges from a salt-free diet, diuretics, transtympanic administration of gentamicin, steroids, or betahistine to different operative procedures. The transtympanic instillation of gentamicin and steroids as well as high-dose, long-term administration of betahistine-dihydrochloride (3×48 mg per day for 12 months) have been reported to have positive effects on the frequency of attacks.

Transtympanic administration of gentamicin

The effect of gentamicin is based on the direct damage it causes to vestibular type 1 hair cells [21]. When this treatment was first introduced, the patients received gentamicin until vestibular function failed. In this way, freedom from attacks was achieved in most cases, but at the cost of a clear inner-ear hypoacusis in more than 50% of the cases. When it was proved that the ototoxic effect of the aminoglycosides began only after a definite delay, the therapy regimen was changed to either single injections, each at least 4 weeks apart, or a single injection and subsequently regular follow-ups. Only if further attacks occurred were more injections given. Two prospective double-blind, randomized, controlled studies have shown efficacy on the symptoms of vertigo [22,23]. These results have been supported by a Cochrane analysis [24]. The fundamental problem of treatment with aminoglycosides is hearing damage, which affects at least 20% of the patients [25]. For this reason, only patients with obvious preexisting hearing damage should in fact receive this treatment. To make matters worse, 30% of patients develop a bilateral Menière's disease after 5 years [26].

Transtympanic administration of glucocorticoids

A controlled, prospective, double-blind study showed an improvement of the attacks of vertigo in 82% as opposed to 57% in the placebo group [27]. According to a Cochrane analysis [28], this study is, to date, the only one that has been performed with precise methods. Thus the indications of the efficacy of transtympanic administration of glucocorticoids are limited.

Comparison between gentamicin and glucocorticoids

In a prospective, controlled, randomized study, the effect of intratympanic gentamicin was compared with that of dexamethasone: gentamicin was superior, reducing vertigo attacks by 93% compared with 61% with dexamethasone [29].

Betahistine

Betahistine is a weak H1 agonist and a strong H3 antagonist. It improves the microcirculation of the inner ear by acting on the precapillary sphincter of the stria vascularis [30] (Figure 27.1). In this way, it can normalize the imbalance between production and resorption of endolymph. Meta-analyses show that betahistine evidently has a prophylactic effect on attacks of Menière's disease [31], although no placebo-controlled, double-blind study has yet

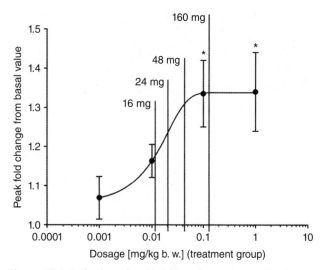

Figure 27.1 Peak values of cochlear blood flow with curve fitted by nonlinear regression and calculated corresponding oral dosage (peak mean $\pm$ SD; *: $p < 0.05$)) showing a sigmoid increase of blood in an animal model. This correlates with the increasing dosages currently used for the treatment of Menière's disease (Source: Ihler *et al.* [30].)

been published. On the basis of clinical experience with a dosing regimen of 3×48 mg betahistine-dihydrochloride per day, an open-pilot long-term study was performed in 112 patients. It showed that the higher doses were significantly superior to the usual dosage of 3×16–3×24 mg per day. After 12 months, the average number of attacks declined from 7.6 month to 4.4 per month in the low-dose group and from 8.8 to 1.0 per month in the high-dose group [32]. If the patients do not respond sufficiently after 3 months on a dose of 3×48 mg per day, it can be successively increased in individual cases up to 480 mg per day [33] or even up to 1440 mg per day in single cases. The goal of therapy is freedom from attacks for at least 6 months; then the dosage can be slowly reduced depending on the course by one tablet every 3 months. This is a long-term treatment, often for many years. Finally, it must, however, be pointed out that up to now no state-of-the-art studies have been published in this field despite the large number of trials. There is an ongoing placebo-controlled dose-finding trial (betahistine-dihydrochloride 16 mg thrice a day versus 48 mg thrice a day versus placebo; the BEMED trial).

Vestibular paroxysmia

Vestibular paroxysmia is characterized by short attacks of rotatory or to-and-fro vertigo. These attacks last for seconds to minutes and may occur up to 30 times a day. Similar to trigeminal neuralgia, hemifacial spasm, or superior oblique myokymia, it is assumed that a neurovascular cross-compression of the eighth cranial nerve is the cause of vestibular paroxysmia [34,35] (Figure 27.2). Therapy with

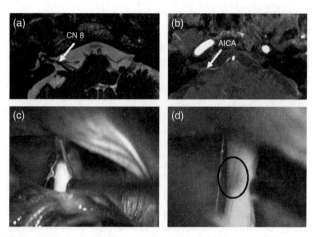

Figure 27.2 Cranial MRI in a patient with vestibular paroxysmia ((a) Constructive interference in steady-state sequence, (b): Time-of-flight) shows contact between the right eighth cranial nerve (CN 8) and the anterior inferior cerebellar artery (AICA). Intraoperative micrographs demonstrate the vascular contact (c) and the considerable compression of the eighth nerve after removal of the arteries (d, circle). (Source: Strupp *et al.* [35]. Reproduced with permission of Wolters Kluwer Health.)

low doses of carbamazepine (200–600 mg per day) reduces the frequency of attacks (provides a positive response useful in the diagnostics of the disease). This was demonstrated in an open trial [36]. In case of intolerance, gabapentin, valproic acid, or phenytoin are possible alternatives. No state-of-the-art studies have been published in this field. There is an ongoing placebo-controlled trial (carbamazepine 400 mg per day versus placebo, the VesPa-trial).

Central vestibular, ocular motor, and cerebellar disorders

In this section, the pharmacological treatment methods of the most important central vestibular, ocular motor, and cerebellar disorders are presented, namely vestibular migraine; episodic ataxia type 2; and downbeat, upbeat, and other forms of nystagmus as well as cerebellar ataxia.

Vestibular migraine

Vestibular migraine is the most common cause of central recurrent attacks of vertigo. Characteristic features include recurrent attacks of various combinations of vertigo, ataxia of stance and gait, visual disorders, and other brainstem symptoms accompanied or followed by occipitally located head pressure, pain, nausea, or vomiting [37]. Treatment is the same as for migraine with aura, that is, for prophylactic therapy, using beta-blockers (metoprolol or propranol), valproic acid, or topiramate for at least 6 months. A few treatment studies on vestibular migraine have been performed. Tricyclic antidepressants in combination with diet showed a good response in a trial on 81 patients [38]. For zolmitriptan, the response rate in acute attacks was 38% vs

22% in a study on 19 patients [39]. Another open trial on 10 patients demonstrated that lamotrigine (100 mg per day as a single dose) had a significant effect on the occurrence of headache and a more marked effect on vertigo [40]. In a retrospective study, the treatment options were evaluated [41]. To date, only the standard treatment of migraine with aura can be recommended for vestibular migraine. There is an ongoing placebo-controlled, multicenter trial (metoprolol 95 mg per day versus placebo; the PROVEMIG trial).

Episodic ataxia type 2 and other cerebellar disorders

Episodic ataxia type 2 (EA 2) is most often caused by mutations of the CACNA1A gene encoding the alpha-subunit of P/Q-type calcium channel [42]. The clinical manifestations of this channelopathy are recurrent bouts of vertigo, ataxic symptoms, and ocular motor disturbances such as downbeat nystagmus [43], often overlapping with migraine [44]. The attacks are often provoked by stress, exertion, or alcohol and usually last hours or days.

Approximately two-thirds of these patients respond to treatment with acetazolamide (250–1000 mg per day) [45], and acetazolamide has been a first-line treatment of EA 2 for many years. However, there are no placebo-controlled trials about the efficacy of this drug. Furthermore, the side effects of acetazolamide (e.g., kidney stones) often limit its therapeutic use.

In 2004, it was shown in an observational study that the potassium-channel blocker 4-aminopyridine (4-AP) reduces the number of attacks of vertigo and was well tolerated [46]. In a randomized, placebo-controlled, double-blind, crossover trial, a significant effect of this agent on the number of attacks and the quality of life was found (Figure 27.3) [47]. These effects of 4-AP on the attacks have been confirmed in several studies with an animal model of EA 2, the tottering mouse [48,49], which also allows the evaluation of the underlying mode of action (see below). More recently, it was also shown in an observational study that the sustained-release form of 4-AP [Ampyra™ (Acorda, USA) or Fampyra™ (Biogen Idec, Europe)] is also effective and well tolerated [50]. The use of 4-AP in a dosage of 5–10 mg three times a day is recommended for the treatment of EA 2. There is an ongoing placebo-controlled trial with the sustained-release form of 4-AP versuss acetazolamide (University of Munich, EAT-2-TREAT).

Cerebellar disorders

Treatment of motor symptoms of degenerative cerebellar ataxia remains difficult. There is consensus that to date, no medication has been proven effective. Aminopyridines and acetazolamide may be the only exceptions, which are beneficial in patients with episodic ataxia type 2; aminopyridines are also effective in a subset of patients

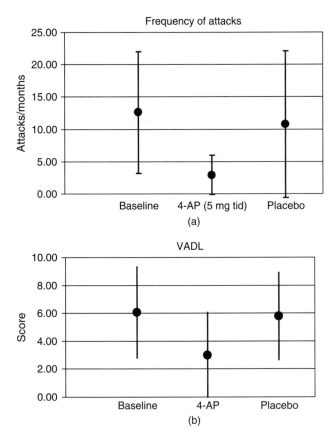

Figure 27.3 Effects of 4-aminopyridine in episodic ataxia type 2.
(a) Number of attacks of ataxia per month. 4-Aminopyridine
significantly reduced the number of attacks of ataxia per month
($p = 0.03$). (b) Patient-reported quality of life (vestibular disorders
activities of daily living scale (VDADL) score as a measure of the burden
of disease). 4-Aminopyridine significantly reduced the VDADL score
($p = 0.022$). (Source: Data from Strupp *et al.* [47].)

presenting with downbeat nystagmus (for Ref. see [51]). In
a retrospective case series, patients with cerebellar ataxic gait
due to different etiologies (multisystem atrophy, sporadic
adult-onset ataxia, cerebellar stroke, CACNA1A mutations,
DBN syndrome) also benefited from 4-aminopyridine
[52]. These observations are currently evaluated in a
placebo-controlled trial (the FACEG trial). Recently it
was shown in a case series that the modified amino-acid
acetyl-leucine, which had been used in France since 1957 for
the symptomatic treatment of vertigo, significantly improves
cerebellar ataxia, dysarthrophonia, and limb ataxia in the
affected patients (Figure 27.4) [53].

Nystagmus

Nystagmus can be defined as periodic, most often involuntary, eye movements that normally consist of a slow
(causative or pathological) phase and a quick eye phase,
which brings the eye back to the initial position. Nystagmus
is quite common; its prevalence lies around 0.1% [54]. The
most common forms of acquired nystagmus are downbeat

and upbeat nystagmus. Both can be treated nowadays with
aminopyridines in their capacity as potassium-channel
blockers. More rare forms are congenital nystagmus,
acquired fixation pendular nystagmus, and periodic
alternating nystagmus. If they cause symptoms, mainly
involuntary movement of the visual surrounding (oscillopsia), treatment with memantine or gabapentin should
be tried. To improve treatment of the different forms of
nystagmus, further randomized controlled trials will be
necessary to test different agents on the basis of our current
knowledge of the pathophysiology of nystagmus.

Common, clinically important forms of nystagmus and their therapy

In this section, the most common and clinically most relevant forms of nystagmus and their pathophysiology as well
as current therapy are described. For the frequency of the different forms, see Table 27.2 [55]. In Table 27.3, the features
are summarized. The treatment of nystagmus is based on
four principles: medical treatment, optical devices, surgery to
weaken certain eye muscles, and somatosensory or auditory
stimuli. Medical treatment is the most relevant and successful
means of treatment.

Downbeat nystagmus (DBN)

Downbeat nystagmus (DBN) is the most frequent type
of acquired nystagmus. Affected patients predominantly
suffer from postural imbalance and cerebellar gait ataxia,
as well as oscillopsia with reduced visual acuity due to
a corrective downward saccade following a spontaneous
upward drift [55–57]. In the majority, it is caused by a
bilaterally impaired function of the cerebellar floccular lobe
[58] due to neurodegenerative disorders.

In a randomized, controlled, crossover trial, the nonselective potassium-channel blocker 3,4-DAP effectively
reduced DBN [59]. Furthermore, 4-AP also alleviates the
symptoms of DBN, particularly in patients with cerebellar
atrophy [60]. Even though 3,4-DAP improved DBN in
patients with spinocerebellar ataxia type 6 (SCA6), there
was no improvement of postural control or other ataxic
symptoms after 1 week of 3,4-DAP (20 mg twice a day)
[61]. The comparison of equal doses of 3,4-DAP with 4-AP
results in a more distinct improvement of DBN following the
administration of 4-AP. Since the latter is lipid-soluble and
crosses the blood–brain-barrier more easily and is evidently
more effective, 4-AP is preferred [62].

A randomized, double-blind, crossover trial of 4-AP in
DBN showed a reduction in slow-phase velocity of DBN by
half and an improvement of visual acuity at a dosage of 5 mg
4-AP four times a day [63]. Furthermore, 4-AP at a dosage of
10 mg four times a day reduced postural sway and improved
motor performance assessed by the timed "get-up-and-go
test." However, there was no subjective improvement,
which may be due to the short half-life of the drug. This

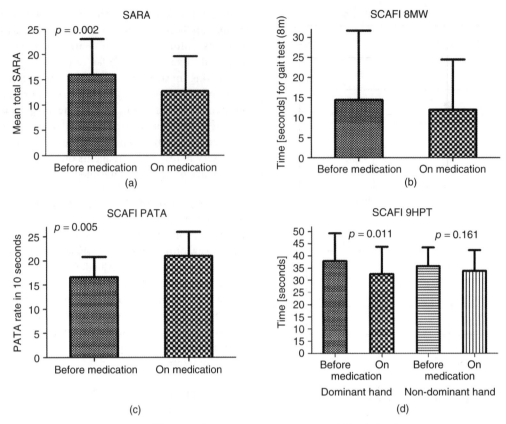

Figure 27.4 Effects of acetyl-dl-leucine (Tanganil™) on cerebellar ataxia. Value changes on (a) Scale for the assessment and rating of ataxia (SARA) and spinocerebellar ataxia functional index (SCAFI) sub-score items in terms of (b) eight-meter walk (8MW), (c) PATA word count in 10 seconds and (d) nine-hole-peg-test (9HPT) of the dominant and nondominant hand before and during the therapy with acetyl-DL-leucine (5 g per day) (mean ± SD) These changes have a significant impact on functioning and quality of life of patients with cerebellar ataxia. (Source: Strupp et al. [53].)

Table 27.2 Frequency of congenital and/or acquired ocular oscillations in a total of 4854 consecutive patients seen in a neurological dizziness unit. DBN was the most frequent fixation nystagmus

Form of central nystagmus	n
Downbeat nystagmus	101
Upbeat nystagmus	54
Central positional nystagmus	26
Acquired endular nystagmus	15
Congenital nystagmus	12
Pure torsional nystagmus	12
See-saw nystagmus	8
Ocular flutter	8
Square wave jerks	7
Opsoclonus	1
Periodic alternating nystagmus	1

Source: Wagner et al. [55]. Reproduced with permission of BMJ.

shortage may be overcome by the sustained-release form of 4-AP which is – in a dosage of 10–20 mg per day – also efficient [64]. Since the latter was only an observational study further trials with the new formulation are needed.

Other drugs have been shown to lack efficacy in DBN (e.g., baclofen) [65]. Finally, it was also demonstrated that 4-AP suppresses central positioning DBN, which correlates with an increased glucose uptake in the ocular motor vermis and the flocculus [66].

In conclusion, based on the current state-of-the-art studies, the use of 4-AP in a dosage of 5 mg two to four times a day is recommended for the treatment of DBN. The sustained-release form Fampyra™ is evidently also efficient.

Chlorzoxazone (CHZ), a nonselective activator of small conductance calcium-activated potassium channels (SK-channels), could be a potentially new therapeutic agent for the symptomatic treatment. In an observational proof-of-concept pilot study [67], slow-phase velocity of DBN, visual acuity, and postural sway showed significant effects.

Mode of action of aminopyridines

Aminopyridines are blockers of the so-called Kv1.5 voltage-activated potassium channels. Thereby, they increase the excitability of neurons. The common mechanism behind the therapeutic influence of aminopyridines lies within

Table 27.3 Summary of the clinical features, pathophysiology, etiology, site of lesion, and current treatment options for common forms of central nystagmus

	Downbeat nystagmus (DBN)	Upbeat nystagmus (UBN)	Acquired pendular nystagmus (APN)	Periodic alternating nystagmus (PAN)	Infantile nystagmus
Direction of nystagmus (quick phase)	Downward, may be diagonal with lateral gaze	Upward	Mainly horizontal, may have vertical and/or torsional components	Horizontal	Mainly horizontal; may have torsional and small vertical components
Waveform (slow phase)	Jerk, constant, increasing, or decreasing slow-phase velocity	Jerk, constant, increasing, or decreasing slow-phase velocity	Pendular, sinusoidal slow-phase velocity	Jerk, mostly constant slow-phase velocity	Accelerating slow-phases; foveation periods when the eye is transiently still
Special features	Increased intensity during lateral and downward gaze; sometimes suppressed by convergence	Increased intensity during upward gaze; may convert to DBN on convergence	Associated with other oscillations (e.g., palate) and with hypertrophic degeneration of the inferior olive	Changes direction every 90–120 seconds	Null zone, in which nystagmus is minimal; often suppressed with convergence
Sites of lesion	Cerebellum (bilateral floccular hypofunction); rarely lower brainstem lesions	Medial medulla, ponto-mesencephalic junction, rarely cerebellum	Pontomedullary, probably affecting components of neural integrator for gaze holding	Cerebellum (nodulus, uvula)	Uncertain; some cases are associated with afferent visual system anomalies
Etiology	Cerebellar tumors, degenerations, and stroke; idiopathic; often associated with bilateral vestibulopathy and neuropathy	Brainstem or cerebellar stroke and tumors; Wernicke's encephalopathy	Multiple sclerosis, oculopalatal tremor due to brainstem or cerebellar stroke	Cerebellar degenerations, cranio-cervical anomalies, multiple sclerosis, cerebellar tumors and stroke	Uncertain; may be associated with afferent visual system anomalies; hereditary in some patients (e.g., FRMD7 mutations)
Treatment	4-Aminopyridine (5–10 mg thrice a day), clonazepam (0.5 mg thrice a day)	Often transient, treatment often not necessary; baclofen (5–10 mg thrice a day), 4-aminopyridine (5–10 thrice a day)	Memantine (10 mg four times a day), gabapentin (300 mg four times a day)	Baclofen (5–10 mg thrice a day)	Gabapentin (300 mg four times a day), memantine (10 mg four times a day)

Source: Strupp *et al.* [2].

the influence on cerebellar Purkinje cells (PCs). In vitro studies with the tottering mouse show that 4-AP increases the excitability of PCs of the guinea pig cerebellum [68] and the precision of pace-making of PCs in a mouse model (tottering mouse) of EA2 [48]; this interpretation, however, is not compatible with a study mathematically modelling the effects of synchronization of PCs [69].

In this mouse model, 4-AP and 3,4-DAP both reduced the frequency of attacks probably by raising the threshold for triggering of attacks [49]. Furthermore, aminopyridines normalize the firing rate and the motor behavior in ataxin-1 mutant mice in vivo [70]. Mice treated early demonstrated better motor function, which may be mediated by a neuroprotective effect due to an enhanced electrical

activity of PCs [70]. Therefore, long-term treatment starting early in the course of neurodegenerative ataxias may help to improve the outcome. Finally, a PET study showed that 4-AP – in parallel to improving DBN – increases the metabolic activity of the flocculus [71]. All these studies give additional support both to the aforementioned hypothesis about the pathophysiology of DBN and the way that aminopyridines act.

Upbeat nystagmus (UBN)

Upbeat nystagmus (UBN), that is, UBN with gaze straight ahead, is an ocular motor disorder that manifests with oscillopsia due to retinal slip of the visual scene and postural instability. It is the second most common cause of acquired nystagmus. UBN usually increases with upgaze. Analogously to DBN, it is associated with impaired upward pursuit. UBN can be caused by lesions in different brainstem and cerebellar regions such as the pontomesencephalic junction, medulla, or cerebellar vermis. Lesions in the pathways mediating upward eye movements, in particular, from the vestibular nuclei through the brachium conjunctivum to the ocular motor nuclei, might result in slow downward drift of the eyes, which is corrected by fast upward movements (for reference see [56]). Other hypotheses are that UBN is caused by an imbalance of vertical vestibulo-ocular reflex tone or a mismatch in the neural coordinate systems of saccade generation and neural velocity-to-position integration.

The symptoms last, as a rule, several weeks but are not permanent in most of the patients. Because the eye movements generally have larger amplitudes, oscillopsia in upbeat nystagmus is very distressing and impairs vision. Upbeat nystagmus due to damage to the pontomesencephalic brainstem is frequently combined with a unilateral or bilateral internuclear ophthalmoplegia, indicating that the MLF is affected. The main etiologies are bilateral lesions in MS, brainstem ischemia or tumor, Wernicke's encephalopathy, cerebellar degeneration, and dysfunction of the cerebellum due to intoxication. One study demonstrated a beneficial effect of baclofen (5–10 mg thrice a day), but this trial was not controlled.

In a single patient with UBN, it was shown that 4-aminopyridine reduces the peak slow-phase velocity in the light from 8.6 to 2.0 deg/s. 4-Aminopyridine did not affect UBN in darkness, but it obviously activated pathways carrying visual information, which could then be used for UBN suppression in the light [72]. Therefore, it was concluded that 4-AP reduces the downward drift in UBN by augmenting smooth pursuit commands. We propose that 4-AP helps to activate parallel pathways that can assume the function of the lesioned structures. 4-AP may strengthen these parallel pathways by increasing the excitability of cerebellar PCs. It may also evoke complex spikes in PCs similar to those elicited by climbing fiber stimulation. In conclusion, placebo-controlled trials are necessary to further evaluate the efficacy of 4-aminopyridine in UBN.

Other forms of nystagmus
Other forms of nystagmus, which are associated with oscillopsia and in some patients with imbalance, are acquired pendular nystagmus, periodic alternating nystagmus, convergence retraction nystagmus, central positioning or positional nystagmus (see above), and see-saw nystagmus. Congenital nystagmus often does not cause any symptoms. Square wave jerks, ocular flutter (mainly horizontal saccades), and opsoclonus (horizontal, vertical, and torsional saccades) belong to the saccadic intrusions or saccadic oscillations and are not classified as a nystagmus. In this section, the features, pathophysiology, and treatment of

congenital nystagmus; periodic alternating nystagmus; and acquired fixation nystagmus are summarized, because they are the clinically most relevant forms (see also Table 27.2).

Acquired pendular nystagmus (APN) and oculopalatal tremor
Acquired pendular nystagmus may have horizontal, vertical, or torsional components. The amplitude varies, and in part the eye movements are not conjugate. The clinical features and associated symptoms, in particular, palatal tremor, often depend on the underlying disease. The three most common causes are multiple sclerosis, brainstem ischemia, and Whipple's disease. In patients with multiple sclerosis, APN has a frequency of 3–6 Hz and is often associated with other central ocular motor disorders such as internuclear ophthalmoplegia or upbeat nystagmus. APN can also be associated with palatal tremor: oculopalatal tremor. In such patients, there is often a synchronization of the nystagmus with the palatal tremor. MRI of patients in the chronic state often reveals a pseudohypertrophy of the inferior olivary nucleus [73]. It is assumed that oculopalatal tremor is caused by damage to the paramedian tract projections and denervation of the dorsal cap of the inferior olive, leading to instability of eye velocity to position integration [74].

Several agents have been recommended for APN. One is trihexiphenidyl [75,76], but a double-blind study demonstrated that only one of six patients responded to this treatment [77]. Memantine, a glutamate antagonist was also recommended [78], but its efficacy has not been proven. There are convincing data for gabapentin from a double-blind study [65]. A significant improvement in visual acuity and reduction of nystagmus was found with gabapentin in 10 out of 15 patients, but not with baclofen. This was confirmed in a more recent examiner-blind crossover trial in patients with multiple sclerosis [79]. The retrobulbar application of botulinum toxin was also recommended, but this was tested in only a small series of patients [80] and was not always successful [81]. From a practical point of view, we now recommend using gabapentin (300–600 mg thrice a day) for acquired pendular nystagmus. Memantine and trihexiphenidyl are second and third choices, respectively.

Periodic alternating nystagmus (PAN)
This form of nystagmus most often beats horizontally and changes its direction every 60–180 seconds. Afflicted subjects complain of oscillopsia. Patients often turn their head in the direction of the quick phase and in this way bring their eyes in the direction of the slow phase of PAN to reduce oscillopsia – in accordance with Alexander's law. The diagnosis requires quite a long examination period, otherwise one might overlook PAN. Similar to many other forms of nystagmus, PAN is most often caused by cerebellar dysfunction, in particular by lesions of the nodulus or the

uvula. These lesions impair the velocity-storage mechanism as was shown in animal experiments and the oscillations are assumed to be caused by an "overcompensation" or instability of the optokinetic–vestibular system [82]. The treatment of choice is the GABA-ergic drug baclofen in a dosage of 5–10 mg thrice a day, which abolishes PAN in most patients [83]. There have been no randomized, controlled trials to date.

Infantile nystagmus

Infantile nystagmus often develops during the first months of life. Some of the cases are familial and genetically heterogeneous. Autosomal-dominant, autosomal-recessive, and X-linked patterns of inheritance have been reported. Linkage analysis suggested the existence of at least three distinct loci for both autosomal-dominant and X-linked forms, although to date only one disease gene was identified on chromosome Xq26.2 (for reference see [84]). Congenital nystagmus is clinically characterized by the following criteria: fixation nystagmus, that is, no decrease of the intensity during fixation; nystagmus most often beating horizontally; large variability of form and form frequency and velocity; intensity depending on gaze position; often a position (the so-called neutral zone) with a minimal intensity which the patient prefers and which leads to an appropriate head turn. Examination with the optokinetic drum often shows an inversion of the direction or during vertical optokinetic stimulation, a diagonal nystagmus. It is important to know that most patients do not have any complaints, namely they have no oscillopsia despite a high intensity of nystagmus. This is most likely due to an impairment of visual motion perception in these subjects. Since most patients do not have any medical complaints, treatment is generally not necessary. In patients with oscillopsia, one might try gabapentin or memantine. In a randomized, controlled, double-blind study, it was demonstrated that memantine at a dosage of 10–40 mg per day (as well as gabapentin at a dosage of 600–2400 mg per day) caused a significant decrease of the intensity of the nystagmus and an increase of visual acuity [85]. This, however, was not associated with visual acuity during regular daily activities or improvement of the patients' disease-related quality of life.

Perspectives

There are still considerable deficits in the pharmacotherapy of most of the vestibular, ocular motor, and cerebellar disorders and nystagmus, in particular, due to the lack of state-of-the-art controlled clinical trials. To overcome these limitations, there are, for instance, at the German Center for Vertigo and Balance Disorders, several ongoing clinical trials on major vestibular and cerebellar disorders, namely benign paroxysmal positioning vertigo, vestibular neuritis, Menière's disease, vestibular paroxysmia, episodic ataxia type 2, and cerebellar ataxias (Table 27.4).

Table 27.4 Current ongoing randomized multicenter investigator initiated clinical trials at the German Center for Vertigo and Balance Disorders, Munich

Peripheral vestibular disorders	
1. BPPV	Vitamin D versus placebo (1000 I.U. vs placebo) VitD@BPPV
2. Vestibular paroxysmia	Carbamazepine (400 mg per day vs placebo) VesPa
3. Menière's disease	Betahistine (placebo vs 48 mg per day vs 144 mg per day) 221 pts. "last out": Nov. 23rd 2013: BEMED
4. Acute vestibular neuritis	Betahistine (144 mg per day vs placebo) BETAVEST (central compensation)
Central disorders	
5. Vestibular migraine	Metoprolol (95 mg per day vs placebo): PROVEMIG
6. Episodic ataxia type 2	Fampridine versus acetazolamide versus placebo: EAT2TREAT
7. Cerebellar gait ataxia	Fampridine versus placebo: FACEG
8. Cerebellar ataxia	Acetyl-DL-leucine versus placebo ALCAT All funded by the Federal Ministry of Research except (7)

Acknowledgements

We thank Judy Benson for copyediting the manuscript. This work was supported by the German Ministry of Education and Research (BMBF), Grant No. 01EO0901 to the German Center for Vertigo and Balance Disorders (IFB^LMU).

References

1 Neuhauser, H.K. (2007) Epidemiology of vertigo. *Current Opinion in Neurology*, **20**(1), 40–46.

2 Strupp, M., Thurtell, M.J., Shaikh, A.G., Brandt, T., Zee, D.S. & Leigh, R.J. (2011) Pharmacotherapy of vestibular and ocular motor disorders, including nystagmus. *Journal of Neurology*, **258**(7), 1207–1222.

3 Huppert, D., Strupp, M., Muckter, H. & Brandt, T. (2011) Which medication do I need to manage dizzy patients? *Acta Oto-Laryngologica*, **131**(3), 228–241.

4 Brandt, T., Dieterich, M. & Strupp, M. (2013) *Vertigo and dizziness - common complaints*, 2nd edn. Springer, London.

5 Strupp, M., Kremmyda, O. & Brandt, T. (2013) Pharmacotherapy of vestibular disorders and nystagmus. *Seminars in Neurology*, **33**(3), 286–296.

6 Sekitani, T., Imate, Y., Noguchi, T. & Inokuma, T. (1993) Vestibular neuronitis: epidemiological survey by questionnaire in Japan. *Acta Oto-laryngologica Supplementum*, **503**, 9–12.

7 Schulz, P., Arbusow, V., Strupp, M., Dieterich, M., Rauch, E. & Brandt, T. (1998) Highly variable distribution of HSV-1-specific

DNA in human geniculate, vestibular and spiral ganglia. *Neuroscience Letters*, **252**(2), 139–142.

8 Arbusow, V., Schulz, P., Strupp, M. *et al.* (1999) Distribution of herpes simplex virus type 1 in human geniculate and vestibular ganglia: implications for vestibular neuritis. *Annals of Neurology*, **46**(3), 416–419.

9 Arbusow, V., Theil, D., Strupp, M., Mascolo, A. & Brandt, T. (2000) HSV-1 not only in human vestibular ganglia but also in the vestibular labyrinth. *Audiology & Neuro-Otology*, **6**(5), 259–262.

10 Theil, D., Arbusow, V., Derfuss, T. *et al.* (2000) Prevalence of HSV-1 lat in human trigeminal, geniculate, and vestibular ganglia and its implication for cranial nerve syndromes. *Brain Pathology*, **11**(4), 408–413.

11 Theil, D., Derfuss, T., Strupp, M., Gilden, D.H., Arbusow, V. & Brandt, T. (2002) Cranial nerve palsies: herpes simplex virus type 1 and varizella-zoster virus latency. *Annals of Neurology*, **51**(2), 273–274.

12 Theil, D., Derfuss, T., Paripovic, I. *et al.* (2003) Latent herpesvirus infection in human trigeminal ganglia causes chronic immune response. *American Journal of Pathology*, **163**(6), 2179–2184.

13 Dutia, M.B. (2010) Mechanisms of vestibular compensation: recent advances. *Current Opinion in Otolaryngology & Head and Neck Surgery*, **18**(5), 420–424.

14 Strupp, M., Zingler, V.C., Arbusow, V. *et al.* (2004) Methylprednisolone, valacyclovir, or the combination for vestibular neuritis. *New England Journal of Medicine*, **351**(4), 354–361.

15 Goudakos, J.K., Markou, K.D., Franco-Vidal, V., Vital, V., Tsaligopoulos, M. & Darrouzet, V. (2010) Corticosteroids in the treatment of vestibular neuritis: a systematic review and meta-analysis. *Otology & Neurotology*, **31**(2), 183–189.

16 Karlberg, M.L. & Magnusson, M. (2011) Treatment of acute vestibular neuronitis with glucocorticoids. *Otology & Neurotology*, **32**(7), 1140–1143.

17 Fishman, J.M., Burgess, C. & Waddell, A. (2011) Corticosteroids for the treatment of idiopathic acute vestibular dysfunction (vestibular neuritis). *Cochrane Database of Systematic Reviews*, (5), CD008607.

18 Wegner, I., van Benthem, P.P., Aarts, M.C., Bruintjes, T.D., Grolman, W. & van der Heijden, G.J. (2012) Insufficient evidence for the effect of corticosteroid treatment on recovery of vestibular neuritis. *Otolaryngology and Head and Neck Surgery*, **147**(5), 826–831. doi:10.1177/0194599812457557. Epub 2012 Aug 21.

19 Gurkov, R., Flatz, W., Louza, J., Strupp, M. & Krause, E. (2011) In vivo visualization of endolyphatic hydrops in patients with Meniere's disease: correlation with audiovestibular function. *European Archives of Oto-Rhino-Laryngology*, **268**(12), 1743–1748.

20 Yeh, T.H., Herman, P., Tsai, M.C., Tran-Ba-Huy, P. & Van-den-Abbeele, T. (1998) A cationic nonselective stretch-activated channel in the Reissner's membrane of the guinea pig cochlea. *American Journal of Physiology*, **274**(3 Pt 1), C566–C576.

21 Carey, J.P., Hirvonen, T., Peng, G.C. *et al.* (2002) Changes in the angular vestibulo-ocular reflex after a single dose of intratympanic gentamicin for Meniere's disease. *Auris Nasus Larynx*, **956**, 581–584.

22 Postema, R.J., Kingma, C.M., Wit, H.P., Albers, F.W. & Van Der Laan, B.F. (2008) Intratympanic gentamicin therapy for control of vertigo in unilateral Menire's disease: a prospective, double-blind, randomized, placebo-controlled trial. *Acta Oto-Laryngologica*, **128**(8), 876–880.

23 Stokroos, R. & Kingma, H. (2004) Selective vestibular ablation by intratympanic gentamicin in patients with unilateral active Meniere's disease: a prospective, double-blind, placebo-controlled, randomized clinical trial. *Acta Oto-Laryngologica*, **124**(2), 172–175.

24 Pullens, B. & van Benthem, P.P. (2011) Intratympanic gentamicin for Meniere's disease or syndrome. *Cochrane Database of Systematic Reviews*, CD008234.

25 Colletti, V., Carner, M. & Colletti, L. (2007) Auditory results after vestibular nerve section and intratympanic gentamicin for Meniere's disease. *Otology & Neurotology*, **28**(2), 145–151.

26 Huppert, D., Strupp, M. & Brandt, T. (2010) Long-term course of Meniere's disease revisited. *Acta Oto-Laryngologica*, **130**(6), 644–651.

27 Garduno-Anaya, M.A., Couthino De, T.H., Hinojosa-Gonzalez, R., Pane-Pianese, C. & Rios-Castaneda, L.C. (2005) Dexamethasone inner ear perfusion by intratympanic injection in unilateral Meniere's disease: a two-year prospective, placebo-controlled, double-blind, randomized trial. *Otolaryngology and Head and Neck Surgery*, **133**(2), 285–294.

28 Phillips, J.S. & Westerberg, B. (2011) Intratympanic steroids for Meniere's disease or syndrome. *Cochrane Database of Systematic Reviews*, (7), CD008514.

29 Casani, A.P., Piaggi, P., Cerchiai, N., Seccia, V., Franceschini, S.S. & Dallan, I. (2012) Intratympanic treatment of intractable unilateral Meniere disease: gentamicin or dexamethasone? A randomized controlled trial. *Otolaryngology and Head and Neck Surgery*, **146**(3), 430–437.

30 Ihler, F., Bertlich, M., Sharaf, K., Strieth, S., Strupp, M. & Canis, M. (2012) Betahistine exerts a dose-dependent effect on cochlear stria vascularis blood flow in Guinea pigs in vivo. *PLoS One*, **7**(6), e39086.

31 Strupp, M., Cnyrim, C. & Brandt, T. (2007) Vertigo and dizziness: Treatment of benign paroxysmal positioning vertigo, vestibular neuritis and Menère's disease. In: Candelise, L. (ed), *Evidence-based Neurology - Management of Neurological Disorders*. Blackwell Publishing, Oxford, pp. 59–69.

32 Strupp, M., Hupert, D., Frenzel, C. *et al.* (2008) Long-term prophylactic treatment of attacks of vertigo in Meniere's disease--comparison of a high with a low dosage of betahistine in an open trial. *Acta Oto-Laryngologica*, **128**(5), 520–524.

33 Lezius, F., Adrion, C., Mansmann, U., Jahn, K. & Strupp, M. (2011) High-dosage betahistine dihydrochloride between 288 and 480 mg/day in patients with severe Meniere's disease: a case series. *European Archives of Oto-Rhino-Laryngology*, **268**(8), 1237–1240.

34 Brandt, T. & Dieterich, M. (1994) Vestibular paroxysmia: vascular compression of the eighth nerve? *Lancet*, **343**, 798–799.

35 Strupp, M., von Stuckrad-Barre, S., Brandt, T. & Tonn, J.C. (2013) Teaching NeuroImages: Compression of the eighth cranial nerve causes vestibular paroxysmia. *Neurology*, **80**(7), e77.

36 Hufner, K., Barresi, D., Glaser, M. *et al.* (2008) Vestibular parox-ysmia: Diagnostic features and medical treatment. *Neurology*, **71**(**13**), 1006–1014.

37 Lempert, T., Olesen, J., Furman, J. *et al.* (2012) Vestibular migraine: Diagnostic criteria. *Journal of Vestibular Research*, **22**(**4**), 167–172.

38 Reploeg, M.D. & Goebel, J.A. (2002) Migraine-associated dizzi-ness: Patient characteristics and management options. *Otology & Neurotology*, **23**(**3**), 364–371.

39 Neuhauser, H., Radtke, A., von Brevern, M. & Lempert, T. (2003) Zolmitriptan for treatment of migrainous vertigo: A pilot randomized placebo-controlled trial. *Neurology*, **60**(**5**), 882–883.

40 Bisdorff, A.R. (2004) Treatment of migraine related vertigo with lamotrigine an observational study. *Bulletin de la Société des Sciences Médicales du Grand-Duché de Luxembourg*, (**2**), 103–108.

41 Baier, B., Winkenwerder, E. & Dieterich, M. (2009) "Vestibu-lar migraine": Effects of prophylactic therapy with various drugs. A retrospective study. *Journal of Neurology*, **256**(**3**), 436–442.

42 Ophoff, R.A., Terwindt, G.M., Vergouwe, M.N. *et al.* (1996) Familial hemiplegic migraine and episodic ataxia type-2 are caused by mutations in the Ca2+ channel gene CACNL1A4. *Cell*, **87**(**3**), 543–552.

43 Jen, J.C. (2008) Hereditary episodic ataxias. *Annals of the New York Academy of Sciences*, **1142**, 250–253.

44 Jen, J.C. & Baloh, R.W. (2009) Familial episodic ataxia: a model for migrainous vertigo. *Annals of the New York Academy of Sciences*, **1164**, 252–256.

45 Jen, J., Kim, G.W. & Baloh, R.W. (2004) Clinical spectrum of episodic ataxia type 2. *Neurology*, **62**(**1**), 17–22.

46 Strupp, M., Kalla, R., Dichgans, M., Freilinger, T., Glasauer, S. & Brandt, T. (2004) Treatment of episodic ataxia type 2 with the potassium channel blocker 4-aminopyridine. *Neurology*, **62**(**9**), 1623–1625.

47 Strupp, M., Kalla, R., Claassen, J. *et al.* (2011) A randomized trial of 4-aminopyridine in EA2 and related familial episodic ataxias. *Neurology*, **77**(**3**), 269–275.

48 Alvina, K. & Khodakhah, K. (2010) The therapeutic mode of action of 4-aminopyridine in cerebellar ataxia. *Journal of Neuroscience*, **30**(**21**), 7258–7268.

49 Weisz, C.J., Raike, R.S., Soria-Jasso, L.E. & Hess, E.J. (2005) Potassium channel blockers inhibit the triggers of attacks in the calcium channel mouse mutant tottering. *Journal of Neuroscience*, **25**(**16**), 4141–4145.

50 Claassen, J., Teufel, J., Kalla, R., Spiegel, R. & Strupp, M. (2013) Effects of dalfampridine on attacks in patients with episodic ataxia type 2: an observational study. *Journal of Neurology*, **260**(**2**), 668–669.

51 Ilg, W., Bastian, A.J., Boesch, S. *et al.* (2014) Consensus paper: Management of degenerative cerebellar disorders. *Cerebellum*, **13**(**2**), 248–268.(Published on-line in November 2013).

52 Schniepp, R., Wuehr, M., Neuhaeusser, M. *et al.* (2012) 4-Aminopyridine and cerebellar gait: A retrospective case series. *Journal of Neurology*, **259**(**11**), 2491–2493.

53 Strupp, M., Teufel, J., Habs, M. *et al.* (2013) Effects of acetyl-DL-leucine in patients with cerebellar ataxia: A case series. *Journal of Neurology*, **260**(**10**), 2556–2561.

54 Stayte, M., Reeves, B. & Wortham, C. (1993) Ocular and vision defects in preschool children. *British Journal of Ophthalmology*, **77**(**4**), 228–232.

55 Wagner, J.N., Glaser, M., Brandt, T. & Strupp, M. (2008) Downbeat nystagmus: aetiology and comorbidity in 117 patients. *Journal of Neurology, Neurosurgery and Psychiatry*, **79**(**6**), 672–677.

56 Leigh, R.J. & Zee, D. (2006) *The Neurology of Eye Movements*, 4 edn. Oxford University Press, Oxford, New York.

57 Hufner, K., Stephan, T., Kalla, R. *et al.* (2007) Structural and functional MRIs disclose cerebellar pathologies in idiopathic downbeat nystagmus. *Neurology*, **69**(**11**), 1128–1135.

58 Kalla, R., Deutschlander, A., Hufner, K. *et al.* (2006) Detection of floccular hypometabolism in downbeat nystagmus by fMRI. *Neurology*, **66**(**2**), 281–283.

59 Strupp, M., Schuler, O., Krafczyk, S. *et al.* (2003) Treat-ment of downbeat nystagmus with 3,4-diaminopyridine: A placebo-controlled study. *Neurology*, **61**(**2**), 165–170.

60 Kalla, R., Glasauer, S., Buttner, U., Brandt, T. & Strupp, M. (2007) 4-aminopyridine restores vertical and horizontal neural integrator function in downbeat nystagmus. *Brain*, **130**(**Pt 9**), 2441–2451.

61 Tsunemi, T., Ishikawa, K., Tsukui, K., Sumi, T., Kitamura, K. & Mizusawa, H. (2010) The effect of 3,4-diaminopyridine on the patients with hereditary pure cerebellar ataxia. *Journal of Neuro-logical Sciences*, **292**(**1–2**), 81–84.

62 Kalla, R., Spiegel, R., Claassen, J. *et al.* (2011) Comparison of 10-mg doses of 4-aminopyridine and 3,4-diaminopyridine for the treatment of downbeat nystagmus. *Journal of Neuro-Ophthalmology*, **31**(**4**), 320–325.

63 Claassen, J., Spiegel, R., Kalla, R. *et al.* (2013) A randomised double-blind, cross-over trial of 4-aminopyridine for downbeat nystagmus--effects on slowphase eye velocity, postural stability, locomotion and symptoms. *Journal of Neurology, Neurosurgery and Psychiatry*, **84**(**12**), 1392–1399.

64 Claassen, J., Feil, K., Bardins, S. *et al.* (2013) Dalfampridine in patients with downbeat nystagmus--an observational study. *Journal of Neurology*, **260**(**8**), 1992–1996.

65 Averbuch-Heller, L., Tusa, R.J., Fuhry, L. *et al.* (1997) A double-blind controlled study of gabapentin and baclofen as treatment for acquired nystagmus. *Annals of Neurology*, **41**(**6**), 818–825.

66 Kremmyda, O., Zwergal, A., la, F.C., Brandt, T., Jahn, K. & Strupp, M. (2013) 4-Aminopyridine suppresses positional nystagmus caused by cerebellar vermis lesion. *Journal of Neurology*, **260**(**1**), 321–323.

67 Feil, K., Claassen, J., Bardins, S. *et al.* (2013) Effect of chlor-zoxazone in patients with downbeat nystagmus: a pilot trial. *Neurology*, **81**(**13**), 1152–1158.

68 Etzion, Y. & Grossman, Y. (2001) Highly 4-aminopyridine sensi-tive delayed rectifier current modulates the excitability of guinea

pig cerebellar Purkinje cells. *Experimental Brain Research*, **139**(4), 419–425.

69 Glasauer, S., Rössert, C. & Strupp, M. (2011) The role of regularity and synchrony of cerebellar Purkinje cells for pathological nystagmus and episodic ataxia type 2. *Annals of the New York Academy of Sciences*, **1233**, 162–167. doi:10.1111/j.1749-6632.2011.06149.x.

70 Hourez, R., Servais, L., Orduz, D. *et al.* (2011) Aminopyridines correct early dysfunction and delay neurodegeneration in a mouse model of spinocerebellar ataxia type 1. *Journal of Neuroscience*, **31**(33), 11795–11807.

71 Bense, S., Best, C., Buchholz, H.G. *et al.* (2006) 18F-fluorodeoxyglucose hypometabolism in cerebellar tonsil and flocculus in downbeat nystagmus. *Neuroreport*, **17**(6), 599–603.

72 Glasauer, S., Strupp, M., Kalla, R., Buttner, U. & Brandt, T. (2005) Effect of 4-aminopyridine on upbeat and downbeat nystagmus elucidates the mechanism of downbeat nystagmus. *Annals of the New York Academy of Sciences*, **1039**, 528–531.

73 Deuschl, G. & Wilms, H. (2002) Clinical spectrum and physiology of palatal tremor. *Movement Disorders*, **17**(**Suppl 2**), S63-6..:S63–S66.

74 Shaikh, A.G., Hong, S., Liao, K. *et al.* (2010) Oculopalatal tremor explained by a model of inferior olivary hypertrophy and cerebellar plasticity. *Brain*, **133**(**Pt 3**), 923–940.

75 Herishanu, Y. & Louzoun, Z. (1986) Trihexyphenidyl treatment of vertical pendular nystagmus. *Neurology*, **36**(1), 82–84.

76 Jabbari, B., Rosenberg, M., Scherokman, B., Gunderson, C.H., McBurney, J.W. & McClintock, W. (1987) Effectiveness of trihexyphenidyl against pendular nystagmus and palatal myoclonus: evidence of cholinergic dysfunction. *Movement Disorders*, **2**(2), 93–98.

77 Leigh, R.J., Burnstine, T.H., Ruff, R.L. & Kasmer, R.J. (1991) Effect of anticholinergic agents upon acquired nystagmus:

A double blind-study of trihexyphenidyl and tridehexethyl chloride. *Neurology*, **41**, 1737–1741.

78 Starck, M., Albrecht, H., Pollmann, W., Straube, A. & Dieterich, M. (1997) Drug therapy for acquired pendular nystagmus in multiple sclerosis. *Journal of Neurology*, **244**(1), 9–16.

79 Starck, M., Albrecht, H., Pollmann, W., Dieterich, M. & Straube, A. (2010) Acquired pendular nystagmus in multiple sclerosis: an examiner-blind cross-over treatment study of memantine and gabapentin. *Journal of Neurology*, **257**(3), 322–327.

80 Starck, M., Albrecht, H., Pollmann, W., Dieterich, M. & Straube, A. (2010) Acquired pendular nystagmus in multiple sclerosis: an examiner-blind cross-over treatment study of memantine and gabapentin. *Journal of Neurology*, **257**(3), 322–327.

81 Tomsak, R.L., Remler, B.F., Averbuch-Heller, L., Chandran, M. & Leigh, R.J. (1995) Unsatisfactory treatment of acquired nystagmus with retrobulbar injection of botulinum toxin. *American Journal of Ophthalmology*, **119**(4), 489–496.

82 Leigh, R.J., Robinson, D.A. & Zee, D.S. (1981) A hypothetical explanation for periodic alternating nystagmus: instability in the optokinetic-vestibular system. *Annals of the New York Academy of Sciences*, **374**, 619–635.

83 Stahl, J.S., Plant, G.T. & Leigh, R.J. (2002) Medical treatment of nystagmus and its visual consequences. *Journal of the Royal Society of Medicine*, **95**(5), 235–237.

84 Self, J. & Lotery, A. (2007) A review of the molecular genetics of congenital idiopathic nystagmus (CIN). *Ophthalmic Genetics*, **28**(4), 187–191.

85 McLean, R., Proudlock, F., Thomas, S., Degg, C. & Gottlob, I. (2007) Congenital nystagmus: randomized, controlled, double-masked trial of memantine/gabapentin. *Annals of Neurology*, **61**(2), 130–138.

CHAPTER 28

Neuro-ophthalmology

Martin Sutton-Brown[1] and Jason J. S. Barton[2]
[1]*Department of Medicine (Neurology), University of British Columbia, Vancouver, Canada*
[2]*Departments of Medicine (Neurology), Ophthalmology and Visual Sciences, Psychology, University of British Columbia, Vancouver, Canada*

Introduction

Neuro-ophthalmology encompasses a broad range of neurological disease affecting vision. This chapter focuses on three frequent causes of visual loss. Optic neuritis is the most common acute optic neuropathy in the young and the first symptom in half of the patients with multiple sclerosis: best practices for its management have largely been defined by the Optic Neuritis Treatment Trial (ONTT). Anterior ischemic optic neuropathy (AION) is the most common acute optic neuropathy in the elderly. Identifying which subjects have arteritis is a challenge and has been the subject of many studies. Non-arteritic AION has a higher incidence, and there has been substantial work and discussion around its prognosis for vision, recurrence, and possible treatment.

Optic neuritis

Optic neuritis is acute inflammation of the optic nerve. It is the third most frequent initial symptom of multiple sclerosis. Conversely, about half of patients with optic neuritis will eventually develop multiple sclerosis. A small fraction of the remaining half will have one of the several other rare causes, which are not pursued unless the history, exam findings, or clinical course are atypical. Optic neuritis has assumed great significance as a model for multiple sclerosis because detailed, objective measures are possible for both visual function and the structural changes with neuronal loss, using optic coherence tomography.

Because of its quality and size, the ONTT is the benchmark for the natural history, investigation, and treatment of optic neuritis [1]. Excluding older studies that used ACTH, there are three other randomized, placebo-controlled trials [2–4], the largest with 66 subjects. Their findings are generally similar to those of the ONTT. Overviews have been performed by a meta-analysis, a Cochrane review, and a practice parameter of the American Academy of Neurology

[5–7]. The meta-analysis [7] combined a heterogeneous set of studies with different interventions and populations with multiple sclerosis, in contrast to the isolated optic neuritis presentations evaluated in the ONTT. The Cochrane review [5] limited its analysis to studies with populations similar to those in the ONTT, but could include only one other trial. The practice parameter did not do a meta-analysis across trials [6].

Do corticosteroids improve the rate of recovery or long-term visual prognosis of optic neuritis?

The ONTT studied 457 patients of ages between 18 and 46 years, with ≤8 days of symptoms. These subjects were randomized to three treatment arms: placebo ($n = 150$), 1 mg/kg of body weight per day of oral prednisone for 14 days ($n = 156$), and 250 mg of intravenous methylprednisolone four times a day for 3 days followed by oral prednisone for 11 days ($n = 151$). Seventy-seven percent of patients were female and 85% were Caucasian. Recovery began in the first 2 weeks in most: 79% in the placebo group, 92% in the intravenous methylprednisolone group, and 92% in the prednisone group. Most of the improvement in visual acuity happened in the first month, with median acuity better than 20/25 by 2 weeks after evaluation in all three groups [8]. On perimetry, the rate of return to normal visual sensitivity was more rapid in the first month in those receiving intravenous methylprednisolone than in the placebo group [1]. A post hoc analysis suggested that accelerated recovery was most pronounced in patients with visual acuity worse than 20/200. Similarly, the meta-analysis for lack of functional improvement at 1 month favored intravenous methylprednisolone over placebo, with an odds ratio of 0.49 [7]. By contrast, oral prednisone did not benefit visual field measures, contrast sensitivity, or visual acuity. At 6 months, though, the adjusted relative "risk" for returning to normal with intravenous methylprednisolone versus placebo was only 1.09 for visual fields and 1.07 for acuity, indicating no benefit of intravenous methylprednisolone at that point. Follow-up at 15 years confirmed a lack of difference in visual function between treatment groups [9]. Of note, 63% of patients continued to have visual complaints despite excellent recovery to acuities of 20/25 or better, reflecting the relative insensitivity of clinical measures of visual function [10].

Thus, intravenous methylprednisolone sped recovery in the first month but showed no long-term effect at 6 months, while oral prednisone at the dose used had no effect on vision. More rapid improvement may be important to some patients, as long as the potential adverse effects are acceptable. However, patients with mild visual loss (acuity < 20/40) already have an excellent prognosis and have little to gain visually from treatment.

As is typical after all treatment studies, alternative dosing regimes are being used in practice without evidence [11]. This includes 1 g IV daily as a single dose or as five doses, the elimination of the 11 days of oral prednisone following intravenous dosing, treatment beginning outside of the 2-week window after onset and use of high doses of oral prednisone alone. The latter reflects data that the bioavailability of 1250 mg of oral prednisone is equivalent to that of 1mg of intravenous methylprednisolone [12]. The efficacy of high-dose oral steroids in multiple sclerosis may be settled soon by the OMEGA Trial [13].

The most common side effects of steroids in these patients were hypertension, cardiac arrhythmia, weight gain, sleep disturbance, metallic taste, a fuller face, and facial acne [7]. Other statistically significant adverse effects were insomnia, mood changes, facial flushing or hot flashes, gastrointestinal symptoms, and weight gain [1,4,14]. In the ONTT, only 2 of the 151 patients had to discontinue methylprednisolone, due to depression or pancreatitis [1].

What is the risk of developing multiple sclerosis after an attack of optic neuritis? Does the choice of treatment affect the risk of developing multiple sclerosis?

The risk of clinically definite multiple sclerosis increases as time passes after an attack of optic neuritis. In the ONTT, taking all groups together, conversion to multiple sclerosis was 30% at 5 years, 38% at 10 years, and 50% at 15 years [15].

The ONTT showed that this risk is modulated by results of the MRI scan at presentation (Figure 28.1). At 5 years, patients with a normal MRI had a 16% risk of a diagnosis of multiple sclerosis, while those with one or two demyelinating lesions had a 37% risk and those with three or more lesions had a 51% risk [16]. By 10 and 15 years, the difference between single and multiple lesions was no longer significant. At 15 years, one or more lesions conferred a risk of multiple sclerosis of 72%, compared to only 25% in patients with a normal baseline MRI [15,17]. In the interval between

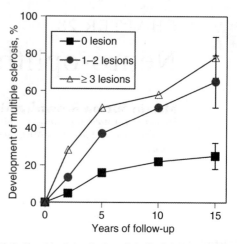

Figure 28.1 The risk of developing clinically definite multiple sclerosis after an initial episode of optic neuritis in the ONTT. Patients are divided into groups based on the presence of lesions on their initial MRI scan of the brain. By 10–15 years, the difference between those with one or two lesions and those with three or more lesions is no longer statistically significant.

10 and 15 years, only 1 of 191 patients with a normal baseline MRI converted to a diagnosis of multiple sclerosis.

At this final 15-year analysis, no other clinical factors were predictive of multiple sclerosis in the patients with abnormal MRI [15]. Among those with a normal MRI scan, females had 3.57 times greater risk of multiple sclerosis (29% vs 8% for males), while a preceding viral illness or lack of disc edema increased the risk by 2.5 times.

The prognostic value of cerebrospinal fluid analysis was not specifically evaluated in the ONTT. Lumbar puncture was optional and only completed in 31.5% of cases [18]. A meta-analysis of 10 prospective studies evaluated oligoclonal bands in 646 patients followed for a mean of 5.5 years (range 1–12.9 years) across studies [19]. This showed a mean sensitivity of 88.5% and specificity of 57%. Evaluating their summary data in a manner analogous to the ONTT showed a 53% chance of developing multiple sclerosis in those 385 patients with positive oligoconal bands (positive predictive value), versus 12% chance in those 216 patients without bands (i.e., negative predictive value of 88%). This is very similar to the predictive values of three or more MRI lesions (51%) versus no lesions (16%) at the 5-year mark of the ONTT. However, oligoclonal banding and MRI lesions are not independent factors. The ONTT showed that 73% of patients with an abnormal MRI have oligoclonal bands whereas only 28% of those with normal MRI do [20]. In fact, oligoclonal bands contributed prognostic information only in those with a normal MRI: in this group, positive predictive value was 27% and negative predictive value was 96% for developing multiple sclerosis by 5 years [21]. Hence, patients with both normal MRI and no oligoclonal bands have an extremely low likelihood of multiple sclerosis. However, lack of standardized methods and diagnostic criteria are practical concerns that may limit the utility of cerebrospinal fluid analysis [19,22].

The impact of treatment on the rate at which patients were diagnosed with multiple sclerosis was also examined by the ONTT. Of the 389 patients in the 2-year analysis of the ONTT cohort, 16.7% in the placebo group converted to clinically definite multiple sclerosis, compared to 7.5% in the intravenous methylprednisolone group and 14.7% in the oral prednisone group [23]. By 10 years, there was no difference in the risk between the treatment arms, with a cumulative risk of 38% [17]. This short-term reduction in risk for conversion to clinically definite multiple sclerosis has not been replicated outside the ONTT [7].

Oral prednisone at the dose used in the ONTT had no beneficial effect on early recovery. In fact, it has been asserted that it may even be harmful [24]. First, it appeared to increase the relative risk of recurrent or contralateral optic neuritis by a factor of 1.79 at 6 months [1]. Again, this has not been replicated by others [7]. Second, it also appeared to increase the risk of developing clinically definite multiple sclerosis at the 2-year mark, when the adjusted rate ratio of *not* converting was 0.38 [23], although this was no longer evident at the 3-year mark [25]. It is not clear why oral prednisone might increase the risk of subsequent optic neuritis or earlier conversion to multiple sclerosis. Beck *et al.* [26] postulated possible mechanisms of immune modulation based on dose. However, a Cochrane review of oral versus intravenous steroids for relapses in multiple sclerosis found no evidence of increased relapse rate with either [27].

The ONTT also evaluated the long-term likelihood of disability, using the Expanded Disability Scale Score (EDSS). Most patients at both 10 and 15 years of follow-up had minimal disability, with 65% having a score of >3.0 and only 12–17% having a score ≤6.0 [15,28]. Lesions on MRI did not affect disability rates. Another study of 143 patients followed for a median of 6 years found that spinal cord lesions at presentation or new T2 lesions on follow-up MRI more than 3 months later were most predictive of disability, though enhancing lesions or infratentorial lesions at baseline also carried some risk [29].

What investigations are necessary for optic neuritis?

Optic neuritis is a clinical diagnosis. Typical symptoms are monocular color vision loss and decreased acuity that worsen over a few days, eye pain that worsens with movement, and a relative afferent pupil defect on examination [30]. The optic discs appear normal in 65% of patients, the so-called "retrobulbar" form of optic neuritis. Thirty-five percent have "anterior optic neuritis" or "papillitis," with modest optic disc edema [1]. A few may have a mild uveitis. Automated perimetry of the central 30 degrees of vision shows diffuse loss in 48% [31], though this can often turn out to be a large cecocentral scotoma on full-field perimetry. Significant improvement within a few weeks supports the diagnosis.

Cases that follow this profile are almost always due to multiple sclerosis or possibly a monophasic, idiopathic inflammatory event [15]. Only 2 of 457 patients enrolled in ONTT had another cause of optic neuropathy, due to a connective tissue disease [1,11]. Hence, it is no longer recommended that antinuclear antibody, fluorescent treponemal antibody absorption, chest radiography or lumbar puncture be obtained in patients with typical optic neuritis [11]. MRI should be focused on the brain to stratify the risk of multiple sclerosis rather than on the orbit to look for other causes of optic neuropathy. The history and examination should exclude atypical features and the patients reassessed to confirm the expected course of improvement within 4–6 weeks. Unusual features should prompt investigations for less common causes of optic neuritis.

Arteritic anterior ischemic optic neuropathy

AION is an infarct of the optic disc, which is supplied by the posterior ciliary arteries. Arteritic AION is due to vasculitis, most often giant cell arteritis in the elderly. Arteritic AION is six times less common than non-arteritic AION [32]. Patients with arteritis are at risk of contralateral visual loss or ischemia in other organs, such as the brain, heart, and intestines, which may be prevented by treatment with steroids. While there are no natural history data on untreated arteritis, follow-up studies show that treated patients have similar mortality rates to controls [33]. Efficacy of steroid treatment has not been rigorously documented and likely never will be. Use of steroids rests solely on an historical observation that none of 55 treated patients developed bilateral blindness whereas 6 of 53 historical controls did [34]. Nevertheless, the consensus is that timely diagnosis is important. This depends on clinical suspicion supported by laboratory investigations and ultimately a biopsy specimen.

What are the best diagnostic clues for arteritis as a cause of AION?

Initial statistical considerations of the diagnosis of giant cell arteritis suggested that meeting at least three of five criteria (Table 28.1) gave a sensitivity of 93% and a specificity of 91% [35]. However, this formulation is awkward as it incorporates the current gold standard for diagnosis, the biopsy. In most subsequent analyses, consideration has focused on the ability of different features to predict a positive biopsy.

One large retrospective review [36,37] and two comprehensive meta-reviews [33,38] provide the best overview of the utility of the symptoms, signs, and investigations in predicting a positive biopsy. These reveal four interesting

Table 28.1 Traditional criteria for diagnosing giant cell arteritis

Age > 50 years
New localized headache
Temporal artery abnormality (tenderness, absent pulse)
ESR > 50 mm/hour, Westergren method
Temporal artery biopsy showing mononuclear cells or granulomatous
    inflammation

observations. First, the absence of any particular clinical feature is not helpful in excluding the diagnosis. Second, jaw claudication, temporal artery pain, and a palpably abnormal temporal artery are the best clinical predictors of a positive biopsy. Third, among investigations, the platelet count is more useful than the ESR. Fourth, a "normal" ESR[1] is more helpful in excluding disease than an increased ESR is in increasing suspicion, except when the ESR is markedly elevated (>100 mm/hour).

These meta-reviews provided likelihood ratios that are convenient for establishing the probability of arteritis in any given patient. Multiplying the prevalence of arteritis in their age cohort by the product of all the applicable likelihood ratios gives the odds that the disease is present (Table 28.2). This can then be used to determine the appropriate investigations in an algorithm – see example, bottom of Table 28.2 [40,41].

Since increased ESR can occur with many conditions, there is a need for tests with better specificity. Even though one study found that C-reactive protein (CRP) at the usual criterion of 0.5 mg/dL also had a low specificity of 82%, a requirement for *both* ESR and CRP to be elevated for a positive result yielded a specificity of 98% [42]. In this study, this Boolean "AND" logic did not cause the sensitivity to drop below that of the ESR alone, because the sensitivity of the CRP was 100%. A cut-off of 2.45 mg/dL was also advocated as giving the best odds ratio of 3.2. However, in this study of 43 patients with biopsy-proven arteritis, the controls were patients with other ophthalmic conditions not requiring biopsy. Hence the relevance of this analysis to patients suspected of arteritis can be questioned. A more recent review of CRP in 591 biopsied patients with a prevalence of arteritis of 16% reported an odds ratio for CRP > 2.45 mg/dL of 5.3 [43]: Our analysis of their data shows sensitivity of 0.80 and specificity of only 0.57. By our calculation, their likelihood ratios for ESR are similar to those in the reviews [33,38], and show that platelets and CRP derive their utility from their negative likelihood ratios being superior to those of ESR (Table 28.3).

There have been a few other studies of other potential diagnostic markers, many reviewed elsewhere [44]. A

[1] In 27,912 adults, age-adjusted normal values are <age/2 for men and <(age + 10)/2 for women [39], but many studies do not define their criteria.

meta-analysis of ultrasound of the temporal arteries in 2036 patients of 23 studies suggested that the presence of a dark halo, stenosis, or occlusion of the temporal arteries yielded a sensitivity of 87% and specificity of 96% [45]. A single study of MRI angiography in 64 patients suggested sensitivity of 80% and specificity of 96% [46]. A meta-analysis of PET scans for FDG uptake by larger arteries in six studies involving a total of 81 arteritic patients and 182 controls showed a sensitivity of 80% and specificity of 89% [47]. If the reportedly high specificity of imaging findings are confirmed, the diagnostic algorithm may evolve into (1) application of tests with high sensitivity to exclude patients with a very low probability of disease (e.g., normal platelets and ESR with few suspicious symptoms), then (2) applying to the remainder tests with high specificity (e.g., ultrasonography or MR angiography). Biopsy should then only be required on those with negative results on the specific tests, with patients with positive results proceeding directly to treatment.

When, how much, and how many arteries to biopsy?

An intriguing issue with any gold standard is its validity. By usual definition, a gold standard has 100% specificity, but its sensitivity can be questioned: that is, how often does this eventually prove to have missed the diagnosis? A Bayesian analysis using data of 439 biopsies from four studies of the discordance of simultaneous bilateral biopsies [37,48–50] suggested that the sensitivity of a unilateral biopsy is 87%, with a prevalence of arteritis of 24% in patients referred for biopsy [40]. If we update this with data from another recent study of 132 patients [51], the sensitivity is 86.5% and prevalence is 29%.

The literature has discussed two practical factors that may contribute to false-negative results: prolonged steroid treatment before biopsy, and small pathologic specimens that may miss patchy disease, the so-called "skip lesions" [52]. The impetus for early biopsy rests on an old retrospective observation that 50 of 61 biopsies of untreated patients were positive, compared to 30 of 51 in patients treated for up to a week, and 4 of 20 treated for more than a week [53]. All patients were presumed to have arteritis by clinical criteria alone, which is problematic: in addition, no clinical details were provided, and hence we do not know if urgently biopsied patients were the ones with higher likelihood of arteritis, as found by other studies [54]. The dose of prednisone was not stated, and the findings are confounded by the fact that biopsies were short in general, and longer in the untreated group (7.9 mm vs 6.2 mm in treated). A subsequent retrospective review of 1113 biopsies with a prevalence of arteritis of 33% found positive results in 67% of the 122 patients biopsied after less than a month of steroids, compared to 34% of the 106 with longer treatment duration [36]: again, this may simply reflect the fact that

Table 28.2 Using age, symptoms, and signs to determine the probability of giant cell arteritis

Age	Pre-test odds			Likelihood ratios (LR)	
	Prevalence (*p*,%)	Pre-test odds = $p/(1-p)$		Positive LR	Negative LR
			Symptoms		
55–59	0.02	0.0002	Jaw claudication	4.026	0.766
60–64	0.05	0.0005	Temporal artery pain	2.259	0.639
65–69	0.14	0.0014	Diplopia	1.99	0.955
70–74	0.31	0.0031	Fever	1.377	0.905
75–79	0.61	0.0061	Any visual symptom	1.301	0.917
80–84	0.86	0.0087	Weight loss	1.3	0.923
85–89	1.1	0.0111	Polymyalgia rheumatica	1.265	0.914
			Myalgia	1.245	0.798
			Headache	1.217	0.748
			Arthralgia	1.139	0.992
			Anorexia	0.949	1.032
			Fatigue	1.2	0.94
			Signs:		
			Palpably abnormal temporal artery	3.083	0.486
Post-test odds = product of all applicable LRs			Scalp tenderness	1.696	0.903
* pre-test odds			Optic atrophy or edema	1.6	0.8
Post-test probability = post-test odds/			Any fundoscopic abnormality	1.1	1
(1 + posttest odds)			Synovitis	0.41	1.1

With visual loss, if post-test probability (%) on the basis of symptoms and signs is:

<0.70	Observe
0.70 to 3.0	Platelet count: if negative observe, if positive do biopsy
4 to 13	Unilateral temporal artery biopsy
14 to 40	ESR: if low do unilateral, if high do bilateral temporal artery biopsy
45 to 60	Bilateral temporal artery biopsy
65 to 85	Platelet count: if negative, biopsy bilaterally, if positive, treat

Example: 85 year old woman, pre-test odds = 0.0111

If she has (1) visual loss, (2) jaw claudication, (3) temporally artery pain, (4) new headache but (5) no weight loss and exam shows (6) abnormal temporal artery,

then post-test odds = 1.301 × 4.026 × 2.259 × 1.217 × 0.923 × 3.083 × 0.0111 = 0.456

and post-test probability = 0.456/(1 + 0.456) = 31.3%

recommendation = temporal artery biopsy, unilateral if ESR low, bilateral if ESR high.

highly suspicious cases were biopsied earlier. On a finer temporal scale, two reviews of 98 [55] and 535 patients [54] found no difference in the prevalence of positive results between those treated before biopsy for 1 week, 2 weeks, or more than 2 weeks, with the latter study reaching this conclusion after adjusting for other clinical variables. A small attempt at a prospective randomized trial of early versus late biopsy in 11 patients still found positive results in 6 of 7 patients biopsied after 4–6 weeks of treatment [56]. Even though all of these studies are limited by the small number of patients with delayed biopsies, the best evidence [54] suggests that the pathology is relatively unaffected by intervals between treatment and biopsy of up to a month.

Even though there are no controlled studies – comparing examinations of different lengths in the same sample – observations consistently imply that longer biopsies are better. In one review, positive results were reported in 32% of 101 biopsies more than 1 cm in length, but in only 14% of 35 biopsies less than 1 cm, with an odds ratio of 2.9 [57]. Another review of 1520 biopsies reported an odds ratio for a positive result of 5.7 for 1674 biopsies of more than 0.5 cm compared to 68 biopsies smaller than that, but little difference for various biopsy lengths of more than 0.5 cm [58]. Conversely, at least four studies have reported that positive biopsies are 20–40% longer than negative ones [55,57,59,60] (Table 28.4). None of these studies controlled

Table 28.3 Likelihood ratios for giant cell arteritis from tests

Laboratory tests	Positive LR	Negative LR
From Niederkohr and Levin [38]		
ESR < 50 mm/hour	0.551	1.581
ESR = 50 to 100 mm/hour	1.095	0.963
ESR > 100 mm/hour	2.466	0.775
Anemia	1.221	0.923
Thrombocytosis	5.982	0.565
From Walvick and Walvick [43]		
ESR < 47 mm/hourr	0.639	1.127
ESR = 47–107 mm/hour	0.939	1.109
ESR > 107 mm/hour	2.335	0.853
CRP > 2.45 mg/dL	1.869	0.356
Platelets > 400,000/μl	2.36	0.667

Table 28.4 Biopsy length in patients with negative versus positive results

	Negative biopsy		Positive biopsy	
	n	Length (mm)	n	Length (mm)
Sudlow [59]	135	8.6	50	10.6
Taylor-Gjevre et al. [57]	98	16.9	38	20.7
Goslin and Chung [60]	29	12.9	18	18.4
Chmelewski et al., [55]	68	18.4	30	24.4

for the possibility that physicians targeted the patients with a more suspicious clinical story for longer biopsies.

Bilateral sequential or simultaneous biopsies have been proposed. How much does a second biopsy add? Our updated analysis of [40] shows a discordant rate (where one biopsy is negative and the other positive) of 6.8%. If the decision about which side to biopsy is random, then half of these (3.4%) would have been missed by a unilateral biopsy. However, that decision is not usually random, and it is plausible that yields are higher on the clinically suspicious side. Unfortunately, none of the studies of simultaneous biopsy provide that data. Regarding the decision to perform a second biopsy after a first negative one, our updated analysis indicates a negative predictive value of a single biopsy of 95%: thus 5% of patients with a negative biopsy will prove ultimately to have arteritis. If we assume the same sensitivity of 86% for the second biopsy, then about 4.6% of second biopsies will yield a positive result if all cases with a negative first biopsy are subjected to a second one. Again, the second biopsy may be less sensitive if taken from a less clinically suspicious side: hence 4.6% may be an overestimate.

Given these figures, the value of a second sequential biopsy needs to be improved by targeting it to subjects with a higher pre-biopsy probability of arteritis. For example, in a subset of patients whose likelihood ratios from clinical features and laboratory investigations in Tables 28.2 and 28.3 indicate a 70% probability of arteritis, 60% of initial biopsies, and 21% of second sequential biopsies will return as positive. This is why one algorithm [38] recommends bilateral biopsy only for those subjects with a high likelihood of disease.

Non-arteritic anterior ischemic optic neuropathy

Non-arteritic AION is the most common acute optic neuropathy in the elderly [61], with an incidence of 2–10/100,000 people per year [32,62]. It presents with sudden monocular vision loss, which about two-thirds of patients note on awakening, and without pain, though 10% may note mild eye or head ache. The key findings on examination are a relative afferent pupil defect and optic disc edema, which lasts on average about 8 weeks [63]. One must question the diagnosis if no disc swelling is seen within 1–2 months after onset, as non-arteritic posterior ischemic optic neuropathy is rare outside of special circumstances of diffuse hypoperfusion, such as shock or postoperative visual loss.

The pathophysiology of non-arteritic AION is assumed to be ischemia from failure of the microvascular supply of the optic nerve head, rather than embolic disease to large arteries [64,65]. About 50–60% of patients have diabetes and/or hypertension [66,67]. These chronic factors may operate partly by impairing vascular autoregulation. A small crowded optic disc, more common in Caucasians and hyperopes, may render the nerve vulnerable to a "compartment syndrome," promoting a vicious cycle between edema and ischemia [68]. Nocturnal hypotension may be an acute precipitating factor, given that many patients awake with visual loss, though small studies have not verified this [69]. A role for venous insufficiency has also been proposed, but this hypothesis requires more data [70].

What is the prognosis for vision loss in non-arteritic AION, and can treatment help?

While the visual defect is maximum at or near the time of onset in most patients, a minority progresses over the first 3–6 weeks [71,72]. In the Ischemic Optic Neuropathy Decompression Trial (IONDT), about 25% of affected eyes had some documented decline of visual acuity within the first month [67]. This is similar to a report in 27 patients that 22% of eyes worsened in the first 2 months by either two lines of visual acuity or 2dB of mean sensitivity on automated perimetry [73].

Improvement can occur in the months that follow. Smaller studies first suggested rates of improvement of 13–24% over the years [73,74]. The best data come from two large studies (Figure 28.2). In a large untreated cohort of 281 eyes followed for at least 6 months [63], 29% of those with initial acuity worse than 20/40 improved acuity by at least three lines, while 11% worsened. In a smaller subset of 59 eyes assessed in the first 2 weeks with acuity of worse than 20/70, 25 (41%) had improved at 6 months whereas 9 (19%) had worsened. These last subset figures are similar to the data of the untreated control group in the IONDT, which required acuity to be worse than 20/64 at entry. In this study, of the 122 eyes assessed at 6 months, 42.6% had improved acuity by three or more lines while 14.8% had worsened [75]. Both of these studies showed no improvement beyond 6 months. Changes on visual fields were more modest. Goldman perimetric results were improved in 26% and worse in 15% of the 105 eyes with moderate to severe vision loss at 6 months [63]. In the IONDT, automated perimetry showed that central fields had improved in 21% and worsened in 9.5% of 179 eyes at 12 months [76]. The latter study also showed that the degree of improvement was modest, generally in the range of 1–2dB of mean sensitivity.

Many approaches have been tried to improve vision in AION [77]. These have generally involved one of four strategies: improving vascular or oxygen supply, reducing the effects of disc edema, improving residual neural function, or enhancing neural plasticity (Table 28.5). However, most studies are observations in a small series of cases without controls, with few if any attempts at replication or larger studies, and will not be discussed further.

Table 28.5 Strategies used in studies of treatment for non-arteritic AION

---

a. Enhancing vascular or oxygen supply
  Aspirin
  Anticoagulation
  Urokinase
  Norepinephrine
  Vasodilators, systemic
  Vasodilators, retrobulbar injection
  Hyperbaric oxygen
  Heparin-induced extracorporeal LDL/fibrinogen precipitation
b. Reducing optic disc edema or its effects
  Steroids
  Triamcinolone, intravitreal
  Anti-vascular endothelial growth factor antibodies, intravitreal
  Optic nerve sheath fenestration
  Optic neurotomy
  Vitrectomy
c. Enhancing neural function
  Diphenylhydantoin
d. Enhancing neural plasticity/survival
  Levo-dopa
  Brimonidine, topical
  Trans-corneal electrical stimulation
  Cytidine-5′-diphosphocholine

For vascular approaches, a retrospective case–control study comparing 23 patients who used aspirin before and during the course of AION with 55 patients who did not use it failed to find an effect on acuity or mean deviation on automated perimetry [78]. A prospective randomized study of 40 patients found no change in acuity or visual evoked potentials but some improvement in mean visual sensitivity on automated perimetry after 3 months of heparin-induced extracorporeal LDL/fibrinogen precipitation started within 2 weeks of onset [79]. However, a key problem was the failure to study patients at a later time point. This was underlined by another prospective randomized study of 20 patients undergoing LDL apheresis, which found transient benefit in mean visual sensitivity at the end of treatment, but not 6 months later [80]. They postulated that this might reflect short-term enhancement of blood flow in the posterior ciliary arteries.

By far the main target of treatment studies has been the optic disc edema. The IONDT was a randomized study of optic nerve sheath fenestration involving 418 subjects [75]. It was motivated by observations that fenestration might improve vision in AION patients with a progressive course [81–83]. The rationale was that fenestration might reduce the exacerbation of ischemia by disc edema, a hypothesis questioned by others [84,85]. The IONDT was stopped prematurely because an interim analysis showed worse outcome in the treated patients. Even though the IONDT included all AION patients, it failed to find any interaction with clinical course to suggest benefit in those with the progressive variant. Other observations have both failed to find benefit in progressive AION [86,87] and documented spontaneous improvement with this variant [88]. More recently, there has been interest in transvitreal optic neurotomy as a means of decompressing the swollen nerve at the lamina cribrosa. An uncontrolled observation in 7 patients [89] was followed by a scantily described randomized but probably unblinded trial in 16 patients [90]. Interpreting the claim of benefit is complicated by the fact that most patients had acuity of count fingers before and after treatment, that some patients in both treatment and observation arms had unusually dramatic improvement, and that there was no description of perimetric method or analysis.

The use of corticosteroids in non-arteritic AION remains controversial. In a large sequential cohort of patients who either declined or opted for steroids, there was a significant reduction in the duration of optic disc edema in 237 patients started on treatment within 2 weeks ($P < 0.0001$) [91]. A second study of 613 patients of this cohort reported the effect on visual function [92]. Among those with visual acuity of 20/70 or worse, there was improvement in 70% of those taking prednisone within 2 weeks of onset, versus 40% of those who declined treatment. Even though the numbers of subjects are impressive, the lack of blinding or randomized assignment has left the field divided on the efficacy of this treatment [93].

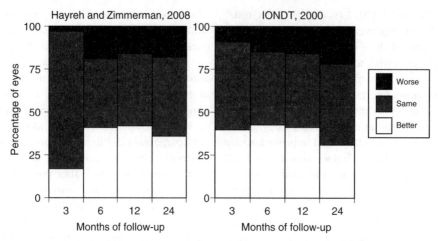

Figure 28.2 The course of vision after onset in an eye affected by non-arteritic anterior ischemic optic neuropathy, in a large observational study in the left graph, and a prospective study in the right graph. Slightly under half of subjects have some improvement by 3–6 months, with no further improvement beyond that point.

Regarding neural strategies, two small prospective randomized studies failed to find visual enhancement by diphenylhydantoin started 3 months after onset [94] or neuroprotection from topical brimonidine started in the first week [95]. A small prospective randomized trial of levodopa started many months after onset of AION reported benefit [96], as did a retrospective case–control study by the same group of levodopa within 1.5 months of onset [97]. However, these results have been hotly debated on methodological grounds [98–100] and were not replicated in a second small prospective randomized trial of late use [101]. Recently, a randomized prospective trial in 26 patients of a 2-month course of cytidine-5′-diphosphocholine begun 6 months after onset of AION-reported benefit in acuity that was sustained 4 months after treatment and up to a year [102]. A number of electrophysiological measures also showed benefit, but perimetry was not performed.

What is the prognosis for second-eye involvement in non-arteritic AION, and can treatment help?

Initially, a large observational study of 388 patients estimated that about 34% of patients developed second-eye involvement by 5 years after the first episode [66]. However, others [103] have pointed out that this may have been an overestimate, because of inclusion of subjects seen for the first time after the second eye had already been affected. In the prospective follow-up of the IONDT, the risk of recurrent AION in the same eye was less than 5% while the contralateral eye was affected in 15% at 5 years, with half occurring in the first year [104]. This is similar to the results of 278 untreated patients in a retrospective review, which estimated a 5-year rate of AION in the second eye of 12–19%, depending on whether patients lost to follow up were included as presumed without recurrence [103]. In both the IONDT [104] and the large observational study

[66], risk of AION in the second eye was increased by diabetes but unaffected by hypertension, the latter finding also noted in another small retrospective series of 100 patients [105]. Male gender was associated with increased risk in the observational study [66] but not in the IONDT [104] or the other retrospective review [103]. In the IONDT, risk was also increased if visual acuity was worse than 20/200 in the first eye, but unaffected by smoking [104].

While there are no prospective trials, aspirin was not found to be an important factor in the risk of recurrence in the observational arm of the IONDT trial [104] or in the large retrospective cohort study [103,104]. A smaller retrospective study reported that the incidence of AION developing in the second eye after 2 years was 17% among those who used aspirin ($n = 33$) and 53% in those who did not: the latter risk raises questions about the results because it contrasts with much lower rates reported by other larger studies [66,103,104].

Whether better control of possible risk factors such as diabetes, hypertension, or sleep apnea makes any difference to the risk of involvement of the second eye is not known. In addition, there remains a question of whether non-arteritic AION is a harbinger of future cardiovascular or cerebrovascular disease, given that the majority of these patients have one or more vascular risk factors [66,67]. In one report, 13 of 71 patients died from these causes over a mean period of 5 years, about 2.5 times expected for the general population [74]. However, this analysis does not clarify whether AION confers any additional risk beyond that for diabetes and hypertension.

Acknowledgement

JB was supported by a Canada Research Chair and the Marianne Koerner Chair in Brain Diseases.

References

1 Beck, R.W. *et al.* (1992) A randomized, controlled trial of corticosteroids in the treatment of acute optic neuritis. The Optic Neuritis Study Group. *New England Journal of Medicine,* **326(9)**, 581–588.

2 Kapoor, R. *et al.* (1998) Effects of intravenous methylprednisolone on outcome in MRI-based prognostic subgroups in acute optic neuritis. *Neurology,* **50(1)**, 230–237.

3 Wakakura, M. *et al.* (1999) Multicenter clinical trial for evaluating methylprednisolone pulse treatment of idiopathic optic neuritis in Japan. Optic Neuritis Treatment Trial Multicenter Cooperative Research Group (ONMRG). *Japanese Journal of Ophthalmology,* **43(2)**, 133–138.

4 Sellebjerg, F. *et al.* (1999) A randomized, controlled trial of oral high-dose methylprednisolone in acute optic neuritis. *Neurology,* **52(7)**, 1479–1484.

5 Vedula, S.S. *et al.* (2007) Corticosteroids for treating optic neuritis. *Cochrane Database of Systematic Reviews,* **1**.: CD001430

6 Kaufman, D.I., et al., Practice parameter: the role of corticosteroids in the management of acute monosymptomatic optic neuritis. report Of the quality standards subcommittee of the american academy of neurology(1). *American Journal of Ophthalmology,* 2000. **130(4)**: 541.

7 Brusaferri, F. & Candelise, L. (2000) Steroids for multiple sclerosis and optic neuritis: a meta-analysis of randomized controlled clinical trials. *Journal of Neurology,* **247(6)**, 435–442.

8 Beck, R.W., Cleary, P.A. & Backlund, J.C. (1994) The course of visual recovery after optic neuritis. Experience of the Optic Neuritis Treatment Trial. *Ophthalmology,* **101(11)**, 1771–1778.

9 Optic Neuritis Study Group (2008) Visual function 15 years after optic neuritis: a final follow-up report from the Optic Neuritis Treatment Trial. *Ophthalmology,* **115(6)**, 1079–1082.e5.

10 Cleary, P.A. *et al.* (1997) Visual symptoms after optic neuritis. Results from the Optic Neuritis Treatment Trial. *Journal of Neuro-Ophthalmology,* **17(1)**, 18–23.; quiz 24-8.

11 Volpe, N.J. (2008) The optic neuritis treatment trial: a definitive answer and profound impact with unexpected results. *Archives of Ophthalmology,* **126(7)**, 996–999.

12 Morrow, S.A. *et al.* (2004) The bioavailability of IV methylprednisolone and oral prednisone in multiple sclerosis. *Neurology,* **63(6)**, 1079–1080.

13 Lublin, F. (2007) *Oral Megadose Corticosteroids Therapy of Acute Exacerbations of Multiple Sclerosis (OMEGA).*

14 Chrousos, G.A. *et al.* (1993) Side effects of glucocorticoid treatment. Experience of the Optic Neuritis Treatment Trial. *JAMA,* **269(16)**, 2110–2112.

15 Optic Neuritis Study Group Multiple sclerosis risk after optic neuritis: final optic neuritis treatment trial follow-up. *Archives of Neurology,* 2008. **65(6)**:727–732. doi: 10.1001/archneur.65.6.727.

16 Optic Neuritis Study Group (1997) The 5-year risk of MS after optic neuritis. Experience of the optic neuritis treatment trial. *Neurology,* **49(5)**, 1404–1413.

17 Beck, R.W. *et al.* (2003) High- and low-risk profiles for the development of multiple sclerosis within 10 years after optic neuritis: experience of the optic neuritis treatment trial. *Archives of Ophthalmology,* **121(7)**, 944–949.

18 Optic Neuritis Study Group (1991) The clinical profile of optic neuritis. Experience of the Optic Neuritis Treatment Trial. *Archives of Ophthalmology,* **109(12)**, 1673–1678.

19 Skov, A.G., Skov, T. & Frederiksen, J.L. (2011) Oligoclonal bands predict multiple sclerosis after optic neuritis: a literature survey. *Multiple Sclerosis,* **17(4)**, 404–410.

20 Rolak, L.A. *et al.* (1996) Cerebrospinal fluid in acute optic neuritis: experience of the optic neuritis treatment trial. *Neurology,* **46(2)**, 368–372.

21 Cole, S.R. *et al.* (1998) The predictive value of CSF oligoclonal banding for MS 5 years after optic neuritis. Optic Neuritis Study Group. *Neurology,* **51(3)**, 885–887.

22 Link, H. & Huang, Y.M. (2006) Oligoclonal bands in multiple sclerosis cerebrospinal fluid: an update on methodology and clinical usefulness. *Journal of Neuroimmunology,* **180(1-2)**, 17–28.

23 Beck, R.W. *et al.* (1993) The effect of corticosteroids for acute optic neuritis on the subsequent development of multiple sclerosis. The Optic Neuritis Study Group. *New England Journal of Medicine,* **329(24)**, 1764–1769.

24 Beck, R.W. (1992) The optic neuritis treatment trial. Implications for clinical practice. Optic Neuritis Study Group. *Archives of Ophthalmology,* **110(3)**, 331–332.

25 Beck, R.W. (1995) The optic neuritis treatment trial: three-year follow-up results. *Archives of Ophthalmology,* **113(2)**, 136–137.

26 Beck, R.W. & Trobe, J.D. (1995) The Optic Neuritis Treatment Trial. Putting the results in perspective. The Optic Neuritis Study Group. *Journal of Neuro-Ophthalmology,* **15(3)**, 131–135.

27 Burton, J.M. *et al.* (2009) Oral versus intravenous steroids for treatment of relapses in multiple sclerosis. *Cochrane Database of Systematic Reviews,* **3**.: CD006921.

28 Beck, R.W. *et al.* (2004) Neurologic impairment 10 years after optic neuritis. *Archives of Neurology,* **61(9)**, 1386–1389.

29 Swanton, J.K. *et al.* (2009) Early MRI in optic neuritis: the risk for disability. *Neurology,* **72(6)**, 542–550.

30 Hickman, S.J. *et al.* (2002) Management of acute optic neuritis. *Lancet,* **360(9349)**, 1953–1962.

31 Keltner, J.L. *et al.* (1993) Baseline visual field profile of optic neuritis. The experience of the optic neuritis treatment trial. Optic Neuritis Study Group. *Archives of Ophthalmology,* **111(2)**, 231–234.

32 Johnson, L.N. & Arnold, A.C. (1994) Incidence of nonarteritic and arteritic anterior ischemic optic neuropathy. Population-based study in the state of Missouri and Los Angeles County, California. *Journal of Neuro-Ophthalmology,* **14(1)**, 38–44.

33 Smetana, G.W. & Shmerling, R.H. (2002) Does this patient have temporal arteritis? *JAMA,* **287(1)**, 92–101.

34 Birkhead, N.C., Wagener, H.P. & Shick, R.M. (1957) Treatment of temporal arteritis with adrenal corticosteroids; results

in fifty-five cases in which lesion was proved at biopsy. *Journal of the American Medical Association*, **163**(10), 821–827.

35 Hunder, G.G. *et al.* (1990) The American College of Rheumatology 1990 criteria for the classification of giant cell arteritis. *Arthritis and Rheumatism*, **33**(8), 1122–1128.

36 Younge, B.R. *et al.* (2004) Initiation of glucocorticoid therapy: before or after temporal artery biopsy? *Mayo Clinic Proceedings*, **79**(4), 483–491.

37 Boyev, L.R., Miller, N.R. & Green, W.R. (1999) Efficacy of unilateral versus bilateral temporal artery biopsies for the diagnosis of giant cell arteritis. *American Journal of Ophthalmology*, **128**(2), 211–215.

38 Niederkohr, R.D. & Levin, L.A. (2005) Management of the patient with suspected temporal arteritis a decision-analytic approach. *Ophthalmology*, **112**(5), 744–756.

39 Miller, A., Green, M. & Robinson, D. (1983) Simple rule for calculating normal erythrocyte sedimentation rate. *British Medical Journal (Clinical Research Ed.)*, **286**(6361), 266.

40 Niederkohr, R.D. & Levin, L.A. (2007) A Bayesian analysis of the true sensitivity of a temporal artery biopsy. *Investigative Ophthalmology & Visual Science*, **48**(2), 675–680.

41 Niederkohr, R.D. & Levin, L.A. (2012) Author response: bayesian estimation of sensitivity of temporal artery biopsies. *Investigative Ophthalmology & Visual Science*, **53**(2), 586.

42 Hayreh, S.S. *et al.* (1997) Giant cell arteritis: validity and reliability of various diagnostic criteria. *American Journal of Ophthalmology*, **123**(3), 285–296.

43 Walvick, M.D. & Walvick, M.P. (2011) Giant cell arteritis: laboratory predictors of a positive temporal artery biopsy. *Ophthalmology*, **118**(6), 1201–1204.

44 Kermani, T.A. and K.J. Warrington, Recent advances in diagnostic strategies for giant cell arteritis. *Current Neurology and Neuroscience Reports*, 2011 **12**(2):138–144. doi: 10.1007/s11910-011-0243-6.

45 Karassa, F.B. *et al.* (2005) Meta-analysis: test performance of ultrasonography for giant-cell arteritis. *Annals of Internal Medicine*, **142**(5), 359–369.

46 Bley, T.A. *et al.* (2007) Diagnostic value of high-resolution MR imaging in giant cell arteritis. *AJNR - American Journal of Neuroradiology*, **28**(9), 1722–1727.

47 Besson, F.L. *et al.* (2011) Diagnostic performance of (1)F-fluorodeoxyglucose positron emission tomography in giant cell arteritis: a systematic review and meta-analysis. *European Journal of Nuclear Medicine and Molecular Imaging*, **38**(9), 1764–1772.

48 Pless, M. *et al.* (2000) Concordance of bilateral temporal artery biopsy in giant cell arteritis. *Journal of Neuro-Ophthalmology*, **20**(3), 216–218.

49 Danesh-Meyer, H.V. *et al.* (2000) Low diagnostic yield with second biopsies in suspected giant cell arteritis. *Journal of Neuro-Ophthalmology*, **20**(3), 213–215.

50 Ponge, T. *et al.* (1988) The efficacy of selective unilateral temporal artery biopsy versus bilateral biopsies for diagnosis of giant cell arteritis. *Journal of Rheumatology*, **15**(6), 997–1000.

51 Breuer, G.S., Nesher, G. & Nesher, R. (2009) Rate of discordant findings in bilateral temporal artery biopsy to diagnose giant cell arteritis. *Journal of Rheumatology*, **36**(4), 794–796.

52 Klein, R.G. *et al.* (1976) Skip lesions in temporal arteritis. *Mayo Clinic Proceedings*, **51**(8), 504–510.

53 Allison, M.C. & Gallagher, P.J. (1984) Temporal artery biopsy and corticosteroid treatment. *Annals of the Rheumatic Diseases*, **43**(3), 416–417.

54 Achkar, A.A. *et al.* (1994) How does previous corticosteroid treatment affect the biopsy findings in giant cell (temporal) arteritis? *Annals of Internal Medicine*, **120**(12), 987–992.

55 Chmelewski, W.L. *et al.* (1992) Presenting features and outcomes in patients undergoing temporal artery biopsy. A review of 98 patients. *Archives of Internal Medicine*, **152**(8), 1690–1695.

56 Ray-Chaudhuri, N. *et al.* (2002) Effect of prior steroid treatment on temporal artery biopsy findings in giant cell arteritis. *British Journal of Ophthalmology*, **86**(5), 530–532.

57 Taylor-Gjevre, R. *et al.* (2005) Temporal artery biopsy for giant cell arteritis. *Journal of Rheumatology*, **32**(7), 1279–1282.

58 Mahr, A. *et al.* (2006) Temporal artery biopsy for diagnosing giant cell arteritis: the longer, the better? *Annals of the Rheumatic Diseases*, **65**(6), 826–828.

59 Sudlow, C. (1997) Diagnosing and managing polymyalgia rheumatica and temporal arteritis. Sensitivity of temporal artery biopsy varies with biopsy length and sectioning strategy. *BMJ*, **315**(7107), 549.

60 Goslin, B.J. & Chung, M.H. (2011) Temporal artery biopsy as a means of diagnosing giant cell arteritis: is there overutilization? *American Surgeon*, **77**(9), 1158–1160.

61 Hayreh, S.S. (1981) Anterior ischemic optic neuropathy. *Archives of Neurology*, **38**(11), 675–678.

62 Hattenhauer, M.G. *et al.* (1997) Incidence of nonarteritic anterior ischemic optic neuropathy. *American Journal of Ophthalmology*, **123**(1), 103–107.

63 Hayreh, S.S. & Zimmerman, M.B. (2008) Nonarteritic anterior ischemic optic neuropathy: natural history of visual outcome. *Ophthalmology*, **115**(2), 298–305. e2.

64 Repka, M.X. *et al.* (1983) Clinical profile and long-term implications of anterior ischemic optic neuropathy. *American Journal of Ophthalmology*, **96**(4), 478–483.

65 Hayreh, S.S. (2011) Management of ischemic optic neuropathies. *Indian Journal of Ophthalmology*, **59**(2), 123–136.

66 Beri, M. *et al.* (1987) Anterior ischemic optic neuropathy. VII. Incidence of bilaterality and various influencing factors. *Ophthalmology*, **94**(8), 1020–1028.

67 The Ischemic Optic Neuropathy Decompression Trial Research Group (1995) Optic nerve decompression surgery for nonarteritic anterior ischemic optic neuropathy (NAION) is not effective and may be harmful. *JAMA*, **273**(8), 625–632.

68 Beck, R.W., Servais, G.E. & Hayreh, S.S. (1987) Anterior ischemic optic neuropathy. IX. Cup-to-disc ratio and its role in pathogenesis. *Ophthalmology*, **94**(11), 1503–1508.

69 Landau, K. *et al.* (1996) 24-hour blood pressure monitoring in patients with anterior ischemic optic neuropathy. *Archives of Ophthalmology*, **114**(**5**), 570–575.

70 Levin, L.A. & Danesh-Meyer, H.V. (2008) Hypothesis: a venous etiology for nonarteritic anterior ischemic optic neuropathy. *Archives of Ophthalmology*, **126**(**11**), 1582–1585.

71 Borchert, M. & Lessell, S. (1988) Progressive and recurrent nonarteritic anterior ischemic optic neuropathy. *American Journal of Ophthalmology*, **106**(**4**), 443–449.

72 Kline, L.B. (1988) Progression of visual defects in ischemic optic neuropathy. *American Journal of Ophthalmology*, **106**(**2**), 199–203.

73 Arnold, A.C. & Hepler, R.S. (1994) Natural history of nonarteritic anterior ischemic optic neuropathy. *Journal of Neuro-Ophthalmology*, **14**(**2**), 66–69.

74 Sawle, G.V., James, C.B. & Russell, R.W. (1990) The natural history of non-arteritic anterior ischaemic optic neuropathy. *Journal of Neurology, Neurosurgery and Psychiatry*, **53**(**10**), 830–833.

75 (2000) Ischemic optic neuropathy decompression trial: Twenty-four-month update. *Archives of Ophthalmology*, **118**(**6**), 793–798.

76 Scherer, R.W. *et al.* (2008) Visual fields at follow-up in the Ischemic Optic Neuropathy Decompression Trial: evaluation of change in pattern defect and severity over time. *Ophthalmology*, **115**(**10**), 1809–1817.

77 Atkins, E.J. *et al.* (2010) Treatment of nonarteritic anterior ischemic optic neuropathy. *Survey of Ophthalmology*, **55**(**1**), 47–63.

78 Botelho, P.J., Johnson, L.N. & Arnold, A.C. (1996) The effect of aspirin on the visual outcome of nonarteritic anterior ischemic optic neuropathy. *American Journal of Ophthalmology*, **121**(**4**), 450–451.

79 Haas, A. *et al.* (1997) Application of HELP in nonarteritic anterior ischemic optic neuropathy: a prospective, randomized, controlled study. *Graefes Archive for Clinical and Experimental Ophthalmology*, **235**(**1**), 14–19.

80 Guerriero, S. *et al.* (2009) LDL apheresis in the treatment of non-arteritic ischaemic optic neuropathy: a 6-month follow-up study. *Eye (London, England)*, **23**(**6**), 1343–1344.

81 Sergott, R.C. *et al.* (1989) Optic nerve decompression may improve the progressive form of nonarteritic ischemic optic neuropathy. *Archives of Ophthalmology*, **107**(**12**), 1743–1754.

82 Kelman, S.E. & Elman, M.J. (1991) Optic nerve sheath decompression for nonarteritic ischemic optic neuropathy improves multiple visual function measurements. *Archives of Ophthalmology*, **109**(**5**), 667–671.

83 Spoor, T.C., Wilkinson, M.J. & Ramocki, J.M. (1991) Optic nerve sheath decompression for the treatment of progressive nonarteritic ischemic optic neuropathy. *American Journal of Ophthalmology*, **111**(**6**), 724–728.

84 Hayreh, S.S. (1990) The role of optic nerve sheath fenestration in management of anterior ischemic optic neuropathy. *Archives of Ophthalmology*, **108**(**8**), 1063–1065.

85 Sadun, A.A. (1993) The efficacy of optic nerve sheath decompression for anterior ischemic optic neuropathy and other optic neuropathies. *American Journal of Ophthalmology*, **115**(**3**), 384–389.

86 Jablons, M.M. *et al.* (1993) Optic nerve sheath fenestration for treatment of progressive ischemic optic neuropathy. Results in 26 patients. *Archives of Ophthalmology*, **111**(**1**), 84–87.

87 Glaser, J.S., Teimory, M. & Schatz, N.J. (1994) Optic nerve sheath fenestration for progressive ischemic optic neuropathy. Results in second series consisting of 21 eyes. *Archives of Ophthalmology*, **112**(**8**), 1047–1050.

88 Aiello, A.L., Sadun, A.A. & Feldon, S.E. (1992) Spontaneous improvement of progressive anterior ischemic optic neuropathy: report of two cases. *Archives of Ophthalmology*, **110**(**9**), 1197–1199.

89 Soheilian, M. *et al.* (2003) Transvitreal optic neurotomy for nonarteritic anterior ischemic optic neuropathy. *Retina*, **23**(**5**), 692–697.

90 Soheilian, M. *et al.* (2008) Histopathologic evaluation of optic neurotomy with microvitreoretinal blade or excimer laser in cadaver eyes. *Ophthalmic Surgery, Lasers & Imaging*, **39**(**1**), 35–39.

91 Hayreh, S.S. & Zimmerman, M.B. (2007) Optic disc edema in non-arteritic anterior ischemic optic neuropathy. *Graefes Archive for Clinical and Experimental Ophthalmology*, **245**(**8**), 1107–1121.

92 Hayreh, S.S. & Zimmerman, M.B. (2008) Non-arteritic anterior ischemic optic neuropathy: role of systemic corticosteroid therapy. *Graefes Archive for Clinical and Experimental Ophthalmology*, **246**(**7**), 1029–1046.

93 Lee, A.G. & Biousse, V. (2010) Should steroids be offered to patients with nonarteritic anterior ischemic optic neuropathy? *Journal of Neuro-Ophthalmology*, **30**(**2**), 193–198.

94 Ellenberger, C. Jr., (1974) R.M. Burde, and J.L. Keltner, Acute optic neuropathy. Treatment with diphenylhydantoin. *Archives of Ophthalmology*, **91**(**6**), 435–438.

95 Wilhelm, B., Ludtke, H. & Wilhelm, H. (2006) Efficacy and tolerability of 0.2% brimonidine tartrate for the treatment of acute non-arteritic anterior ischemic optic neuropathy (NAION): a 3-month, double-masked, randomised, placebo-controlled trial. *Graefes Archive for Clinical and Experimental Ophthalmology*, **244**(**5**), 551–558.

96 Johnson, L.N., Gould, T.J. & Krohel, G.B. (1996) Effect of levodopa and carbidopa on recovery of visual function in patients with nonarteritic anterior ischemic optic neuropathy of longer than six months' duration. *American Journal of Ophthalmology*, **121**(**1**), 77–83.

97 Johnson, L.N. *et al.* (2000) Levodopa may improve vision loss in recent-onset, nonarteritic anterior ischemic optic neuropathy. *Ophthalmology*, **107**(**3**), 521–526.

98 Hayreh, S.S. (2000) Does Levodopa improve visual function in NAION? *Ophthalmology*, **107**(**8**), 1434–1438.

99 Cox, T.A. (2000) Does levodopa improve visual function in NAION? *Ophthalmology*, **107**(**8**), 1431.

100 Beck, R.W. (2000) Does Levodopa improve visual function in NAION? *Ophthalmology*, **107**(**8**), 1431–1434.; discusson 1435–1438.

101 Simsek, T., Eryilmaz, T. & Acaroglu, G. (2005) Efficacy of levodopa and carbidopa on visual function in patients with non-arteritic anterior ischaemic optic neuropathy. *International Journal of Clinical Practice*, **59**(3), 287–290.

102 Parisi, V. *et al.* (2008) Cytidine-5′-diphosphocholine (Citicoline): a pilot study in patients with non-arteritic ischaemic optic neuropathy. *European Journal of Neurology*, **15**(5), 465–474.

103 Beck, R.W. *et al.* (1997) Aspirin therapy in nonarteritic anterior ischemic optic neuropathy. *American Journal of Ophthalmology*, **123**(2), 212–217.

104 Newman, N.J. *et al.* (2002) The fellow eye in NAION: report from the ischemic optic neuropathy decompression trial follow-up study. *American Journal of Ophthalmology*, **134**(3), 317–328.

105 Kupersmith, M.J. *et al.* (1997) Aspirin reduces the incidence of second eye NAION: a retrospective study. *Journal of Neuro-Ophthalmology*, **17**(4), 250–253.

CHAPTER 29

Therapeutic connection in neurorehabilitation: theory, evidence and practice

Nicola M. Kayes, Kathryn M. McPherson, and Paula Kersten
Centre for Person Centred Research, Health and Rehabilitation Research Institute, School of Clinical Sciences, AUT University, Auckland, New Zealand

Background

Medical advances have resulted in many more people surviving the initial insult of neurological injury or illness. However, many of those who survive are inevitably left living with a range of significant disabling consequences. Evidence now suggests that the potential for recovery following a neurological event is far greater than previously thought possible due to cellular regeneration [1] and also that those with chronic neurological conditions have greater rehabilitation potential [2]. Despite this, we frequently fail to see knowledge advance in neurorehabilitation translate to better outcomes for those living with neurological impairment.

For success, neurorehabilitation frequently requires intensive effort over long intervals on the part of the patient and his/her family [3,4]. However, while increasing attention has been given to the efficacy of specific interventions, less-explicit attention has been given to patient engagement in those interventions as a vital component for a good outcome. Failure to achieve anticipated outcomes may be put down to the patient being 'unmotivated' [5], 'non-compliant' [6] or 'not ready' [7] implying these are states over which only the patient has control. However, there is increasing theoretical debate about whether such concepts are internal, or rather a consequence of a range of other factors, such as impairment in executive functioning [5,8–10], the therapeutic process [11], or indeed a psychological response to a life-changing event [12,13]. These explanations suggest something more complex (and more able to be influenced) than patient choice. They highlight a role, even a responsibility on the part of the clinician, to actively draw on strategies to facilitate patient engagement in their rehabilitation to optimise outcome.

A traditional approach would suggest the role of psychology in neurorehabilitation to be neuropsychological testing or the psychological treatment of commonly diagnosed mental health disorders. However, there is growing recognition of the relevance a number of psychological theories and models have for the everyday rehabilitation practitioner. One area, in particular, that has received a great deal of theoretical and empirical attention in psychotherapy and related fields that may have relevance to neurorehabilitation is the role of the patient–practitioner relationship (referred to throughout this chapter as *therapeutic connection*). The therapeutic connection has long been considered a key contributor to treatment effect in psychotherapy and related fields with research consistently linking it to outcome [14–17]. Indeed, Bordin proposed *'the working alliance'* between clinician and patient to be *'the key to outcome'* [18], p.252. By comparison, empirical work aiming to explore the therapeutic connection in rehabilitation is less well established [11] though Schontz and Fink were one of the first to explore the role of rapport in rehabilitation as far back as 1957 [19]; a first step in considering the role of therapeutic connection in a rehabilitation setting.

While work *explicitly* exploring the therapeutic connection in rehabilitation has been limited, both practitioners [20–25] and patients consistently identify it as critical [26–30]. Physiotherapists, for example, have identified the patient-practitioner relationship to be more important to treatment success than the treatment itself [25], and the ability to develop a collaborative relationship and prioritise centrality of the patient to be the hallmark of an 'expert' practitioner [21]. In occupational therapy, acknowledgement of the role of the patient–practitioner interaction is quite

Evidence-Based Neurology: Management of Neurological Disorders, Second Edition. Edited by Bart M. Demaerschalk and Dean M. Wingerchuk.
© 2015 John Wiley & Sons, Ltd. Published 2015 by John Wiley & Sons, Ltd.

explicit with the phrase 'therapeutic use of self' commonly referred to in principles of practice to denote mindfulness of establishing optimal therapist–client connections in practice [23]. Research exploring patient perspectives of quality care has indicated the need for balance between technical competence and 'humanness' [26]. Similarly, a recent review of patient satisfaction in musculoskeletal physiotherapy found therapist characteristics, such as professionalism, competence, friendliness, caring and communication, highly associated with patient satisfaction [31]. The therapeutic connection has also been linked with improved outcomes in a range of conditions [32–38]. Hall's review in 2010 synthesised findings from 13 prospective rehabilitation studies, concluding that aspects of the therapist–patient relationship were linked to treatment adherence, patient satisfaction, and improvements in a range of outcomes including pain, depression and physical function [35]. In a series of studies we have undertaken, findings suggest that explicit emphasis on establishing such a connection may enhance longevity of rehabilitation outcome [39–42]. The body of evidence highlighting the potential importance of a therapeutic connection for perceived quality care and engagement in rehabilitation, and also outcome is growing. In this chapter we aim to more specifically critically explore theory and evidence for therapeutic connection in a neurorehabilitation setting and discuss key implications for practice.

Defining therapeutic connection

As discussed in our recent article in Disability and Rehabilitation on this topic [11], many terms have been used to describe the patient-practitioner relationship, including therapeutic alliance [17], working alliance [18,43], therapeutic relationship [22,44], therapist–patient interaction [45], therapeutic bond [46] and helping alliance [47]. Such terms are frequently used interchangeably despite carrying different meanings. Some place more emphasis on the affective relationship and bond between patient and therapist (therapeutic relationship, therapeutic bond), while others place emphasis on the interaction and concordance between patient and therapist (working alliance, helping alliance). Indeed, such terms have also been variably defined. For example, Gartland defines the therapeutic relationship as 'a means of communication wherein both therapist and patient interact to achieve a therapeutic goal' (p.26) focussing on aspects relating to the interaction between patient and therapist [44]. By contrast, Cole and McLean refer to 'a trusting connection and rapport established between therapist and client through collaboration, communication, therapist empathy and mutual understanding and respect' (p.44), incorporating both the relational and interactive components of the relationship [48]. Arguably, what sets rehabilitation apart from other health disciplines is that it requires active participation on the part of the patient, as

opposed to the patient being a more passive recipient of services. In her paper in 1999, Bellner supports this notion suggesting that occupational and physical therapy outcomes depend on the patient's 'collaboration, cooperation and participation' (p.56) and that part of the rehabilitation professionals' responsibility is to activate the patient's own resources, therefore requiring a 'therapeutic' interaction to take place [49]. In our recent work exploring engagement in stroke rehabilitation from the perspectives of patients, their family and rehabilitation practitioners, we identified 'connection' to be crucial, with one participant stating 'there needs to be some connectivity there' [50]. We have opted to use the phrase 'therapeutic connection' throughout this chapter as it seems to capture these ideologies, as well as encompassing both the relational and interactional aspects of the rehabilitation partnership. We use this phrase through the remainder of this chapter except where explicitly referring to work where another phrase was adopted to stay true to the nature of what is being reported.

Framing clinical questions

Rehabilitation following a neurological event (such as stroke or traumatic brain injury) occurs over a long interval with people frequently accessing rehabilitation services (often intermittently) many years following injury/diagnosis. Establishing a good therapeutic connection early in the rehabilitation process may play a key role in sustaining patient engagement in rehabilitation over the long term. However, there are many complexities inherent in neurological conditions which may compromise a therapeutic connection (or ability to establish a connection), such as deficits in neurobehavioural functioning, cognition, self-awareness and communicative ability. Exploring evidence regarding therapeutic connection, specifically in the context of neurorehabilitation, should advance our understanding of the role that therapeutic connection plays and aspects which may be unique to the neurorehabilitation setting. This will enhance the neuropractitioners' ability to optimise and draw on therapeutic connection as a resource in practice. Scoping revealed a growing body of empirical work exploring therapeutic connection in neurorehabilitation. However, to our knowledge this evidence has not been synthesised to date. We aim to synthesise existing evidence with a focus on the following four clinical questions:

1 What does the evidence say about the association between therapeutic connection and outcome in neurorehabilitation?
2 What is the theoretical basis for research exploring therapeutic connection in neurorehabilitation?
3 How important is the therapeutic connection with family for outcome in neurorehabilitation?
4 How do the cognitive, neurobehavioural and communication sequelae commonly inherent in brain injury impact on the development of a therapeutic connection?

Approach to searching the evidence

A pragmatic approach to searching the evidence was adopted. EBSCO health databases were searched using keywords for therapeutic connection (such as 'working alliance', 'therapeutic relationship', 'therapeutic alliance', 'patient–practitioner interaction/relationship' and 'patient–therapist interaction/relationship') AND keywords for neurorehabilitation (such as 'neuro-rehabilitation' and 'neurological rehabilitation'). Keywords for 'stroke' and 'brain injury' were also incorporated into this search using the Boolean operator 'OR' to combine with 'neurorehabilitation' given they represent a large proportion of the neurorehabilitation population. The search was carried out in 2012 and limited to articles published from 2000 onwards as scoping indicated that the vast majority of relevant research was published after this time. Titles and abstracts were screened for relevance and the full text obtained for all articles identified as probably or possibly relevant. Papers were included if they explored therapeutic connection (independent variable) in relation to outcome (dependent variable) in the context of neurorehabilitation, whether or not this was the primary aim of the study and regardless of the outcome of interest. Reference lists for relevant review papers were screened for additional articles not already identified in the database search. No additional articles were identified via this approach. A number of excluded articles were retained if they added contextual information relevant to any one of the clinical questions identified above. Figure 29.1 presents details of search results and reasons for exclusion.

1. What does the evidence say about the association between therapeutic connection and outcome in neurorehabilitation?

Eight studies were identified which explored the relationship between aspects of therapeutic connection and outcome in neurorehabilitation. They included the work of three groups of researchers and six independent data sets. Table 29.1 provides a summary of included studies.

Of the eight studies, there was one prospective study using a historical control design [32]. The remaining seven studies were cohort studies. The prospective, historical control study aimed to explore the effectiveness of an interdisciplinary team intervention aiming to improve therapeutic alliance. The intervention consisted of three components: (1) one family meeting, (2) nine sessions of monthly in-services for clinical staff focused on strategies for building therapeutic alliance and (3) each member of the team completing working alliance surveys (WASs), developed for the purpose of this study, on a weekly basis for each client to keep clinicians oriented to the concept and for use as reflective tool. In addition to these ratings, the patient, a family member, and the neuropsychologist on the team rated alliance using the California Psychotherapy Alliance Scales (CALPAS [51]) at

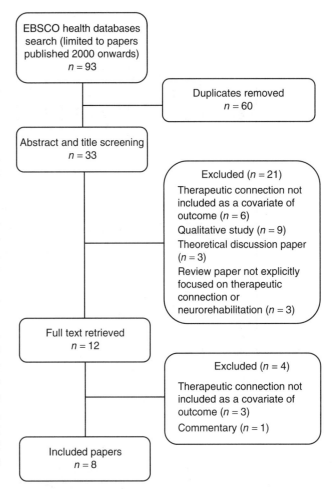

Figure 29.1 Summary of search findings.

2 weeks post discharge for inclusion in study analyses. They reported no significant differences between groups on the CALPAS for patient, family or neuropsychologist alliance ratings, though higher ratings by the neuropsychologist using the CALPAS were associated with lower levels of emotional distress and family discord, as well as improvements in productivity status across the two groups. It is possible that the lack of between-group difference is due to limitations of the historical control design where the control group is not derived from the same population as that of the intervention group and where it is difficult (if not impossible) to prevent bias due to the lack of assurance regarding comparability of groups. This highlights the complexity of exploring the effectiveness of an intervention targeting a change in process or change in clinician behaviour where a traditional randomised controlled trial is not possible due to inevitable contamination across groups, or indeed where there are ethical issues associated with having a control group that does not explicitly aim to establish a therapeutic connection.

Another reason for the lack of between-group differences may be the timing of CALPAS ratings that were carried out

Table 29.1 Summary of included studies

Reference	Design and intervention	Participants	Measures	Assessment points	Findings	Comments
Evans et al., 2008 [32]	Prospective with two consecutive samples – historical control (CNT) and treatment (TX) CNT – Post-acute brain injury rehabilitation (PABIR) TX – PABIR + interdisciplinary team intervention to improve TA	TBI CNT (n = 69) TBI TX (n = 35)	• California Psychotherapy Alliance Scales (CALPAS) – client, family and therapist (neuropsychologist only) perceptions • Awareness Questionnaire • Centre for Epidemiologic Studies Depression Scale • Family Assessment Device • Disability Rating Scale • Productivity Status – 'Productive' (work, school, independent homemaker) and 'Non-productive' • WA Surveys (WAS) – completed weekly by each treatment team member; scores over first 3 months were averaged for analysis; TX group only due to being part of the intervention	Alliance, awareness, family discord and depression at 2 weeks post admission to PABIR Disability rating and productivity at discharge	No significant between-group differences on CALPAS ratings for clients, families or therapists Better WAS and CALPAS therapist ratings were significantly associated with lower levels of emotional distress and family discord (p < 0.05) Higher team WAS ratings of alliance were associated with programme completion (p < 0.01) and productive status (p = 0.05); CALPAS therapist ratings were also associated with productivity status (p = 0.002)	Inclusion of a team-based working alliance rating (WAS) a novel approach though validity of approach not established Historical cohort design a limiting factor CALPAS ratings at two weeks post admission and only by neuropsychologist may have impacted lack of between-group differences Higher ratings of TA by patients and family (in comparison to therapist ratings) may result in ceiling effects making it more difficult to detect associations
Klonoff et al., 2001 [36]	Cohort Adult day hospital for neurorehabilitation; length of treatment (months): 6 (mean) and 0.8–18 (range)	TBI (n = 113) CVA (n = 38) Other neurological insult (n = 13)	• WA – staff ratings for both patients and their families; average of all WA ratings while in the programme and WA at discharge • Productivity – 'Productive' (full or part-time work/ school, volunteer, home-maker) and 'Non-productive' (retired, unemployed).	3 months, 1-, 3-, 5-, 7-, 9- and 11-year intervals When patients were contacted at multiple follow-up points, outcome data were utilised for the time furthest from discharge.	All WA ratings were significantly higher for patients in the 'productive' group. Patients WA; p = 0.006 (average), p = 0.002 (discharge) Families WA; p = 0.004 (average), p = 0.045 (discharge).	Lack of clarity: how WA was rated Staff-only ratings of WA Sample size reduced over follow-up period

Klonoff et al., 2007 [56]*	Cohort	Cognitive retraining in the context of an adult day hospital for neurorehabilitation	TBI (n = 65) CVA (n = 22) Other neurological insult (n = 14)	• WA – staff ratings on a 100-point scale for both patients and their families collected monthly • Cognitive retraining tasks (Matching shapes, Digit symbol Level 1, Block design level 1 and word fluency) • Cognitive Retraining Behaviour Checklist (CRBC) • Work/School status – categorised into one of five outcomes: (1) gainful, same as pre-injury without modifications; (2) gainful, same as pre-injury with some modification; (3) gainful, different and below pre-injury status; (4) volunteer role; (5) not working	Mean scores across programme as well as discharge scores for WA Initial, last, best and mean scores for cognitive retraining tasks	No significant relationship between WA and work/school status WA was significantly associated with a range of variables on the CRBC including but not limited to 'timeliness', 'level of organisation', 'ability to see the big picture', 'use of compensatory strategies' A number of CRBC variables significantly predicted work/school status	WA rating not validated Staff-only ratings of WA
Klonoff et al., 2010 [55]*	Cohort	Cognitive retraining in the context of an adult day hospital for neurorehabilitation	TBI (n = 65) CVA (n = 29) Other neurological insult (n = 13)	• WA – staff ratings on a 100-point scale for both patients and their families collected monthly • Cognitive retraining tasks (Matching shapes, Digit symbol Level 1, Block design level 1 and word fluency) • Cognitive Retraining Behaviour Checklist (CRBC) • Driving status – categorised into one of two outcomes: (1) cleared to drive; (2) not cleared to drive	Mean scores for WA Initial, last, best and mean scores for cognitive retraining tasks	Participants who were cleared to drive had higher mean and discharge WA scores (p < 0.01) Higher mean WA scores were significantly associated with a range of CRBC variables including 'timeliness', 'use of compensatory strategies', 'communication pragmatics', 'level of distractibility' and 'ability to see the big picture'	WA rating not validated Staff-only ratings of WA

(continued overleaf)

Table 29.1 (continued)

Reference	Design and intervention	Participants	Measures	Assessment points	Findings	Comments
Schönberger et al., 2006 [54]	Cohort Neuropsychological outpatient rehabilitation programme; ~14 weeks	Traumatic brain injury (n = 26) CVA (n = 58) Other neurological insult (n = 14)	• WA and patient compliance – rating completed for all patients by senior neuropsychologist and senior physiotherapist retrospectively between 18 months and 4 years after patients finished the programme • Employment – categorised into one of five categories 'competitive', 'retraining', 'supported', 'voluntary', 'unemployed' • Physical training – categorised into one of three categories 'no training', 'leisure physical activity or infrequent physical training', 'at least weekly physical training'	WA scores dichotomised into 'good or excellent' and 'poor or fair' Compliance coded into three categories: 'low', 'average' and 'high'	Discrepancy between neuropsychologist and physiotherapist ratings of WA and compliance with the neuropsychologist being more positive WA and compliance significantly related ($p < 0.001$) WA related to employment at follow-up (neuropsychologist < 0.01; physiotherapist 0.05)	WA and compliance ratings not validated WA rated retrospectively and may be subject to recall bias Staff-only ratings of WA
Schönberger et al., 2006 [52]*	Cohort Neuropsychological outpatient rehabilitation programme; ~14 weeks	Traumatic brain injury (n = 27) Cerebrovascular accident (n = 49) Other neurological insult (n = 10)	• Working Alliance Inventory (WAI) – completed by patients and their primary therapists • Awareness and compliance – therapist ratings on a 7-point likert scale	2, 6, 10 and 14 weeks into the programme	Significant improvements on the task, bond and total WAI therapist scores over time, but not for patient scales Patients rated WA more positively on all scales and time points WA with a bi-frontal or right hemisphere injury was rated lower on all therapist WAI scales at 2 weeks, but not at later time points Patient WAI (bond) significantly predicted awareness ($p < 0.05$)	Awareness and compliance ratings not validated Specifically interested in the bond component of Bordin's WA theory

| Schönberger et al., 2006[43]* | Cohort | Neuropsychological outpatient rehabilitation programme; ~14 weeks | TBI ($n=27$) CVA ($n=49$) Other neurological insult ($n=10$) | • Working Alliance Inventory (WAI) – completed by patients and their primary therapists • Awareness and compliance – therapist ratings on a 7-point likert scale • European Brain Injury Questionnaire (EBIQ) • Overall success of collaborative work – client rating on a 5-point scale | 2, 6, 10 and 14 weeks into the programme | Patient WAI (bond) correlated with compliance ($r=0.30$, $p<0.05$) Awareness and Patient WAI (bond) accounted for 56% of variance in compliance ($p<0.001$); only awareness contributed significantly to the prediction. A mediating relationship was observed, i.e. that patients perceived emotional bond with their therapist affects patient awareness which in turn fosters compliance. Any relationship between brain injury-related problems (measured by the EBIQ) and WAI ratings (patient and therapist) disappeared when patient awareness was accounted for Patient WAI (bond) scores at t2 and t3 (mid-therapy) were predictive of reduction in depression ratings ($R=0.68$, $p<0.001$) WAI (bond) scores at t4 (end of treatment) were significantly associated with overall patient and therapist success ratings | Awareness and compliance ratings not validated |

(continued overleaf)

Table 29.1 (*continued*)

Reference	Design and intervention	Participants	Measures	Assessment points	Findings	Comments
Sherer et al., 2007 [59]	Cohort Post-acute brain injury rehabilitation (PABIR)	TBI (n = 69)	• California Psychotherapy Alliance Scales (CALPAS) • Prigatano Alliance Scale • Awareness Questionnaire • Centre for Epidemiologic Studies Depression Scale • Family Assessment Device • Disability Rating Scale • Productivity Status – 'Productive' (work, school, independent homemaker) and 'Non-productive'	Alliance, awareness, family discord and depression at 2 weeks post admission to PABIR Disability rating and productivity at discharge	Patient and therapist perceptions of TA were significantly associated ($r = 0.53$, $p = 0 < 0.001$ and $r = 0.46$, $p = <0.001$; Family perceptions of TA were not associated with patient or therapist ratings Discrepancy between family and therapists on ratings of patient function and higher levels of family discord were associated poorer TA Family and patient perceptions of stronger TA were predictive of a greater likelihood of productive outcome at discharge Stronger patient ratings of TA were associated with greater risk of dropout TA not associated with overall patient functional status at discharge	TA ratings at 2 weeks post admission may have impacted findings Higher ratings of TA by patients and family (in comparison to therapist ratings) may result in ceiling effects making it more difficult to detect associations

CVA-Cerebrovascular Accident; TA-Therapeutic Alliance; TBI-Traumatic Brain Injury; WA-Working Alliance

[a] These two studies share the same data set

at 2 weeks post admission and may not have allowed time to establish a therapeutic connection, or at least for the intervention to have markedly influenced this process. Indeed, Schönberger et al.'s findings suggest that therapist ratings improve over time [52]. To further explore the potential benefit of the intervention on therapeutic connection, the researchers averaged the weekly WAS ratings completed in the first 3 months of the intervention period for the team. Similar to the neuropsychologist ratings of alliance, better team WAS scores were associated with lower levels of emotional distress and family discord and improvements in productivity status. Furthermore, higher team WAS ratings were linked to higher rates of programme completion. An interesting trend was observed in relation to WAS ratings across the course of the study with better working alliance reported in the last 3 months relative to the first 3 months of the study (consistent with Schönberger et al.'s findings outlined above). This may be an indicator of the time it takes to develop a therapeutic connection in the context of neurorehabilitation. However, the authors of this work suggest that this may also reflect an improvement over time in awareness and skill regarding therapeutic connection and associated strategies for practice. This is consistent with Summers and Barber who reviewed evidence regarding therapeutic alliance skill development in psychotherapy and concluded that while some aspects of therapeutic alliance are more teachable than others and/or subject to influence by a range of factors, therapeutic alliance is a skill that can be developed through training and which improves with 'accumulated clinical hours, and more complex case conceptualisations' [53], p.162.

Six of the seven cohort studies reported higher ratings of therapeutic connection being associated with improved outcomes including productivity [36,54], cognitive retraining tasks [55,56], driving status [55], awareness [52], compliance [52,54], depression [43] and client ratings of collaborative success [43]. Of particular interest is the work carried out by Klonoff et al. [36] who explored outcome up to 11 years post-discharge from an adult day hospital for neurorehabilitation (ADHNR). Klonoff et al. reported higher staff working alliance ratings to be associated with better long term vocational outcomes indicating that the quality of the working alliance may impact outcome for many years following discharge from formal rehabilitation services. Later work by the same group reported interesting findings regarding the relationship between working alliance and outcome on cognitive retraining tasks [55,56], linking better ratings of working alliance with the development of important meta-cognitive skills frequently impaired by neurological illness or injury. While in this later work working alliance was not directly associated with school or work status, improvements in meta-cognitive skills were, suggesting that the relationship between working alliance and meta-cognitive skill may interact to enhance the relationship between meta-cognitive skill and school or work status [56]. Development of key self-regulatory skills may be crucial to psychosocial adjustment and to successful reintegration into the community following a neurological event [57,58]. As such, these findings offer some important insight into potential value of investing in skill development for clinicians with a focus on process variables such as working alliance to optimise rehabilitation outcome. One cohort study [59] reported more mixed results regarding therapeutic alliance and outcome variables. This study found that family and patient perceptions of stronger therapeutic alliance (measured at two weeks post admission) were predictive of a greater likelihood of productive outcome at discharge, but were not associated with overall patient functional status. In addition, stronger patient ratings of therapeutic alliance were associated with greater risk of dropout.

The measures most frequently adopted in the research reported here are the CALPAS [51] and Working Alliance Inventory (WAI [60]). Both have been singled out as strong measures of therapeutic alliance in terms of their conceptual basis, validity and reliability in a psychotherapy setting [17,61]. However, both measures were developed explicitly for use in psychotherapy (where the concept of therapeutic alliance first originated) and so may not capture aspects unique to therapeutic connection in neurorehabilitation. Indeed, the conceptual basis of the WAI has been challenged in the context of physiotherapy and rehabilitation in recent years [35,62,63]. The development of measures more specific to the concept of therapeutic connection in rehabilitation would likely allow for a greater advancement of knowledge in this field regarding the role that therapeutic connection plays in outcome following a neurological event. Another important aspect of measurement to note from these studies is exactly *whose* perspective is being explored. For example, four of the eight studies presented in Table 29.1 only included clinician ratings of therapeutic connection. This makes interpretation of findings, particularly with respect to possible causality, more difficult. For example, is the association between working alliance and compliance such that a better working alliance enhances compliance or is it simply that therapists perceive the quality of their working relationships to be better with the 'good patient'. More research exploring therapeutic connection from the perspectives of *all* stakeholders in the rehabilitation process (i.e. patient, family and clinician) would allow for more explicit exploration as to whether particular perspectives matter more in terms of predicting outcome (this links to the third clinical question addressed below). Similarly, some more work to explore therapeutic connection at different time points in the rehabilitation continuum will add to our understanding of key time points in the rehabilitation process as well as offer some insight into the time it takes to develop a strong therapeutic connection with patients post admission to neurorehabilitation services.

One clear limitation of the existing literature is that while it offers broad support for the relationship between therapeutic connection and outcome, there is no insight as to what might be the key active ingredients (e.g. trust, empathy and rapport). A better understanding of those aspects of therapeutic connection considered to be most crucial (or which mix) as a covariate of outcome in neurorehabilitation will allow for more targeted professional education and training [11]. While there is clearly scope for further work in this area, the evidence presented suggests that the therapeutic connection may play a key role in influencing outcome following neurorehabilitation.

2. What is the theoretical basis for research exploring therapeutic connection in neurorehabilitation?

Having a clear idea of the theoretical basis which underpins current evidence can help to elucidate the mechanisms through which therapeutic connection may impact outcome as well as aid critical reflection regarding the application of key ideas to the neurorehabilitation context and setting. Table 29.2 displays the terms adopted in the eight included studies as well as the operational definition provided and the source of that definition.

From Table 29.2 it is clear that the existing literature almost exclusively draws on Bordin's Theory of Working Alliance [18]. The only other operational definition drawn on came from Prigatano *et al.* who were one of the first to operationally define working alliance and incorporate a measure of working alliance into their research in neurorehabilitation in 1994 [37]. However, their operational definition was mostly focused on behavioural indicators of alliance on the part of the patient, such as high rates of attendance, signs of preparation for therapy time and so on. This may be conceptually missing the mark given it is not clear whether the behavioural indicators they propose are truly representative of therapeutic connection. Further, there is little acknowledgement of the role the clinician may have in the development of that therapeutic connection. It is important to note that both research groups, who drew from this definition in their early work, went on to draw from Bordin's theory in subsequent work, suggesting they recognised the limitations inherent in that operational definition.

In his theory, Bordin argues a 'working alliance' comprises three core features: *goals, tasks* and *bonds*. *Goals* refer to the goals of therapy with the extent to which they are mutually agreed upon by the therapist and patient being a key characteristic of a strong working alliance. *Tasks* are the behaviours or activities of therapy that will serve to accomplish the therapy goals. *Bonds* refer to the personal and emotional attachment between therapist and patient and includes, but is not limited to, mutual trust and confidence. Bordin argues that the quality of the working alliance is a function of the concordance and agreement on tasks and goals and the strength of the emotional bond between the two parties. The proposed interdependent nature of the working alliance was a departure from previous understandings of the working alliance [60]. The development of the WAI measure underpinned by Bordin's conceptualisation of working alliance has made this theory both accessible to researchers (to advance knowledge regarding the role of working alliance in outcome following neurorehabilitation) and clinicians (as a tool to critically reflect on the state of the working alliance in practice). Indeed, Kissinger argues that this model may provide a useful framework for working with people with traumatic brain injury, and provides a case example of how this might take place in our practice [64].

While Bordin's theory clearly has relevance to neurorehabilitation, a number of other theories and models relevant to therapeutic connection have been proposed in the psychotherapy, counselling and related literature which may have relevance. There are two theories, in particular, which offer a different and arguably useful perspective to that of Bordin's theory for neurorehabilitation. In their 1985 article [65], Gelso and Carter draw on the earlier work of Greeson (1967) to argue for a distinction between three components of the therapeutic relationship in psychotherapy: the working alliance, the transference relationship and the real relationship. They build on Greeson's earlier work, arguing that not only is the therapeutic relationship marked by three distinct components, but that all are prevalent in every patient–therapist relationship; the salience of each varying throughout an encounter and/or period of therapy. By focussing exclusively on Bordin's theory (focussing only on 'working alliance'), we may miss other key components. The transference relationship has its roots in psychoanalytic theory and at risk of oversimplifying, essentially refers to the idea that feelings, behaviours and attitudes relevant to a traumatic event experienced by patients in the past are displaced onto the therapist [65]. Whilst we defer (and refer) to Gelso and Carter for a more in-depth discussion of the complexities of the transference relationship, what bears consideration in the context of neurorehabilitation is their argument that transference occurs in all therapeutic relationships, and in fact in *all* relationships. Further, how the therapist manages this when it happens can impact both the process and outcome of therapy. Whilst the language around transference may on first reading sound far removed from the patient experience in neurorehabilitation, evidence suggests a neurological insult to be a traumatic event for people [12,13]. The 'real relationship' consists of participants (therapist and patients) 'genuine and realistic perceptions of and reactions to each other' [65], p.185. The real relationship refers to the personal relationship that exists between therapist and patient, which manifests itself from their first meeting [66,67]. It is an acknowledgement that quite aside from any therapeutic interaction or working alliance that might exist; both therapist and patient

Table 29.2 Overview of terms adopted and related definitions for included studies

Reference	Term adopted	Definition provided	Definition underpinned by
Evans *et al.*, 2008 [32]	Therapeutic alliance	'Collaboration between the client and therapist in their efforts to combat the client's problems. Therapeutic alliance is determined by the following: (1) client and therapist agreement on tasks of therapy, (2) client and therapist agreement on the goals of therapy and (3) the interpersonal bond between the client and therapist'. (p.329)	Bordin's Theory of Working Alliance [18]
Klonoff *et al.*, 2001 [36]	Therapeutic alliance	'Operationally defined as observing a high rate of attendance, signs of preparation for therapy time, progressive verbal agreement between therapist and patient regarding goals of therapy, and level of realistic appreciation for accomplishments'. (p.414)	Prigatano *et al.* [37]
Klonoff *et al.*, 2007 [56]	Working alliance	'The quality of the relationship between staff and the patient/family, encompassing levels of trust and respect in communications, openness and honesty in dialogue and acceptance of feedback; the level of patient/family follow-through on agreed upon tasks; and agreement on therapeutic goals'. (p.1099)	Bordin's Theory of Working Alliance [18]
Klonoff *et al.*, 2010 [55]	Working alliance	'Specific subcomponents of working alliance are the rapport or relationship between the patient and therapists, the degree of follow-through with specific tasks and procedures associated with the rehabilitation process and the level of concordance between the patient and treatment team on therapeutic goals'. (p.67)	Bordin's Theory of Working Alliance [18]
Schönberger *et al.*, 2006 [54]	Working alliance	'Operationally defined as (1) percentage of patient attendance, (2) quality of verbal agreement between therapist and patient as to a course of action, (3) patient appreciation of accomplishments and services and (4) patient engagement'. (p.302)	Prigatano *et al.* [37]
Schönberger *et al.*, 2006 [52] Schönberger *et al.*, 2006 [43]	Working alliance	'A combination of (1) the agreement between client and therapist on goals, (2) their agreement on how to achieve these goals (common work on tasks) and (3) the development of a personal bond between client and therapist'. (p.445)	Bordin's Theory of Working Alliance [18]
Sherer *et al.*, 2007 [59]	Therapeutic alliance	'Collaboration between the client and therapist in their efforts to combat the client's problems. Therapeutic alliance is determined by: (1) client and therapist agreement on tasks of therapy, (2) client and therapist agreement on the goals of therapy and (3) the interpersonal bond between the client and therapist'. (p.663)	Bordin's Theory of Working Alliance [18]

are real people and therefore will necessarily develop a personal relationship. This raises a number of questions in the context of neurorehabilitation. For example, can one truly distinguish between the working alliance and the real relationship in neurorehabilitation? If both do exist, do they exist independent of the other or are they interdependent? Is one any more important than the other (i.e. could the real relationship be a necessary component of the working alliance)?

Pinsof's Integrative Systems Perspective of the therapeutic alliance may also have some relevance in the context of neurorehabilitation. The Integrative Systems Perspective [68] suggests that therapy is the interaction between *therapist* and *patient systems*. The therapy system comprises anyone involved in therapy provision and includes, but is not limited to the therapists themselves. From a neurorehabilitation perspective, the *therapist system* could include, for example, any members of the therapy team, rehabilitation assistants, the receptionist, service manager and so on. Similarly, the *patient system* includes anyone who may be 'part of the presenting problem or the solution to the problem' [68], p.174. Pinsof highlights that it is unlikely that all those in the therapist system and patient system will interact directly and so he also distinguishes between direct and indirect therapist systems, and likewise direct and indirect patient systems and that people can shift between direct and indirect systems. Therefore, for example, a family member may be physically present for a session (and therefore form part of the direct patient system) and not for the next (in which case they form part of the indirect patient system). In other words, just because someone is not directly involved in a therapeutic episode at a given time he/she can still form part of the broader system and exert influence over the system, a concept Pinsof refers to as *mutual causality*. Mutual causality refers to the notion that 'every subsystem within a system influences every other subsystem bidirectionally and recursively' [68], p.175. Pinsof argues that this systems perspective offers a new way of thinking about the therapeutic alliance, where the therapeutic alliance is no longer between two individuals, but rather between and within therapist and patient systems. He argues that the alliance may develop and be impacted across multiple layers including between individuals, between interpersonal subsystems of both the therapist and patient systems, between the whole system (i.e. between the whole therapist system and the whole patient system) and within systems (i.e. between individuals or subsystems *within* the therapist system or *within* the patient system). While this presents a complex picture, it has congruence with the reality of neurorehabilitation in that it is complex and involves a number of players at any one time across the care continuum, which may serve to influence the therapeutic connection.

In summary, while existing work draws primarily on Bordin's Theory of Working Alliance as a conceptual framework, a number of other theories exist that may augment our understanding of therapeutic connection in neurorehabilitation. Future work should explore the potential application of these in a neurorehabilitation setting. It should be noted however that, like existing measures of therapeutic connection, these theories were devised in the context of psychotherapy and as such should be applied with caution without further testing regarding their validity. By comparison, research aiming to advance our conceptual understanding of therapeutic connection specific to the neurorehabilitation setting, or indeed rehabilitation more broadly, has been limited. Developing a better conceptual understanding of therapeutic connection as it relates to neurorehabilitation more explicitly will serve to provide a clear basis for future research and practice in this field.

3. How important is the therapeutic connection with family for outcome in neurorehabilitation?

Even though rehabilitation interventions target individual patients, they rarely exist in isolation, most commonly inhabiting a broader family and social context. As such, those that surround the individual play a role in both supporting (and possibly hindering) the rehabilitation process. One of the key questions that arise when considering Pinsof's Integrative Systems Perspective described earlier is the impact the therapeutic connection between the therapist and other parties in the *patients system* have on outcomes in neurorehabilitation, including family. Only two of the articles reviewed sought family perceptions of therapeutic connection [32,59]. Sherer et al. found that while patient and therapist ratings of therapeutic alliance were significantly associated, family perceptions were not associated with either [59]. This is in contrast to Evans et al. who found no significant difference between patient, therapist and family ratings of therapeutic alliance [32]. In both studies, family rated the therapeutic alliance the highest, followed by patients and then therapists. Sherer et al. found that discrepancy between family and therapists regarding ratings of patient functioning, and higher levels of family discord, were both associated with poorer clinician rated therapeutic alliance. Similarly, Evans et al. found that better team WAS and CALPAS-therapist scores were significantly associated with lower levels of family discord.

While the evidence is limited, these findings highlight the potential for family involvement (or the nature of their involvement and their relationship to the patient) to compromise the strength of the therapeutic connection with family discord, and discrepancy between family and therapist's perspectives of function both identified as a possible threat. McLaughlin and Carey suggest that the relationship between family and practitioners in brain injury rehabilitation is inevitably adversarial as both are doing their jobs [69]. Families may see the rehabilitation team as getting in the way of their loved one getting the rehabilitation he/she needed, or the families may be dealing with their own grief for the loss of the loved one they once knew (commonly referred to as ambiguous loss [12]); and the rehabilitation team and associated processes may be an outlet for that.

Levack et al. interviewed clinicians to explore how they talked about involving family in goal setting in the context of adult rehabilitation of acquired brain injury [70]. They found that clinicians actively limited involvement of family in goal planning sessions where they perceived there might be tensions similar to those described by McLaughlin and Carey [69]. Findings from Sherer and Evan's studies suggest that while this strategy may eliminate the problem in the immediate future, there is a risk it may contribute to the development of a poor therapeutic connection between the family and therapist which in turn may impact detrimentally on the therapeutic connection with the patient.

In summary, while evidence is limited, family involvement in rehabilitation and the dynamics of families in this context appears to play a part in the development of therapeutic connection. Future research should explore the possible application of Pinsof's Integrated Systems Perspective of therapeutic alliance to explore how different *systems*, within and between *patient* and *therapist systems*, interact to optimise therapeutic connection and outcome in neurorehabilitation.

How do the cognitive, neurobehavioural and communication sequelae commonly inherent in brain injury impact on the development of a therapeutic connection?

There has been some interest in the literature regarding the degree to which it is possible to establish a therapeutic connection with brain-injured patients, or whether cognitive, neurobehavioural and communication sequelae inhibit this process [71]. Judd and Wilson carried out an open-ended survey with psychologists, psychotherapists and counsellors involved in psychotherapy services for brain-injured patients to explore their perspectives regarding the challenges of forming a working alliance with people with TBI. Challenges identified included a range of cognitive (lack of insight, impaired memory, inflexible thinking, poor attention/concentration, language difficulties), behavioural (disinhibited behaviour) and emotional (emotional ability) factors. Impaired memory, lack of insight and inflexible thinking were the most commonly reported challenges. This is consistent with Schönberger *et al.* who found a tendency for therapist ratings of alliance at 2 weeks post admission to be lower for right hemisphere and bi-frontal injuries [52]. However, the relationship between therapist ratings of alliance and injury localisation did not endure at 6, 10 and 14 weeks into the rehabilitation programme. This could either be an indication of improvements in the symptoms associated with these injuries and therefore the impact of them becoming less and less over time, or that following the initial rehabilitation period, therapists were more able to adopt strategies to overcome the impact of those symptoms on the working alliance.

Schönberger *et al.* explored the relationship between attention, memory function and higher cognitive function and patient and therapist working alliance at 2, 6, 10 and 14 weeks post admission to neurorehabilitation [72]. While there were some significant findings, correlations were weak overall broadly indicating that it is entirely possible to develop a good working alliance in the face of even severe cognitive deficits. An interesting finding from Schönberger *et al.*'s study is that there is a discrepancy between therapists and patients regarding what aspects contributed to a better working alliance and at which stage in the rehabilitation process. For example, for patients, good performance on memory tests was negatively correlated with working alliance at 2 weeks post admission, while cognitive function was not related to patients ratings of working alliance at any time point. There are a number of explanations for this. Schönberger *et al.* propose that (1) people with more memory deficits need a stronger alliance and (2) those with better cognitive functioning expect more

from the rehabilitation process and the collaborative work that entails. By contrast, better performance on memory tests were positively associated with therapist ratings of working alliance later in the rehabilitation period (10 and 14 weeks) and higher scores on only selected measures of cognitive function were related to higher therapist ratings of working alliance across all time points but particularly in the later time points.

The participants in Judd and Wilson's study [71] identified a range of strategies they used to overcome the challenges of developing a working alliance including education and information, behavioural experiments, memory aids, involving family and behavioural management. Schönberger *et al.* [72] argue that the relatively weak correlations found in their study may indicate that while it is possible that cognitive deficits do indeed present as a therapeutic challenge, in most instances therapists appear to be able to manage these via the range of strategies identified in Judd and Wilson's study so that they do not impact on the development of a working alliance.

Chapter summary

In this chapter, we have reviewed existing literature regarding four key questions associated with therapeutic connection in neurorehabilitation including the relationship between therapeutic connection and outcome, the theoretical basis for work to date and the role of family and deficits commonly present following a neurological event. We found better ratings of therapeutic connection to be associated with a range of important outcomes, including lower levels of emotional distress and family discord, improvements in productivity status, performance on cognitive retraining tasks, driving status, awareness, compliance, depression and higher rates of programme completion. A particularly interesting finding is the potential for better ratings of therapeutic connection to be associated with the development of key meta-cognitive skills frequently impaired by neurological illness or injury; arguably one of the most crucial outcomes for longer term benefit following neurorehabilitation [57,58]. While further work is needed, our findings also indicate that family members may have an influencing role in successful development of a therapeutic connection. In addition, existing evidence supports the development of a therapeutic connection even in the face of severe cognitive deficit. There are some limitations to existing work in terms of the measures adopted and theoretical basis, both of which are borrowed from psychotherapy and related fields and therefore may be conceptually missing the mark in the context of neurorehabilitation. In addition, while there is broad support for therapeutic connection, some further work regarding *whose* perspective matters most in relation to outcome (i.e. patient, therapist or family) and what core components (or which mix) of therapeutic connection are most crucial would advance our understanding of this important covariate of outcome and allow for more targeted training for practitioners working in a neurorehabilitation setting.

Conclusion

An ageing population and more people surviving initial injury/illness and living with residual disability mean that the number of people accessing neurorehabilitation services is growing. Optimising rehabilitation services for enduring health outcomes is therefore crucial. However, strategies efficacious in research settings often fail to translate to effective strategies in real world practice [7,73–75]. The evidence presented in this chapter reports therapeutic connection to account for significant variability in a range of neurorehabilitation outcomes and therefore may be key to seeing positive outcomes from research translate and endure in the real world. While there are some key areas identified earlier where more research is needed, the evidence presented suggests a greater focus on establishing a therapeutic connection as a legitimate intervention in neurorehabilitation is clearly warranted. Indeed, not doing so may mean we fail to tap into the true potential of therapeutic connection as a covariate of outcome.

References

1   McDonald, J.W. 3rd, Sadowsky, C.L. & Stampas, A. (2012) The changing field of rehabilitation: Optimizing spontaneous regeneration and functional recovery. *Handbook of Clinical Neurology*, **109**, 317–336.

2   Learmonth, Y.C., Paul, L., Miller, L., Mattison, P. & McFadyen, A.K. (2011) The effects of a 12-week leisure centre-based, group exercise intervention for people moderately affected with multiple sclerosis: A randomized controlled pilot study. *Clinical Rehabilitation*, **26**(7), 579–593.

3   Di Carlo, A. (2009) Human and economic burden of stroke. *Age and Ageing*, **38**(1), 4–5.

4   Schönberger, M., Ponsford, J., Olver, J. & Ponsford, M. (2010) A longitudinal study of family functioning after TBI and relatives' emotional status. *Neuropsychological Rehabilitation*, **20**(6), 813–829.

5   Maclean, N. & Pound, P. (2000) A critical review of the concept of patient motivation in the literature on physical rehabilitation. *Social Science and Medicine*, **50**, 495–506.

6   Boucher, T., Connolly, S., Pierce, E. & Hewitt, G. (2003) Patient compliance: Comparison of patient and staff perceptions. *International Journal of Therapy and Rehabilitation*, **10**(3), 94–99.

7   van den Broek, M.D. (2005) Why does neurorehabilitation fail? *The Journal of Head Trauma Rehabilitation*, **20**(5), 464–473.

8   Maclean, N., Pound, P., Wolfe, C. & Rudd, A. (2000) Qualitative analysis of stroke patients' motivation for rehabilitation. *BMJ*, **321**(7268), 1051–1054.

9   Siegert, R.J. & Taylor, W.J. (2004) Theoretical aspects of goal-setting and motivation in rehabilitation. *Disability and Rehabilitation*, **26**(1), 1–8.

10 Wiles, R., Cott, C. & Gibson, B.E. (2008) Hope, expectations and recovery from illness: A narrative synthesis of qualitative research. *Journal of Advanced Nursing*, **64**(6), 564–573.

11 Kayes, N.M. & McPherson, K.M. (2012) Human technologies in rehabilitation: 'Who' and 'How' we are with our clients. *Disability and Rehabilitation*, **34**(22), 1907.

12 Landau, J. & Hissett, J. (2008) Mild traumatic brain injury: Impact on identity and ambiguous loss in the family. *Families, Systems & Health*, **26**(1), 69–85.

13 Levack, W.M.M., Kayes, N.M. & Fadyl, J.K. (2010) Experience of recovery and outcome following traumatic brain injury: A metasynthesis of qualitative research. *Disability and Rehabilitation*, **32**(12), 986.

14 Horvath, A.O. (2001) The alliance. *Psychotherapy: Theory, Research, Practice, Training*, **38**(4), 365–372.

15 Horvath, A.O. & Symonds, B.D. (1991) Relation between working alliance and outcome in psychotherapy: A meta-analysis. *Journal of Counseling Psychology*, **38**(2), 139–149.

16 Lambert, M.J. & Barley, D.E. (2001) Research summary on the therapeutic relationship and psychotherapy outcome. *Psychotherapy: Theory, Research, Practice, Training*, **38**(4), 357–361.

17 Martin, D.J., Garske, J.P. & Davis, M.K. (2000) Relation of the therapeutic alliance with outcome and other variables: A meta-analytic review. *Journal of Consulting and Clinical Psychology*, **68**(3), 438–450.

18 Bordin, E.S. (1979) The generalizability of the psychoanalytic concept of the working alliance. *Psychotherapy*, **16**(3), 252–260.

19 Shontz, F.C. & Fink, S.L. (1957) The significance of patient-staff rapport in the rehabilitation of individuals with chronic physical illness. *Journal of Consulting Psychology*, **21**(4), 327–334.

20 Gordon, S., Hamer, P. & Potter, M. (2003) The difficult patient in private practice physiotherapy: A qualitative study. *The Australian Journal of Physiotherapy*, **49**(1), 53–61.

21 Jensen, G.M., Gwyer, J. & Shepard, K.F. (2000) Expert practice in physical therapy. *Physical Therapy*, **80**(1), 28.

22 Leach, M.J. (2005) Rapport: A key to treatment success. *Complementary Therapies in Clinical Practice*, **11**(4), 262–265.

23 Punwar, A.J. & Peloquin, S.M. (2000) *Occupational therapy: principles and practice*. Lippincott Williams & Wilkins, Philadelphia.

24 Roberts, L. & Bucksey, S.J. (2007) Communicating With Patients: What Happens in Practice? *Physical Therapy*, **87**(7), 957.

25 Stenmar, L. & Nordholm, L.A. (1994) Swedish physical therapists' beliefs on what makes therapy work. *Physical Therapy*, **74**(11), 1034.

26 Fadyl, J.K., McPherson, K.M. & Kayes, N.M. (2011) Perspectives on quality of care for people who experience disability. *BMJ Quality & Safety*, **20**(1), 87–95.

27 Hargreaves, S. (1982) The relevance of non-verbal skills in physiotherapy. *The Australian Journal of Physiotherapy*, **28**(4), 19–20.

28 Hills, R. & Kitchen, S. (2007) Satisfaction with outpatient physiotherapy: Focus groups to explore the views of patients with acute

and chronic musculoskeletal conditions. *Physiotherapy Theory and Practice*, **23**(**1**), 1.

29 Potter, M., Gordon, S. & Hamer, P. (2003) The physiotherapy experience in private practice: The patients' perspective. *The Australian Journal of Physiotherapy*, **49**(**3**), 195–202.

30 Rademakers, J., Delnoij, D. & de Boer, D. (2011) Structure, process or outcome: Which contributes most to patients' overall assessment of healthcare quality? *BMJ Quality & Safety*, **20**(**4**), 326–331.

31 Hush, J.M., Cameron, K. & Mackey, M. (2011) Patient satisfaction with musculoskeletal physical therapy care: A systematic review. *Physical Therapy*, **91**(**1**), 25–36.

32 Evans, C.C., Sherer, M., Nakase-Richardson, R., Mani, T. & Irby, J.J.W. (2008) Evaluation of an Interdisciplinary team intervention to improve therapeutic alliance in post-acute brain injury rehabilitation. *The Journal of Head Trauma Rehabilitation*, **23**(**5**), 329–338.

33 Ezrachi, O., Ben-Yishay, Y., Kay, T., DiUer, L. & Rattok, J. (1991) Predicting employment in traumatic brain injury following neuropsychological rehabilitation. *The Journal of Head Trauma Rehabilitation*, **6**(**3**), 71–84.

34 Guidetti, S., Asaba, E. & Tham, K. (2009) Meaning of context in recapturing self-care after stroke or spinal cord injury. *American Journal of Occupational Therapy*, **63**(**3**), 323–332.

35 Hall, A.M., Ferreira, P.H., Maher, C.G., Latimer, J. & Ferreira, M.L. (2010) The Influence of the Therapist-Patient Relationship on Treatment Outcome in Physical Rehabilitation: A Systematic Review. *Physical Therapy*, **90**(**8**), 1099–1110.

36 Klonoff, P.S.L.D.G.H.S.W. (2001) Outcomes from milieu-based neurorehabilitation at up to 11 years post-discharge. *Brain Injury*, **15**(**5**), 413–428.

37 Prigatano, G.P., Klonoff, P.S., O'Brien, K.P. *et al.* (1994) Productivity after neuropsychologically oriented milieu rehabilitation. *The Journal of Head Trauma Rehabilitation*, **9**(**1**), 91–102.

38 Strauser, D.R., Lustig, D.C., Chan, F. & O'Sullivan, D. (2010) Working alliance and vocational outcomes for cancer survivors: An initial analysis. *International Journal of Rehabilitation Research*, **33**(**3**), 271–274.

39 Bright, F.A.S., Boland, P., Rutherford, S.J., Kayes, N.M. & McPherson, K.M. (2012) Implementing a client-centred approach in rehabilitation: An autoethnography. *Disability and Rehabilitation*, **34**(**12**), 997.

40 Kayes, N.M. (2011) *Physical activity engagement in people with Multiple Sclerosis [PhD]*. AUT University, Auckland.

41 Kayes NM, McPherson KM, Taylor D, Schluter PJ. *The Facilitating Activity for well-Being (FAB) Programme: A pilot study of a new approach to engaging people with Multiple Sclerosis (MS) in goal-directed physical activity*. AFRM/NIRR/NZRA Rehabilitation Conference; 2009; Queenstown, New Zealand.

42 McPherson, K.M., Kayes, N.M., Weatherall, M. & on behalf of all members of the Goals SR Research Group (2009) A pilot study of self-regulation informed goal setting in people with traumatic brain injury. *Clinical Rehabilitation*, **23**(**4**), 296–309.

43 Schönberger, M.F.T.W. (2006) Subjective outcome of brain injury rehabilitation in relation to the therapeutic working alliance, client compliance and awareness. *Brain Injury*, **20**(**12**), 1271–1282.

44 Gartland, G.J. (1984) Teaching the therapeutic relationship. *Physiotherapy Canada*, **36**, 24–28.

45 Cahill, J., Barkham, M., Hardy, G. *et al.* (2008) A review and critical appraisal of measures of therapist-patient interactions in mental health settings. *Health Technology Assessment*, **12**(**24**), 3–9.

46 Saunders, S.M., Howard, K.I. & Orlinsky, D.E. (1989) The therapeutic bond scales: Psychometric characteristics and relationship to treatment effectiveness. *Psychological Assessment*, **1**(**4**), 323–3230.

47 De Weert-Van Oene, G.H., De Jong, C., Jorg, F. & Schrijvers, G. (1999) Measurements, instruments, scales, and tests: The helping alliance questionnaire: Psychometric properties in patients with substance dependence. *Substance Use & Misuse*, **34**(**11**), 1549–1569.

48 Cole, M.B. & McLean, V. (2003) Therapeutic relationships re-defined. *Occupational Therapy in Mental Health*, **19**(**2**), 33–56.

49 Bellner, A. (1999) Senses of responsibility: A challenge for occupational and physical therapists in the context of ongoing professionalization. *Scandinavian Journal of Caring Sciences*, **13**(**1**), 55–62.

50 Bright F, Kayes NM, Cummins C, McPherson KM, Worrall L. *"There needs to be some connectivity there": The role of therapeutic connections in facilitating engagement in rehabilitation*. New Zealand Rehabilitation Conference; 2013; Rutherford Hotel, Nelson, NZ.

51 Gaston, L. & Marmar, C.R. (1994) The California Psychotherapy Alliance Scales. In: Horvath, A.O. & Greenburg, L.S. (eds), *The Working Alliance: Theory, Research and Practice*. John Wiley & Sons, New York, pp. 85–108.

52 Schönberger, M., Humle, F. & Teasdale, T.W. (2006) The development of the therapeutic working alliance, patients' awareness and their compliance during the process of brain injury rehabilitation. *Brain Injury*, **20**(**4**), 445–454.

53 Summers, R.F. & Barber, J.P. (2003) Therapeutic alliance as a measurable psychotherapy skill. *Academic Psychiatry*, **27**(**3**), 160–165.

54 Schönberger, M.F.P.T. (2006) Working alliance and patient compliance in brain injury rehabilitation and their relation to psychosocial outcome. *Neuropsychological Rehabilitation*, **16**(**3**), 298–314.

55 Klonoff, P.S., Olson, K.C., Talley, M.C. *et al.* (2010) The relationship of cognitive retraining to neurological patients' driving status: The role of process variables and compensation training. *Brain Injury*, **24**(**2**), 63–73.

56 Klonoff, P.S., Talley, M.C., Dawson, L.K. *et al.* (2007) The relationship of cognitive retraining to neurological patients' work and school status. *Brain Injury*, **21**(**11**), 1097–1107.

57 Ownsworth, T. & Fleming, J. (2005) The relative importance of metacognitive skills, emotional status, and executive function in psychosocial adjustment following acquired brain injury. *The Journal of Head Trauma Rehabilitation*, **20**(**4**), 315–332.

58 Hart, T. & Evans, J. (2006) Self-regulation and goal theories in brain injury rehabilitation. *The Journal of Head Trauma Rehabilitation*, **21**(**2**), 142–155.

59 Sherer, M., Evans, C.C., Leverenz, J. *et al.* (2007) Therapeutic alliance in post-acute brain injury rehabilitation: Predictors of strength of alliance and impact of alliance on outcome. *Brain Injury*, **21**(7), 663–672.

60 Horvath, A.O. & Greenberg, L.S. (1989) Development and validation of the working alliance inventory. *Journal of Counseling Psychology*, **36**(2), 223–233.

61 Elvins, R. & Green, J. (2008) The conceptualization and measurement of therapeutic alliance: An empirical review. *Clinical Psychology Review*, **28**(7), 1167–1187.

62 Besley, J., Kayes, N.M. & McPherson, K.M. (2011) Assessing therapeutic relationships in physiotherapy: Literature review. *New Zealand Journal of Physiotherapy*, **39**(2), 81–91.

63 Besley, J., Kayes, N.M. & McPherson, K.M. (2011) Assessing the measurement properties of two commonly used measures of therapeutic relationship in physiotherapy. *New Zealand Journal of Physiotherapy*, **39**(2), 75–80.

64 Kissinger, D.B. (2008) Traumatic brain injury and employment outcomes: Integration of the working alliance model. *Work*, **31**(3), 309–317.

65 Gelso, C.J. & Carter, J.A. (1985) The relationship in counseling and psychotherapy: Components, consequences, and theoretical antecedents. *The Counseling Psychologist*, **13**(2), 155–243.

66 Gelso, C.J. (2009) The time has come: The real relationship in psychotherapy research. *Psychotherapy Research*, **19**(3), 278–282.

67 Gelso, C.J. (2009) The real relationship in a postmodern world: Theoretical and empirical explorations. *Psychotherapy Research*, **19**(3), 253–264.

68 Pinsof, W.M. (1994) An integrative systems perspective on the therapeutic alliance: Theoretical, clinical and research implications. In: Horvath, A.O. & Greenburg, L.S. (eds), *The Working Alliance: Theory, Research and Practice*. John Wiley & Sons, New York, pp. 173–195.

69 McLaughlin, A.M. & Carey, J.L. (1993) The adversarial alliance: Developing therapeutic relationships between families and the team in brain injury rehabilitation. *Brain Injury*, **7**(1), 45–51.

70 Levack, W., Siegert, R., Dean, S. & McPherson, K. (2009) Goal planning for adults with acquired brain injury: How clinicians talk about involving family. *Brain Injury*, **23**(3), 192.

71 Judd, D. & Wilson, S.L. (2005) Psychotherapy with brain injury survivors: An investigation of the challenges encountered by clinicians and their modifications to therapeutic practice. *Brain Injury*, **19**(6), 437–449.

72 Schönberger, M., Humle, F. & Teasdale, T.W. (2007) The relationship between clients' cognitive functioning and the therapeutic working alliance in post-acute brain injury rehabilitation. *Brain Injury*, **21**(8), 825–836.

73 Camp, C.J. (2001) From efficacy to effectiveness to diffusion: Making the transitions in dementia intervention research. *Neuropsychological Rehabilitation*, **11**(3), 495–517.

74 Cheeran, B., Rothwell, J., Rudd, A. *et al.* (2009) The future of restorative neurosciences in stroke: Driving the translational research pipeline from basic science to rehabilitation of people after stroke. *Neurorehabilitation and Neural Repair*, **23**(2), 97.

75 Glasgow, R.E., Lichtenstein, E. & Marcus, A.C. (2003) Why don't we see more translation of health promotion research to practice? Rethinking the efficacy-to-effectiveness transition. *American Journal of Public Health*, **93**(8), 1261.

Telemedicine feature

PART 4

Telemedicine feature

30

CHAPTER 30

Evidence-based teleneurology practice

William D. Freeman[1], Kevin M. Barrett[2], Kenneth A. Vatz[3], and Bart M. Demaerschalk[4]

[1]Departments of Neurology, Critical Care and Neurosurgery, Mayo Clinic Florida, Jacksonville, FL, USA
[2]Department of Neurology, Mayo Clinic, Jacksonville, FL, USA
[3]Department of Neurology, CommunityHealth, Chicago, IL, USA
[4]Department of Neurology, Mayo Clinic, Phoenix, Arizona, USA

Introduction to the chapter

Teleneurology is a subset of telemedicine, which uses a real-time audiovisual technology to provide a doctor–patient interaction or evaluation for medical decision-making or recommendations [1]. *Telestroke* is a subset of teleneurology, and it specifically evaluates a patient for stroke. Literature continues to grow on the subject of telemedicine and telestroke. [2] The evidence regarding teleneurology and telestroke is reviewed here.

The demand for teleneurology and telestroke services has been fueled in part by a relative shortage of neurological subspecialists in rural and underserved regions [3–6]. The administration of intravenous (IV) recombinant tissue plasminogen activator (rtPA) for acute ischemic stroke is considered a medical emergency with timely evaluation for eligible patients within 3 hours of stroke onset. This issue is further compounded by Emergency Department physicians feeling uncomfortable administering IV-rtPA alone and without neurology input [7]. This has lead to relatively low rates of rtPA utilization (approximately 2–5%) at underserved hospitals even among potentially eligible stroke patients [6]. Teleneurological evaluation of stroke patients is reported to increase IV-rtPA utilization rates [8,9].

Methodology

We performed PubMed and Cochrane database literature searches using the search terms, "teleneurology," "telestroke," "telemedicine," and/or "neurology" specific to this chapter. We reviewed the literature provided and the abstracts for relevance among these categories for this chapter, which were approximately 74 (telestroke), 22 (teleneurology), and 195 (telemedicine and neurology). There was only one Cochrane statement germane to

telemedicine feasibility with other hits being irrelevant to teleneurology (e.g., mobile phone messaging for diabetes). The GRADE system was utilized to rank the level of evidence [10] which uses the following definitions in grading the quality of the evidence: *high* = further research is very unlikely to change the confidence in the estimate of effect; *moderate* = further research is likely to impact the confidence in the estimate of effect and may change the estimate of the effect; *low* = further research is very likely to have important changes on the confidence and estimate of effect; *very low* = any estimate of effect is uncertain. Recommendations are weighted and operationally defined by the GRADE system, where the *net benefit* is defined as when the intervention clearly does more good than harm; *trade-offs* defined as when important considerations must be taken into account between benefits and harms; *uncertain trade-offs* defined as when it is unclear whether the intervention does more good than harm; and *no net benefit* defined when the intervention does not result in more good than harm.

Clinical Questions

Question 1: Is teleneurology feasible and safe?

Teleneurology literature has various levels of quality of evidence and various neurological disease states studied. Feasibility and relative safety is reported among different neurological patient subtypes including Alzheimer's, neuro-ophthalmology, neurophysiology, epilepsy, Parkinson's, and stroke patients in both inpatient and outpatient settings [11–23]. However, only a high degree of evidence exists by the GRADE level of evidence system for feasibility and safety of evaluating new neurological outpatients [16], patients with Parkinson's disease [17], and patients with acute stroke (telestroke) [24,25] based on the presence of randomized controlled trials or critical appraisal. In

Evidence-Based Neurology: Management of Neurological Disorders, Second Edition. Edited by Bart M. Demaerschalk and Dean M. Wingerchuk.
© 2015 John Wiley & Sons, Ltd. Published 2015 by John Wiley & Sons, Ltd.

particular, telestroke has multicenter network trials such as TEMPiS [24,25] and STRokE DOC [26,27].

(a) GRADE level of evidence: There is a sufficient and high level of evidence that the intervention of teleneurology itself is feasible and safe for those disease models described earlier, particularly telestroke evaluation of intravenous tPA [28–32]. There are serious limitations in the evidence for new outpatient evaluations due to lack of hands on examination similar to a live examination and lack of other validating studies.

(b) Recommendations: Teleneurology has important trade-offs to be considered, namely the infrastructure and technology to accomplish the technically sophisticated audiovisual evaluation, which must be weighed against the apparent safety and feasibility of providing access to subspecialist who can provide diagnostic information and potentially useful recommendations or treatment (e.g., IV rtPA for acute stroke) to patients in rural and underserved areas [33,34].

Question 2: Is teleneurology "cost-effective"?

There is considerable heterogeneity regarding the different modes of technology used to deliver Teleneurology [4,30]. In addition, at the time of this review, there were only three cost-related or cost-effective studies published on Telestroke [6,35,36].

(a) GRADE level of evidence. There is low level of evidence with regard to cost-effectiveness of telestroke, and thus further research is likely to have important changes on the confidence and estimate of effect. There is essentially very low evidence for teleneurology in general outside of telestroke, and thus assessment of effect is uncertain.

(b) Recommendations: With regard to cost-effectiveness of teleneurology, *uncertain trade-offs* are apparent since it is unclear whether the intervention provides efficacy more than "costs." However, this is mostly due to the lack of published literature measuring the effect.

Question 3: How does teleneurology exam compare to the complete neurological bedside exam?

There are limited data that directly compare the full neurological examination to the Teleneurology examination [4]. The best studied examination comparison is the NIH Stroke scale (NIHSS) examination, which has good inter-rater reliability and agreement.

(a) GRADE level of evidence: There is a low level of evidence that directly compares the complete neurological examination to the Teleneurology examination, perhaps partly due to the lack of physical examination by the audiovisual environment or grading of the "virtual examiner" against the onsite examiner of the same patient. Telestroke, however, using the NIH stroke scale has a high level of evidence showing good agreement between the local-site examiner and the remote examiner scores [37,38].

(b) Recommendations: With regard to the level of agreement of examination of the physical neurological exam versus that of teleneurology, *uncertain trade-offs* are apparent since it is unclear if the teleneurological examination is equal to the full direct physical neurological examination. However, this is mostly likely due to the lack of literature comparing the full neurological examination against the teleneurological examination. With regards to telestroke examination, using the NIH Stroke scale, there are *trade-offs* to be considered that must be taken into account between potential benefits and harms, namely the potential benefit of the patient having a neurologist examine the patient and potentially helping the patient with acute stroke by giving IV-rtPA, versus the same situation in which there is a stroke mimic disorder such as post-ictal state that cannot be measured by the NIH stroke scale adequately.

Question 4: Can teleneurology affect patient outcomes?

There is evidence regarding patient outcomes for telestroke, but little evidence about outcomes for teleneurology [39–42].

(a) GRADE level of evidence: There is a medium level of evidence by randomized clinical trials, but primarily aimed at rtPA utilization rates or other indirect patient outcome measures [41,42]. There are also studies that show telestroke centers can later meet criteria for being a "stroke center" or equivalent [43,44].

(b) Recommendations: There are uncertain trade-offs to consider with teleneurology in terms of providing access to a specialist and diagnosis and recommendations, against the perceived long-term patient outcomes. For telestroke, there are trade-off benefits for rtPA and patient outcomes

Chapter summary

Teleneurology appears safe and feasible to those centers that have the resources which can provide care, and appears to help rural and underserved areas which would be impossible for any neurologist. While there are certain technical limitations, computers and the Internet speeds continue to improve, and the devices that perform teleneurology or telestroke are becoming smaller and more portable. More research is needed on teleneurology patient outcomes and telestroke as well as cost-efficacy of this in relation to patient care.

Acknowledgements

The authors report none.

Disclosures

The authors report no conflict of interest or funding for this manuscript.

References

1 Patterson, V. (2005) Teleneurology. *Journal of Telemedicine and Telecare*, **11**(**2**), 55–59.

2 Capampangan, D.J., Wellik, K.E., Bobrow, B.J. *et al.* (2009) Telemedicine versus telephone for remote emergency stroke consultations: a critically appraised topic. *The Neurologist*, **15**(**3**), 163–166.

3 Freeman, W.D. & Vatz, K.A. (2010) Future of Neurology. *Neurologic Clinics*, **28**(**2**), 537–561.

4 Freeman WD, Barrett KM, Vatz KA, Demaerschalk B. Future Neurohospitalist: Teleneurohospitalist. *Neurohospitalist*. 2012;2(**4**):132–143. doi: 10.1177/1941874412450714..

5 Wang, S., Gross, H., Lee, S.B. *et al.* (2004) Remote evaluation of acute ischemic stroke in rural community hospitals in Georgia. *Stroke*, **35**(**7**), 1763–1768.

6 Wiborg, A. & Widder, B. (2003) Teleneurology to improve stroke care in rural areas: The Telemedicine in Stroke in Swabia (TESS) Project. *Stroke*, **34**(**12**), 2951–2956.

7 Scott, P.A., Xu, Z., Meurer, W.J., Frederiksen, S.M. *et al.* (2010 Sep) Attitudes and beliefs of Michigan emergency physicians toward tissue plasminogen activator use in stroke: baseline survey results from the increasing Stroke Treatment through interactive behavioral Change Tactic (INSTINCT) trial hospitals. *Stroke*, **41**(**9**), 2026–2032. Epub 2010 Aug 12.

8 Kleindorfer, D., Xu, Y., Moomaw, C.J., Khatri, P., Adeoye, O. & Hornung, R. (2009) US geographic distribution of rt-PA utilization by hospital for acute ischemic stroke. *Stroke*, **40**, 3580–3584.

9 Henninger, N., Chowdhury, N., Fisher, M. & Moonis, M. (2009) Use of telemedicine to increase thrombolysis and advance care in acute ischemic stroke. *Cerebrovascular Diseases*, **27**(**Suppl 4**), 9–14.

10 Atkins, D., Best, D., Briss, P.A., Eccles, M. *et al* (2004) Grading quality of evidence and strength of recommendations. *BMJ*, **328**, 1490.

11 Duncan, C., Dorrian, C., Crowley, P., Coleman, R. & Patterson, V. (2010) Safety and effectiveness of telemedicine for neurology outpatients. *Scottish Medical Journal*, **55**(**1**), 3–5.

12 Ahmed, S.N., Mann, C., Sinclair, D.B. *et al.* (2008) Feasibility of epilepsy follow-up care through telemedicine: a pilot study on the patient's perspective. *Epilepsia*, **49**(**4**), 573–585.

13 Breen, P., Murphy, K., Browne, G. *et al.* (2010) Formative evaluation of a telemedicine model for delivering clinical neurophysiology services part II: the referring clinician and patient perspective. *BMC Medical Informatics and Decision Making*, **10**, 49.

14 Biglan, K.M., Voss, T.S., Deuel, L.M. *et al.* (2009) Telemedicine for the care of nursing home residents with Parkinson's disease. *Movement Disorders*, **24**(**7**), 1073–1076.

15 Bremner, F., Kennedy, C., Rees, A., Acheson, J. & Murdoch, I. (2002) Usefulness of teleconsultations in neuro-ophthalmology. *Journal of Telemedicine and Telecare*, **8**(**5**), 305–306.

16 Chua, R., Craig, J., Wootton, R. & Patterson, V. (2001) Randomised controlled trial of telemedicine for new neurological outpatient referrals. *Journal of Neurology, Neurosurgery and Psychiatry*, **71**, 63–66.

17 Dorsey, E.R., Deuel, L.M., Voss, T.S. *et al.* (2010) Increasing access to specialty care: A pilot, randomized controlled trial of telemedicine for Parkinson's disease. *Movement Disorders*, **25**(**11**), 1652–1659. doi:10.1002/mds.23145

18 Harvey, R., Roques, P.K., Fox, N.C. & Rossor, M.N. (1998) CANDID–Counselling and Diagnosis in Dementia: a national telemedicine service supporting the care of younger patients with dementia. *International Journal of Geriatric Psychiatry*, **13**(**6**), 381–388.

19 Hubble, J.P. (1992) Interactive video conferencing and Parkinson's disease. *Kansas Medicine*, **93**(**12**), 351–352.

20 Hubble, J.P., Pahwa, R., Michalek, D.K., Thomas, C. & Koller, W.C. (1993) Interactive video conferencing: a means of providing interim care to Parkinson's disease patients. *Movement Disorders*, **8**(**3**), 380–382.

21 Jabre, J.F., Stalberg, E.V. & Bassi, R. (2000) TeleMedicine and Internet EMG. *Supplements to Clinical Neurophysiology*, **53**, 163–167.

22 Samii, A., Ryan-Dykes, P., Tsukuda, R.A., Zink, C., Franks, R. & Nichol, W.P. (2006) Telemedicine for delivery of health care in Parkinson's disease. *Journal of Telemedicine and Telecare*, **12**(**1**), 16–18.

23 Paiva, T., Coelho, H., Araujo, M.T. *et al.* (2001) Neurological teleconsultation for general practitioners. *Journal of Telemedicine and Telecare*, **7**(**3**), 149–154.

24 Audebert, H.J., Kukla, C., Clarmann von Claranau, S. *et al.* (2005) Telemedicine for safe and extended use of thrombolysis in stroke: the Telemedic Pilot Project for Integrative Stroke Care (TEMPiS) in Bavaria. *Stroke*, **36**(**2**), 287–291.

25 Audebert, H.J., Schenkel, J., Heuschmann, P.U., Bogdahn, U. & Haberl, R.L. (2006) Effects of the implementation of a telemedical stroke network: the Telemedic Pilot Project for Integrative Stroke Care (TEMPiS) in Bavaria, Germany. *Lancet Neurology*, **5**(**9**), 742–748.

26 Gross, H., Hall, C.E., Wang, S. *et al.* (2006) Prospective reliability of the STRokE DOC Wireless/Site Independent Telemedicine System. *Neurology*, **66**(**3**), 460.

27 Meyer, B.C., Raman, R., Hemmen, T. *et al.* (2008) Efficacy of site-independent telemedicine in the STRokE DOC trial: a randomised, blinded, prospective study. *Lancet Neurology*, **7**(**9**), 787–795.

28 Hess, D.C., Wang, S., Hamilton, W. *et al.* (2005) REACH: clinical feasibility of a rural telestroke network. *Stroke*, **36**(**9**), 2018–2020.

29 Choi, J.Y., Porche, N.A., Albright, K.C., Khaja, A.M., Ho, V.S. & Grotta, J.C. (2006) Using telemedicine to facilitate thrombolytic therapy for patients with acute stroke. *Joint Commission Journal on Quality and Patient Safety*, **32**(**4**), 199–205.

30 Demaerschalk, B.M., Bobrow, B.J., Raman, R. *et al.* (2010) Stroke team remote evaluation using a digital observation camera in Arizona: the initial mayo clinic experience trial. *Stroke*, **41**(**6**), 1251–1258.

31 Shafqat, S., Kvedar, J.C., Guanci, M.M., Chang, Y. & Schwamm, L.H. (1999) Role for telemedicine in acute stroke. Feasibility and reliability of remote administration of the NIH stroke scale. *Stroke*, **30**(**10**), 2141–2145.

32 Pervez, M.A., Silva, G., Masrur, S. *et al.* (2010) Remote supervision of IV-tPA for acute ischemic stroke by telemedicine or telephone before transfer to a regional stroke center is feasible and safe. *Stroke*, **41**(**1**), e18–e24.

33 Hess, D.C., Wang, S., Gross, H., Nichols, F.T., Hall, C.E. & Adams, R.J. (2006) Telestroke: extending stroke expertise into underserved areas. *Lancet Neurology*, **5**(**3**), 275–278.

34 Khan, K., Shuaib, A., Whittaker, T. *et al.* (2010) Telestroke in northern alberta: a two year experience with remote hospitals. *Canadian Journal of Neurological Sciences*, **37**(**6**), 808–813.

35 Demaerschalk, B.M., Hwang, H.M. & Leung, G. (2010) Cost analysis review of stroke centers, telestroke, and rt-PA. *The American Journal of Managed Care*, **16**(**7**), 537–544.

36 Craig, J., Chua, R., Russell, C., Patterson, V. & Wootton, R. (2000) The cost-effectiveness of teleneurology consultations for patients admitted to hospitals without neurologists on site. 1: A retrospective comparison of the case-mix and management at two rural hospitals. *Journal of Telemedicine and Telecare*, **6**(**Suppl 1**), S46–S49.

37 Handschu, R., Littmann, R., Reulbach, U. *et al.* (2003) Telemedicine in emergency evaluation of acute stroke: interrater agreement in remote video examination with a novel multimedia system. *Stroke*, **34**(**12**), 2842–2846.

38 Handschu, R., Scibor, M., Willaczek, B. *et al.* (2008) Telemedicine in acute stroke: remote video-examination compared to simple telephone consultation. *Journal of Neurology*, **255**(**11**), 1792–1797.

39 Amarenco, P. & Nadjar, M. (2007) Telemedicine for improving emergent management of acute cerebrovascular syndromes. *International Journal of Stroke*, **2**(**1**), 47–50.

40 Tatlisumak, T., Soinila, S. & Kaste, M. (2009) Telestroke networking offers multiple benefits beyond thrombolysis. *Cerebrovascular Diseases*, **27**(**Suppl 4**), 21–27.

41 Schwab, S., Vatankhah, B., Kukla, C. *et al.* (2007) Long-term outcome after thrombolysis in telemedical stroke care. *Neurology*, **69**(**9**), 898–903.

42 Vespa, P.M., Miller, C., Hu, X., Nenov, V., Buxey, F. & Martin, N.A. (2007) Intensive care unit robotic telepresence facilitates rapid physician response to unstable patients and decreased cost in neurointensive care. *Surgical Neurology*, **67**(**4**), 331–337.

43 Smith, E.E., Dreyer, P., Prvu-Bettger, J. *et al.* (2008) Stroke center designation can be achieved by small hospitals: the Massachusetts experience. *Critical Pathways in Cardiology*, **7**(**3**), 173–177.

44 Audebert, H.J., Wimmer, M.L., Hahn, R. *et al.* (2005) Can telemedicine contribute to fulfill WHO Helsingborg Declaration of specialized stroke care? *Cerebrovascular Diseases*, **20**(**5**), 362–369.

Index

Evidence-Based Neurology: Management of Neurological Disorders, Second Edition. Edited by Bart M. Demaerschalk and Dean M. Wingerchuk.
© 2015 John Wiley & Sons, Ltd. Published 2015 by John Wiley & Sons, Ltd.